SPINAL TRAUMA

SPINAL TRAUMA

Thomas J. Errico, M.D.

Department of Orthopaedics
New York University Medical Center
New York, New York

R. David Bauer, M.D.

Department of Orthopaedics
Davis-Monthan Air Force Base
Tucson, Arizona

Theodore Waugh, M.D.

Department of Orthopaedics
New York University Medical Center
New York, New York

WITH 35 CONTRIBUTORS

Illustrations by
Keelin Murphy

J. B. LIPPINCOTT COMPANY
PHILADELPHIA

Grand Rapids   New York   St. Louis
San Francisco   London   Sydney   Tokyo

Acquisitions Editor: Darlene Barela Cooke
Editorial Assistant: Maria A. D'Arcangelo
Project Editor: Melissa B. McElroy
Indexer: Victoria Boyle
Art Director: Susan Hess Blaker
Production Manager: Caren Erlichman
Production Coordinator: Sharon McCarthy
Compositor: Tapsco, Incorporated
Printer/Binder: Arcata Graphics/Halliday

1 3 5 6 4 2

Library of Congress Cataloging in Publication Data

Spinal trauma / [edited by] Thomas J. Errico, R. David Bauer, Theodore Waugh; with 28 contributors.
    p. cm.
  ISBN 0-397-50983-9
  1. Spine—Wounds and injuries. 2. Spine—Wounds and injuries—Surgery. I. Errico, Thomas J. II. Bauer, R. David. III. Waugh, Theodore R.
  [DNLM: 1. Spinal Cord Injuries. 2. Spinal Injuries. 3. Spine—surgery. WE 725 S7543]
  RD533.S675 1990
  617.5'6044—dc20
  DNLM/DLC
  for Library of Congress   89-13295
                                                       CIP

To my surgical mentors for their patience and inspiration. To my family for their constant support and advice. Most importantly to my wife and children for their unending love.

Thomas J. Errico

To my family for their support, and to my teachers for their help and guidance.

R. David Bauer

CONTRIBUTORS

Jung H. Ahn, M.D.

Assistant Professor of Clinical Rehabilitative Medicine
New York University School of Medicine
New York, NY
Project Director
New York Regional Spinal Cord Model System

R. David Bauer, M.D.

Department of Orthopaedics
Davis-Monthan Air Force Base
Tucson, AZ

Drew A. Bednar, M.D., C.M., FRCSC

Attending Orthopaedic Surgeon
Hamilton General and Civic Hospital
Associate Professor
Orthopaedic Surgery
McMaster University
Hamilton, Ontario, Canada

Jean Pierre Benazet, M.D.

Chef de Clinique
Faculté de Medicine
Pitié-Saltpétrière
Paris, France

Professor Raymond Roy-Camille

Professor of Orthopaedic Surgery and Traumatology
Pietie-Salpetriene
Chief of Orthopaedic Surgery and Traumatology
Hospital de la Pitie
Paris, France

Levon M. Capan, M.D.

Associate Professor of Clinical Anesthesia
New York University Medical Center
Associate Director of Anesthesia
Bellevue Hospital Center
New York, NY

Allen L. Carl, M.D.

Assistant Professor
Orthopaedic Surgery
Albany Medical College
Albany, NY

Russell Crider, M.D.

Clinical Instructor of Orthopaedic Surgery
University of California, San Diego
San Diego, CA

Thomas J. Errico, M.D.

Assistant Professor
Department of Orthopaedics
New York University Medical Center
New York, NY

Stephen I. Esses, M.D., M.S.C., FRCSC, F.A.A.O.S.

Toronto General Hospital
Toronto, Ontario, Canada

Hossein Firooznia, M.D.

Professor of Clinical Radiology
New York University Medical Center
New York, NY

Thomas F. Gleason, M.D.

Assistant Clinical Professor
Department of Othopaedics
University of Illinois, Chicago
Chicago, IL

Cornelia Golimbu, M.D.

Clinical Associate Professor of Radiology
New York University Medical Center
New York, NY

Vincent J. Gulfo, M.D.

Rehabilitative Medicine
New York University Medical Center
New York, NY

Kurt A. Jellinger, M.D.

Professor of Neurology and Neuropathology
University of Vienna School of Medicine
Director
Ludwid Boltzmann Institute of Clinical Neurobiology
    and Department of Neurology
Lainz Hospital
Vienna, Austria

John P. Kostuik, M.D., FRCSC

Professor of Orthopaedic Surgery
University of Toronto
Head, Combined Division of Orthopaedic Surgery
Toronto General/Mt. Sinai General Hospital
Head, Spinal Unit
Toronto General Hospital
Toronto, Ontario, Canada

Justin Lamont, M.D.

Assistant Professor
Department of Orthopaedics
New York University Medical Center
New York, NY

Matt J. Likauec, M.D.

Assistant Professor of Neurosurgery
Case Western Reserve University
Cleveland, OH

Mark Lorenz, M.D.

Assistant Professor
Department of Orthopaedics
Loyola University
Chicago, IL

Timothy J. Massey, M.D.

Assistant Professor of Orthopaedics
University of Illinois, Chicago
Chicago, IL

Christian Mazel, M.D.

Chef de Clinique
Faculté de Medicine
Pitié-Saltpétrière
Paris, France

Stanford M. Miller, M.D.

Assistant Professor of Clinical Anesthesiology
New York University School of Medicine
Attending Anesthesiologist
New York University Medical Center
Attending Anesthesiologist
Bellevue Hospital Center
New York, NY

George S. Miz, M.D.

Department of Orthopaedic Surgery
Michael Reese Hospital and Medical Center
Chicago, IL

Ismael Montane, M.D.

Mount Sinai Medical Center
Clinical Assistant Professor
Orthopaedics and Rehabilitation
University of Miami School of Medicine
Miami, FL

James A. O'Neill, M.D.

Orthopaedic Surgeons
Associates of Lima Ohio
St. Rita's Medical Center
Lima Memorial Hospital
Lima, OH

Kent M. Patrick, M.D.

Sutter Community Hospital
Sacramento, CA

Avinash Patwardhan, Ph.D.

Associate Professor
Department of Orthopaedics
Loyola University
Chicago, IL

John G. Peters, M.D.

Clinical Fellow in Spine Surgery
Cleveland Metropolitan General Hospital
Case Western Reserve University
Cleveland, OH

Andrew E. Price, M.D.

New York University Medical Center
Department of Orthopaedics
New York, NY

Nahvash Rafii, M.D.

Clinical Associate Professor of Radiology
New York University Medical Center
New York, NY

Gerard Saillant, M.D.

Professeur
Faculté de Medicine
Pitié-Saltpétrière
Paris, France

Richard M. Sommer, M.D.

Chief, Anesthesiology
Manhattan V.A. Medical Center
Assistant Professor of Anesthesiology
New York University School of Medicine
New York, NY

R. Geoffrey Wilber, M.D.

Assistant Professor of Orthopaedics
Case Western Reserve University
Cleveland, OH

Wise Young, M.D., Ph.D.

Director of Neurosurgery
Research Laboratories
Associate Professor of Physiology and Biophysics
New York University
New York, NY

Michael R. Zindrick, M.D.

Spinal Cord Unit
Hines Veterans Administration Hospital
Hines, IL
Assistant Clinical Professor
Loyola University Medical Center
Maywood, IL

FOREWORD

For too many years most emergency rooms and trauma centers have referred patients with spinal trauma to orthopaedic surgeons if there was no neurological deficit and to neurosurgeons if there was. The result has not been optimal patient care. Frequently the orthopaedist has been inordinately concerned with the stability of the vertebral column which he would correct by increasingly complex internal fixation, with fatal disregard for important neurologic structures. Similarly the neurologic surgeon in his concern for the spinal cord and nerve roots has tended to ignore stability in an attempt to provide immediate relief of pressure, sometimes increasing the instability and the problems of long-range rehabilitation as a consequence. Today the lines between neurologic and orthopaedic surgical management have become less distinct, with both groups becoming sensitive to the needs of all aspects of spinal fractures. We believe it is no longer acceptable to have a disproportionately greater concern for one area than the other.

For these reasons, at New York University-Bellevue Medical Center, where we receive a large number of all spinal trauma patients in the greater New York area, both surgical specialties work together to provide comprehensive and optimal surgical care of the patient. To this end we have set up a fellowship program that encompasses both departments with equal emphasis, so that those trained in this program will be complete spinal surgeons and true representatives of the evolving discipline of neuro-orthopaedics. This book attempts to address the issues of spinal trauma using this approach.

Joseph Ransohoff, M.D.

Theodore R. Waugh, M.D., Ph.D., F.R.C.S.(C).

PREFACE

Increasingly the patient with a traumatic or pathologic fracture of the spine requires a multidisciplinary approach to treatment. Physicians need a common knowledge of both disciplines and must share their expertise with one another. As sophistication increases, the search for newer and better surgical techniques becomes more intense. Not only does this quest cross traditional disciplinary lines but international lines as well. The international experience with spinal treatment has grown until today it cannot be ignored. This book attempts to present a foundation of traditional information and integrate it with newer viewpoints not only from North America but from Europe as well.

The text strives to build in the reader a multi-disciplinary platform of knowledge including topics from anesthesiology, biomechanics, neurosciences, orthopaedics, pathology, radiology, and rehabilitation. The *general consideration* chapters attempt to provide an unbiased view of the world experience and current knowledge of management of traumatic injuries. Subsequent specific technique-oriented chapters are designed to present new concepts for the surgeon to integrate into his surgical armamentarium. No method is supported over another; each is presented with its inherent strong points and weak points.

The sections on spinal cord injury have been exhaustively prepared to provide a basic understanding of the intricacies of cord injury. Hopefully an understanding of the microdynamics of spinal cord injuries will lend insight to the physician dealing with the macromecanics of spinal column injuries.

A *special considerations* section has also been included. Sections on infections and on pathologic fractures due to tumors were included to show how they are similar and dissimilar to acute traumatic injuries. The remaining chapters were selected to shed light on specific critical aspects of spinal trauma.

This book should prove useful to medical students, residents, orthopaedists, neurosurgeons, physiatrists, and anesthesiologists alike. With a common background of information, the multidisciplinary approach to treatment can hopefully be enhanced.

Thomas J. Errico, M.D.

CONTENTS

THORACIC AND LUMBAR SPINE

SACRAL SPINE

SPINAL CORD INJURY

SPECIAL CONSIDERATIONS

1

HISTORICAL PERSPECTIVES OF SPINAL TRAUMA

Ismael Montane

EARLY TREATMENT

The Edwin Smith surgical papyrus is the oldest description of spinal cord injury in recorded history. Dated almost 5000 years ago, it described vertebral fractures as an "ailment not to be treated." This pessimistic attitude persisted until the Greek "Golden Era," when more modern teachings of medicine were introduced. Hippocrates is credited with advancing the treatment of spinal injuries. His method, which was used for centuries, achieved vertebral reduction and alignment by use of axial distraction while an anterior force was applied to the gibbus. The patient, placed prone on an extension bench, was distracted by simultaneous traction applied to the shoulders and hips. The physician either sat or stood on the gibbus until the deformity was reduced. Other physicians used a crossbar to apply direct pressure to the gibbus and thereby correct the deformity.

These forceful methods persisted through the Middle Ages with few modifications. Illustrations of these techniques appeared in manuscripts published in the 16th century (Figs. 1-1, 1-2). Both paralyzed and nonparalyzed patients were treated by these or even more brutal methods, such as those employed by Jean Francis Calot in the late 1800s. He described the manipulation of paralyzed patients with his fists in an attempt to correct the spinal deformity.

DEVELOPMENT OF MODERN METHODS

During the first half of this century, more modern methods of treatment of patients with spinal cord injury were developed. With the introduction of radiology, a greater understanding of the pathophysiology of vertebral fractures became possible. This led to advances in both conservative and operative management of patients with spinal cord injuries.[4,7,8,12,18,19,34,40]

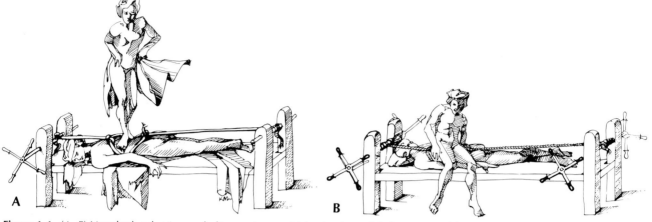

Figure 1-1. (*A, B*) Vertebral reduction and alignment was obtained using axial distraction while an anterior force was applied to the gibbus. The patient was placed prone on the extension bench, and distracted by simultaneous traction applied to the shoulders and hips. The physician then either sat or stood on the gibbus.

NONSURGICAL MANAGEMENT

Postural reduction by forced hyperextension of the spine was reported by several authors.[6,7,8,14] This was followed by hyperextension body casts applied from the symphysis pubis to below the clavicles. However, problems with pressure sores in patients with insensate skin soon limited their use, prompting the development of alternative management techniques for the spinal cord-injured individual.

During the 1940s several spinal cord injury centers were established in England to care for veterans and civilians who had sustained vertebral fractures with paralysis. The experience obtained from the management of a large number of patients with spinal cord injury allowed the development of gentler forms for achieving and maintaining spinal reduction. Guttman,[19] at Stoke Mandeville Hospital, obtained reduction using pillow packs or sorbo-rubber packs. The patient was lifted and turned by the nursing staff every 2 hours, so that when in the supine position, he would lie directly on the packs. In patients with neck injuries, cervical traction was added to facilitate postural reduction. Using these techniques, Guttman and other authors have reported a gradual correction of spinal alignment.[5,6,7,14,24,25] Once radiographic evidence of union occurred, the patient was permitted to sit in a light plastic body jacket or cervical collar.

In 1947, Stanger[36] reported a series of 43 patients with thoracolumbar and lumbar fracture-dislocations who were treated by either surgical or nonsurgical methods. He found a high incidence of late spinal deformity in patients who had radiologic evidence of a previous reduction with spinal realignment.

Nicoll,[32] in 1949, classified thoracolumbar fractures as being either stable or unstable depending on the integrity of the posterior interspinous ligaments. He considered an intact ligament to denote spinal stability, in which case further spinal reduction and immobilization were unnecessary. With rupture of the interspinous ligament he recommended postural reduction and cast immobilization. However, some patients were noted to develop late kyphotic deformities despite a previous anatomic reduction. This prompted renewed interest in the operative stabilization of vertebral fractures.

SURGICAL TECHNIQUES

Paul of Aegina performed the first surgical procedure for spinal cord injury in the 7th century. There are no other reports of spinal instrumenta-

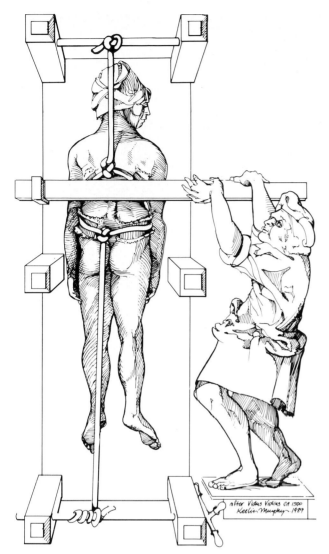

Figure 1-2. A crossbar was used to apply direct pressure to the gibbus and thereby correct the deformity. (Vidus Vidius: Chirurgia, è Graeco in Latinum Connersa. Paris, 1544)

tion until the second half of the 18th century, when interspinous wiring techniques for the management of cervical and thoracolumbar fractures were developed. These techniques failed largely because a concomitant spinal fusion was not performed.

In 1911, Hibbs[21] and Albee[3] reported using tibial bone graft for the fusion of scoliosis. With improved techniques of spinal fusion Albee[2] expanded its use, and in 1940 recommended open reduction and fusion of fracture-dislocations of the spine. He did not use internal fixation. Wilson,[42] in 1940, introduced the technique of stabilizing the fractured spine by plates. This method did not gain widespread acceptance until 1953, when Holdsworth and Hardy[23] improved the technique by using metal plates secured to the spinous processes with transfixing bolts.

Holdsworth and Hardy[23] revolutionized the management of vertebral fracture-dislocations in the second half of this century. They based their methods on their review of more than 1000 patients treated for traumatic paraplegia or quadriplegia at Sheffield Spinal Injuries Centre. They classified fractures into stable or unstable injuries according to the integrity of the posterior ligamentous complex. Stable fractures included compression and bursting fractures with an intact posterior ligamentous complex. Unstable injuries included pure dislocations, tension fractures, and rotational fracture-dislocations, also called slice fractures. After longer follow-up, they found that some of the patients initially presumed to have stable injuries developed progressive angulation with severe deformities.

Holdsworth[22,23] advocated open reduction and internal fixation with plates attached to the spinous processes. The purpose was to restore alignment and provide an optimal environment for maximum neurologic recovery. He recommended instrumenting one or two levels above and below the fracture, and limited the use of plates largely to thoracolumbar fracture-dislocations. He recommended 3 months of bedrest with periodic turning. Initially, Holdsworth and Hardy reported favorable results using these techniques. However, after longer follow-up they noted that many patients developed loosening of the plates with subsequent redislocation. This was particularly true with the use of the long, straight Meurig–Williams plates.

Additionally, Holdsworth[22] cautioned against routine laminectomy in patients with neurologic injury. His research demonstrated failure of significant neurologic recovery following laminectomy. In patients who were followed for longer periods he observed an increased potential for the development of late spinal deformity and further neurologic injury.

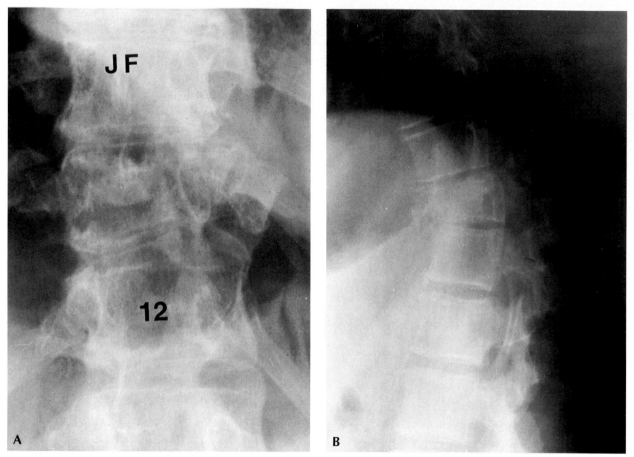

Figure 1-3. This 56-year-old man fell 20 feet from a tree. He sustained a fracture-dislocation of T-11–T-12 without neurological injury. (A) Anteroposterior radiograph shows compressing of the interior end-plate of T-11 with disruption of the right-sided facets. (B) Lateral radiograph shows anterior compression T-11 with an acute kyphosis of the thoracolumbar junction.

INSTRUMENTATION TECHNIQUES

In 1958, Harrington[14] first applied dual-distraction rod instrumentation for the treatment of thoracolumbar spine fracture-dislocations. His method employed Hippocrates' principles of vertebral reduction. Axially directed forces created at the end vertebrae instrumented restored vertebral length, while anatomic reduction of the gibbus was effected by anteriorly directed forces created as the rods pushed the apical laminae forward. Harrington recommended insertion of the hooks two intact laminae above and below the fractured segment.

Harrington rod instrumentation rapidly gained widespread acceptance, with many authors advocating its use for the treatment of thoracolumbar and lumbar injuries (Fig. 1-3).[9,13,17,37,43] Its indiscriminate use for all types of fractures led several authors to report instrument failure secondary to either hook dislodgment or cut-out at the superior hook site, especially when the rods were not contoured to reconstruct the normal sagittal spinal alignment. Purcell and associates[33] performed Harrington rod instrumentation on fresh cadaver spines. They found that increased stability was obtained by hook placement three laminae above and two laminae below the unstable segment. This

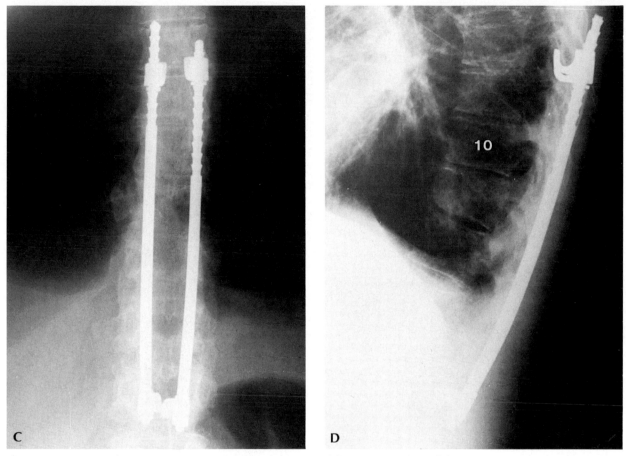

Figure 1-3. (*Continued*). (*C*) Upon surgery complete dislocation of the T-11–T-12 facets bilaterally was observed. Harrington rod instrumentation from T-8 to L-2 with fusion was used to stabilize the spine. (*D*) Note correction of the kyphotic deformity and restoration of vertebral height.

provided increased stability particularly in the flexion mode, and decreased the probability of superior hook failure.

In 1982, Luque and associates[28a] described segmental spinal instrumentation using Luque-rods secured with sublaminar wires. This method of segmental stabilization was initially developed to facilitate postoperative care for patients with paralytic spinal deformities. Luque rod instrumentation soon began to be used for the treatment of other spinal disorders, including spinal fractures. Biomechanical studies have demonstrated that Luque rod instrumentation provides very rigid stabilization with good flexion and rotational con-

trol.[41] Its strongest indication is the stabilization of severe thoracolumbar fracture-dislocations in which there has been a disruption of the anterior longitudinal ligament. Telescoping of the instrumented vertebral segments may occur and its use in burst fractures may result in increased retropulsion of bone and disk fragments within the canal with further encroachment of the neural tissues.

Several authors[1,11,39] have subsequently combined the instrumentation techniques developed by Harrington and Luque to obtain increased stability of distraction instrumentation of spinal fractures. With sublaminar wiring of distraction rods, secure segmental fixation is achieved (Fig. 1-4). Decreased instrumentation failure from hook dislodgment or cut-out by combining these techniques has been demonstrated both experimentally and clinically.

MANAGEMENT OF LUMBAR SPINE FRACTURES

The management of lumbar fractures incorporates two basic principles: the preservation of lumbar lordosis and the preservation of all possible free-motion segments below the fused spinal segment. Of the two, preservation of lumbar lordosis is the most important. In 1977, Moe and Denis[31] reported the iatrogenic loss of lumbar lordosis that resulted from the use of straight Harrington distraction rods in the lumbar spine. Failure to preserve lumbar lordosis produced a crouched gait with abnormal or impaired ambulation, especially in those patients who had neurologic injuries.[20,31] To preserve lumbar lordosis they recommended the use of square-ended rods contoured to recreate normal lordosis.[32,42] Edwards,[16] prompted by the technical difficulties involved in Harrington rod instrumentation of the lumbar spine, developed polypropylethelene spacers. These spacers effectively increased lumbar lordosis by applying direct pressure to the apical laminae. Un-

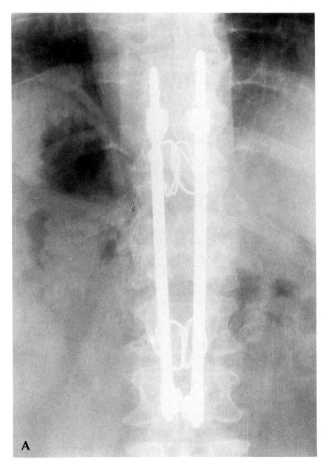

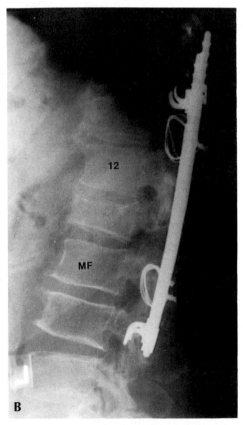

Figure 1-4. This 55-year-old man sustained a fracture-dislocation of T-12–L-1 with complete paraplegia as a result of a boating accident. Anteroposterior (A) and lateral (B) postoperative radiographs show Harrington rods in place with restoration of the normal spinal alignment. Note augmentation of fixation by sublaminar wires one level above and below the fractured segment.

fortunately, both the Moe and Denis and the Edwards techniques still require placement of the inferior hooks two laminae below the fractured segment, thereby sacrificing mobile lumbar segments. Several authors have addressed this problem by "rodding long and fusing short," with subsequent removal of the rods 1 year after surgery. However, degeneration of the articular cartilage of the facets and spontaneous fusion have been reported in both experimental models and clinical settings.[24]

In an attempt to preserve motion segments, several other techniques were developed. Screw fixation of the lumbar spine was initially performed by King[26] in 1944 and Boucher[10] in 1955. They described oblique transfacet fixation and fusion. However, a high incidence of nerve injury and a high rate of pseudarthrosis forced the abandonment of these techniques. In 1970, Roy-Camille[35] described segmental fixation of the lumbar spine using transpedicular and interfacet fixation. During the last decade, other authors have used interpeduncular osteosynthesis for the stabilization of lumbar fractures.[29,38,44] Initially, they recommended instrumenting two levels above and below the fractured segment. More recently, with improved interpeduncular fixation devices, secure rigid fixation has been achieved by instrumenting only one level above and below the fractured segment.[44]

Alternatively, external spinal skeletal fixation has been used in Switzerland since 1977 for the reduction and stabilization of thoracolumbar and lumbar fractures.[30] Transpedicular insertion of Schanz screws linked by an adjustable connecting device is used to obtain reduction and maintain spinal alignment. Simultaneous screw fixation of the facet joints improves the stability of the spinal construct and consequently the degree of neurologic recovery in patients who have sustained incomplete spinal cord injuries. However, if rigid stabilization is not obtained in unstable injuries, the result is dislodgment of the bone graft or pseudarthrosis.

These problems have prompted several investigators to develop anterior spinal fixation devices. Dunn[15] designed an implant system to rigidly fix thoracolumbar and lumbar fractures. This anterior device rigidly fixes the spine at a single level above and below the level of injury. The system consists of two rods linked by vertebral body bridges. Instrumentation and fusion at only two spinal motion units allows preservation of more mobile lumbar segments. Kostiuk[27,28] and Kaneda[25] have also developed anterior spinal implants for the stabilization of bursting fractures of the thoracolumbar and lumbar spine. They have reported that anterior instrumentation effectively stabilizes the fractured segment and allows a better environment for neurologic recovery.

SUMMARY

Spinal cord injuries have occurred throughout recorded history. Due to the dismal outcome that followed these injuries, for centuries patients were treated by benign neglect. Hippocrates studied the pathophysiology of vertebral fractures and established the principles of vertebral reduction and spinal realignment, which are still used today.

During this century, spinal cord injury centers have been established to provide comprehensive care for patients with vertebral fractures and dislocations. The concentration of a large number of patients in these centers has resulted in more modern management of spinal cord injuries. Additionally, posterior and anterior surgical techniques of spinal stabilization with instrumentation and fusion have been developed to facilitate care, preserve existing neurologic function, and allow a better environment for neurologic recovery.

REFERENCES

1. Akbarnia BA, Fogarty JP, Tayob AA: Contoured Harrington instrumentation in the treatment of unstable spinal fractures: The effect of supplementary sublaminar wires. Clin Orthop 189:186–194, 1984
2. Albee FH: Bone Graft Surgery. New York, Appleton, 1940
3. Albee FH: Transplantation of a portion of the tibia into the spine for Pott's disease: A preliminary report. JAMA 57:885, 1911
4. Bailey RW, Badgley CE: Stabilization of the cervical spine by anterior fusion. J Bone Joint Surg [Am] 42:565–594, 1960

5. Beatson TR: Fractures and dislocations of the cervical spine. J Bone Joint Surg [Br] 45:21–35, 1963

6. Bedbrook GM: Pathological principles in the management of spine cord trauma. Paraplegia 4:43–56, 1966

7. Bedbrook GM: Spinal injuries with tetraplegia and paraplegia. J Bone Joint Surg [Br] 61:267–284, 1979

8. Bohlman HH: Acute fractures and dislocations of the cervical spine: An analysis of three hundred hospitalized patients and review of the literature. J Bone Joint Surg [Am] 61:1119–1142, 1979

9. Bohlman HH: Treatment of fractures and dislocations of the thoracic and lumbar spine. J Bone Joint Surg [Am] 67:165–169, 1985

10. Boucher HH: A method of spinal fusion. J Bone Joint Surg [Br] 41:248, 1959

11. Bryant CE, Sullivan A: Management of thoracic and lumbar spine fractures with Harrington distraction rods supplemented with segmental wiring. Spine 8:532–537, 1983

12. Cheshire DJE: The stability of the cervical spine following the conservative treatment of fractures and fracture dislocations. Paraplegia 7:192–203, 1969

13. DeWald RL: Burst fractures of the thoracic and lumbar spine. Clin Orthop 189:150–161, 1984

14. Dickson JH, Harrington PR, Erwin WD: Results of reduction and stabilization of the severely fractured thoracic and lumbar spine. J Bone Joint Surg [Am] 60:799–805, 1978

15. Dunn HK: Anterior stabilization of thoracolumbar injuries. Clin Orthop 189:116–124, 1984

16. Edwards CC, Griffith P, Levine AM, DeSilva JB: Early clinical results using the spinal rod sleeve method for treating thoracic and lumbar injuries. Orthopaedic Transactions 6:345, 1982

17. Flesch JR, Lieder LL, Erickson DL et al: Harrington instrumentation and spine fusion for unstable fractures and fracture dislocations of the thoracic spine. J Bone Joint Surg [Am] 59:143–153, 1977

18. Frankel HL, Hancock DO, Hyslop G et al: The value of postural reductions in the initial management of closed injuries of the spine with paraplegia and tetraplegia. Paraplegia 7:179–192, 1969

19. Guttman L: Surgical aspects of the treatment of traumatic paraplegia. J Bone Joint Surg [Br] 31:399–403, 1949

20. Hasday CA, Passoff TL, Perry J: Gait abnormalities arising from iatrogenic loss of lumbar lordosis secondary to Harrington instrumentation in lumbar fractures. Spine 8:501–511, 1983

21. Hibbs PA: An operation for progressive deformities. NY State J Med 93:1013, 1911

22. Holdsworth F: Fractures, dislocations and fracture-dislocations of the spine. J Bone Joint Surg [Am] 52:1534–1551, 1970

23. Holdsworth FW, Hardy A: Early treatment of paraplegia from fractures of the thoracolumbar spine. J Bone Joint Surg [Br] 35:540–550, 1953

24. Kahanovitz N, Bullough P, Jafcobs RR: The effect of internal fixation without arthrodesis on human facet joint cartilage. Clin Orthop 189:204–208, 1984

25. Kaneda K, Abume K, Fujiya M: Burst fractures of thoracolumbar and lumbar spine with neurologic involvement: Anterior decompression and fusion with instrumentation. Presented at the meeting of the Scoliosis Research Society, Denver, Colorado, September, 1982

26. King D: Internal fixation for lumbosacral fusion. Am J Surg 66:357, 1944

27. Kostuik JP: Anterior fixation for fractures of the thoracic and lumbar spine with or without neurologic involvement. Clin Orthop 189:103–115, 1984

28. Kostuik JP: Anterior spinal cord decompression for lesions of the thoracic and lumbar spine: Techniques new methods of internal fixation results. Spine 8:512–531, 1983

28a. Luque ER, Cassis N, Ramirez-Wiella G: Segmental spinal instrumentation in the treatment of fractures of the thoracolumbar spine. Spine 7:312–317, 1982

29. Luque ER: Interpeduncular segmental fixation. Clin Orthop 203:54–57, 1986

30. Magerl F: Stabilization of the lower thoracic and lumbar spine with external skeletal fixation. Clin Orthop 189:125–141, 1984

31. Moe JH, Denis F: The iatrogenic loss of lumbar lordosis. Orthopaedic Transactions 1:131, 1977

32. Nicoll EA: Fractures of the dorso-lumbar spine. J Bone Joint Surg [Br] 31:376–394, 1949

33. Purcell GA, Markof KL, Dawson EA: Twelfth thoracic-first lumbar vertebral mechanical stability of fractures after Harrington rod instrumentation. J Bone Joint Surg [Am] 63:71, 1981

34. Rogers WA: Treatment of fracture dislocations of the cervical spine. J Bone Joint Surg 24:245–258, 1942

35. Roy-Camille R, Saillant G, Mazel C: Internal fixation of the lumbar spine with pedicle screw plating. Clin Orthop 203:7–17, 1986

36. Stanger JK: Fracture-dislocation of the thoracolumbar spine with special reference to reduction by open and closed operations. J Bone Joint Surg 29:107–118, 1947

37. Stauffer ES: Internal fixation of fractures of the thoracolumbar spine. J Bone Joint Surg [Am] 66:1136–1138, 1984

38. Steffee AD, Biscup RS, Sitkowski DJ: Segmental spine plates with pedicle screw fixation: A new internal fixation device for disorders of the lumbar and thoracolumbar spine. Clin Orthop 203:45–53, 1986

39. Sullivan JA: Sublaminar wiring of Harrington distraction rods for unstable thoracolumbar spine fractures. Clin Orthop 189:178–185, 1984

40. Watson-Jones SR: Fractures and Other Bone and Joint Injuries, p. 211. Baltimore, Williams & Wilkins, 1940

41. Wenger DR, Carollo JJ, Wilderson JA et al: Laboratory testing of segmental spinal instrumentation versus traditional Harrington instrumentation for scoliosis treatment. Spine 7:265–269, 1982

42. Wilson PD, Straub LR: Lumbosacral fusion with metallic plate fixation. Am Acad Orthop Instr Course Lectures 9:53, 1952

43. Yosipovitch Z, Robin GC, Makin M.: Open reduction of unstable thoracolumbar spinal injuries and fixation with Harrington rods. J Bone Joint Surg [Am] 59:1003–1015, 1977

44. Zuckerman J, Hsu K, White A, Wynne G: Early results of spinal fusion using variable spine plating system. Spine 13:570–579, 1988

2

RADIOGRAPHIC DIAGNOSIS OF FRACTURE-DISLOCATIONS OF THE SPINE

Hossein Firooznia
Mahvash Rafii
Cornelia Golimbu
Vincent J. Gulfo

The clinical and radiographic diagnosis of fracture-dislocations of the spine is difficult. There are a number of reasons for this. First, the anatomy of the spine is intricate. The spine consists of curvilinear and overlapping surfaces, with complex and varied articulations between adjacent vertebrae. The vertebrae are not only anatomically different in the cervical, thoracic, and lumbar segments of the spine, but each vertebra is also shaped differently from the ones caudad and cephalad to it within the same segment. Mastering the three-dimensional anatomy of the spine and its contents is an arduous and challenging task.

Second, it is often difficult, if not impossible, to project the various components of the vertebrae on conventional radiography free from the adjacent structures of the spine. Conventional tomography overcomes some of these difficulties, and when indicated, is helpful in delineation of the precise anatomy of the spine. However, the most significant advance in radiographic diagnosis of disorders of the spine was achieved when computed tomography (CT) and subsequently magnetic resonance imaging (MRI) were introduced into clinical practice. Their use made it possible to generate cross-sectional images in virtually any plane desired, eliminating the confusing superimposition of the image of adjacent structures.

Computed tomography is particularly helpful for an axial delineation of the anatomy and pathology of the spinal canal, vertebral arch, and vertebral elements. Because CT relies on absorption of roentgen rays by the tissues in its path, it is most helpful in delineation of structures containing calcification, dense osteosclerotic bone, and cortical bone, which is a major component of the vertebral arch and vertebral elements and forms an envelope surrounding the peripheral margin of the vertebral bodies.

Magnetic resonance imaging is most useful in evaluation of the soft-tissue content of the spine, particularly the spinal cord and spinal nerves. It is also useful for a long-segment, overall evaluation of the alignment of the spine and for evaluating the alignment, size, and configuration of the spinal canal as well as the intervertebral disks and paravertebral soft tissues. The ability to directly generate coronal and sagittal sections of the spine and its contents is a distinct advantage of MRI.

The following is a brief description of the radiologic diagnosis of fracture-dislocations of the spine. For a comprehensive study of spinal anatomy, the reader is referred to classic textbooks of anatomy and to more recent CT and MRI correlative studies with microsectional anatomy of the spine. An excellent and exhaustive study of roentgen anatomy of the spine by means of conventional radiography as well as of conventional radi graphic diagnosis of fracture-dislocations of the spine may be found in a classic textbook by Gehweiler and associates.[12] Computed tomography of spinal trauma will be briefly discussed in this chapter. Magnetic resonance imaging of trauma to the spine is covered in Chapter 3.

RADIOGRAPHIC EXAMINATION OF THE ACUTELY INJURED PATIENT

Emergency care and subsequent management of patients with injury to the spine requires medical personnel with specialized training. Proper care of the patient starts at the scene of the accident and includes extrication of the patient from the accident scene, handling of the patient during transport to a suitable trauma center, and medical care and life-support assistance in the receiving facility.

The radiographic examination of these patients, who may have significant neurologic deficit, may be unconscious, or may suffer from multi-system injury, presents a distinct challenge. Every trauma center must have a protocol for evaluation of patients with multi-organ injury that includes the radiographic examination of the patient. This protocol should specify the kind of radiographic views that must be obtained in these patients to assure that no significant injury goes unrecognized. Although it is the duty of the radiologist to ensure that a proper and pertinent radiographic examination of the spine is performed, nevertheless, the timing and the extent of the radiographic examina-

tion must fit into the overall protocol for the clinical care of these patients. It is obvious that the welfare of the patient, not the beauty of the radiographic images, is the most important issue.

The critical condition of some patients with spinal injury and the need for surgical and medical intervention to save the patient's life necessitates a flexible protocol. Some institutions have multiple protocols depending on the clinical status of the patient and the nature and extent of suspected organ injuries. Protocols for the care of these critically ill patients must be developed jointly by emergency room nurses, emergency care physicians, trauma surgeons, radiologists, orthopedists, and neurosurgeons.

RADIOGRAPHIC TECHNIQUE

Patients with injury to the spine are usually in the supine position on a spinal board, with sandbags on either side of the neck and skull, when radiographic examination begins. They may already be in traction. It is possible to obtain a fairly complete radiographic examination of the cervical, thoracic, and lumbar spine with the patient in this position, without moving the patient, by use of a portable x-ray unit.

Cervical Spine

Gehweiler and associates[12] recommend the following six views of the cervical spine. In our experience, their technique has proven to be of great value:

1. Cross-table lateral view with a grid cassette
2. Right and left 30-degree oblique views. The roentgenogram tube is angled toward the head of the patient. The central beam enters just behind the larynx. A nongrid cassette is placed flat on the stretcher as close to the neck as possible.
3. Anteroposterior view of the lower cervical spine. The central ray must have an angle of 20 degrees with the vertical in a cranial direction.
4. Anteroposterior view of the atlanto-axial complex through the open mouth, if possible.

5. Anteroposterior vertebral arch view with the central beam angled 25 to 30 degrees toward the feet.

The cross-table lateral view of the cervical spine is the single most important projection of the spine in these patients. Approximately two thirds of all fracture-dislocations of the cervical spine are detectable on the lateral radiograph of the spine. Because fracture-dislocations of C-6, C-7, and T-1 vertebrae are quite common, it is imperative that the lateral view of the cervical spine demonstrate these vertebrae. In some patients the shoulders obscure the lower cervical vertebrae. In these patients, the shoulders should be pulled down. To do this two assistants, each holding one of the patient's wrists, pull the shoulders gently down, while the neck is kept in traction. Alternatively, traction may be applied on the arm by means of canvas straps on the patient's wrists, over padding, as described by McRae.[21] It may be necessary to obtain a swimmer's view of the spine. A cross-table swimmer's view should be sufficiently well exposed to visualize the lower cervical and upper thoracic vertebrae.

If sufficient radiographic information is not obtained, and the condition of the patient permits, there should be no hesitation in performing tomography of the spine.

Thoracic and Lumbar Spine

The following two projections are the minimum radiographic views of the thoracic and lumbar spine, and can be obtained in all patients in the supine position on a stretcher:

1. Anteroposterior projection of the spine. It may be necessary to perform multiple anteroposterior projections to encompass the entire suspected area of pathology. Depending on the curvature of the spine, i.e., kyphosis or lordosis, it may be necessary to angle the central roentgen beams toward the patients's feet or head in order to obtain true en-face views of the body of the vertebrae. In some patients, anteroposterior angled views may show the vertebral arch to better advantage.
2. Cross-table lateral view of the spine. Once

again, multiple lateral views may have to be obtained for proper evaluation of the entire length of the thoracic and lumbar spine.

If sufficient information is not obtained on these studies, further radiographic examination should be performed as clinically indicated. In all instances, the extent of radiographic examination should be tailored to the patient's clinical situation and the usefulness of the information obtained for management of the patient.

ROUTINE RADIOGRAPHIC EXAMINATION OF THE SPINE

It is obvious that when the initial clinical examination in the emergency room indicates that the patient is a candidate for a routine radiographic examination, this examination should be tailored to the patient, taking into consideration the probable injury to the spine.

CERVICAL SPINE

A routine, or standard radiographic examination of the cervical spine (Figs. 2-1 to 2-9) usually consists of:

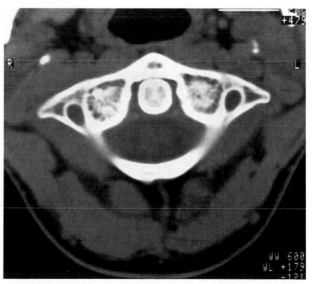

Figure 2-1. Normal C-1–C-2: Axial CT through the atlas and odontoid process. Note the normal relationship of the odontoid process to the anterior arch of the atlas and spinal canal.

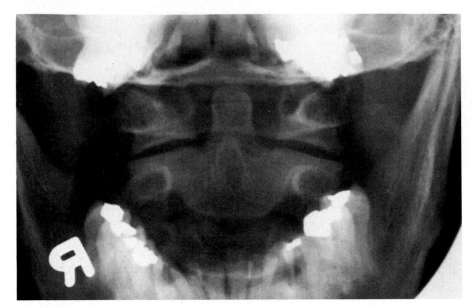

Figure 2-2. Normal C-1–C-2: Anteroposterior, open-mouth view of the atlanto-axial complex. Note the normal relationship between the articular facets of C-1 and C-2 and the exact alignment of the lateral surface of the lateral masses of C-1 with the corresponding part of C-2.

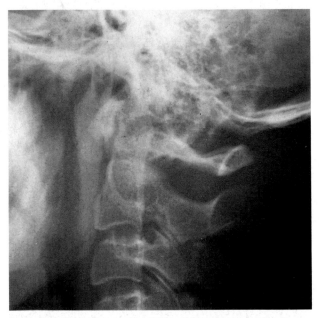

Figure 2-3. Lateral view of the C-1–C-2 region.

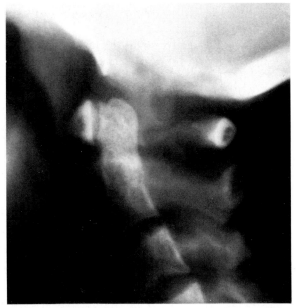

Figure 2-4. Midline tomogram of the C-1–C-2 region. Note the normal relationship of the odontoid process to the anterior arch of C-1. The joint space (predental space) between the odontoid process and the anterior arch of C-1 is observed. Note the relationship of the odontoid process to the spinal canal.

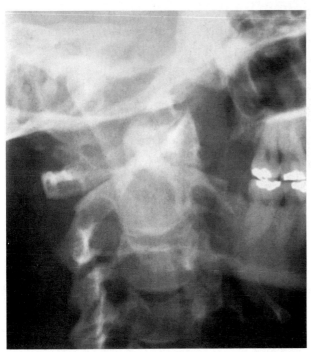

Figure 2-5. Normal oblique projection of the C-1–C-2–C-3 region. In some patients, the body of C-2 and the odontoid process are better visualized on the oblique projection of the cervical spine.

1. Anteroposterior view of the atlanto-axial complex through the open mouth or with the jaw in motion.
2. Anteroposterior view of the lower cervical spine, preferably angled 20 degrees cephalad.
3. Lateral projection of the cervical spine.
4. Right and left oblique projections.

We prefer to obtain the lateral and oblique projections of the cervical spine with the patient in the erect position. The patient may sit on a stool. The shoulders should be dropped down. In patients with a short neck and/or stout shoulders this study should be performed with the patient holding a weight in his hands to help lower the shoulders. The lateral projection should, at the least, show all seven cervical vertebrae and, if possible, the first and second thoracic vertebrae. In some patients this is not possible. In these patients, a 10- to 15-degree oblique view of the cer-

vicothoracic region should be performed. With the patient sitting on a stool or standing up, the central beam should be directed at the cervicothoracic junction. The patient is then turned 10 to 15 degrees from the lateral position, the arm closest to the cassette is raised and the hand is placed on the head, and the other arm is pulled down with the help of a weight held in the hand.[22] This

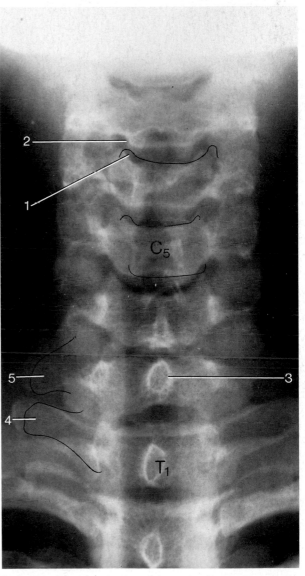

Figure 2-6. Frontal projection of the cervical spine. (1) Uncinate process. (2) Luschka (uncovertebral) joint. (3) Spinous process of C-7. (4) Transverse process of T-1. (5) Transverse process of C-7.

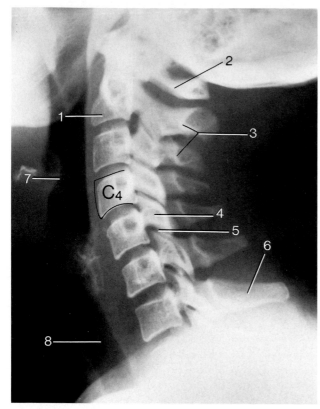

Figure 2-7. Normal lateral projection of the cervical spine. (1) Body of C-2. (2) Posterior arch of C-1. (3) Spinal–laminal junction forming the posterior wall of the spinal canal. (4) Articulating pyramid of C-5. (5) C-5–C-6 facet joint. (6) Spinous process of C-7. (7) Hyoid bone. (8) Trachea.

projection may have to be repeated with slightly different oblique angulations. In most instances, the lower cervical and upper thoracic bodies are seen to better advantage on the oblique views.

Other Views of the Cervical Spine

Because of the complexity of the anatomy of the cervical vertebrae and overlapping of multiple structures, in a significant number of patients with injuries to the cervical spine, it may be impossible to visualize the exact site and nature of the pathology. For this reason, a number of other views of the cervical spine have been recommended by various investigators.

McRae[21] considers frontal and lateral stereoscopic views of the cervical spine to be essential.

Gehweiler[12] and Abel[1] have used 13 projections of the cervical spine to fully visualize the morphology of each vertebra. The projections are:

1. Anteroposterior view of the atlas–axis through the open mouth.
2. Anteroposterior view of the lower cervical spine.
3. Lateral projections in neutral, flexion, and extension positions.

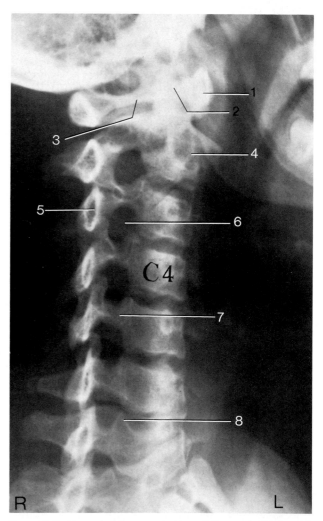

Figure 2-8. Normal oblique projection of the cervical spine. (1) Anterior arch of C-1. (2) Odontoid process. (3) Posterior arch of C-1. (4) Body of C-2. (5) Lamina of C-3 seen on end. (6) Right neural foramen between C-3 and C-4. (7) Right pedicle of C-5. (8) Right uncinate process of C-7.

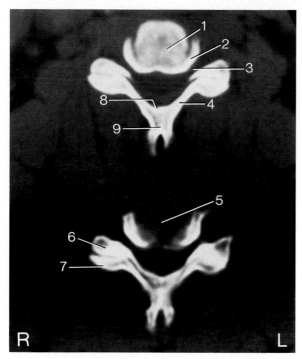

Figure 2-9. Normal CT of C-5 and C-5–C-6 disk. (1) Inferior end-plate of C-5. (2) Left uncinate process of C-6. (3) Neural foramen. (4) Lamina. (5) C-5–C-6 intervertebral disk. (6) Superior articular process of C-6. (7) Inferior articular process of C-5. (8) Spinal–laminal junction and cortex of the posterior wall of the spinal canal. (9) Spinous process.

4. 45 degree right and left oblique projections.
5. 20-degree right and left oblique projections.
6. Posteroanterior arch views.
7. Right and left posterior oblique vertebral arch views.
8. Semiaxial view of the atlas.

We have found that around-the-clock oblique projections centered on the C-1–C-2 region are occasionally very helpful in patients with suspected injuries to this region.

It is obvious that these extensive series of the cervical spine cannot be performed on a routine basis on all patients suspected of cervical spine trauma. In our experience, several of these views have to be repeated with different angulations and different exposure factors, even in the hands of the most experienced technologists and when technically up-to-date radiographic equipment is used.

In our experience the procedure takes at least 1 hour, often longer, and may still not show the full extent of the pathology, particularly when encroachment into the spinal canal is present or when small fractures of the posterior arch and articular pillars are present.

We believe these specialized views, as well as other special views of the spine, should only be used when there is a definite clinical indication for the presence of a fracture or dislocation of the cervical spine and yet the routine radiographic examination is apparently normal and a high-resolution CT examination of the cervical spine, supplemented by tomography if needed, reveals no indication for a fracture or dislocation. Clinical indications include pain and disability following injury to the cervical spine, evidence of motor and sensory deficit, and other findings.

We prefer CT as a problem-solving modality for suspected fracture-dislocations of the cervical spine to the specialized views of the spine just described. However, in traumatic lesions of the atlanto-axial region and in some patients with moderate compression fractures of the vertebral bodies, conventional tomography may have to be performed in addition to CT. In our experience, it is the rare patient in whom various fractures of the cervical spine, particularly those affecting the articular pyramids and the vertebral arch, are not discovered on high-resolution CT.

We have examined 13 patients with undiagnosed fracture-dislocations on routine cervical spine views in whom both the specialized views mentioned above as well as a high resolution CT examination of the cervical spine were performed. In six patients, conventional tomography was also performed. Although most of the clinically significant fracture-dislocations of the spine were seen on both CT and the specialized views, the recognition was clearly easier on CT examination. Additionally, in seven patients one or two small fractures of the margins of the articular pillars, pedicles, foramen transversarium, and the posterior surface of the vertebral body were discovered on CT, but escaped detection on the specialized views. In no patient was a fracture noted on the specialized views that was not noted on the CT examination. Based on our experience with these patients as well as our review of CT examination of more than 400 patients with fracture-dislocations of the cervical spine, we believe that CT, supplemented by conventional tomography if necessary, is the procedure of choice in patients with suspected occult traumatic injuries of the cervical spine.

We prefer CT because it is easier to identify and characterize most fracture-dislocations, there is no need for a technician with specialized training in spinal trauma radiography, the examination time is significantly shorter, the cost is less, and radiation exposure to the patient is a fraction of that delivered by the specialized views described.

THORACIC SPINE

The following views are obtained as clinically indicated (Figs. 2-10 to 14):

1. Anteroposterior view.
2. Lateral view of the thoracic spine.
3. Lateral swimmer's view of C-7 and the T-1–T-3 region.
4. Lateral, slightly oblique view of the upper thoracic spine. (This projection is the same as the lateral-oblique projection of the lower cervical spine already described.)

Because the thoracic spine usually has a kyphotic curvature, it may become necessary to obtain multiple frontal projections with slight angulations of the central beam when studying specific vertebral bodies. Although oblique projections are not ordinarily obtained, in many instances these are very helpful.

The first three to four thoracic vertebrae are difficult to visualize on conventional radiography. Consequently, significant pathology of these vertebrae may go unnoticed. We believe that CT is the procedure of choice for evaluation of this region. Although conventional tomography can be performed in frontal projection for this region, conventional radiography and tomography in lateral projection are not ideal for this region.

LUMBAR SPINE

The routine views (Figs. 2-15, 2-16, 2-17) of the lumbar spine are the following:

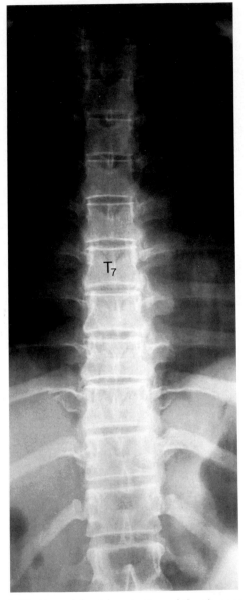

Figure 2-10. Normal frontal projection of the thoracic spine. Note poor visualization of T-1, T-2, and T-3. The pedicles of the thoracic vertebrae may appear thin and inconspicuous on the frontal projection. The posterior arch cannot be evaluated on this view. The costovertebral articulations are also poorly visualized.

1. Anteroposterior view of the lumbar spine.
2. Lateral view of the lumbosacral spine.
3. Spot lateral view of the L-4–L-5–S-1 region.
4. Right and left oblique views of the lumbar spine.

anteroposterior view of the lumbar spine with the central ray angled cranially would show the bodies of these vertebrae to better advantage. The oblique projections of the lumbar spine are particularly useful for demonstration of the facet joints, superior and inferior articular processes, and laminae. However, because the angle of inclination of the facet joints is not the same throughout the lumbar spine, an additional oblique projection with a different angle may be necessary.

(Text continued on p. 22)

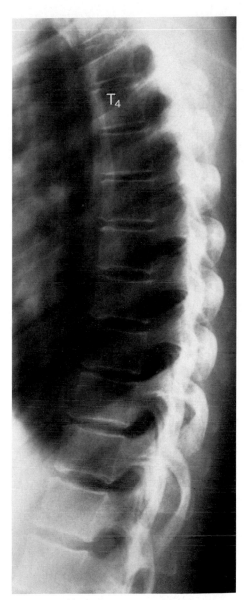

Figure 2-11. Normal lateral projection of the thoracic spine. The vertebral bodies and the intervertebral disks are well seen on this projection. The right and left pedicles are superimposed. The posterior arch is almost completely obscured by the superimposed image of the ribs.

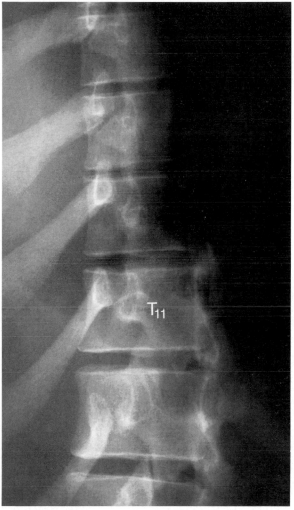

Figure 2-12. Normal oblique projection of the lower thoracic spine. The costovertebral articulations are better visualized on this projection. However, a definitive evaluation usually requires a CT examination.

In many patients the bodies of L-5 and occasionally L-4 are not well seen on routine anteroposterior views of the lumbar spine. This is because the longitudinal axis of these two vertebrae is not perpendicular to the roentgen beam. An

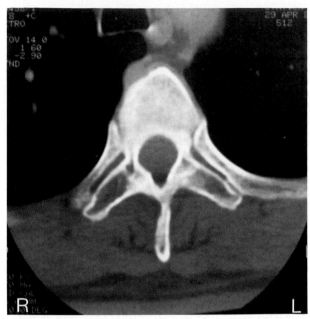

Figure 2-13. Normal CT examination through T-5 reveals the articulation of the ribs with the vertebral body (costocentral) and with the transverse process (costotransverse).

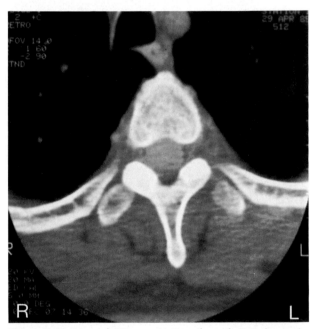

Figure 2-14. Normal CT examination through T-5 shows the thoracic neural foramen.

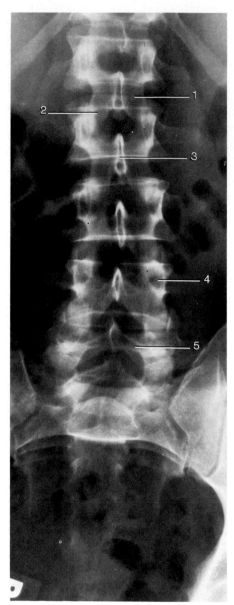

Figure 2-15. Normal frontal (anteroposterior) projection of the lumbar spine. (1) Lamina of L-1. (2) Inferior articular process of L-1. (3) Spinous process of L-2. (4) Pedicle of L-4. (5) Lamina of L-5. The body of L-5 is not visualized because of lordosis.

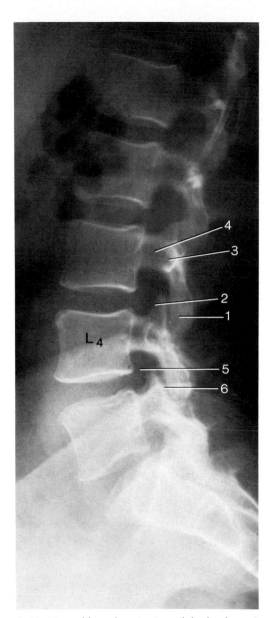

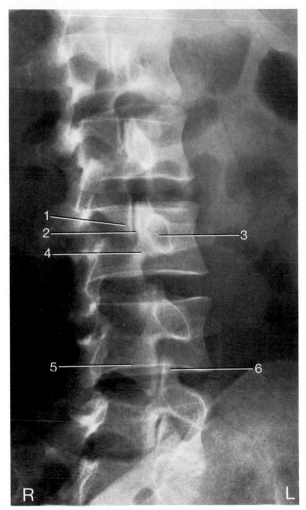

Figure 2-16. Normal lateral projection of the lumbar spine. (1) Inferior articular process of L-3. (2) Superior articular process of L-4. (3) Transverse process of L-3 seen on end. (4) Pedicle of L-3. (5) Neural foramen between L-4 and L-5. (6) Facet joint between L-4 and L-5.

Figure 2-17. Normal oblique projection of the lumbar spine. (1) Inferior articular process of L-2. (2) Facet joint between L-2 and L-3. (3) Eye of the "Scotty dog," which is mostly composed of the pedicle at L-1. As one goes toward L-5, the base of the transverse process and pedicle merge and become essentially one structure at L-5. Thus, the eye of the Scotty dog is formed by the base of the transverse process and the pedicle at L-5. (4) Neck of the Scotty dog, which corresponds to the pars interarticularis. (5) Lamina of L-4. (6) Superior articular process of L-5.

As is the case for the cervical spine and thoracic spine, we prefer to use CT as a problem-solving modality in patients with suspected traumatic lesions of the lumbar spine (Fig. 2-18). Most fracture-dislocations of the thoracic spine and lumbar spine are well delineated on CT.

NORMAL ANATOMY AND RADIOGRAPHIC EXAMINATION OF SPINAL PARTS

LANDMARKS OF THE LATERAL PROJECTION OF THE CERVICAL SPINE

The atlanto-axial complex is well visualized on conventional radiography. On anteroposterior open-mouth views or an anteroposterior view obtained with the jaw in motion (chewing), the atlas, odontoid process, and atlanto-axial articulations are well seen. With the head held in a straight position, the odontoid process should be in the midline and the atlas in the coronal position. The atlanto-occipital joints and lateral atlanto-axial joints should be symmetrical, and the articular

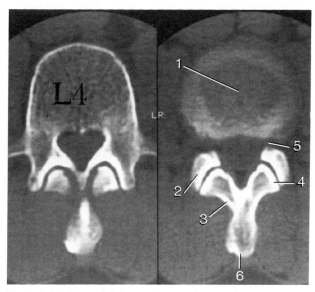

Figure 2-18. Normal CT examination of L-4 and L-4–L-5 intervertebral disk. (1) L-4–L-5 disk. (2) Superior articular process of L-5. (3) Lamina of L-4. (4) Facet joint formed between the superior articular process of L-5 and the inferior articular process of L-4. (5) Left neural foramen of L-4–L-5. (6) Spinous process of L-4.

facets should match without a noticeable overhanging of their margins. If there is any doubt as to the integrity of these structures, conventional tomography in the frontal and lateral projections should be performed. Conventional tomography is particularly helpful for clarification of deformities of the odontoid process, fractures through the odontoid process or the body of C-2, and in some fractures of the atlas. On the lateral projection, the relationship of the anterior arch of the atlas to the odontoid process and basion is usually well seen. Ordinarily, the body of C-2 and the odontoid process are in a moderate lordotic position as a continuation of the lordosis of the cervical spine. The median atlanto-axial articulation should be carefully evaluated on every lateral radiographic projection of the cervical spine. The joint between the anterior arch of the atlas and the odontoid process is usually visualized as a thin lucent line. The width of this joint, the predental space, should not normally exceed 3 mm in adults.[12,17] In children, up to 5 mm may be normal.

The prespinal soft tissues should be carefully evaluated on lateral projections of the cervical spine. The thickness of the soft tissues anterior to the anterior arch of the atlas and basion is usually in the order of several millimeters to a centimeter or so. Evaluation of the soft tissues of the base of the skull in this region is often difficult on routine lateral projections of the cervical spine. Lateral projections of the nasopharynx with soft-tissue technique and/or tomography may be necessary for this purpose. Evaluation of the soft tissues may be complicated by the presence of inflammation or enlargement of lymph nodes, particularly in children. However, one must be suspicious of any unusual contour of the soft tissues in this region in a traumatized patient. Hematoma and swelling will obviously produce distortion of the contour of the soft tissues. The prespinal soft tissues up to the level of C-4 or so usually present as a smooth, sharply outlined layer of soft-tissue density approximately 4 to 5 mm thick. The anterior surface of this soft-tissue layer is usually perfectly smooth and follows the curvature of the cervical spine. In patients with a retropharyngeal soft-tissue mass, abscess, swelling, or hematoma, this soft-tissue layer is deformed and an area of bulging and thickening may be noted. The retropharyngeal space ordinarily should not be more than 7 mm thick in normal subjects.[12,28] Any widening of the retropharyngeal space beyond 7 mm is suspicious for the presence of swelling or hematoma in a patient with trauma to the cervical spine.

The retrotracheal space extends from the C-4–C-5 region to the base of the neck. The soft tissue in this region may be as thick as the anteroposterior diameter of C-5. If measurement of this region, from the posterior surface of the trachea to the anterior surface of C-6, is greater than 14 mm in children and 22 mm in adults[1] it should be considered abnormal. In patients with trauma to the cervical spine this finding is suspicious for the presence of swelling, edema, and bleeding.

Another normal landmark of the lateral projection of the cervical spine is the prevertebral fat stripe.[12,27] On properly exposed lateral projections of the cervical spine a thin layer of lucency corresponding to the prevertebral fat stripe is noted a few millimeters anterior to the anterior surface of the cervical vertebral bodies. The prevertebral fat stripe is a thin layer of fatty tissue that parallels the course of the anterior longitudinal ligament of the spine. It is usually visualized well in the midportion of the cervical spine. At the level of C-6 or so the prevertebral fat stripe may no longer be visible. It may be noted to extend anteriorly into the base of the neck. Displacement of the prevertebral fat stripe is an important radiographic sign of soft-tissue swelling or bleeding in the prevertebral space. According to Gehweiler,[12] displacement of this landmark on the lateral radiograph, even when there is no widening of the prevertebral soft tissues, is a reliable indirect clue to the presence of underlying hemorrhage and/or edema.

JOINTS OF THE CERVICAL SPINE

The occipital bone articulates with the atlas with the aid of biconvex occipital condyles, which are situated on the anterolateral margins of the foramen magnum. The atlas has a pair of matching upper articular facets for articulation with the occipital bone. These articulations are not usually well seen on conventional anteroposterior projections. They are visualized on tomography and on reformatted images of CT examination of this region.

The atlanto-axial complex has three articulations. The median articulation is between the odontoid process and the anterior arch of the atlas. Laterally, the inferior articulating facets of the atlas articulate with the superior articulating facets of the axis on either side. The odontoid process is held in place by the transverse ligament of the atlas, which proceeds from one side of this bony ring to the other, dividing the spinal canal of the atlas into a smaller cylindrical socket in front for the odontoid process and a much larger passage posteriorly for the spinal cord.[14] For its size, the transverse ligament of the atlas is said to be one of the strongest ligaments in the body.[14] As it bulges backward around the odontoid process, it is joined superiorly and inferiorly in the midline by longitudinal bands. These structures together form the cruciate ligament. There is a small ligament extending from the tip of the odontoid process to the basion, the so-called apical ligament. The odontoid process is separated from the spinal canal by the tectorial membrane, which is the continuation of the posterior longitudinal ligament.

Apophyseal Joints (Facet Joints)

The neural arches of the cervical vertebrae articulate with the vertebrae above and below via specific articulating facets on either side of the midline. On either side, there is one superior and one inferior articulating facet. The bony mass bearing these facets is called the articular process or articular pyramid of the cervical spine. The articular processes are situated posterolaterally, arising from the pedicle. The articular facets slant inferiorly and posteriorly in the cervical spine. As viewed on the lateral projection, the posterior surface of the articular pyramid projects slightly posterior to the midpoint of the anteroposterior diameter of the spinal canal. The facet joints of the cervical spine are synovial joints and their articular surfaces are covered by hyaline cartilage (Figs. 2-19 to 2-22).

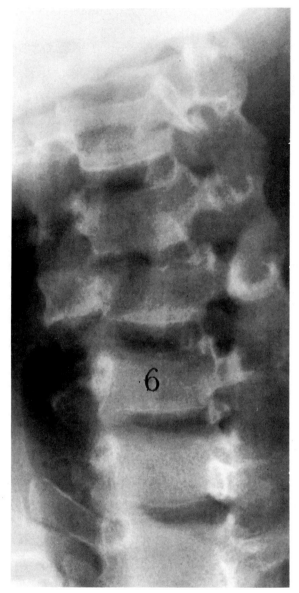

Figure 2-19. Fracture through the right articular pyramid, pedicle, and lamina of C-4 and C-5, and subluxation of C-4 on C-5. Frontal projection of the cervical spine reveals slight scoliosis and malalignment of C-4 relative to C-5. There is a slight rotation of C-4 and C-5 to the left. There is deformity of the right lateral border of the body of C-5 and its junction with its pedicle, articulating pyramids, and transverse process.

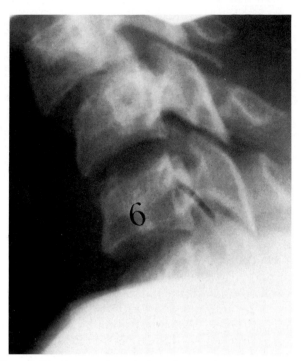

Figure 2-20. Fracture through the right articular pyramid, pedicle, and lamina of C-4 and C-5, and subluxation of C-4 on C-5. Lateral projection reveals subluxation of C-4 on C-5 with a small avulsion fracture of the cortex in the anterior margin of the superior end-plate of C-5.

Luschka Joints

On anteroposterior views of the cervical spine of adults, one notes a bony projection arising from the lateral border of the superior end-plate of C-3–T-1. There are matching slanting facets on the lateral margins of the inferior end-plates of C-2–C-7. On the lateral projection, one notes that a bony ridge or thin wall extends along the anteroposterior length of the lateral margin of the superior end-plate of C-3–C-7. On CT one notes that these thin bony processes curve around the posterolateral corners of the end-plates and extend for a few millimeters along the posterior margin of the end-plates. There are slanting facets on the corresponding surface of the inferior end-plates of C-2–C-7. The thin bony process is called the uncinate process or the Luschka process. The articulation with the superior vertebral body is called the uncovertebral joint or the Luschka joint. There is no uniform agreement as to whether

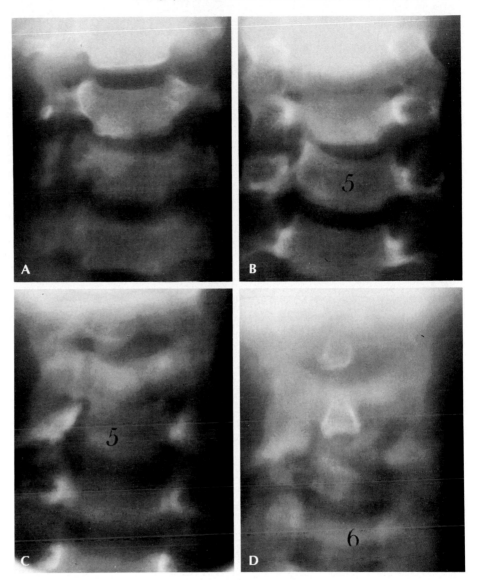

Figure 2-21. Fracture through the right articular pyramid, pedicle, and lamina of C-4 and C-5, and subluxation of C-4 on C-5. (*A*) Anteroposterior tomogram of the cervical spine reveals malalignment of C-4–C-5 vertebral bodies. (*B*) A fracture through the articulating pyramid of C-5 is noted. (*C*) The fracture continues through the base of the pedicle of C-5. (*D*) The fracture continues through the lamina of C-5. There are associated fractures of both right and left laminae of C-4.

these joints are true synovial joints or articulations that do not contain true synovial tissue.

Luschka joints may be affected in inflammatory spondylitis such as psoriatic or rheumatoid arthritis. The joints are also commonly noted to be severely affected with degenerative disease in older persons. An important point in patients with old trauma to the cervical spine is the radiographic presentation of severe degenerative disease of the Luschka joints. Occasionally on a lateral projection of the cervical spine, a horizontal lucent line is projected over the body of the cervical vertebrae, usually C-5 or C-6. This lucent line usually shows fairly marked sclerosis along its superior and inferior margins. In a number of cases this has been mistaken for an old fracture of the vertebrae. However, on careful inspection marked degenerative disease of the Luschka joints is discovered. In these patients the uncinate process forms hypertrophic spurs, which extend in a horizontal fashion laterally. There is a matching hypertrophic osteophyte arising from the inferior end-plate of

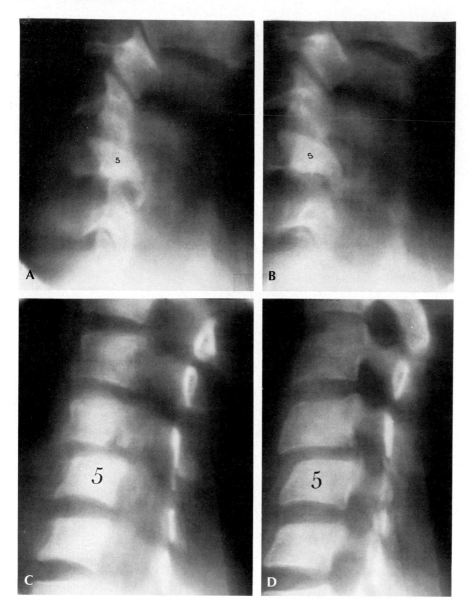

Figure 2-22. Fracture through the right articular pyramid, pedicle, and lamina of C-4 and C-5, and subluxation of C-4 on C-5. (*A*) Lateral tomogram through the lateral portion of the articulating pyramids reveals subluxation of the C-4–C-6 articular processes. (*B*) A fracture of the inferior articular process of C-5 is noted. Note subluxation of C-5–C-6. (*C*) Lateral tomogram reveals fracture of the posterior aspect of the body of C-4 and subluxation of C-4–C-5. (*D*) A small fracture of the superior aspect of the posterior border of the body of C-5 is noted.

the superior vertebral body, also extending laterally. The cleft formed between the two hypertrophic osteophytes is usually situated along the midplane of the vertebral body. On the lateral projection, this cleft is projected on the vertebral body, producing the lucent line described above.

NEURAL FORAMINA (INTERVERTEBRAL FORAMINA)

The cervical neural foramina are best visualized on oblique projections. On CT studies, the inti-

mate relationship of the Luschka process to the anterior and medial aspect of the neural foramina is noted. The articular pyramid and facet joint are situated posterolaterally. The cervical nerve roots occupy the lower one half of the neural foramina.

The cervical intervertebral disks, like the remainder of the spine, consist of an annulus fibrosus and a nucleus pulposus. Anteriorly, a broad ligament, the anterior longitudinal ligament, is attached and merges to the fibers of the annulus fibrosus. Posteriorly, a significantly narrower ligament, the posterior longitudinal ligament, extends from the posterior aspect of the basion (tectorial membrane) to the L-5–S-1 region. The fibers of the posterior longitudinal ligament are attached to the annulus fibrosus.

Disruption of the intervertebral disks may occur in severe hyperextension injury to the cervical spine. In these patients, disruption of the anterior longitudinal ligament may also be present. Traumatic disruption of the intervertebral disks may manifest itself as moderate widening of the intervertebral disks. Such widening may be associated with a vacuum phenomenon on extension of the cervical spine. Disruption of the disk may become evident when a prominent widening of the intervertebral disk is demonstrated.

The articular pyramids and facet joints are best visualized on the lateral projection of the cervical spine. When a question remains as to the integrity of these structures, conventional tomography in the lateral projection is often very useful.

The laminae are visualized on angled anteroposterior arch views. When a question remains as to the integrity of these structures, CT is the procedure of choice.

The spinous process is usually well visualized as a midline structure on anteroposterior projections of the cervical spine. When there is a rotary subluxation of one of the vertebrae, the spinous process is noted to be deviated from the midline.

SPINAL CANAL

The spinal canal is best seen on CT. On the lateral projection of the cervical spine, the posterior border of the vertebrae form the bony cortex of the anterior wall of the spinal canal. These form a continuous and gentle lordotic curve. Posteriorly, the cortex of the posterior bony wall of the spinal canal is noted as a dense line at the base of the spinous process, where the two laminae fuse. The posterior wall of the spinal canal also forms a smooth continuous curve, describing the normal lordosis of the cervical spine.

The average normal sagittal diameter of the spinal canal at C-1 is 22 mm, at C-2 is 20 mm, and at the levels between C-3 and C-7 is 17 mm.[22] Wolf and associates,[30] based on measurement of the cervical bony canal in 200 normal adults, con-

cluded that a sagittal diameter of 10 mm or less due to posterior spurs is likely to be associated with cord compression, but that a sagittal diameter of greater than 13 mm suggests that spur formation alone could not be responsible for cord compression in this area. We believe that a definitive evaluation of the size of the spinal canal with measurement of its surface area should be made on CT. This is usually more reliable than the sagittal diameter of the canal.

JOINTS OF THE THORACIC SPINE

There are 12 thoracic vertebrae. Of these, the first three or four are usually not well visualized on conventional radiographic studies. To overcome the superimposition of the shoulders, the swimmer's view or slight oblique lateral views may be helpful. However, a definitive evaluation of the abnormalities of this region often requires CT. Conventional tomography is helpful in an anteroposterior projection, but it is cumbersome and less diagnostic in the lateral projection.

The thoracic vertebrae articulate with the ribs. There are two facets articulating with the head of the ribs: one posterolaterally on the vertebral body just above the inferior end-plate, the other just below the superior end-plate. There is also a facet on the transverse process for articulation with the tubercle of the ribs. The articulation between the ribs and the thoracic vertebrae is difficult to visualize on conventional radiography and tomography. Computed tomography is ideal for the display of the anatomy in this region.

The facet joints in the thoracic spine are almost in a coronal plane. They are visualized to better advantage on CT. The thoracic spinal canal is usually smaller in surface area than that of the cervical and lumbar spine. Tables of normal transverse diameter of the canal have been published for the thoracic spine. However, we feel that the optimum method for measurement of the surface area of the thoracic canal is afforded by CT.

JOINTS OF THE LUMBAR SPINE

There are five lumbar vertebrae. The lumbar spine has a normal lordotic curvature, and the lumbar vertebral bodies are usually well seen on lateral projections of the lumbar spine. On straight frontal projections of the lumbar spine, the bodies of L-1–L-4 are usually well seen. The body of L-5 may not be well seen because of lordosis. The lumbar pedicles are seen on the frontal projection of the lumbar spine. The facet joints have an oblique orientation, which changes from L-1 to the L-5–S-1 region, and are best seen on oblique projections of the lumbar spine. The oblique projection is also suitable for visualization of the superior and inferior articular facets, pars interarticularis, and laminae. The neural foramina are best seen on the lateral projection.

As in the rest of the spine, evaluation of the size and configuration of the spinal canal is best achieved on CT.

MOTION STUDIES OF THE SPINE

Traditionally, flexion and extension views of the spine have been obtained for evaluation of instability of the spine. We believe a better understanding of instability is achieved if motion studies of the spine are performed under direct fluoroscopic control, and recorded on a videotape. These studies should be performed with a physician familiar with the patient in attendance.

The occipital–atlanto-axial articulation qualifies as a universal joint because flexion, extension, lateral flexion, and rotation all occur in this region.[12] Approximately 25 degrees of anteroposterior movement (nodding motion) occurs between the occiput, atlas, and axis. Approximately one half of the nodding motion occurs between the occipital bone and atlas and the other half occurs between the atlas and axis. When the skull rotates, the atlas goes with the occiput and the occiput–atlas unit rotates on the axis. Approximately 40 to 45 degrees of rotating motion occurs at this level. If the skull is turned more than 45 degrees, the remainder of rotation occurs in the rest of the cervical spine.[12,14] The extent of the rotation permitted by the atlanto-axial complex and by the remainder of the cervical spine necessitates a relatively loose articular capsule for the

atlanto-axial articulations as well as the facet joints of the cervical spine.

Flexion–extension studies of the cervical spine are helpful in detection of instability of the atlanto-axial articulation, which may occur secondary to traumatic injury of the transverse ligament of the atlas. In patients with rheumatoid arthritis, ankylosing spondylitis, psoriatic arthritis, and similar disorders, there may be extensive erosive changes of the odontoid process as well as disruption of the ligaments, leading to subluxation at the atlanto-axial articulation. Traumatic injuries of the cervical spine are more likely to lead to complete disruption of the transverse ligament and to atlanto-axial dislocation in these patients. In patients with extensive inflammatory facet joint disease, flexion–extension studies of the cervical spine may show multiple areas of malalignment of the cervical spine before bony ankylosis occurs. Similarly, in advanced stages of inflammatory arthritis, bending motions to the right and to the left may reveal abnormal motion of the vertebral bodies.

Motion studies may also be used for evaluation of instability of the thoracic and lumbar spine. These may be performed with the patient in the erect or recumbent position, as dictated by clinical findings. Whenever possible, these studies should be performed with the patient in a standing position.

Stability of the spine may also be evaluated following surgical fusion and stabilization of the spine. Any abnormal motion at the site of fusion or above or below it may be observed using these studies.

Occasionally an abnormal motion occurs during the course of flexion or extension, as visualized on fluoroscopy, and may go unrecognized if only endpoint flexion and extension radiographs are obtained. It is helpful to record the fluoroscopic image of the motion on a suitable medium such as videotape because this offers an opportunity to study the motion of the spine as many times as necessary, without exposing the patient to further radiation. An added advantage is the opportunity to restudy the examination for detection of unsuspected abnormalities of motion or to compare it with a follow-up examination.

TOMOGRAPHY OF THE SPINE

Tomography of the spine is useful for clarification of fracture-dislocations of the spine when this diagnosis is not evident on conventional radiography (Figs. 2-19 to 2-22). Tomography is particularly useful for evaluating fracture-dislocations of the atlanto-axial articulations, both median and lateral joints, fractures at the base of the odontoid process (Figs. 2-23, 2-24), horizontal fractures and fracture-dislocations of the cervical facet joints.[2,20] However, it must be acknowledged that almost all of these abnormalities may also be eval-

uated on high-resolution CT when thin slices (2 to 3 mm) are used and reformatting in sagittal and coronal planes is performed.[6] Occasionally tomography is needed as a complementary procedure for a definitive clarification of fractures of the base of the odontoid process and fracture-dislocations of the facet joints, particularly facet lock and horizontal fractures of the spine. In patients with fractures of the spine that are in the healing stage, and in postoperative patients in whom bone graft has been used, CT may also be necessary as a complementary procedure to tomography to assess the status of bone formation and healing.

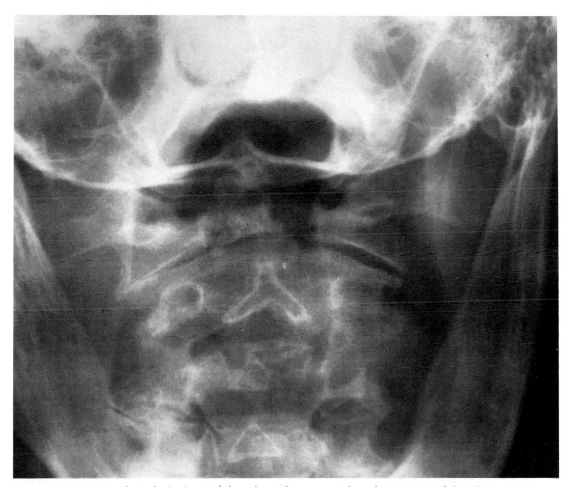

Figure 2-23. Fracture through the base of the odontoid process. A frontal projection of C-1–C-2 reveals a fracture through the base of the odontoid process with displacement of the odontoid process to the right of the midline. Note displacement of the lateral mass of C-1 and overhanging of the lateral margin of C-1 relative to C-2, indicating a lateral C-1–C-2 subluxation on the right side.

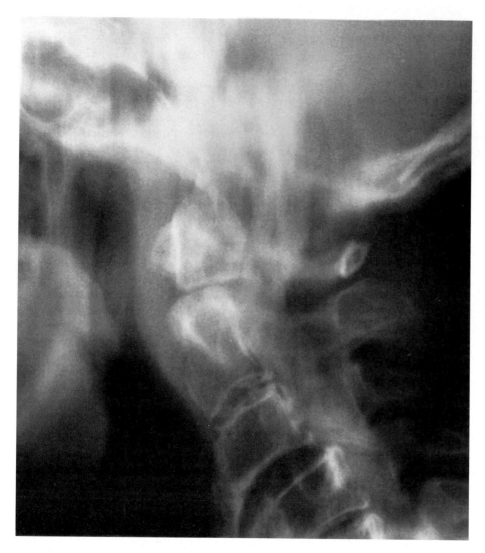

Figure 2-24. Fracture through the base of the odontoid process. Lateral tomogram of C-1–C-2 complex reveals a fracture through the base of the odontoid process with slight posterior displacement. Note that the anterior arch of C-1 is in normal relationship to the odontoid process and it is displaced posteriorly along with the odontoid process.

In the thoracic and lumbar spine, conventional tomography is occasionally needed for clarification of small fractures of the articulating processes, facets, pedicles, and pars interarticularis. In most of these instances, conventional tomography is useful as a complementary procedure to CT.

CT AND CT–MYELOGRAPHY OF THE SPINE

Computed tomography is ideal for evaluation of fracture-dislocations of the spine, particularly for detection of fracture fragments displaced into the spinal canal (Figs. 2-25 to 2-29). The ability to obtain cross-sectional images has eliminated the problem of overlapping of complex and curvilinear contours of the spine. Thus, it has become possible to display directly the spinal canal, neural foramina, and vertebral elements easily and quickly and without moving the patient.[6,15]

The major shortcoming of CT is that large segments of the spine are difficult to evaluate. It is usually not practical to study more than 4 to 5 vertebral bodies. The best studies are usually obtained when the level of injury is known and thin slices with some overlapping are used to facilitate reformatting in sagittal and coronal planes. It is

(Text continued on p. 34)

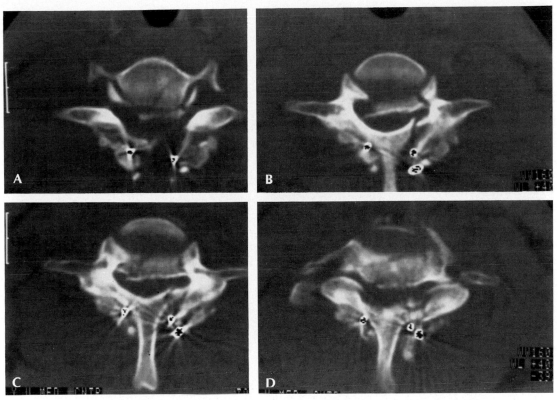

Figure 2-25. Comminuted fracture of the body and vertebral elements, including the posterior arch of C-5. (*A*) An axial slice through C-5 reveals a comminuted fracture of the C-5 vertebral body. There is marked displacement of the posterior fracture fragments into the spinal canal, causing more than 50% stenosis of the canal. A fracture through the left lamina is noted. There are multiple bone chips posterior to the laminae bilaterally, as well as artifacts due to metallic wires used for posterolateral fusion of the spine in this patient. (*B*) Note the fracture through the luschka process on the left side, separation of the posterior cortex of the body and displacement into the spinal canal, and the oblique fracture through the posterior aspect of the vertebral body, bone chips, and metallic wires posterolaterally. (*C*) A comminuted fracture through the body is noted, with marked displacement of the posterior fracture fragment into the spinal canal causing more than 50% stenosis of the spinal canal. There is a comminuted fracture of the lamina on the left side. Note bone chips as well as metallic surgical wires. (*D*) A comminuted fracture of the body of C-5 with displacement of fragments into the spinal canal is noted. There is also a comminuted fracture of the lamina on the left side. Note bone chips and metallic surgical wires.

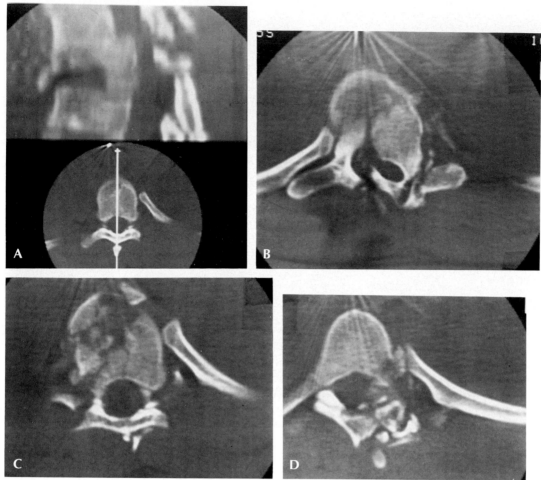

Figure 2-26. Comminuted fracture of T-7 and T-8 vertebral bodies and vertebral elements including the posterior arch, visualized on CT of the spine. (*A*) A sagittal reformatted image reveals displacement of the posterior fracture fragments of the T-8 vertebral body, producing marked stenosis of the spinal canal. (*B*) A comminuted fracture of the body of T-8 is noted. There is also a comminuted fracture through the base of the left transverse process and the posterior arch. There is displacement of the posterior arch anteriorly, causing severe stenosis of the spinal canal. (*C*) A comminuted fracture of the body of T-8 is noted. The spinal canal is normal at this point. (*D*) There is a comminuted fracture of the body of T-8 laterally, extending through the transverse process and the posterior arch and including the left lamina. There is displacement of the left eighth rib anteriorly.

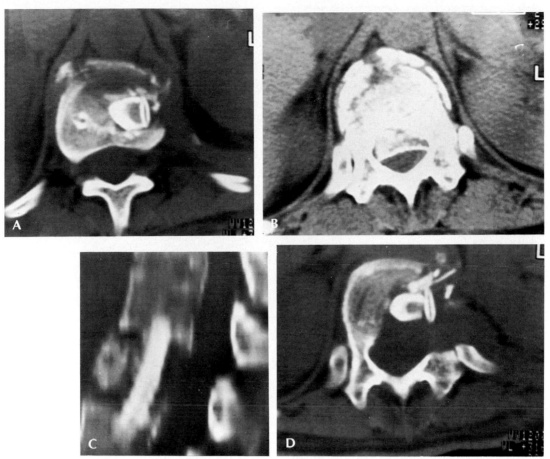

Figure 2-27. Fracture of the T-11 vertebral body. (*A*) Computed tomographic examination reveals the cephalic end of bone graft (ribs) in the body of T-10. (*B*) A comminuted fracture of the body of T-11 with marked displacement of the posterior fracture fragment, producing more than 50% stenosis of the spinal canal, is noted. (*C*) A sagittal reformatted image reveals an interbody bone graft between T-10, T-11 and T-12 following decompression and removal of the displaced posterior fragment of T-11. (*D*) The inferior end of the interbody bone graft in the left side of the body of T-12 is noted. The decompression was performed using a lateral transthoracic approach.

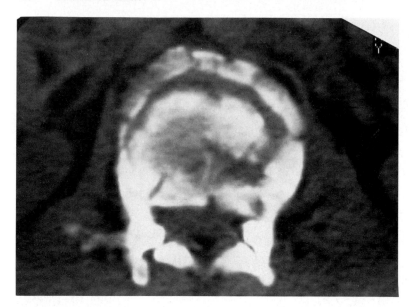

Figure 2-28. Comminuted fracture of L-1. Axial CT reveals a comminuted fracture of the body of L-1 in a young man who jumped from a six-story window. There is moderate displacement of the posterior fragments into the spinal canal.

not usually possible to use CT to screen large segments of the spine.

Depending on the patient's status, a myelogram may also be performed. This is particularly helpful in patients with neurologic deficit. In these patients, CT–myelography offers the ability to visualize potentially reversible compression of the spinal cord. Due to the high contrast sensitivity of CT, small doses of intrathecal contrast medium are usually sufficient to completely opacify the subarachnoid space. The contrast agent may be injected from the lumbar region. However, in patients in whom this is impossible, a C-1–C-2 lateral puncture may be performed with the patient in a supine position. Myelography is also useful in patients with avulsion of spinal nerves. In these patients, various deformities of the root sleeve, usually enlargement, and an arachnoid diverticulum may be noted (Fig. 2-30).

Magnetic resonance imaging is now becoming widely available and is replacing CT and CT–myelography in some patients. MRI has the additional advantage of directly demonstrating the spinal cord in sagittal and coronal planes as well as in axial planes. There are a number of difficulties when using MRI to evaluate an acutely injured patient. However, some of these difficulties are being eliminated with advances in technology. Whether an MRI study or a CT–myelogram should be performed in a patient with fracture-dislocations of the spine and neurologic deficit depends on the circumstances of the patient, the experience of the physicians caring for the patient, and the availability of these modalities.

When CT is used to evaluate traumatic lesions of the occipito-atlanto-axial region, very thin slices (1 to 2 mm) should be obtained for evaluation of the complex anatomy of this region. In the remainder of the cervical spine, 3-mm slices are usually obtained. The physicians must remember that malalignment of the spine may go unrecognized on axial images. Also, an overall evaluation of the spinal canal and alignment of the vertebrae are usually more easily performed on sagittal reformatted images. Coronal and sagittal reformatted images are, therefore, recommended as a routine component of CT for evaluation of traumatic injuries of the spine. One should remember that horizontal fractures and compression fractures of the vertebrae may be missed on axial images; how-

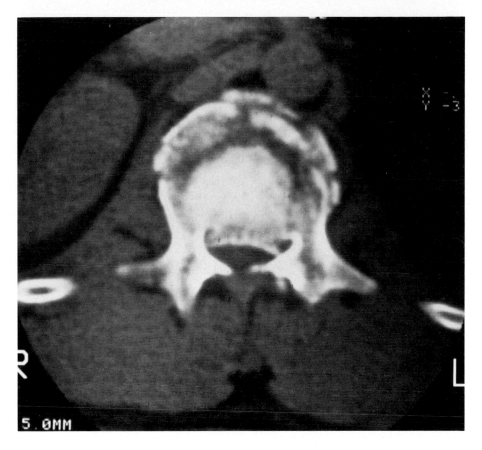

Figure 2-29. Comminuted fracture of the body of L-1. There is marked displacement of the posterior fracture fragment into the spinal canal, causing more than 60% stenosis of the spinal canal.

ever, if a high resolution CT with sufficiently thin slices has been performed, reformatted images usually will show these fractures.

Computed tomography is particularly useful in revealing the extent of displacement of fracture fragments into the spinal canal (Figs. 2-25, 2-27, 2-29). CT–myelography will reveal the extent of compression of the dural sac and of the spinal cord. Another important observation is the discovery of unsuspected fractures of the neural arch on CT. In our experience, in a large number of patients, fractures of the neural arch, which were not seen on conventional radiographic examinations of the spine, were discovered on CT.

Computed tomography is also useful in postoperative patients. In patients with interbody fusion and bone graft, reformatted CT images in sagittal and coronal planes will display the anatomy of the spinal canal and the relationship of the fracture fragments and the bone graft to the spinal canal (Fig. 2-27). In patients with Harrington rod stabilization, although there are artifacts generated by the metallic elements, usually the detail of the anterior portion of the spinal canal and the posterior surface of the vertebral body is well visualized. Thus, occasionally a displaced fragment into the spinal canal, which may be caused by persistent neurologic abnormality, may be discovered. In some patients, the existence of these potentially treatable, posteriorly displaced fracture fragments is not known until a CT examination is performed. In patients with superimposed osteomyelitis following fracture-dislocations of the spine, CT examination may be the first modality leading to a correct diagnosis.

The CT presentation of dislocation of the facets

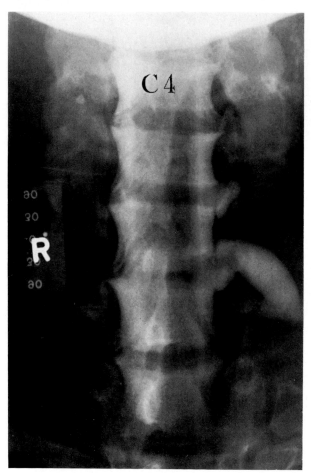

Figure 2-30. Traumatic avulsion of C-6 and C-7 cervical roots on the left side. The anteroposterior projection of a cervical spine myelogram reveals the collection of contrast material in a small diverticulum associated with the C-6 root, and in a much larger diverticulum associated with the C-7 root on the left side. The arachnoid diverticulum formed at the site of avulsion of the left C-7 root extends through the neural foramen. There was associated fracture of the neural arch, which was minimally displaced.

may be confusing. However, comparison of the normal levels with the dislocated level on the axial views is often helpful. The superior facet of the cervical vertebral bodies usually has a flat posterior border, and is normally situated in front of the inferior facet, which has a flat anterior border. When the superior facet, which appears as a frag-

ment of bone with a flat posterior border, is identified posterior to the inferior facet, a locked facet is diagnosed on CT. Reformatted images are often very helpful for a definitive diagnosis.

Another advantage of CT of the spine in patients with spinal trauma is the detection of traumatic disk herniation. This may occur in a bursting fracture of the vertebra when the intervertebral disk herniates into the substance of the vertebral body. It may also be associated with fracture of the posterior aspect of the vertebral body and displacement of a fragment of bone and disk into the epidural space. In some patients, a traumatic herniation of the intervertebral disk may be noted without a significant fracture of the posterior border of the vertebrae.

RADIOGRAPHIC DIAGNOSIS OF SPECIFIC FRACTURE-DISLOCATIONS

FRACTURE-DISLOCATIONS OF THE CERVICAL SPINE

Fracture-dislocations of the upper cervical region may be divided into:

1. Fractures of the atlas.
2. Fractures of the axis.
3. Atlanto-axial fracture-dislocations.

Fractures of the Atlas

The atlas vertebra is situated deep within the soft tissues of the neck. The atlas is usually fractured secondary to indirect blunt trauma. The most common fractures of the atlas are fractures of the anterior or posterior arch and the Jefferson fracture.

Fracture of the Anterior or Posterior Arch. Fractures of the posterior arch of the atlas usually occur through the weakest point of the arch, which corresponds to the groove for the vertebral artery. Fractures of the anterior arch of the atlas are almost as common as posterior arch fractures. In patients with fractures of the anterior arch, other fractures of the cervical spine, particularly fractures of the odontoid process, are often also noted.[12,13]

Detection of a fracture of the posterior or anterior arch of the atlas may be difficult on routine radiographic studies. Often, oblique views of this region are helpful. Computed tomography of this region, using 2- to 3-mm thick slices, is also useful in identification of these fractures.

Jefferson Fracture. This is the so-called bursting fracture of the atlas. It is usually produced by an axial loading force to the skull, such as a blow to the vertex of the head. The axial force causes compression of the atlas between the occipital condyles above and the articular surfaces of the axis below. Usually, one encounters fractures of the anterior and posterior arch simultaneously.[18]

The Jefferson fracture may not be visible on routine lateral radiographs of the cervical spine. However, it is usually well delineated on oblique projections and on open mouth view of the atlanto-axial region. Normally, the lateral margins of the lateral mass of the atlas line up with the corresponding part of the lateral aspect of the axis. In patients with a Jefferson fracture, the axial loading force to the vertex of the skull forces the fractured arch of the atlas laterally. Thus, careful inspection of the atlanto-axial complex on the frontal open-mouth view reveals the lateral masses of the atlas displaced laterally on the axis, producing an overhanging configuration.

If doubt persists as to the exact nature of the fracture, CT using 2- to 3-mm thick slices is recommended in these patients. Computed tomography may also reveal additional unsuspected fractures through the atlas or axis vertebrae. Computed tomography should be performed with contiguous, preferably 2-mm overlapping, slices to facilitate reformatting in sagittal and coronal planes. This is important because horizontal fractures that are in the same plane as the axial slices of CT may be missed on axial images. Jefferson fractures are often well visualized on reformatted images. Additionally, reformatted images in coronal and sagittal planes reveal the three-dimen-

sional anatomy of the spinal canal as well as the relationship of the odontoid process and the anterior arch of the atlas. If there is displacement of a fracture fragment into the spinal canal, this is usually detected on axial images. However, a better overall impression of the extent of encroachment into the canal is obtained on axial and sagittal reformatted images. When the lateral mass of the atlas is displaced more than 6.9 mm relative to the axis, a tear of the transverse ligament of the atlas should be suspected.[7,12]

Fractures of the Axis

Fractures of this vertebra may affect the dens, body, vertebral arch, vertebral elements, or a combination thereof. Fractures of the axis may be associated with atlanto-axial dislocation or may be seen without an associated dislocation.

Atlanto-axial fracture-dislocations are encountered fairly frequently. More than one third of our patients with cervical spinal fractures had fracture-dislocations of the atlanto-axial region. Fractures of the odontoid process may involve the base of this structure, i.e., the junction of the odontoid process and the body of the vertebra (see Figs. 2-23, 2-24). The fracture line may extend through the body inferiorly and laterally. Less commonly, in our experience, the fracture may be higher up, in the midportion or tip of the odontoid process.

Fractures of the body of the axis may be encountered without other associated fractures or may be seen with fractures of the vertebral arch and the dens. Fractures of the vertebral arch may be unilateral or bilateral.

Hangman's Fracture. The so-called Hangman's fracture is encountered when there is a bilateral arch fracture through the pedicles between the posterior arch and the body of axis as well as anterior subluxation of the body of the axis on C-3 (Figs. 2-31, 2-32, 2-33). There is fairly uniform agreement that this fracture is commonly seen with hyperextension injuries. Injuries to the C-2–C-3 disk, the body of C-3, or other fractures

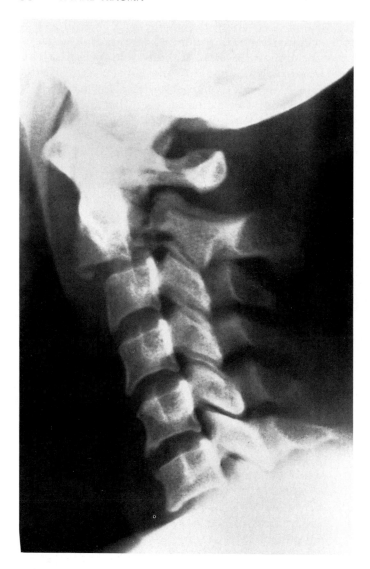

Figure 2-31. Hangman's fracture of the axis. A lateral projection reveals a fracture through the pedicles at the junction with the posterior aspect of the body of C-2. There is anterior displacement of the body of C-2 and narrowing of the C-2–C-3 intervertebral disk. A small fracture from the anterior margin of the inferior end-plate of the body of C-2 is also noted.

of the cervical spine may also be associated with this fracture.[12,14,16]

It is remarkable that a large number of patients with atlanto-axial fracture-dislocations do not have significant neurologic abnormalities. This is partially due to the fact that the cervical spinal canal is quite capacious in this region. Compression of the spinal cord, therefore, occurs only in those with marked distortion of the spinal canal and stenosis produced by these fractures, or in those who suffered momentary compression or shearing of

the spinal cord during the actual moment of accident.

The radiographic diagnosis of fractures of the axis requires meticulous attention to the radiographic anatomy of the atlanto-axial complex on frontal as well as lateral projections. High-quality complex motion tomography in frontal and lateral projections is often necessary for proper delineation of these fractures. Computed tomography is also helpful for evaluation of the status of the spinal canal and delineation of these fractures, partic-

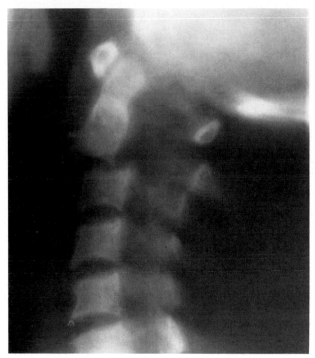

Figure 2-32. Hangman's fracture of the axis. A lateral tomogram reveals anterior displacement of the body of C-2 relative to C-3. Note that the relationship of the anterior arch of the atlas to the odontoid process is normal. The posterior arch of C-2 has remained in normal anatomic relationship to C-3, resulting in widening of the spinal canal at the level of the axis.

and superimposed linear structures caused by various overlying bones, including the occipital bone and the teeth on the atlanto-axoid complex, particularly the odontoid process. Often, a definitive differentiation cannot be made until tomography and/or CT studies of this region have been obtained. Of particular interest are congential anomalies of the odontoid process, congential clefts of C-1, rudimentary C-1, partial or complete fusion of C-1 to the occipital bone, and other anomalies of the axis and the foramen magnum region.

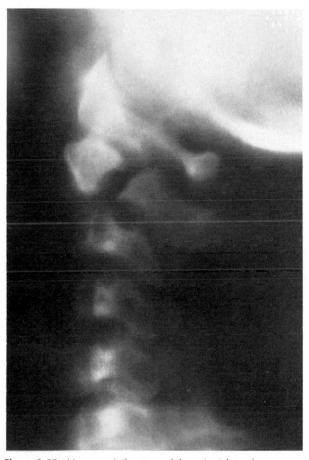

Figure 2-33. Hangman's fracture of the axis. A lateral tomogram obtained on the left side of the midline reveals the fracture of C-2. Note widening at the area of fracture secondary to displacement of the body of C-2 anteriorly while the posterior arch of C-2 has remained in its normal position.

ularly fractures of the vertebral arch. High-resolution CT capable of obtaining 2-mm or so thick slices, if available, may be substituted for tomography. For this purpose, contiguous 2-mm thick slices are obtained and reformatting is performed in sagittal and coronal planes. In patients with atlanto-axial dislocations, fracture fragments displaced into the spinal canal, and neurologic symptomatology, it is important to have all the information that can be obtained regarding the status of the spinal cord. For this purpose, CT–myelography or MRI should be performed, if this modality is available. The true width of the spinal canal, the extent of compression of the spinal cord, and other abnormalities of the spinal canal are delineated by these two modalities.

On conventional radiographic studies, a differentiation has to be made between true fractures

Atlanto-axial Fracture-Dislocations

Atlanto-axial dislocations may occur without an associated fracture or may occur with fractures of the odontoid process or other fractures of the axis. Traumatic atlanto-axial dislocations without an associated fracture are quite uncommon. In our patients there were only two dislocations of this type in 211 fracture-dislocations of the spine. The atlas is kept in anatomic position in relationship to the axis by the strong tranverse ligament. When there is dislocation of the atlas on the axis, almost always anteriorly, a tear of the tranverse ligament must be present.[7] If displacement of the atlas on the axis is severe, the possibility of injury to the spinal cord, which is caught between the posterior arch of the atlas and the odontoid process, should be considered.

Nontraumatic Atlanto-axial Dislocations. The most important conditions to be considered in this category are inflammatory systemic arthritis, pyogenic and tuberculous arthritis, other inflammatory processes, deformities, and congenital anomalies of this region.[12,14]

There are synovial bursae between the odontoid process and the anterior arch of the atlas anteriorly and the tranverse ligament posteriorly. Thus, the odontoid process may show evidence for erosion in patients with longstanding inflammatory arthritis affecting the spine, such as rheumatoid arthritis, psoriatic arthritis, and ankylosing spondylitis. In advanced cases, there is also disruption of the transverse ligament as well as other ligaments. The erosion and destruction of the odontoid process may be very marked (Fig. 2-34). Dislocation of the atlanto-axial articulation may be observed in these patients, particularly when flexion and extension views are obtained. There may also be extensive erosive change of the lateral atlanto-axial articulation, resulting in marked subluxation of the atlas relative to the axis. Similar abnormalities may be noted in association with

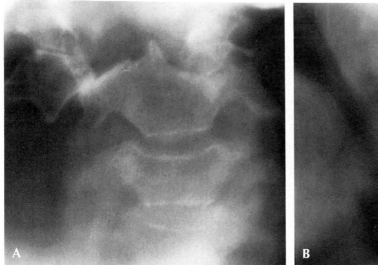 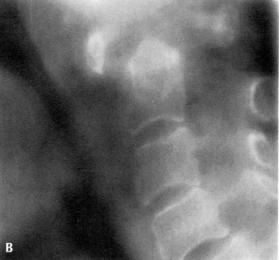

Figure 2-34. Atlanto-axial dislocation secondary to long-standing rheumatoid arthritis. (*A*) Anteroposterior tomography reveals severe erosion of the odontoid process. Only a small segment of the base of the odontoid process is left. There is dislocation of the axis to the left relative to the atlas. Note osteosclerosis of the lateral atlanto-axial articulation on the right side. (*B*) Lateral tomography reveals severe erosion of the odontoid process. Only a small amount of bone is left at the base of the odontoid process. Note the indistinct margins of the remaining base of the odontoid process. There is dislocation of C-1 relative to C-2, producing widening of the predental space. Consequently, there is narrowing of the spinal canal posterior to the odontoid process.

pyogenic infection, tuberculous infection, or other infectious processes of this region.

Of interest is the association of atlanto-axial dislocation with retropharyngeal abscess, mastoiditis, and other inflammatory processes occurring in the structures surrounding the atlanto-axial complex.

The radiographic diagnosis of atlanto-axial dislocation is made when there is an increase in the distance between the odontoid process and the anterior arch of the atlas. The distance between the posterior surface of the anterior arch of the atlas to the anterior surface of the odontoid process is usually less than 3 mm in adults and less than 5 mm in children. If the predental space measures more than this, dislocation of the atlanto-axial articulation is present. The radiographic diagnosis is usually made on the lateral projection if the anterior arch of the atlas is noted to be displaced forward relative to the axis. In doubtful instances, tomography should be performed. Tomography in the frontal projection is also helpful for evaluation of the lateral dislocation of the atlas relative to the axis. Tomography and CT are usually also necessary for a definitive evaluation of deformities and congenital anomalies of the atlas and axis.[12,14,17]

Atlanto-axial Rotary Fixation. Wortzman and Dewar[31] in 1968 described persistent rotation of the atlas–axis and termed it rotary fixation of the atlanto-axial joint. The characteristic clinical presentation is persistent torticollis, usually occurring after trivial trauma or an upper respiratory infection. However, this condition may be seen spontaneously or following orthodontic surgical procedures. The head is usually tilted to one side, rotated to the opposite side, and slightly flexed.

Fielding and Hawkins[8,9] described atlanto-axial rotary fixation in 1977. Fielding recommended cineradiography of the atlanto-axial region in the lateral position for diagnosis of this condition. The radiographic diagnosis of atlanto-axial rotary fixation is made when there is lack of normal motion between the atlas and axis during attempted rotation.

Kowalski and associates[19] described functional CT examination of the atlanto-axial complex for diagnosis of this condition. In this study, motion between the atlas and axis, or return of the rotated atlas to the normal position, was noted in patients with transient torticollis, while no motion between the atlas and axis was noted following attempted rotation of the neck in patients with rotary atlanto-axial fixation.

Other Cervical Spine Fracture-Dislocations

Teardrop Fracture. This is a fracture-dislocation affecting one cervical body, usually in the lower half of the cervical spine (Fig. 2-35). It is caused by a major flexion injury of the cervical spine. The patient usually shows neurologic manifestations of acute anterior cervical cord injury, consisting of quadriplegia with loss of pain, touch, and temperature sensation but with retention of sensation of position, motion, and vibration, which are functions of the posterior column of the spinal cord. This fracture is unstable and is associated with significant soft-tissue injury, including disruption of the posterior longitudinal ligament, intervertebral disk, and anterior longitudinal ligament. Dislocation of the facets associated with relatively marked kyphosis at the level of the fracture-dislocation, with a wide gap between the spinous processes posteriorly indicating disruption of the posterior ligament complex, is also usually noted. The radiographic diagnosis is usually not difficult when the above features are present. The term teardrop refers to the triangular fracture of the anterior and inferior aspect of the vertebral body. The fracture fragment is usually displaced slightly anteriorly and inferiorly, while the remainder of the body is usually displaced posteriorly.[12,16]

Wedge Fracture. This fracture is usually produced during flexion of the cervical spine. The fracture produces a characteristic deformity of the vertebra with loss of the vertebral height anteriorly. There may be no other abnormality associated with this fracture.

Unilateral and Bilateral Facet Lock. When there is dislocation of a facet joint of the cervical spine, the inferior articulating process comes to rest in front of the superior articulating process of the vertebral body below. Bilateral facet locking is usually

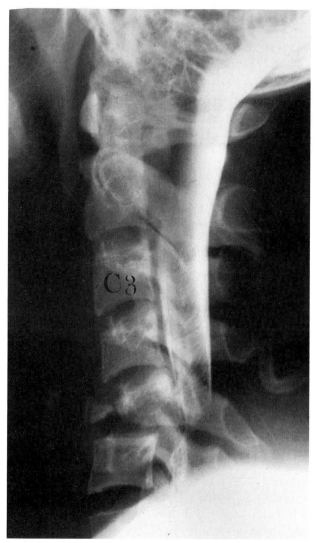

caused by a major hyperflexion injury. This may occur in motor vehicle accidents, mugging, contact sports, and falls. In unilateral facet locking, there is rotation of the involved vertebra and the vertebrae above it away from the midline (Figs. 2-36 to 2-41). In bilateral facet locking (Figs. 2-42, 2-43) there is usually major injury to the posterior ligament complex of the spine and the intervertebral disk. Dislocation of the spine

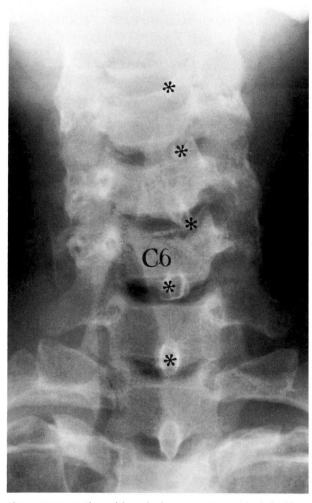

Figure 2-35. Teardrop hyperflexion fracture-dislocation of C-5. A lateral view of a cervical myelography study reveals a comminuted fracture of the body of C-5. The smaller fracture fragments are displaced anteriorly. The remainder of the fractured body of C-5 is displaced markedly posteriorly. A kyphotic curvature with the apex at C-5–C-6 is produced. There is marked compression of the dural sac with near-complete block to the flow of the contrast in the subarachnoid space, and marked compression of the spinal cord. There is marked narrowing of the C-5–C-6 intervertebral disk, indicating disruption of this disk. Marked pre-spinal soft-tissue swelling is also noted. There was no fracture of the posterior arch on CT examination. This patient was quadriplegic almost immediately following a diving accident.

Figure 2-36. Unilateral facet lock, C-5 on C-6 on the left side. A frontal projection reveals displacement of the spinous processes of C-3, C-4, and C-5 vertebrae to the left. The spinous processes are indicated by an asterisk.

processes of the vertebra below. Consequently, the spinal canal is significantly narrowed, because the posterior arch of the dislocated vertebra has now moved more than one half of the anteroposterior diameter of the vertebral body anteriorly.

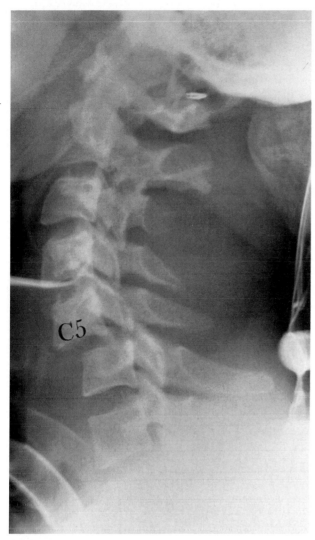

Figure 2-37. Unilateral facet lock, C-5 on C-6 on the left side. A lateral projection reveals dislocation of C-5 on C-6. Note that the left inferior articulating process of C-5 is situated anterior to the superior articulating process of C-6 (facet lock). The facets on the right side are not well seen.

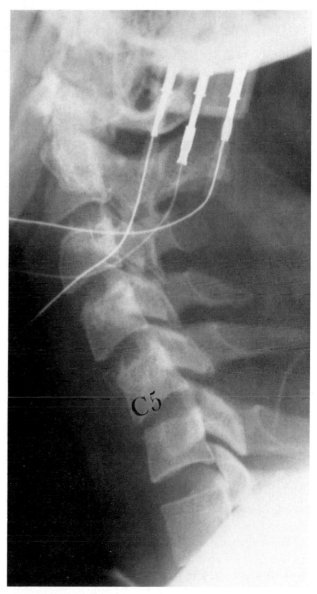

Figure 2-38. Unilateral facet lock, C-5 on C-6 on the left side. Lateral projection of the cervical spine after reduction of facet lock. There is reversal of lordosis at C-5–C-6 associated with deformity of the C-5–C-6 intervertebral disk, indicating injury to this disk. Note the normal relationship of the C-5–C-6 facets.

usually occurs around C-5–C-6 and C-6–C-7. The dislocated vertebral body and the vertebrae above it are forced anteriorly following disruption of the ligamentous structures and intervertebral disks. As the displaced vertebral column attempts to return to its normal position, the inferior articulating processes of the dislocated vertebra are caught and locked in front of the superior articulating

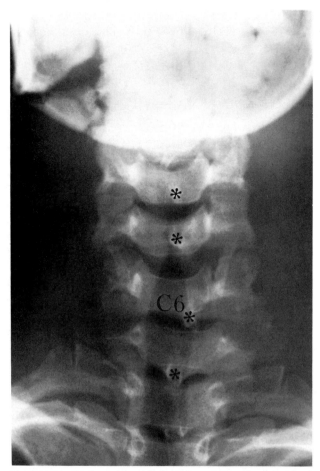

Figure 2-39. Unilateral facet lock, C-6 on C-7 on the left side. A frontal projection of the cervical spine reveals displacement of the spinous process of C-6 to the left. The spinous processes of C-4 and C-5 are only slightly deviated from the midline toward the left side. The spinous processes are marked by asterisks. Note marked asymmetry of the intervertebral disks at C-5–C-6 and C-6–C-7 and a slight malalignment at C-6–C-7, producing slight scoliosis of the cervical spine. A comminuted fracture of the right jaw is noted.

In patients with pre-existing spinal stenosis, the damage to the spinal cord may be extensive.

The radiographic diagnosis of facet locking requires careful attention to detail on frontal, lateral, and oblique projections of the cervical spine. Oblique projections may be obtained, depending on the condition of the patient, in the erect position or in the supine position without moving the patient, as described previously. The diagnosis of

facet locking may not be made if all of the required views are not obtained. In our experience, it is not unusual to see patients with missed diagnosis of facet locking for months, and sometimes years, following the initial injury.

In unilateral facet locking there is anterior displacement of the dislocated vertebra. The inferior articulating process is noted to lie in front of the superior articulating process of the vertebral body below (see Fig. 2-41). This is the opposite of the normal anatomic arrangement of the facets. On the frontal projection, the spinous process of the dislocated vertebra is noted to be deviated toward the side of the lock (see Figs. 2-36, 2-39). If the

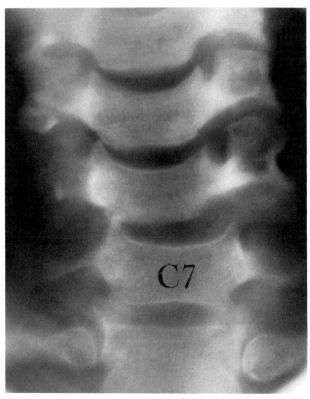

Figure 2-40. Unilateral facet lock, C-6 on C-7 on the left side. Tomography of the cervical spine in anteroposterior projection reveals a slight to moderate subluxation of C-6 to the right relative to C-7. Note a small cortical fracture of the articular facet (uncovertebral or luschka joint) of the base of C-6 on the right side, immediately lateral to the luschka process of C-7. Note marked widening of the luschka joint on the left side at C-6–C-7. A similar subluxation of the C-5–C-6 was also present on the left side, but to a lesser degree.

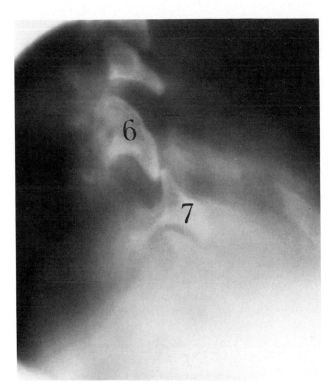

Figure 2-41. Unilateral facet lock, C-6 on C-7 on the left side. Tomography of the spine reveals locking of C-6 and C-7 facets. Note that the inferior articulating process of C-6 is situated in front of the superior articulating process of C-7. This is the reverse of the normal anatomic relationship of these articular processes.

condition of the patient permits, tomography in the lateral projection is ideally suited for this purpose because it reveals the exact anatomic relationship of the dislocated facet joint, as well as associated fractures, to best advantage (see Fig. 2-41). Computed tomography is also helpful for this purpose. This is particularly so if thin slices in a contiguous manner are obtained and reformatting in the parasagittal plane is performed. The dislocated facets and the facet locking can also be identified on axial images of the cervical spine by the characteristic configuration of the facets, as was described previously.

The radiographic diagnosis of bilateral facet locking is also made when displacement of the vertebrae anteriorly and positioning of the inferior articulating process in front of the superior

articulating process of the vertebra below is noted (Figs. 2-42, 2-43). Frontal, lateral, and oblique projections of the cervical spine are necessary in these patients. If the condition of the patient permits, tomography in the lateral projection usually reveals the abnormal relationship of the involved facets to best advantage. Tomography and CT are also helpful in identification of associated fractures.

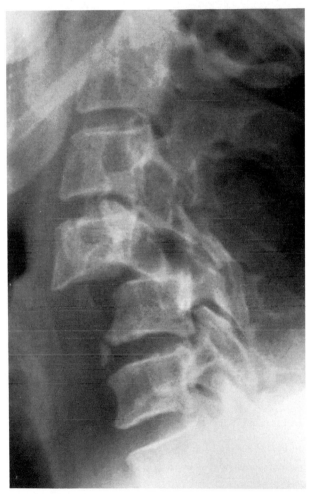

Figure 2-42. Bilateral locking of facets, C-4 on C-5. A lateral projection of the cervical spine reveals anterior displacement of C-4, and the vertebrae above it, on C-5. The C-4–C-5 intervertebral disk is disrupted. A fracture of the cortex of the anterolateral surface of the body of C-5, displaced anteriorly, is noted. Note the position of the inferior articular process of C-5 in front of the superior articular process of C-6. An intercalary bone is present between C-5 and C-6.

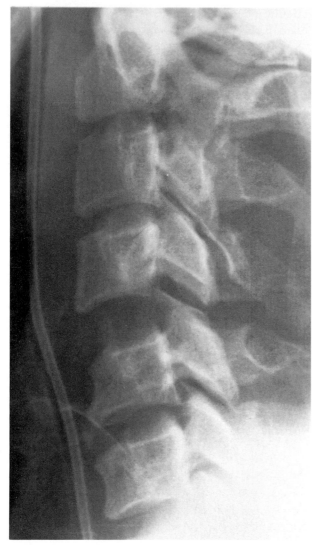

Figure 2-43. Bilateral locking of facets, C-4 on C-5. A lateral projection of the cervical spine after reduction of the C-4–C-5 locked facet reveals a normal relationship between the articular processes of C-4 and C-5. However, note the marked widening of the C-4–C-5 intervertebral disk secondary to disruption of this disk during the injury.

Bursting Fracture of the Lower Cervical Spine. The mechanism of injury in this fracture is similar to that in Jefferson fracture of C-1. Injury is usually in the form of an axial loading force to the vertex of the head with the neck held in an erect position. The force is transmitted through the vertebral bodies to the intervertebral disks. The axial loading force may lead to rupture of the annulus fibrosus, which may cause herniation of the intervertebral disk.

The pathophysiology of this fracture, as described by Roaf[24] and Harris,[16] begins with the intervertebral disk. If the compressive force affecting the intervertebral disk does not result in rupture of the annulus fibrosus, the nucleus pulposus is forced through the inferior end-plate into the body of the vertebra. This results in explosion or bursting of the vertebral body, which causes the comminuted and outwardly displaced bursting fracture of the vertebra. The displacement of fracture fragments is in all directions, including posteriorly into the spinal canal.

The radiographic diagnosis of bursting fracture of the cervical spine is optimally made on CT. This is particularly important for detection of the extent of fracture fragment displacement into the spinal canal. Computed tomography–myelography or MRI is usually necessary to evaluate the extent of compression of the spinal cord by associated fragments of the herniated disk and by bony fracture fragments.

Clay-Shoveler's Fracture. This is an avulsion fracture of the spinous processes of T-1, C-7, or T-2[3] (Fig. 2-44). This fracture is stable and is not usually associated with other fracture-dislocations of the spine.[12,16] The radiographic diagnosis is usually established when a fracture of the spinous process is identified on the lateral projection of the spine. The avulsed fractured fragment is usually noted to be in an oblique horizontal plane, a few millimeters away from the site of avulsion from the spinous process. This fracture should be differentiated from calcification of the nuchal ligament, which is usually situated posteriorly in a vertical position.[3]

Hyperextension Dislocation. This injury is caused by a violent force that causes sudden hyperextension of the head and cervical spine. The injury may cause disruption of the intervertebral disk and displacement of the vertebrae above this disk posteriorly. The anterior longitudinal ligament is usually torn, and the posterior longitudinal ligament is

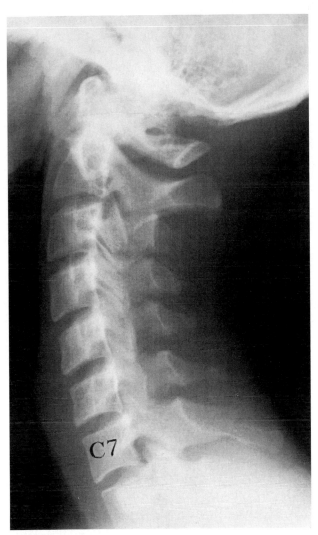

Figure 2-44. Clay-shoveler's fracture. A lateral projection of the cervical spine reveals a fracture of the spinous process of C-7. Note slight displacement of the fracture fragment inferiorly.

appears normal in alignment. However, these patients usually experience an extensive and diffuse prevertebral soft-tissue swelling. With careful examination of the initial radiographs obtained from these patients, we have noted widening, or asymmetry, of the disrupted intervertebral disk, irregularity of the outline, or horizontal fractures through the vertebral end-plates, and small avulsion fractures of the anteroinferior margins of the vertebrae. Occasionally, a small vacuum sign in the interrupted intervertebral disk may be noted.

Atlanto-axial Rotary Fixation. Wortzman and Dewar[31] in 1968 described persistent rotation of the atlas–axis and termed it rotary fixation of the atlanto-axial joint. The characteristic clinical presentation is called persistent torticollis, and usually occurs after trivial trauma or upper respiratory infection. However, this condition may also be seen spontaneously or after orthodontic surgical procedures. The head is usually tilted to one side, rotated to the opposite side, and slightly flexed.

Fielding and Hawkins[7,8] described atlanto-axial rotary fixation in 1977. Fielding recommends cine-radiography of the atlanto-axial region in the lateral position for diagnosis of this condition. The radiographic diagnosis of atlanto-axial rotary fixation is made when there is lack of normal motion between the atlas and the axis during attempted rotation. Kowalski and Associates[19] described functional CT examination of the atlanto-axial complex for diagnosis of this condition. In this study, motion between the atlas and axis, or return of the rotated atlas to the normal position, was noted in patients with transient torticollis, while no motion between the atlas and the axis was noted after attempted rotation of the neck in patients with rotary atlanto-axial fixation.

FRACTURE-DISLOCATIONS OF THE THORACIC AND LUMBAR SPINE

Compression Fracture

The most common fractures of the thoracolumbar region occur when the spine is maintained in a flexed position. This is the natural protective pos-

stripped from the posterior cortex of the vertebrae. The posterior dislocation of the vertebrae results in compression of the spinal cord against the posterior arch of the spine. Consequently, varying degrees of neurologic findings, from transient neurologic deficit to complete quadriplegia, may be noted.[12,16]

The radiographic diagnosis of this severe spinal injury may be difficult. Usually, the spine returns to its normal position after it is dislocated posteriorly. Thus, the bony cervical spine deceptively

ture attained by the body in response to external injury. Compression fractures of the vertebrae are caused by acute flexion of the spine, such as occurs in a fall from a height or when a heavy object falls on the head, shoulders, or back. The resulting fracture depends on the magnitude of the injury. With moderate trauma, there may be buckling of the end-plates, which is characteristically noted in the anterior margins of the superior end-plates. With progressively more severe trauma, various degrees of depression of the end-plate are noted. There may be sharply angulated depression of the end-plate, indicating a severe fracture of the vertebral body. Herniation of the intervertebral disk into the vertebral body may occur and may cause bursting of the vertebral body. The comminuted fracture of the body seen in these patients may be associated with displacement of fracture fragments into the spinal canal and compression of the spinal cord or neural elements. Significant ligamentous injury in fractures of the posterior elements may also be seen in association with comminuted compression fractures of the spine. Dislocation of the vertebral body posteriorly into the spinal canal and moderate kyphotic angulation of the level of the disrupted intervertebral disk may also be seen in these patients.

The radiographic diagnosis of these fractures usually presents no problem if frontal and lateral projections of acceptable quality are available. Computed tomography is usually necessary for evaluation of the spinal canal and detection of displaced fracture fragments into the spinal canal. Fractures of the posterior arch, which are usually difficult to identify on conventional studies, particularly in these patients in whom the highest quality radiographic studies may not be available, are also easily detected on CT. Myelography or MRI is usually necessary to evaluate the extent of compression and injury to the spinal cord.

Fracture-Dislocation of the Vertebral Arch

Fracture of the vertebral pedicles, articulating processes, tranverse processes, laminae, and spinous process are usually difficult to identify on conventional radiographic studies. In our patients, the number of fractures of the posterior arch that were detected in patients with spinal injury in-

creased significantly when we started performing CT of the spine as a routine diagnostic procedure in these patients. Prior to our routine use of CT, we relied heavily on tomography for identification of these fractures. In our experience, high-resolution CT using contiguous slices 5 mm or less in thickness are necessary for this purpose. We perform reformatting in the sagittal and coronal planes for identification of these lesions. Fractures of the tranverse process and spinous process are usually identified on quality conventional radiographic studies of the spine. Conventional radiographic studies and conventional tomography in the oblique projection are often helpful in identification of fractures of the articulating processes as well as the laminae.

Seat Belt Injuries

These are hyperflexion fracture-dislocations of the spine that occur in subjects wearing lap seat belts without a cross-body belt, as was installed in older-model cars. Typically, the upper lumbar bodies are involved in this injury. Gehweiler[12] divides these fracture-dislocations into two categories:

1. Posterior ligament avulsions, in which the apophyseal joints, posterior longitudinal ligament, and intervertebral disk are disrupted without any bony injury, or with avulsion fractures of the articular processes and posterior aspect of the vertebral bodies. This type of injury is more commonly noted in younger persons.
2. Posterior distraction fracture of the vertebral arch, in which a more or less horizontal fracture of the vertebral arch is present. Three variants of this fracture are recognized:
   a. Smith fracture,[26] in which there is a horizontal fracture through the posterior arch but no fracture of the spinous process. However, there is associated rupture of the interspinous and supraspinous ligaments. Fracture of the superior articulating process and a small fracture of the posterosuperior aspect of the vertebral body are also present.

b. Chance fracture,[4] which is similar to the Smith fracture except that the fracture line extends through the spinous process.

c. Horizontal fissure fracture, in which the horizontal arch fracture is extended anteriorly through the vertebral body to produce a complete tranverse fissuring or splitting of the spine.

The radiographic recognition of these fractures may be difficult if properly exposed radiographic studies are not available. Tomography and CT are usually necessary for a definitive identification of the extent and nature of these fractures of the posterior arch in these patients.[4,25,26]

FRACTURE-DISLOCATIONS OF THE SPINE IN ASSOCIATION WITH OTHER DISEASES OF THE SPINE

Osteoporosis

Osteoporosis is a condition in which there is diminution of bone mass per unit volume of bone to a level that bone is prone to spontaneous fractures or fracture following a minor trauma. Osteoporosis is the most common metabolic disease of bone. In the United States, it affects as many as 20% to 30% of white postmenopausal women. If current demographic trends continue, the relative number of elderly persons in the population will steadily increase, and osteoporosis would be expected to be encountered with increasing frequency in the future.

The earliest manifestations of osteoporosis are minimal fractures of the end-plates, causing characteristic deformities; eventually, fractures of the vertebral bodies develop. Fractures of other parts of the skeleton, e.g., the proximal humerus, distal radius, and hip, are also recognized manifestations of osteoporosis.

Bone loss in most forms of osteoporosis probably occurs simultaneously in both trabecular and cortical bone. However, because the rate of trabecular bone loss is several times that of cortical bone, trabecular bone loss is the dominant feature in the early stages of osteoporosis. The vertebral bodies contain significant amounts of trabecular bone and are thus prone to osteoporotic fractures.[11]

The radiographic manifestations of spinal osteoporosis include decreased density of bone and deformities of the end-plates, which eventually lead to biconcave configuration of the vertebrae (fishmouth deformity). In advanced stages, wedge fractures or crush fractures of the vertebrae are noted.

Differentiation between osteoporotic fractures of the vertebrae and fractures occurring in the vertebrae that contain metastasis may be very difficult. As a rule, in osteoporosis there is usually no destructive change of the pedicles or posterior elements and no erosion of the vertebral cortex, findings which may be noted in metastasis.

Metastasis

The axial skeleton is a common site for metastatic disease.[23] Destructive lesions of the bodies of the vertebrae and the vertebral elements are noted in patients with metastasis to the spine. Pathologic compression fractures commonly occur in association with these lesions.

The medical work-up of patients suspected of having spinal metastases should begin with a radionuclide bone scan.[24] Regions of the skeleton showing abnormal increased radioisotope uptake are then usually examined by means of radiography. If a lesion indicative of metastasis is identified, the radiographic work-up of the patient is terminated. In those in whom a reason for the abnormal bone scan is not identified, in the right clinical setting, further investigation to detect the possibility of metastasis is indicated. We use CT of the spine as a problem-solving modality for this purpose. In our experience, CT has been very helpful in detection of metastases to the vertebrae where conventional radiographic studies were nondiagnostic.

We have also used MRI of the spine for this purpose. On MRI, areas of metastasis to the spine appear as zones of low signal intensity on T1 weighted sequences. In the right clinical setting, the MRI presentation of metastasis is suggestive of this diagnosis. An additional advantage of MRI is the ability to visualize enroachment of pathologically fractured vertebrae, or the soft-tissue component of the metastasis, into the epidural space with resultant compromise of the spinal canal and compression of the spinal cord. Formerly, we had to resort to myelography prior to institution of proper therapeutic measures for identification of the site of cord compression in patients with spinal metastasis. At the present time, MRI examination has practically eliminated the need for emergency myelography in these patients.

Spondyloarthropathy and Ankylosing Spinal Hyperostosis

In patients who have inflammatory spondyloarthropathy, e.g., ankylosing spondylitis, psoriatic spondylitis, and related conditions, there may be bony ankylosis of the spine. In these patients the spinal column may behave somewhat like a long solid bone as far as response to trauma is concerned. We have seen patients with spinal ankylosis who show marked displacement at the site of fracture of the spinal column. We have also observed similarly marked displaced fractures of the spine in patients with ankylosing spinal hyperostosis (Forestier disease) or diffuse idiopathic skeletal hyperostosis (DISH). In more than half of our patients with ankylosis of the spine in whom a fracture was noted following a hyperextension injury, associated fractures of the posterior arches of two and sometimes three vertebrae were also noted. Fracture of the posterior arch is a beneficial lesion in these patients because it is helpful in lessening the chance and magnitude of cord compression.

Patients with ankylosis of the cervical spine are in danger of suffering fracture and cord injury during forced extension of the spine. These patients should inform the anesthesiologist or the surgeon before tracheal intubation is attempted. We have seen fractures of the spine and neurologic deficit in patients intubated for general anesthesia when the anesthesiologist had no prior knowledge of ankylosis of the spine.

Spinal Stenosis

Patients with spinal stenosis are particularly in danger of damage to the spinal cord as a complication of fracture-dislocations. Slight or moderate displacements of the vertebrae or protrusion of fracture fragments into the spinal canal, which may be asymtomatic in patients with a relatively large spinal canal, may produce significant compression of the spinal cord and neurologic deficit in patients with spinal stenosis.

Another clinically interesting aspect of spinal stenosis is the patient who is completely or almost completely asymptomatic despite marked spinal stenosis. However, following a minor trauma to the spine without an associated fracture or dislocation, the patient may become quadriplegic or paraplegic. It seems that the spinal cord had significant tolerance to slowly progressive mechanical pressure, as it occurs in slowly progressive spinal stenosis in patients with degenerative disease of the spine or calcification of the posterior longitudinal ligament. In these patients, the spinal cord adjusts to the distorted shape of the stenotic spinal canal and fills most of the available space. However, when there is absolutely no more room left in the canal, any additional encroachment into the canal, for example by swelling and edema secondary to a minor trauma to the spine (even without an associated fracture or dislocation), or a minor disk herniation may just be enough to precipitate cord compression and a major neurologic catastrophy.[10]

A definitive evaluation of the size, configuration, and extent of encroachment into the spinal canal by calcified bony fragments, bony ridges, or calcified ligaments is best achieved on CT. Evaluation of compression of the spinal cord is best achieved on MRI or CT–myelography if MRI is not available.

Spondylolysis

Spondylolysis refers to a defect of the pars interarticularis of the posterior arch of the spine (Fig. 2-45). This defect is seen in the cervical, thoracic, and lumbar spine, although it is by far most commonly noted in the lower lumbar area. In more than two thirds of our patients, the lesion was bilateral. The defect of the pars interarticularis was for a long time considered to be congenital in nature. However, there is now almost unanimous agreement that spondylolysis is a type of stress or fatigue fracture of the pars interarticularis that is

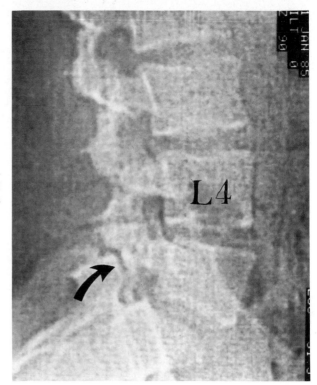

Figure 2-45. Spondylolysis of L-5 associated with L-5–S-1 spondylolisthesis and herniation of the L-5–S-1 intervertebral disk. A lateral CT localizer image of the lumbar spine reveals a defect of the pars interarticularis of the posterior arch of L-5 (*curved arrow*).

caused by repeated mechanical stress placed on this region by walking erect and extending the lumbar spine in lordosis. It is highly likely that the tendency to acquire spondylolysis is inherited.[29]

The radiographic diagnosis of spondylolysis is usually established when a defect of the pars interarticularis is noted on lateral or oblique radiographs of the lumbar spine. In a typical case, there is usually no confusion with an acquired recent fracture of the pars interarticularis. Usually in patients with spondylolysis there is moderate to marked osteosclerosis as well as narrowing of the pars interarticularis region. In patients with acute traumatic fractures occurring in a normal lumbar spine these associated abnormalities should not be present. However, acute trauma occurring in a patient with borderline spondylolysis or prespondylolysis deformity of the pars interarticularis may produce a fracture through this region that is in-

distinguishable from the average case of spondylolysis.

Spondylolisthesis

This condition refers to a slippage of the vertebral column, usually anteriorly but sometimes posteriorly or laterally on the vertebrae below (Figs. 2-46 to 2-48; see Fig. 2-45). Spondylolisthesis may be associated with spondylolysis, or more commonly, with severe degenerative disease of the facet joints.[5]

The radiographic diagnosis usually presents no problem when alignment of the posterior border of the vertebrae are checked against one another. Computed tomography is usually necessary to evaluate the extent of encroachment into the spinal canal and spinal stenosis caused by spondylolisthesis.

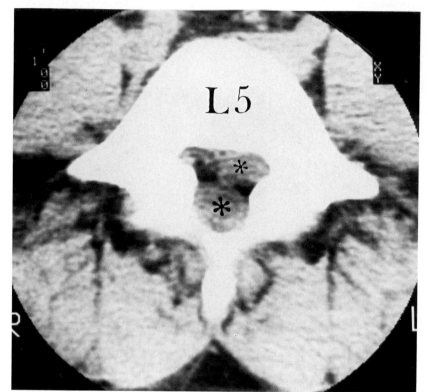

Figure 2-46. Spondylolysis of L-5 associated with L-5–S-1 spondylolisthesis and herniation of the L-5–S-1 intervertebral disk. A CT examination through the body of L-5 reveals widening of the spinal canal anteroposteriorly secondary to spondylolisthesis. The dural sac is indicated by the large asterisks. There is a soft-tissue density on the anterolateral portion of the spinal canal on the left side. This was proved to be a free fragment of a herniated disk at L-5–S-1 that had migrated superiorly and was visualized at the level of the pedicle of L-5. The herniated disk fragment is marked by a small asterisk.

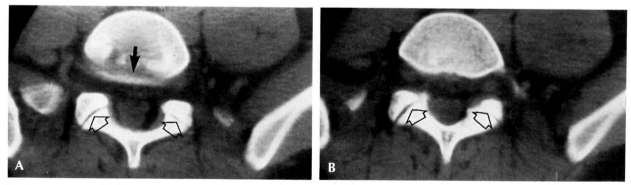

Figure 2-47. Spondylolysis of L-5 associated with L-5–S-1 spondylolisthesis and herniation of the L-5–S-1 intervertebral disk. (*A*) Computed tomographic examination at the level of L-5–S-1 intervertebral disk. The solid arrow points to the cortex of the posterior margin of the superior end-plate of S-1. The broad hollow arrows point to the facet joints. (*B*) This slice is through the inferior portion of the body of L-5, 5 mm below the inferior cortex of the pedicles of L-5. The broad hollow arrows point to the facet joints. Note the widening of the spinal canal due to displacement of the body of L-5 anteriorly.

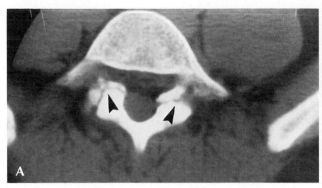 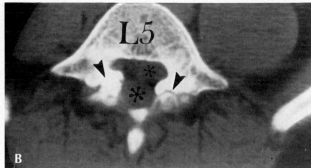

Figure 2-48. Spondylolysis of L-5 associated with L-5–S-1 spondylolisthesis and herniation of the L-5–S-1 intervertebral disk. (*A*) An axial CT slice slightly above *B* reveals distortion and anteroposterior widening of the spinal canal secondary to spondylolisthesis. The arrow heads point to the defects of the pars interarticularis. Note fragmentation of the pars interarticularis in this region. (*B*) An axial slice through the pedicles of L-5 reveals the distorted shape of the spinal canal as well as the increased anteroposterior diameter of the canal secondary to spondylolisthesis. The arrow heads point to the defect and fragmentation of the pars interarticularis. The large asterisk indicates the thecal sac. The small asterisk indicates the free fragment of the herniated disk at L-5–S-1, which is trapped at the level of the pedicle of L-5.

REFERENCES

1. Abel MS: Occult traumatic lesions of the cervical vertebrae. CRC Crit Rev Diagn Imaging 6:469–553, 1975

2. Binet F, Moro JJ, Marangola JP, Hodge CT: Cervical spine tomography in trauma. Spine 2:162–171, 1977

3. Cancelmo JJ: Clay-shoveler's fracture. AJR 115:540–543, 1972

4. Chance GQ: Note on a type of flexion fracture of the spine. Br J Radiol 21:452–453, 1948

5. Epstein BS, Epstein JA, Jones MD: Lumbar spondylolisthesis with isthmic defects. Radiol Clin North Am 15:261–274, 1977

6. Federle MP, Brant-Zawadzki M: Computed Tomography Evaluation of Trauma, pp 106–152. Baltimore, Williams & Wilkins, 1982

7. Fielding JW, Cochran GVB, Lawsing JF, Hohl M: Tears of the transverse ligament of the atlas: A clinical and biomechanical study. J Bone Joint Surg [Am] 56:1683–1691, 1974

8. Fielding JW, Hawkins RJ: Atlanto-axial rotatory fixation. J Bone Joint Surg [Am] 59:37–44, 1977

9. Fielding JW, Hawkins RJ, Hensinger RN, Francis WR: Atlantoaxial rotary deformities. Orthop Clin North Am 9:955–967, 1978

10. Firooznia H, Ahn JH, Rafii M, Ragnarsson RT: Sudden quadraplegia after a minor trauma: The role of pre-existing spinal stenosis. Surg Neurol 23:165–168, 1985

11. Firooznia H, Golimbu C, Rafii M, Schwartz MS: QCT of bone density and its relationship to fracture occurrence and fracture incidence, pp 103–113. In Genant HK (ed): Osteoporosis Update 1987. San Francisco, University of California, 1987

12. Gehweiler JA, Osborne RL, Becker RF: The Radiology of Vertebral Trauma. Philadelphia, WB Saunders, 1980

13. Grogono BJS: Injuries of the atlas and the axis. J Bone Joint Surg [Br] 36:397–410, 1954

14. Hadley LA: Anatomico-Roentogenographic Studies of the Spine. Springfield, IL, Charles C Thomas, 1964

15. Handel SF, Lee Y: Computed tomography of spinal fractures. Radiol Clin North Am 19:69–89, 1981

16. Harris JH, Harris WM (eds): The Radiology of Emergency Medicine, 2nd ed, pp 122–125. Baltimore, Williams & Wilkins, 1981

17. Jackson H: Diagnosis of minimal atlanto axial subluxation. Br J Radiol 23:672–678, 1950

18. Jefferson G: Fracture of the atlas vertebra: Report of four cases and a review of those previously recorded. Br J Surg 7:407–422, 1920

19. Kowalski HM, Cohen WA, Cooper P, Wisoff JH: Pitfalls in the CT diagnosis of atlanto-axial rotary subluxation. AJR 149:595–600, 1987

20. Maravilla KR, Cooper PR, Sklar FH: The influence of thin-section tomography on the treatment of cervical spine injuries. Radiology 127:131–139, 1978

21. McRae DL: The cervical spine and neurologic disease. Radiol Clin North Am 4:145–158, 1966

22. Meschan I: An Atlas of Normal Radiographic Anatomy, 2nd ed, pp 378–439. Philadephia, WB Saunders, 1963

23. Rafii M, Firooznia HF, Golimbu C, Beranbaum E: CT of skeletal metastasis. Seminars in ultrasound, CT and MR 7:372–379, 1986

24. Roaf R: A study of the mechanics of spinal injuries. J Bone Joint Surg [Br] 42:810–823, 1960

25. Rogers LF: The roentgenographic appearance of transverse or chance fracture of the spine: The seat belt fracture. AJR 111:844–849, 1971

26. Smith WS, Kaufer M: Patterns and mechanisms of lumbar injuries associated with lap seat belts. J Bone Joint Surg [Am] 51:239–254, 1969

27. Whalen JP, Woodruff CL: The cervical prevertebral fat stripe: A new aid in evaluation of the cervical prevertebral soft tissue space. AJR 109:445–451, 1970

28. Wholey M, Bruwer AJ, Baker HL: The lateral roentgenogram of the neck. Radiology 71:350–356, 1958

29. Wiltsi LL, Widell GH, Jackson DW: Fatigue fracture: The basic lesion in isthmic spondylolisthesis. J Bone Joint Surg [Am] 57:17–22, 1975

30. Wolf BS, Khilnani M, Malis M: Sagittal diameter of bony cervical spinal canal and its significance. Mt Sinai J Med 23:283–292, 1956

31. Wortzman G, Dewar RP: Rotary fixation of the atlanto-axial joint: Rotational atlanto-axial subluxation. Radiology 90:479–487, 1968

3

MAGNETIC RESONANCE IMAGING IN SPINAL INJURY

R. Geoffrey Wilber
Russell Crider

Magnetic resonance imaging (MRI) represents a major advance in the understanding of spinal pathology. Its early application to the brain, foramen magnum, and spine has clearly demonstrated the ability to show both normal and pathologic states.[1,8,14,15]

Two advances have improved MRI's signal-to-noise ratios over a limited distance and have resulted in images of improved clarity and detail. Early magnetic resonance work in the spine was frustrated by its limited ability for spatial resolution. This was markedly improved by the advent of surface coil technology, which allows for much higher resolution and better images.[4] Surface coils can now produce slices of less than 1 mm with superior resolution. Second, increasing magnet size has shortened scan times and augmented definition. Increase in magnet size to 1.5 tesla allows for shorter scan times but does not necessarily change the signal-to-noise ratios or spatial resolution.

The goal of this chapter is to inform the reader of recent advances in MRI technology that, when used with other imaging modalites, can provide an anatomic assessment of patients with spine and spinal cord injuries. Currently accepted uses and potential future applications of MRI will be discussed.

THEORY

Atomic nuclei with an odd number of protons and/or neutrons produce individual magnetic fields. Most MRI currently uses the proton nucleus of hydrogen for routine clinical imaging.

When protons are placed in a magnetic field they orient their individual magnetic fields along the line of the magnet (like the needle of a compass). In a magnetic field only a small proportion of nuclei will be aligned at any one time. This represents a lower energy state as compared to nonaligned nuclei. A resonant frequency is used to excite nuclei exposed to this magnetic field to induce an antiparallel or high energy state. When the nuclei return to the "resting" state they emit energy that can be detected by a radiofrequency antenna. In heterogeneous materials like the human body these signals can be spatially oriented. The use of computer formatting allows reconstruction of images recognizable anatomically. These images can visualize normal as well as pathologic states, such as the normal spine and spinal trauma. Different sampling techniques and times allow for varying imaging signals (*i.e.*, T1 vs T2 imaging).

CLINICAL APPLICATION

The spine and its contents are composed of bony as well as soft-tissue elements. The soft tissues include the ligaments, intervertebral disks, dural sac, cerebrospinal fluid, nerve roots, spinal cord and blood vessels. Following spinal trauma it is important to define injury to both bony and soft-tissue components.

Integrity of the bone, disks and ligaments determines the stability of the spine. Damage to the spinal cord and nerve roots determines the neurologic status. Assessment of spine trauma involves identifying injury to the various bone and soft tissue elements with particular concern for those circumstances that compromise spine stability and involve compression of neural structures. Magnetic resonance imaging can be applied to evaluate the status of each of the spinal components that provides information on which treatment decisions are based.[11]

An appreciation of bony injury to the spine is vital in the evaluation of both stability and compression of neural elements. Cortical bone does not image well owing to low signal output; however, marrow has an intense signal so that bony injuries manifest by changes in the signal intensity and patterns of the marrow space. This is most apparent on the T1-weighted image in which compression of cancellous bone is readily appreciated. The nonosseous structures also have a unique signal intensity that silhouettes changes in the bone, further defining osseous pathology.

The morphologic changes in both soft-tissue and bony elements can be clearly seen by MRI. This allows for visualization of bony or soft-tissue impingement on the thecal sac. Posterior ligament disruption also can be seen (Figs. 3-1, 3-2).

The status of the ligamentous elements (posterior column) and posterior longitudinal ligament can be inferred, to a certain extent, from the bony configuration seen on plain radiographs. Tomography can also be helpful in predicting this. Magnetic resonance imaging allows a unique view of the posterior elements and allows for direct imaging of ligaments and hematoma[5] (Fig. 3-3). Single- or multiple-level ligament disruption, as well as bony elements, are easily visualized. This is valuable in predicting spinal stability and guiding treatment planning.

The intervertebral disk is well visualized by MRI techniques.[14] Subtle changes in the disk are well described, and they relate primarily to changes in water content of intercellular matrix. In clinical practice MRI is at least comparable to conventional contrast computed tomography in

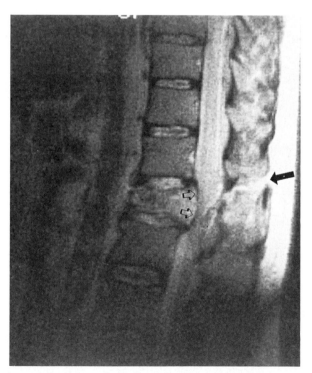

Figure 3-1. Three-column burst fracture at the thoracolumbar junction. Note the significant retropulsion of bone posteriorly. There is marked ligamentous disruption posteriorly (*arrow*).

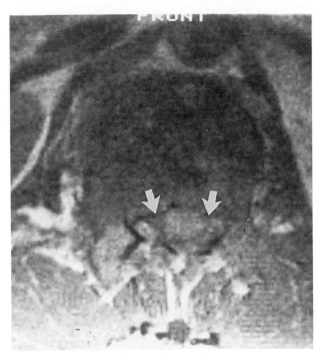

Figure 3-2. Same burst injury as in Figure 3-1. In the axial plane, note the significant disruption of signal intensity from the vertebral body. There is gross retropulsion of bone into the spinal canal (*arrows*).

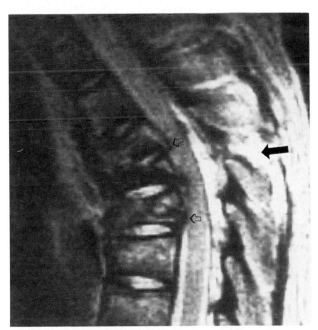

Figure 3-3. Three-level wedge compression fractures in the upper thoracic spine. There is gross disruption of the ligaments posteriorly (*large arrow*). There is mild compression of the spinal cord anteriorly along with kyphotic deformity (*small arrows*).

demonstrating intervertebral disk disease. Changes in disk water content with disruption and degeneration are better seen with **MRI** than with any other imaging technique.

Disk protrusions can be accurately localized using sagittal and transaxial images. Furthermore, **MRI** defines the relationship of retropulsed disk or bone fragments to the posterior longitudinal ligament, which is of major significance in predicting the success of specific treatment options (Fig. 3-4). In the presence of kyphotic or translational deformity **MRI** can establish the contribution of disk pathology to underlying neural compression (Fig. 3-5).

In contrast to myelography, which may demonstrate complete blockage or obliteration of the dye column (Fig. 3-6), **MRI** provides precise definition of those anatomic structures causing neural compression (Figs. 3-6, 3-7). Also, **MRI** will reveal pathology not visualized below the level of a complete myelographic block.

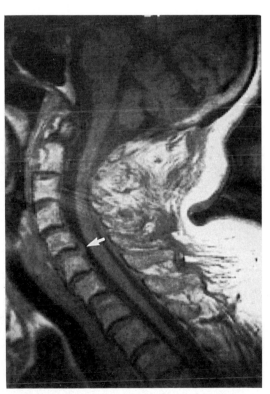

Figure 3-4. Subluxation at the C-5–C-6 level with gross disk protrusion present under the posterior longitudinal ligament. The posterior elements appear intact.

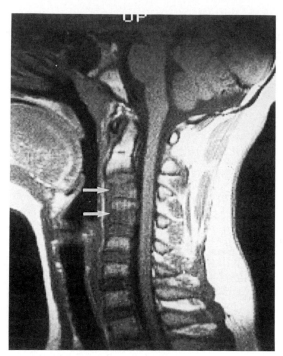

Figure 3-5. Two-level compression fracture involving the C-3 and C-4 vertebral bodies. There is preservation of the middle column. Notice the decreased signal intensity of the fractured vertebral bodies (*arrows*).

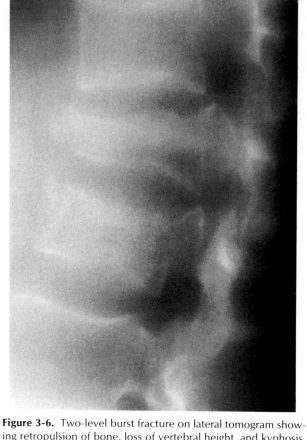

Figure 3-6. Two-level burst fracture on lateral tomogram showing retropulsion of bone, loss of vertebral height, and kyphosis.

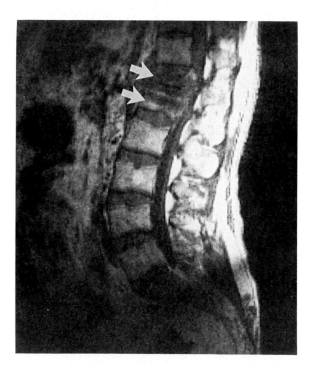

Figure 3-7. Two-level stable burst fracture at T-12 and L-1. There is disruption of the anterior and medial columns. The posterior elements are normal.

MRI will be useful in elucidating the pathoanatomy of the often described yet poorly defined whiplash injury. This modality will be important in treatment as well as in medicolegal implications. Clinical studies with regard to this injury are pending.

Evaluation of neural injury is currently made by clinical or postmortem examination. There is evidence that anatomic definition of neurologic injuries may be possible with MRI.[2]

Kulkarni and associates[9] have proposed a method of evaluating spinal cord injuries. Three distinct patterns of injury were described:

Type I shows central hypointensity of hemorrhage and surrounding hyperintensity or edema.

Type II shows cord enlargement and an area of hyperintensity or edema extending superiorly and inferiorly.

Type III shows a small central area of hypointensity or hemorrhage surrounded by hyperintensity or edema.

These investigators concluded that the best prognostic findings were those of spinal cord edema and the worst were those of hemorrhage within the spinal cord.

The status of nerve roots and the patency of neural foramina can be easily evaluated on the off-center sagittal view as well as in the cross-sectional view (Fig. 3-8). Localization of the anatomic site of neural compression in a partial neurologic injury allows accurate planning of surgical approaches and treatment. Magnetic resonance imaging can accurately demonstrate canal compromise (Fig. 3-9).

REGIONAL ROLE OF MAGNETIC RESONANCE IMAGING IN SPINAL INJURIES

The cervical spine can be divided into two distinct anatomic areas for classification of injury patterns: the upper cervical spine (occiput to C-2) and the lower cervical spine (C-2–T-1). Magnetic resonance imaging has a clear-cut application in both areas.[10,13]

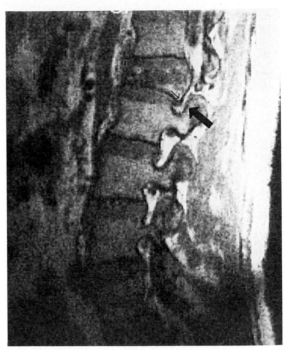

Figure 3-8. Foraminal view of the lumbar spine. Narrowing of the neural foramina is seen on this T1 weighted image (*arrow*).

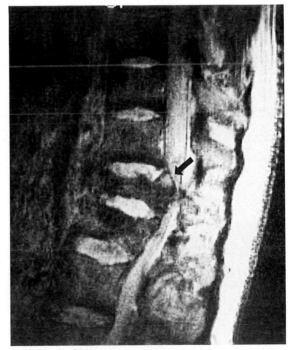

Figure 3-9. Burst fracture with marked canal compromise on a T2 weighted image. There is disk protrusion, causing part of the compression (*arrow*).

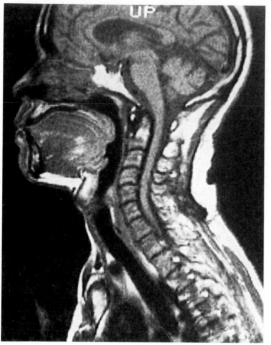

Figure 3-10. Sagittal T1 view of the cervical spine. There is normal alignment with cervical–cranial structures. The prevertebral soft tissues are seen with no evidence of swelling.

The most common injuries in the upper cervical spine include odontoid fractures, Jefferson fractures, traumatic spondylolisthesis of C-2 (hangman's fracture), and disruption of the ligamentous complex of the atlanto-axial joint. The ligamentous structures in the upper cervical spine are well visualized by **MRI**, as are the spinal contour and soft tissue swelling of the retropharyngeal space. The brainstem and upper spinal cord are seen in proper relationship to the surrounding structures (Fig. 3-10).

Dynamic flexion/extension sagittal studies are easily accomplished by **MRI** (Figs. 3-11, 3-12). They allow for determination of instability patterns and degree of compression of neurologic elements. This can facilitate planning of stabilization procedures and has particular application to late instability patterns.

The upper cervical spine is poorly visualized by traditional radiographic techniques. **MRI** has allowed for accurate demarcation of both bony and

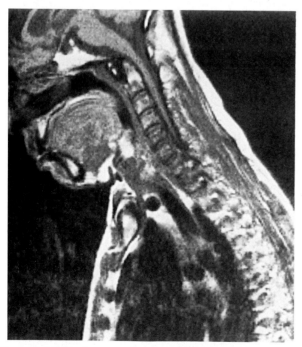

Figure 3-11. Flexion sagittal view of the normal cervical spine.

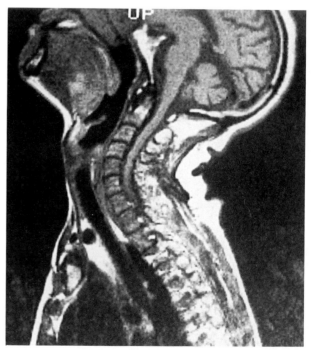

Figure 3-12. Extension sagittal view of the normal cervical spine.

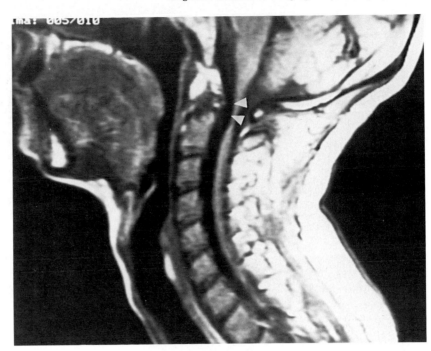

Figure 3-13. Chronic nonunion of the odontoid process is present with cord compression. There is anterior compression by the tissue at the nonunion site (*arrowheads*).

soft-tissue elements that escape precise definition using other imaging techniques (Fig. 3-13).

There were early problems in imaging patients with traction devices and halo vests. Recently, nonferrous cervical traction units, tongs, and halo apparatuses, which can all be left in place during cervical or cranial MRI, have been developed.

In the lower cervical spine MRI shows the alignment of the spinal column (See Fig. 3-10). A compression fracture of C-3 without posterior ligamentous disruption is seen in Figure 3-5. There is some mild compression of the thecal sac at the apex of the kyphotic deformity.

The integrity of supporting ligamentous structures can be determined in the cervical spine using MRI. In remote injuries ligamentous laxity with resultant instability patterns can be recognized. This is best seen by sagittal imaging views (Figs. 3-14, 3-15). Subluxation, unilateral facet dislocation, and bilateral facet dislocation are easily recognized by contrasting T1- and T2-weighted images (Fig. 3-16).

A problem area in conventional imaging of the spine is the cervicothoracic junction, which is

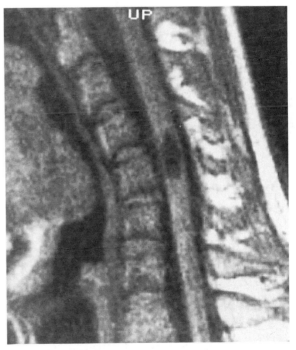

Figure 3-14. Post-traumatic syringomyelia is present at the site of a previous teardrop fracture. This patient presented with a progressive neurologic deficit many years after his injury.

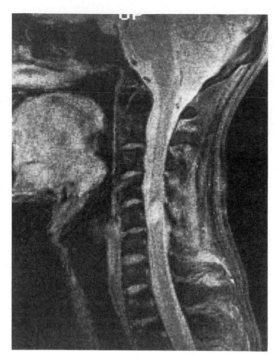

Figure 3-15. T2 weighted view of syringomyelia seen in Figure 3-14.

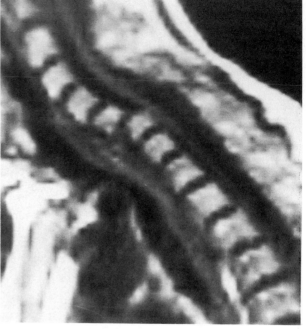

Figure 3-16. Complete fracture-dislocation of C-6 on C-7. There is marked compression of the spinal cord. Plain films were of poor quality due to the patient's high shoulder profile.

often obscured by the ribs and shoulder girdle. Radiography using a swimmer's view, tomography, and computed tomographic scanning with sagittal reconstruction can be helpful. Magnetic resonance imaging, however, gives clear sagittal images of the cervicothoracic junction (Figs. 3-17, 3-18).

As suggested previously, there appears to be a relationship between the acute MRI image of the injured spinal cord and ultimate neurologic recovery. According to Kulkarni and associates, a T1-weighted MRI image done within 24 hours of injury has value in predicting intraneural hemorrhage and edema.[9] In their study neurologic recovery of patients with major cord hemorrhage was poor. Recovery of function in patients with cord edema was better. A small amount of hemorrhage with surrounding edema was suggestive of intermediate recovery.

In a similar manner the thoracic spine is clearly seen by MRI, which is a major advance in visualizing pathologic processes, especially disk herniataion. The anterior position of the spinal cord is

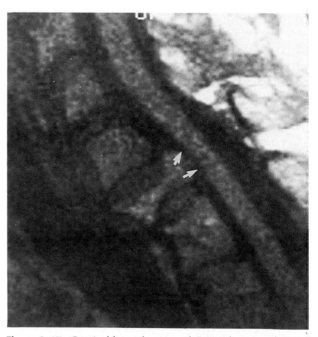

Figure 3-17. Cervical burst fracture of C-7 with retropulsion of bone onto the spinal canal. The spinal cord is in direct continuity with the bone fragments (*arrows*).

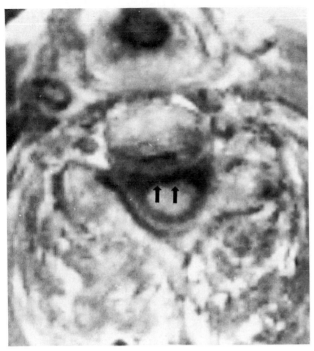

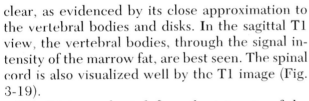

Figure 3-18. Axial view of the cervical spine at the neural foramina level. A disk bulge is seen (*arrows*). The adjacent soft-tissue structures (i.e., trachea, carotid arteries, vertebral arteries) are seen.

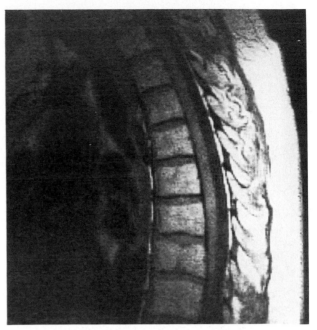

Figure 3-19. T1 weighted image of the thoracic spine. The anterior and posterior elements are normal. The cord is seen anteriorly in the dural sac.

clear, as evidenced by its close approximation to the vertebral bodies and disks. In the sagittal T1 view, the vertebral bodies, through the signal intensity of the marrow fat, are best seen. The spinal cord is also visualized well by the T1 image (Fig. 3-19).

The T2 image best defines the integrity of the disk as well as CSF space (Fig. 3-20). Axial imaging techniques show the costovertebral joint, anterior vascular structures, spinal cord, and dural sac (Fig. 3-21).

The three-column theory of fracture stability is discussed in Chapter 8. The MRI image is uniquely able to demonstrate the integrity of the bone and ligamentous portions of these columns. A simple compression fracture will involve only the anterior spinal column. In a stable bursting fracture, failure of both the anterior and middle columns occurs while the posterior ligamentous structures and laminae remain intact. Retropulsion of bone usually occurs at the level of pedicles (Figs. 3-22, 3-23, 3-24).

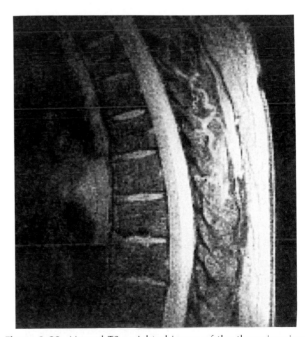

Figure 3-20. Normal T2 weighted image of the thoracic spine. The cerebrospinal fluid has an increased signal intensity as do the disk spaces.

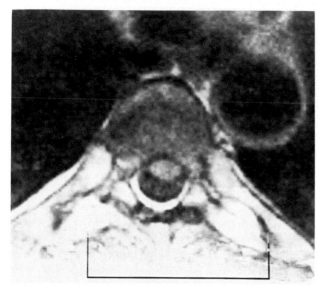

Figure 3-21. Normal axial image of the thoracic spine. The spinal cord is seen anteriorly within the canal. The view is through the midpedicle level.

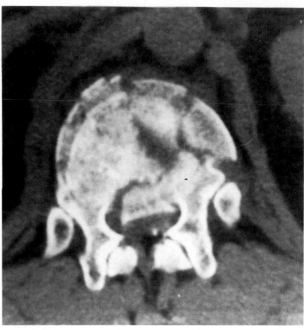

Figure 3-23. L-1 burst fracture seen on CT/myelogram with retropulsion of bone fragments. The posterior elements appear normal.

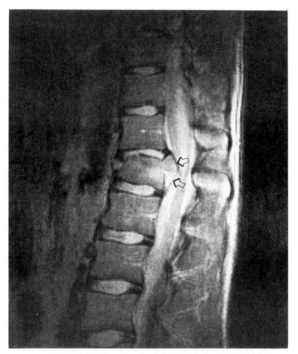

Figure 3-22. Stable burst fracture in the lower thoracic spine. There is canal compromise with evidence of an intact posterior longitudinal ligament (*arrows*). The posterior elements are normal.

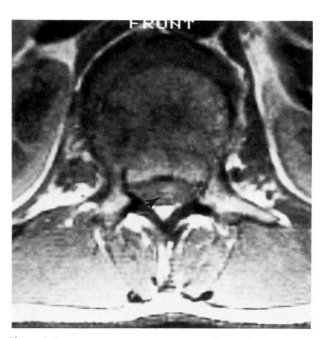

Figure 3-24. Magnetic resonance image of same burst fracture as in Figure 3-23. This shows the bony impingement as well as the position of the conus medullaris in the dural sac (*arrow*).

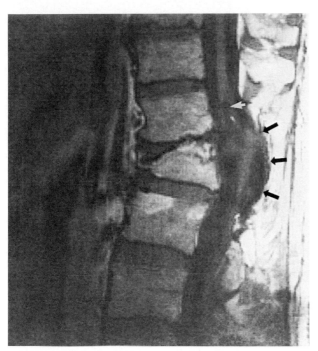

Figure 3-25. Burst fracture with continuing neurologic anterior compression, previously treated with a laminectomy. Note posterior scar (*black arrows*) as well as cystic change within the cord (*white arrow*).

Ligamentous injury to the thoracolumbar spine can usually be seen on MRI; therefore, MRI is helpful in guiding surgical approaches and treatment. Previous examples in this chapter show posterior column disruption (Figs. 3-1, 3-3, 3-16).

Dural compression can easily be seen on MRI, whether it is caused by disk, bone, or hemorrhage (Figs. 3-25, 3-27, 3-28). This is especially true in the previously operated back (Fig. 3-26). Similarly, MRI can be used postoperatively to access surgical decompression of the spinal cord and nerve roots (Figs. 3-29, 3-30).

Improved visualization of the previously operated spine can be achieved using MRI with specific enhancing agents.[7,17] The use of weakly paramagnetic compounds such as gadolineum has been shown to be quite useful in differentiating scar and recurrent disk herniation. These studies also seem to increase the overall definition of the paraspinal and intraspinal tissues and may in the future be-

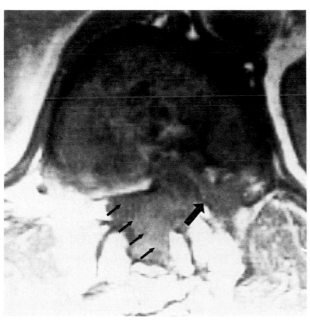

Figure 3-26. Continuing neural compression from bone and disk (*large arrow*). Postlaminectomy scar formation is seen (*small arrows*).

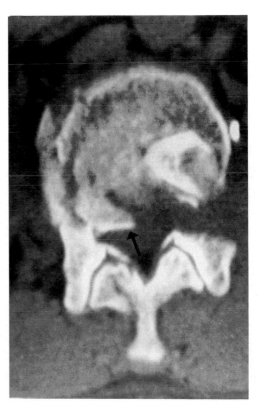

Figure 3-27. Burst fracture following anterior decompression, with residual neural compression by bone fragments (*arrow*). Iliac crest bone is in place.

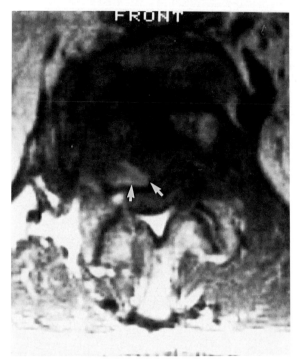

Figure 3-28. Magnetic resonance image of the same the level as Figure 3-27, showing residual anterior compression (*arrows*).

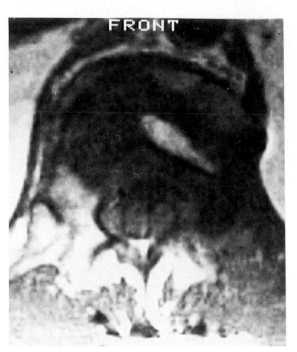

Figure 3-30. Axial view of the same patient as in the three previous Figures following further decompression. Complete anterior decompression is present. The iliac crest bone graft is seen as an area of increased signal intensity.

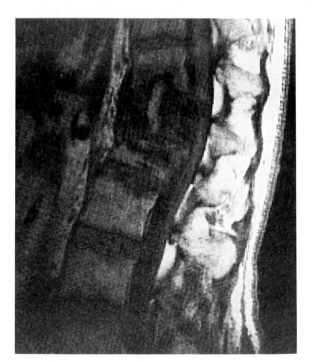

Figure 3-29. Sagittal image of the same patient as in Figures 3-27 and 3-28 following more radical decompression. The bone graft is in place and residual kyphosis is seen. The canal itself is not well visualized.

come standard aspects of **MRI** spinal studies. They have been shown to be quite useful in defining intraneural pathology, especially neoplastic conditions. Contrasted **MRI** may provide better definition of neurologic injury, which would help the clinician predict the outcome from spinal cord injury.

Newer approaches of **MRI** using three-dimensional reconstruction and thin slices allow for better understanding of spinal pathology and can act as an accurate guide in planning surgical approaches.

Post-traumatic changes of the injured spinal cord have been well described. Post-traumatic syringomyelia, myelomalacia, and cyst formation can cause significant late neurologic loss. Magnetic resonance imaging has clear advantages over conventional techniques for diagnosing these conditions.[16,19]

Management of the patient during **MRI** evaluation of the spine presents challenging problems for the treating physician. The strong magnetic field and the time-consuming nature of the study interfere with conventional monitoring equipment. The long tunnel can cause problems with ventilating assistance, traction, and stabilization. Techniques to circumvent these problems are well described.[3,6,12,18]

SUMMARY

Magnetic resonance imaging of the spine, although still in its infancy, offers definite advantages over conventional approaches to the traumatized spine. It is noninvasive, does not carry the risk of ionizing, and does not involve the frequent repositioning required by myelography. It appears to be predictive of injuries to the bone, ligaments, disk, and neural elements. It is at least as accurate as conventional imaging techniques for most areas of spinal involvement. It is superior to conventional techniques for lesions of the craniocervical junction as well as the cervicothoracic region.

Magnetic resonance imaging is currently the only imaging technique available that is able to show the neurologic elements and their degree of injury. It seems to have a predictive value in neurologic recovery. It is the study of choice in demonstrating post-traumatic cysts and syringomyelia.

Magnetic resonance imaging, although less than 10 years old, offers many advantages over conventional radiographic techniques. Future developments can only be expected to increase the efficacy of this imaging technique.

REFERENCES

1. Cammoud P, Seibert C, Morgan C et al: Magnetic resonance imaging (MRI) of the spine and spinal cord. Magn Reson Imaging 3:192, 1985
2. Carvlin M, McGrath J, Grossman R et al: Hemorrhage and edema in acute spinal cord compression: Demonstration by MR imaging. Radiology 161:387-390, 1986
3. Dunn V, Coffman C, McGowadi J et al: Mechanical ventilation during magnetic resonance imaging. Magn Reson Imaging 3:169-177, 1985
4. Edelman RR, Shonkimas GM, Stark DD et al: High-resolution surface coil imaging of lumbar disc disease. AJNR 6:479-485, 1985
5. Emery SE, Pathria M, Wilber RG et al: MRI of post-traumatic ligament injury. Presented at the meeting of the American Academy of Orthopaedic Surgery, Las Vegas, Nevada, 1989
6. Geiger R, Casloebl H: Anesthesia in an NMR scanner. Anesth Analg 64:622-623, 1984
7. Hueftle M, Modic M, Ross J et al: Post-operative MR imaging with Gd-DTPA. J Rad 167:817-824, 1988
8. Hyman RA, Edwards JH, Vacirla SJ, Sein HL: 0.6T MR imaging of the cervical spine: Multislice and multiecho techniques. AJNR 6:229-236, 1985
9. Kulkarni M, McArdle C, Kopanicky D et al: Acute spinal cord injury: MR imaging at 1.5T. Radiology 164:837-843, 1987
10. McAffee P, Bohlman H, Han J, Salvagno R: Comparison of nuclear magnetic resonance imaaging and computed tomography in the diagnosis of upper cervical spinal cord compression. Spine 11:295-304, 1944
11. McArdle C, Crofford M, Mirfarhraee M et al: Surface coil MR of spinal trauma: Preliminary experience. AJNR 7:885-893, 1944
12. McArdle C, Wright J, Prevost W et al: MR imaging of the acutely injured patient with cervical traction. Radiology 159:273-274, 1986
13. Mirvis S, Geisler F, Jelinek J et al: Acute cervical spine trauma: Evaluation with 1.5T MR imaging. Radiology 166(3):807–816, 1988
14. Modic MT, Pavlicek W, Weinstein MA et al: Magnetic resonance imaging of intervertebral disk disease. Radiology 141:103-111, 1984
15. Norman D, Mills CM, Brant-Zawadzki M et al: Magnetic resonance imaging of the spinal cord and canal: Potentials and limitation. AJR 141:1147-1152, 1983
16. Quencer R, Sheldon J, Post M et al: Magnetic resonance imaging of the chronically injured cervical spinal cord. AJNR 7:357-464, 1986
17. Ross J, Masaryk T, Modic M et al: Lumbar spine: Postoperative assessment with surface-coil MR imaging. Radiology 164:851-860, 1987
18. Roth J, Nugent M, Gray J et al: Patient monitoring during magnetic resonance imaging. Anesthesiology 62:80-83, 1985
19. Yeates A, Zawadzki M, Norman O et al: Nuclear magnetic resonance imaging of syringomyelia. AJNR 4:234-237, 1983

CERVICAL SPINE

4

CERVICAL SPINE INJURIES

R. David Bauer

Thomas J. Errico

Few diseases or injuries have greater potential for producing devastating effects on life and on the quality of life than cervical spine injuries. Since antiquity, the diagnosis of a broken neck has always carried a bad prognosis.[233] Cervical spine injuries are among the most serious injuries that can result from falls, industrial accidents, motor vehicle collisions, penetrating trauma, and athletic activities. There is a high risk of quadraparesis in recreational sports, such as diving.[96,101,143,144] Cervical spine fractures are the most frequent neck injury in severely injured automobile accident victims, especially for those occupants who do not wear shoulder and lap belt restraints.[51,77,117] The spectrum of injury these fractures can cause ranges from minor neck pains to quadraplegia and death.[53,252]

As of 1980, there were between 120,000 and 150,000 individuals with spinal cord injuries living in the United States. Approximately 10,000 new injuries occur each year. The cervical spine is the most frequently injured region of the spine.[87] The highest proportion of injury is sustained by the younger segment of the population, especially those in the 15- to 35-year age range.[105]

Diagnostic strategy in the detection of cervical spine injuries is directed toward the evaluation of bony or ligamentous instabilities, and the presence of or potential for neurologic injury. Management of these injuries consists of early recognition of injury with prompt and effective immobilization of the spine. The goals of treatment should also stress the prevention of complications. The ultimate goal is the anatomic reconstruction of the cervical spine so that it is able to carry weight, be fully mobile, and be free of pain. In addition, the facilitation of nursing and the possibility of early mobilization of tetraplegics should be high priorities.[1]

PATIENT EVALUATION

When the patient first arrives in the emergency area, the first priority is to **diagnose and care for**

associated life-threatening injuries. Many patients with cervical spine injuries have sustained other significant injuries that can lead to their demise. Treating physicians must be aware of this possibility and follow established trauma protocols.[9,77,228] Airway, ventilation, and circulation are evaluated and treated as necessary. A quick initial survey of the patient detects life-threatening emergencies. A neurologic examination demonstrates the presence and extent of neurologic injury. Intra-abdominal injuries must be ruled out, by peritoneal lavage if necessary,[197] and injuries to the face, skull, and extremities must be evaluated. Only 16% of patients with cervical fractures have no evidence of other injury. Almost one quarter have other "minor" injuries, such as facial and scalp lacerations and contusions, or general body lacerations and abrasions. A substantial number of patients with facial or severe body trauma have undiagnosed cervical spine injuries.[197]

The diagnosis of cervical spine injuries must begin with the suspicion that such an injury has occurred. Patients with head, neck, facial, and multiple injuries must be suspected of cervical spine instability. All patients involved in motor vehicle accidents and other multiple-trauma victims should be immobilized[52,192] and treated as though they had an unstable cervical spine until proven otherwise. Patients who have received contact injuries to the head or neck should be suspected of having cervical spine injuries. All complaints of neck pain in these patients, no matter how trivial, should be evaluated aggressively. Similarly, patients who complain of weakness, hypoesthesias, dysethesias, or paresthesias in the upper or lower extremities should be suspected of having a spinal cord injury. All patients whose level of consciousness is altered by head injury, shock, or intoxication should also be suspected of having been injured in this manner.[3,15,42,56] The absence of mental status changes, craniofacial injuries, range of motion abnormalities, and focal neurologic findings, however, is not uncommon, and their absence should not lower the examiner's index of suspicion.[36,251]

Injuries can be exacerbated during transport to and early treatment in the hospital. As many as 10% of all patients with spinal injuries will develop new and progressive neurologic deficits during the initial stage of management, often from a failure to recognize the presence or severity of the bony injury.[56,192,201] Therefore, a high index of suspicion for cervical spine injury must be maintained in the emergency area.

Historical information, which may be provided by emergency crews initially assisting the victim, is important in the evaluation of the patient. Was the patient thrown from a vehicle? Did he strike his head? Were there signs of paralysis at the time of injury? Was the patient able to move his hands or feet at the scene, and later lose that ability? Did the patient lose consciousness?[233] The answers to these questions frequently aid the examiner in determining the mechanism and severity of injury, and may suggest other possible injuries. Inspection of the face and head may reveal abrasions, contusions, or lacerations. Anterior head and facial wounds may be indicative of hyperextension injury, while posterior wounds may be consistent with flexion type injuries.[140]

A thorough neurologic examination should be performed to determine a baseline of injury, and should be repeated at intervals to detect the waxing or waning of the neurologic status. The level of injury is defined as the lowest spinal cord segment with *intact* motor and sensory function. Spinal injury at the T-1 level will result in incomplete loss of function of the intrinsic hand muscles, while injury at C-8 will result in paralysis of the interossei and lumbrical muscles. Injury at C-7 paralyzes the triceps and limits active elbow extension, while injury at C-6 affects the biceps and weakens elbow flexion. Injury at C-5 further weakens elbow flexion and paralyzes the deltoid. The diaphragm is innervated from C-3–C-5, and injuries in this region will weaken it to varying degrees.

The sensory examination is likewise dermatomic: T-1 supplies the undersurface of the proximal arm, C-8 the ulnar palm and the last two digits, C-7 the middle finger and midpalm, C-6 the radial digits and palm. The fifth cervical vertebra supplies the shoulder, while the area under the clavicle is supplied by C-4. The fourth cervical vertebra supplies the lower neck and C-2 supplies the upper neck (Fig. 4-1).[56] Muscle strength, cutaneous pain sensation, position sensation, and deep tendon reflexes are carefully evaluated and recorded.[249]

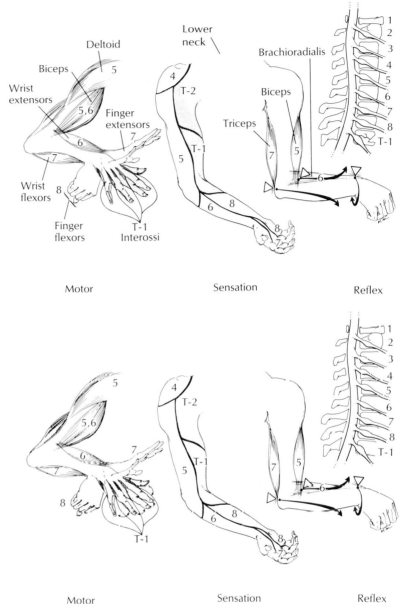

Figure 4-1. Segmental motor and sensory examination C-3 to T-1. The diaphragm is innervated from C-3 to C-5, and injuries in this region will weaken it to varying degrees. C-2 supplies sensation to the upper neck, while C-3 supplies the lower neck. The area under the clavicle is supplied by C-4. C-5 supplies sensation to the shoulder area, and a C-5 injury will weaken elbow flexion and paralyze the deltoid. Injury at C-6 will affect the biceps and weaken elbow flexion, causing numbness in the radial digits and palm. C-7 supplies sensation to the middle finger and midpalm, and motor function to the triceps, and injury at this level limits active elbow extension. Injury at C-8 will result in paralysis of the interossei and lumbricals, reducing sensation in the ulnar palm and the last two digits. Spinal injury at the T-1 level will result in incomplete loss of function of the intrinsic hand muscles with compromise of sensation on the undersurface of the proximal arm.

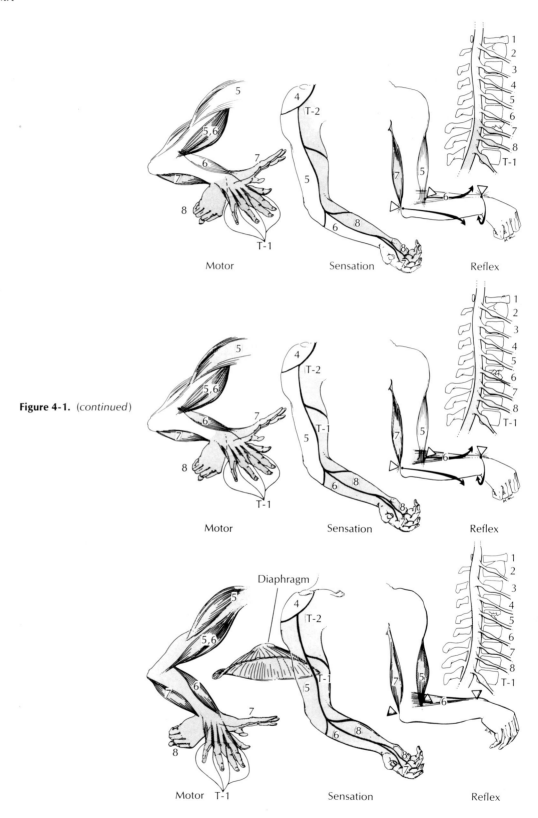

Figure 4-1. (*continued*)

Motor   Sensation   Reflex

Motor   Sensation   Reflex

Diaphragm

Motor   T-1   Sensation   Reflex

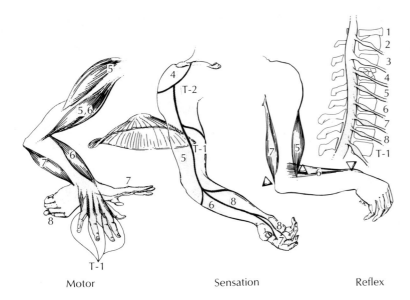

Motor   Sensation   Reflex

Figure 4-1. (*continued*)

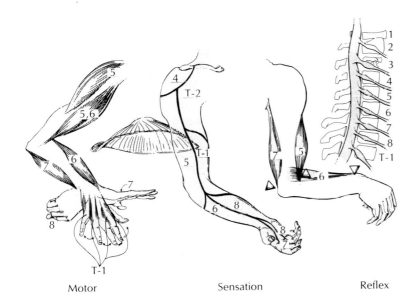

Motor   Sensation   Reflex

NEUROLOGIC INJURY

Cervical spine injuries are potentially devastating events. Both the potential for and propensity toward neural injury are caused by the instability of the supporting structures. Canal size is important in the determination of injury. While the midsagittal diameter of the *cord* does not tend to differ between individuals, the midsagittal diameter of the *canal* can vary depending on the person's sex, age, and body habitus.[74,77] Smaller canals have a significantly higher incidence of severe neurologic trauma while larger canals allow protection from injury.

Vascular insufficiency resulting from direct pressure on the spinal cord or roots is the principal cause of neural injury. Experiments on impact injury have demonstrated that trauma causes mechanical destruction as well as hemorrhage of neuronal elements. This results in decreased vascular perfusion, tissue hypoxia, edema, and further necrosis. Rapid inhibition of neural function occurs. By 6 hours after trauma, axoplasmic transport has ceased.[254]

The histologic picture of cord tissue has been studied extensively in animal studies. Seconds after trauma to the cord, flame hemorrhages appear in the gray matter and pia-arachnoid. Within 10 minutes, they have spread to the white matter and begin to affect the microcirculation of the cord.[2,65] Hemorrhage within the central gray matter spreads to the outer periphery of the white matter within 4 hours, resulting in irreversible cystic degeneration and neurolysis. After 24 hours, cord necrosis begins and complete lesions remain unchanged.[165]

Most patients develop incomplete neurologic injuries with mixed motor and sensory deficits. Incomplete lesions are defined by the preservation of function more than one level below the injury. Examples of incomplete lesions are those with sacral sparing (the preservation of perianal sensation and rectal tone), preserved distal motor or sensory function, or intact somatosensory-evoked potentials distal to the lesion.[56,216] Somatosensory-evoked potentials can be used early in the evaluation of the injured patient if obtained within 48 hours of injury.[272] They are more sensitive than a neurologic examination in detecting any retained neural function. Although they are approximately 85% predictive for later return of neural function, somatosensory-evoked potentials cannot predict the amount of recovery.[204,232,272] Progressive normalization of the wave form is a sensitive early indicator of favorable prognosis,[204] although it is not unusual for the somatosensory-evoked potential to deteriorate or disappear soon after injury.[272] Its absence at the time of injury, however, does not preclude later return of neural function in a patient with an incomplete injury.[232]

If a patient sustains immediate paralysis at the time of injury and has no sign of distal sparing, he may have a complete cord lesion. Classically, as soon as spinal shock is over, heralded by the return of the bulbocavernosus reflex (elicited by pulling the glans penis, tapping the clitoris, or tugging on an indwelling urinary catheter and obtaining a rectal sphincter response), a definitive diagnosis can be made. If the reflex has returned and complete paralysis continues, there will be no neural recovery.[121,233] The somatosensory-evoked potential is absent in patients with complete motor and sensory loss.[109,204]

Neurologic injury to the cervical cord may result in either complete or partial loss of sympathetic nervous system control to vital functions. This occurs because a major portion of the sympathetic autonomic nervous system is located at the upper thoracic cord. In neurogenic shock, peripheral vasomotor integrity is lost as a result of the sudden interruption of sympathetic vasomotor control. Peripheral vasodilation occurs, resulting in hypotension and decreased body temperature. The loss of sympathetic fibers innervating the myocardium allows vagal nerve override and bradycardia, further compounding the hypotension.[165] Neurogenic shock further decreases capillary perfusion to the injured cord. This added ischemia may further embarrass the spinal cord.

When there is incomplete motor or sensory loss, the neurologic examination may reveal a specific pattern of damage. "Cord syndromes" are caused by injury to specific fiber tracts, and the damage can be predicted by knowledge of the cross-sectional anatomy of the cord. In general, the major motor pathways descend in the anterior half of the spinal cord, while the sensory tracts are located in the posterior and lateral aspects of the spinal cord (Fig. 4-2).

Anterior cord syndromes are caused by damage to the ventral aspect of the spinal cord, involving mainly the spinothalamic (pain and temperature) and corticospinal (motor function) tracts. This usually results in immediate partial or complete paralysis with loss of pain and temperature sensation. There is preservation of proprioception, vibration sense, and deep pressure sensation.[85,131] Trauma occurs either to the anterior spinal artery or the ventral aspect of the spinal cord, or both. This is the most common syndrome seen, usually due to a flexion injury to the cervical spine. It may be associated with a retropulsed disk, fracture-dislocation, or vertebral bursting fracture. The prognosis for neurologic recovery in this syndrome is guarded. Preservation of the spinothalamic tract, with preservation of pinprick sensation, is a favorable prognostic sign.[165]

Central cord syndromes are usually caused by expanding hematomas of the central cord, causing compression of the adjacent pyramidal fibers.[121,131,157,170,213,214] Central cord syndromes can be seen in younger patients after acute hyperextension trauma.[157] These syndromes, however, are most commonly seen in older patients, especially those with degenerative changes, narrowed spinal canals, and osteophytic ridges, following severe extension injuries.[56,170,214] The hallmark of the central cord syndromes is greater motor impairment of the upper than the lower extremities, with bladder dysfunction and varying degrees of sensory loss below the level of the lesion,[165] although the only presenting sign may be a burning sensation in the hands. Fine finger movements are the first motor function affected and last to recover. Lower extremity fibers are privileged by their lateral position and recover first. Bladder function also recovers early. A varying degree of recovery is possible, but many patients are left with permanent neurologic deficits.[56,254]

The mechanism of the *Brown–Sequard syndrome* is poorly understood, but is probably related to rotational dislocation or subluxation injuries or to unilateral pedicle and laminar injuries. There is motor weakness on the side of the lesion and decreased pain and temperature sensation on the side contralateral to the injury, beginning one or two segments below the level of injury. Significant neurologic recovery often occurs.[56,131,254]

The *posterior cord syndrome* is marked by loss of position and vibration sense distal to the lesion caused by involvement of the posterior columns. Rarely seen, it is usually associated with extension injuries.[56,85,254]

Fitting a patient's pattern of injury into one of these neurologic syndromes may help establish a prognosis for the patient.

DETECTION OF CERVICAL SPINE INJURY

A patient sent for radiographic evaluation with the suspicion of cervical spine injury should be treated in the radiography suite as though the fracture or subluxation exists.[56] Immobilization of the neck should be continued, and the roentgen studies initiated on the patient's stretcher. The presence of a soft or semirigid collar does not guarantee immobilization of the spine.[11,52,192] A routine series of high-quality films should be obtained, including anteroposterior and lateral views, the open-mouth view (to visualize the odontoid), and a detailed, overpenetrated lateral view (allowing better definition of bony injuries at the expense of soft-tissue definition).[68,114,140,162,196,254]

Delayed recognition of cervical injuries is a significant problem, occurring in more than 20% of cervical spine injuries in a recent study.[196] Delayed recognition can lead to the emergence or exacerbation of neurologic deficits.[191,195,196] The inability to appreciate injuries can occur after failure to take appropriate radiographs or failure to correctly interpret them.[17,50,191,195,196] Failure to appreciate the severity of injury occurs most often in the presence of mild neural deficits or in the neurologically intact patient.[195,196] The presence of alcohol, multiple spinal injuries, and altered levels of consciousness all tend to delay diagnosis.[50,196] Routine cervical spine radiographs must be obtained in all patients with multiple trauma or head injuries, and in all intoxicated or obtunded patients with a history of a fall.

PLAIN FILM EVALUATION

Radiographic evaluation should begin with the lateral view. This view is a rapid and effective way of evaluating cervical spine injuries. A lateral radiograph is satisfactory only if all seven cervical vertebrae are visualized. Before a patient can be moved, or a protective collar removed, all seven cervical vertebrae *must* be clearly visualized as normal. If the lateral film is normal and the patient's neurologic examination is normal, the remainder of the standard films are obtained without moving the patient's head.[41,225] The lateral radiograph alone can detect only 75% to 85% of all cervical spine injuries.[23a,208,238] Injuries in the C-1–C-2 region are easily missed on the lateral view.[238] When the open-mouth odontoid view and the supine anteroposterior view are added, the accuracy rises to almost 100%. Any area that is

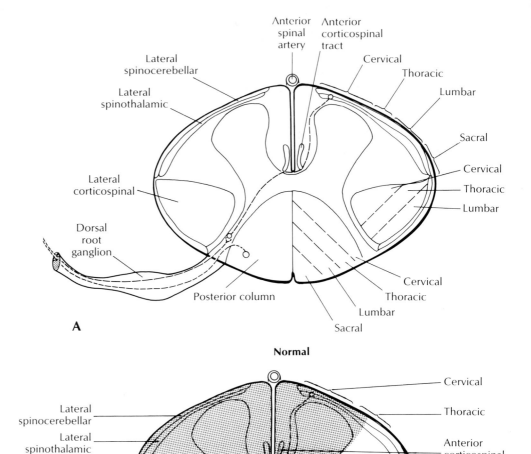

Figure 4-2. With incomplete motor or sensory injury, neurologic examination may reveal a ''cord syndrome,'' due to injury to specific fiber tracts. The damage can be predicted by knowledge of the cross-sectional anatomy of the cord. (A) The major motor pathways descend in the anterior half of the spinal cord, while the sensory tracts are located in the posterior and lateral aspects of the spinal cord. (B) *Anterior cord syndromes* are caused by damage to the ventral aspect of the spinal cord; they involve mainly the spinothalamic (pain and temperature) and corticospinal (motor function) tracts. Such damage results in immediate partial or complete paralysis with loss of pain and temperature sensation but with preservation of proprioception, sense of vibration, and deep pressure sensation.

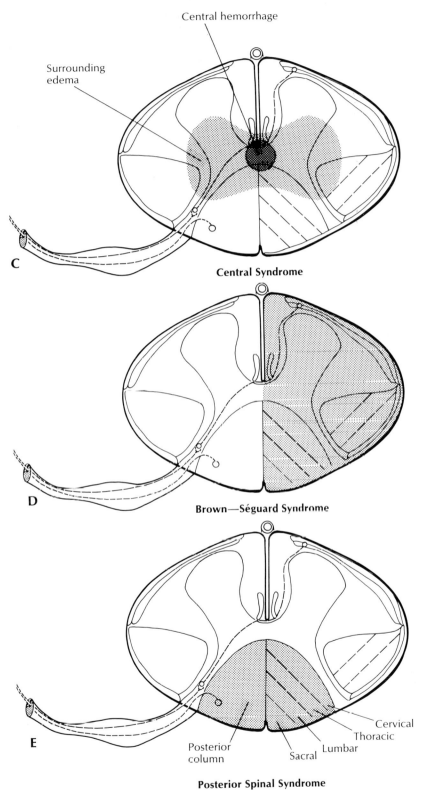

Central hemorrhage

Surrounding
edema

C

Central Syndrome

D

Brown—Séguard Syndrome

E

Posterior
column

Sacral

Lumbar

Cervical

Thoracic

Posterior Spinal Syndrome

Figure 4-2. *(continued) (C) Central cord syndromes* cause greater motor impairment of the upper than the lower extremities, with bladder dysfunction and varying degrees of sensory loss below the level of the lesion. *(D) Brown–Séguard syndrome* causes a motor weakness on the side of the lesion and decreased pain and temperature sensation on the side contralateral to the injury, beginning one or two segments below the level of injury. *(E)* The *posterior cord syndrome* is marked by loss of position and sense of vibration distal to the lesion. It is caused by involvement of the posterior columns.

inadequately demonstrated on the three-view spinal series should be examined by computed tomography (CT).[3,15,23a,203,208,238]

Routine lateral radiographs frequently fail to show the cervicothoracic junction due to overlapping shoulder shadows. This is especially true if the patient is bull-necked, heavily built with well-developed shoulders, or uncooperative. Since the incidence of isolated C-7 injury may be as high as 30%, other techniques should be used when C-7 is not demonstrated on the lateral view. Radiographs can be obtained with the head steadied in a halter and the arms pulled downward by an assistant. A "swimmer's," or Twining view, is obtained by centering the roentgen tube above the shoulder to the opposite shoulder (away from the film), pointed towards the patient's axilla nearest the film, with the roentgen tube angled 10 to 15 degrees toward the head.[15,78,85,185,196]

Soft tissues often provide significant information on the lateral radiograph with regard to localization of cervical spine trauma. At the anteroinferior margin of C-3 a retropharyngeal (or prevertebral) width of greater than 5 mm may be indirect evidence of either hemorrhage or edema. Hematoma in the C-1–C-4 region is closely related to fractures of the anterior elements of the spine, but may rarely result from avulsion of the anterior longitudinal ligament without fracture of the body. Relatively small hematomas are encountered with odontoid fractures and compression fractures.[57,63,102,149,186,240] In children, the prevertebral soft tissue should measure one third of the thickness of C-2. Care should be taken in interpreting this sign because crying or talking increases the space.[85] This measurement is not valid in the presence of endotracheal or nasogastric tubes.[240]

On the lateral radiograph, loss of the lordotic curve is usually indicative of muscle spasm; however, this may be a subtle sign of instability after flexion injury. Abnormalities in the alignment of the spinous processes should be sought.[118,160] Interpretation of changes in cervical lordosis is highly uncertain. The patient's chin must be depressed prior to taking the film in order to obtain a meaningful evaluation. Lateral flexion–extension views should be performed on all individuals presenting with loss or reversal of the lordotic curve

as their only radiographic abnormality. In the absence of severe degenerative disk disease, there should be straightening of the kyphotic curve in hyperextension and accentuation of the curve in flexion. A full range of motion indicates that the reversal of lordosis is normal for the individual.[228]

Evaluation of the bony anatomy should be made in a routine and organized manner. The tips of the spinous processes form a gentle longitudinal curve, as do the anterior and posterior portions of the vertebral bodies.[62] The spino-laminar line is found at the junction of the lamina and spinous process. A gentle curve, parallel to the others, is formed by joining these. Interruption of these curves represents a fracture or subluxation of the spine. One should then inspect the vertebral bodies for obvious fractures and for the presence of angulation. The spinous processes should also be evaluated for any loss of parallelism, and the disk spaces evaluated for uniformity of height and width.[17,267] Degenerative changes may cause confusion in diagnosis of acute traumatic changes due to abnormalities of the disk spaces and vertebral shapes. These changes should be evaluated by CT to differentiate them from traumatic injury.[136,185,192]

The open-mouth view is necessary in the evaluation of the C-1–C-2 articulation.[227,238] Fractures of the odontoid process are most easily identified by this view. Attention should be paid to the lateral masses of C-1 and their positions relative to the body of C-2. Changes in this relationship can be indicative of rotatory instability as well as disruption of the bony and ligamentous structures. Other fractures of the atlas may be visualized on this view.

Oblique films may be obtained to evaluate the apophyseal joints. Localization of unilateral facet dislocation or fracture may be accomplished in this manner. In addition, oblique views may confirm relocation of jumped facets. Computed tomography, however, may be more helpful in this regard.[85,167,228,264,270]

When evaluating a patient in whom cervical injury is suspected, one must be cognizant of the fact that injuries to disks and ligaments are *not* documented by standard radiographs. Pathologic studies have shown that a normal radiograph cannot necessarily be equated with normal anatomy.[271] Special studies may be necessary to rule out injuries.

DYNAMIC STUDIES

Flexion–extension films may be obtained as part of the initial evaluation. These films may demonstrate displacement that is not visualized on plain films. They are used primarily to evaluate instability caused by occult ligamentous injury. Flexion–extension views should not be obtained if there is objective evidence of neurologic, bony, or soft-tissue injury. The patient should position himself without the assistance of either technicians or physicians. False negative films may be obtained as a result of pain and muscle spasm. This may preclude definitive, early use of this technique. As soon as cervical spasm subsides, these films should be pursued if indicated.[3,85,228]

Alternatively, the "stretch test" can be obtained to evaluate the competency of the posterior ligaments. The examination is performed while traction is applied to the head, usually by a cloth cervical halter. An initial lateral radiograph is obtained and cleared as normal. Traction is then begun with a fairly light weight (usually 15 lb, though the initial weight and increments can be changed depending on the level of the lesion and the tolerance of the spine).[166] Traction is increased incrementally (usually 5 or 10 lb at a time) with repeated radiologic and neurologic evaluations. This radiologic examination should be obtained only with a physician in attendance. Any change in alignment or separation of vertebral bodies in indicative of damage to posterior structures. Any change in neurologic status or abnormal separation of anterior or posterior elements constitutes a positive examination, and the test is stopped.[7,255,261,260]

SPECIAL STUDIES

The use of CT and planar tomography in the diagnosis of cervical trauma is a necessity. Plain films have been shown to underestimate the presence and severity of spinal fractures at all levels. Computed tomographic scans are especially useful for lesions that are not visible on plain films. Computed tomography allows a thorough evaluation of

obscure fractures of the posterior elements, exposing the patient to less radiation and maintaining the supine position.[3,15]

Computed tomography provides an accurate display of cross-sectional anatomy at any level. In addition, it accurately displays soft-tissue structures and allows visualization of the bony limits of the spinal canal in the axial plane. It is superior to other diagnostic procedures in demonstrating impingement on the neural canal. Reformatting of CT images can allow heightened awareness of the three-dimensional geometry of fractures, although information can be lost if the patient has moved. A major drawback of reformatting is that it can produce a "pseudofracture" where none actually exists.[33,57,135] Three-dimensional CT scanning is becoming increasingly available, and can demonstrate injuries with amazing clarity.[269]

Although CT has replaced tomography in many instances, lateral tomography remains the most useful mode for evaluating odontoid fractures and other anterior atlantal fractures that are parallel to the plane of the CT scan.[114] Lateral tomography is also better than CT in the evaluation of posterior facet fractures. Plain anteroposterior and lateral radiographs are obtained to ascertain the site of bone and spinal cord pathology. This precise localization facilitates targeting of the CT scanner, and ensures that a lesion is not missed.[147]

MYELOGRAPHY

Myelography is indicated for optimum visualization of compression of the spinal cord after trauma. A lateral C-1–C-2 puncture and injection of water-soluble nonionic contrast material can be performed with the patient supine. Because the material is completely miscible with cerebrospinal fluid, the spinal cord is easily seen whether there is blockage or not. Myelography alone is rarely indicated, and should primarily be used in conjunction with CT.[3]

Computed tomography with myelographic contrast in place is more accurate than CT alone or myelography alone[57,105] in the demonstration of intraspinal pathology. The main indication for CT–myelography in acute spinal injury is an incomplete lesion of nonosseous origin. This includes lesions caused by disk herniation or hematoma in the spinal canal, which are not easily distinguished on CT scanning.[3]

MAGNETIC RESONANCE IMAGING

The advent of magnetic resonance imaging has added a new and powerful tool to the armamentarium of the diagnostician. It provides exquisite details of both musculoskeletal soft tissues and neural structures in the sagittal, coronal, and axial planes, and enhances the ability to make diagnoses in a wide variety of spinal disorders.[3]

The use of magnetic resonance imaging in acute spinal trauma is not clear cut. Its use in this situation requires overcoming certain technical hurdles. Ferromagnetic objects cannot be placed close to the scanner: this includes respirators, oxygen tanks, and most traction devices.[3] Transferring patients in and out of the scanner while maintaining cervical traction may also be problematic. However, once these obstacles have been overcome, the images obtained may be very helpful. Disk herniation associated with dislocations may be discovered, thus preventing neurologic injury during reduction maneuvers. Early evidence demonstrates that patterns representative of different cord injuries may be of prognostic value with regard to neural recovery.[31,145,161]

DIAGNOSTIC STRATEGY

In the patient with a normal physical examination but an abnormal lateral film, radiographic examination should proceed cautiously. The patient's spine must be stabilized, and static examinations should be performed first. Any bony abnormality on the initial studies should be further evaluated with CT. If there are further indications, a contrast-enhanced CT scan may be obtained.

In patients with neurologic deficits, the sequence and goals of the diagnostic evaluation may be different. In patients with complete lesions, radiologic evaluation should be limited to defining the pathologic bony anatomy, as significant neurologic recovery rarely occurs. A CT–myelogram is not indicated. Patients with incomplete lesions, who demonstrate preservation of some motor or sensory function, should be worked up speedily and aggressively to evaluate and precisely define the presence of spinal cord compression.

When both the lateral radiograph and the neurologic examination are abnormal in the patient with incomplete lesions, the patient should be placed immediately into tongs (the halo device may be applied initially if it is anticipated that this will be part of a patient's definitive care) with traction to maintain overall alignment. Further studies are now obtained as indicated,[140] including CT and myelography via cisternal puncture.

In the patient with evidence of head and neck injury, a normal lateral radiograph but an abnormal neurologic examination with incomplete neural loss presents a diagnostic problem. Possible diagnoses include osteophytic protrusion into a small canal, leading to contusion of the cord without fracture or subluxation; an intervertebral disk herniation that cannot be demonstrated on plain films; or spontaneous reduction of the spinal subluxation that created the cord injury.[56] Computed tomography–myelography must be obtained in order to visualize the intraspinal pathology.[56,57,140] If these studies are insufficient to determine the etiology of the insult, controlled flexion–extension films may be obtained to rule out subluxation.[56]

Multiple-level fractures occur more than 5% of the time, and the second level is overlooked in more than two thirds of original assessments.[141] Most of the lesions occur at opposite ends of the cervical spine, and neurologic changes may occur because the injury is missed.[41] The presence of any spinal fracture at any level should prompt the surgeon to rule out a noncontiguous fracture.[239]

CONSIDERATION OF PEDIATRIC PATIENTS

Epiphyseal lines can mimic fractures. With very few exceptions, the neck has obtained an adult form in children older than 8 years of age, and the normal epiphyseal lines are no longer a problem. Prior to that time, the injured child's neck can be a diagnostic dilemma even for the most experienced physicians. In general, epiphyseal plates are smooth and regular, and can be found in predictable locations accompanied by subchondral sclerotic lines. Fractures are irregular, without sclerosis, and are generally in unpredictable locations.[57]

The child's cervical spine, especially in the upper levels, is much more mobile than the adult spine. Normal ligamentous laxity permits considerable excursion at the atlas anteriorly and posteriorly. In flexion, an atlas–dens interval of up to 4 mm may be normal. In extension, the atlas may appear to sublux cephalad on the dens.[9,114,222]

Pseudosubluxation, usually at the C-2–C-3 or C-3–C-4 levels, commonly causes concern. This is attributed to a combination of ligamentous laxity, a relatively horizontal orientation of the facet joints, and lesser development of the uncinate processes in the younger child. In the fully flexed neck, 3 to 4 mm of anterior displacement of one body on the subjacent body may be seen. The posterior boundaries of the neural canal, the spino-laminal junction line, normally will align in an almost straight fashion. This can be used to distinguish normal alignment from a pathologic situation.[6,9,114,222]

Normal anterior wedging of the immature vertebral body can produce the appearance of a compression fracture. Spinous process growth centers can resemble avulsion fractures.[222] Serious ligamentous disruptions can be detected by an increase in the interspinous distance, loss of parallelism between articular processes, and posterior widening of the disk spaces.[184] Careful attention to these details and matching of roentgen irregularities with clinical symptoms should prevent over- or undertreatment.[6,194]

INITIAL CARE AND PREVENTION OF COMPLICATIONS

Care and evaluation of the injured patient begins at the scene of the accident. Ambulance technicians are trained to assess patients for cervical spine trauma and to provide emergency splinting. Correct transportation procedures must be followed. As many as 10% to 25% of cervical spine injuries resulting in permanent neurologic deficit were caused by improper handling of the patient during extrication, transport, and initial evaluation.[159,201] Patients are to be transported from the scene in a "scoop"[165] with cervical immobilization, preferably with the head sandbagged as well.[159,228] The presence of a soft cervical collar does not guarantee that the cervical cord is protected or immobilized,[127,128,159,228] and one should not be lulled into a false sense of complacency merely by the presence of a collar. All transfers must be accomplished without movement of the head and neck. The patient must be moved without rotation of the head and neck until spinal injury has been ruled out or treated appropriately.

PULMONARY CARE

It cannot be overemphasized that when the patient with cervical spine injuries arrives in the hospital's emergency area, the first priority is always to diagnose and care for associated life-threatening injuries. Respiratory function should be carefully evaluated. An impaired level of consciousness may be the result of shock or cranial injury, or it may be the result of ingestion of a toxic substance (which may have caused the accident), contributing to respiratory depression. Airway obstruction caused by debris or injury to the nose, mouth, or trachea should be evaluated and treated. Injury to the neck or chest that would complicate respiration, such as a flail chest or tension pnuemothorax, should be searched for and treated.[132,228]

Patients should be in the supine position during evaluation. Later, patients should be moved from the supine position to both decubitus positions and also to the almost-prone position to assist in clearing secretions. Humidified air or oxygen will keep secretions moist and easier to mobilize. Patients should be maintained in an intensive care setting following injury to enable frequent suction and close observation.[132]

Among the earliest critical decisions is whether to intubate the patient. If possible, intubation should be withheld until a lateral radiograph has been obtained and cleared.[228] If it is not possible to wait, blind nasotracheal intubation with the neck in the neutral position, or tracheostomy should be performed. An elective intubation in the face of an unstable cervical spine can be performed with flexible bronchoscopy.[32,132]

After injury, the patient's vital capacity may be markedly reduced due to the loss of lower intercostal and abdominal muscles. The diaphragm may be partially paralyzed.[14,132,235] The decreased ability to cough and clear secretions further limits lung capacity, and is the leading cause of respiratory failure. Repeated pulmonary function tests and arterial blood gasses should be performed. Prophylactic intubation or tracheostomy should be performed if the patient is tiring or the arterial blood gas is deteriorating below acceptable levels (especially if the P_{CO_2} has risen above 45 mm Hg). Frequent suctioning and bronchoscopy are essential to clear mucous plugs.[235] In addition, mucolytic agents may be helpful.[132]

A nasogastric tube should be inserted in patients with complete lesions to prevent emesis and aspiration. It will reduce gastric dilation in patients who may be dependent on diaphragmatic breathing.[132,228,234] Later, the nasogastric tube is useful in the monitoring of gastric pH and the administration of antacids to prevent the formation of stress ulcers.

CIRCULATION

Preservation of normotension is important in patients with cervical spine injury. Neurogenic shock, characterized by hypotension and bradycardia, should be attended to early. Large-bore intravenous catheters should be inserted in all patients, and volume expansion with albumin, dextran, or (preferably) Ringer's lactate solution begun. Blood loss should be monitored and replaced, preferably by transfusion of type-specific or cross-matched blood to maintain oxygen-carrying potential.[228]

Bradycardia occurs as a result of traumatic quadraplegia, usually secondary to unopposed vagal tone. The cervical sympathetic chain has been separated from the chest cavity, and the sympathetic input no longer reaches the heart. While bradycardia is self-limited, with pulses returning to normal within 3 to 5 weeks, patients exhibiting reduced pulse have a higher mortality rate than those with a normal pulse.[14,159,268]

An indwelling urinary catheter should be inserted to monitor fluid balance. Measurements of central venous pressure may be unreliable in the face of acute injury. One must be careful that patients do not become fluid-overloaded when sympathetic tone returns. If this occurs, treatment with diuretics is essential.[235]

DEEP VENOUS THROMBOSIS AND THROMBOEMBOLISM

Deep venous thrombosis is a relatively frequent phenomenon in patients with cervical cord injuries, with an incidence from 20% to 100%, depending on the aggressiveness of diagnosis.[23,112,175] It is caused by a combination of factors. Trauma induces a state of hypercoagulability,[23] and a reduced blood flow state exists secondary to the loss of the calf pump.[189] Stasis is further compounded by the pressure of the calves on the bed.[189] Pulmonary embolism also occurs in approximately 5% of patients with cervical spine injury. Both deep venous thrombosis and pulmonary embolism usually occur within the first 2 weeks after injury.[23]

Deep venous thrombosis does not present in the same fashion in the neurologically injured patient as it does in the intact patient. The first sign is usually subtle, mild, unilateral edema. Detection of this edema is difficult, especially in the presence of atrophic changes. Daily measurement of the calves for the first 3 weeks after injury may be useful. In patients with suspected deep venous thrombosis, confirmation is obtained by Doppler and venographic studies.[23]

Prophylaxis against deep venous thrombosis is essential, given its prevalence and the difficulty of its detection. Prompt initiation of either minidose (5000 units subcutaneously every 12 hours)[23] or adjusted dose[106] heparin or elastic, intermittent compression stockings[245] are the modalities most effective in this situation.

PREVENTION OF SKIN BREAKDOWN

Maintenance of the integrity of the skin is one of the most overlooked aspects of spinal injury. With loss of skin sensation and ability to move, a neurologically impaired patient is at great risk for skin breakdown. This can occur if patients are allowed to remain in the same position for more than 2 hours. The skin must also be examined at frequent intervals for areas of irritation, and bony prominences must be padded.[235]

TREATMENT OF CORD INJURY WITH EXPERIMENTAL MODALITIES

The use of steroids to decrease cord edema and to prevent neural injuries from completing is controversial.[165] There is no general agreement between those who report a beneficial effect and those who find paradoxical or no apparent improvement following administration of steroids after cord trauma.

The mechanism of reported protection is unclear but may be related to several factors, including reduction of exudation of leukocytes and plasma constituents, maintenance of cellular membrane integrity to prevent excessive swelling of cells, maintenance of electrolyte balance and plasma glucose levels, inhibition of lysosomal release from granulocytes, inhibition of phagocytosis, and stabilization of the membranes of the intracellular lysosomes.[65,165] In a study using cats, high doses were reported to reduce the spread of morphologic damage and prevent loss of axonal conduction and reflex activity.[65] Another study reported an increase in blood flow to the damaged cord.[273] De la Torre considers it "understandable and perhaps even justifiable" to use steroids in patients with acute spinal trauma until further data has been accumulated.[65]

Osmotic diuretics, such as mannitol, have been suggested to be useful in cord trauma,[105] as they are in head trauma. There are, however, complications to their use. When they succeed in mobilizing extracellular fluid, they appear not to affect the cord–blood barrier. Mannitol has the further complication of producing a sudden hypokalemia. In de la Torre's opinion, osmotic diuretics probably should not be used in spinal cord trauma.[65]

Naloxone has been used with success in cats in whom experimental spinal cord injury has been produced.[65] The return of motor control in animals treated with naloxone was associated with preservation of spinal cord blood flow (which was shown to be reduced in the controls)[89] and preservation of somatosensory-evoked potentials.[274] A dose-related response has been reported in humans.[88]

GENERAL TREATMENT CONSIDERATIONS

The goals of treatment in cervical spine injury vary with the specific type of injury. The two main considerations are spinal stability and neurologic functioning. Obviously, the two factors are intimately related. With a neurologically intact pa-

tient immediate and long-term stability must be provided to prevent neurologic deterioration. With the neurologically impaired patient stability must be provided not only to prevent deterioration but to allow potential recovery to occur.

Patients with incomplete neurologic injury require consideration beyond immediate and long-term stabilization of the bony–ligamentous complex. Potentially remediable areas of neural compression due to bony fragments, disk material, dislocations, or subluxations must be identified and addressed.

Traction is an important modality in the initial treatment of cervical spine injuries associated with gross malalignment. It is useful for reduction of subluxations and dislocations, and it serves to protect the spine from further injury. If gross malalignment is not present, skull traction may not be necessary.

Emergency surgery is rarely indicated in cervical spine trauma.[165] Deterioration in neurologic status calls for emergent myelography or CT scanning. Surgical treatment can then be considered based on the lesions found. The one clear indication for emergent intervention is a civilian (low velocity) pistol wound to the anterior neck with associated tracheal or esophageal injuries. These require débridement, establishment of long term airway control, and prevention of mediastinal infection or esophageal fistula formation. Because of the life-threatening nature of the injury, the wound in the spinal canal is never approached.[165,250] Surgical débridement is not indicated for clean posterior wounds with immediate, complete neurologic loss.[165]

STABILITY OF THE CERVICAL SPINE

It is important to define whether a patient's spine is unstable after an accident. Such a decision can profoundly affect patient care: Misjudgment can result in death or neurologic injury on the one hand, or unnecessary surgery with its attendant risks on the other. Stability of the cervical spine is determined by the integrity of the ligaments and bones of the spine.

Instability can be functionally defined as a weakness of the intervertebral bonds that render the spine unable to withstand physiologic loads tolerable to the normal spine. This implies actual or potential abnormal excursion of one segment on another and therefore potential or actual compromise or irritation of neural elements. In addition, there should be no development of incapacitating deformity or pain from structural changes.[85,260] The percentage of patients with untreated, late instability after cervical spine injury has been found to range from 17%[47] to 42%[26].

The process of determining whether a given patient's spine is potentially unstable at the time of injury is controversial. There are various signs of instability that should be sought on the plain films:

1. "Fanning" of the spinous processes in excess of what is observed at the adjacent levels, with or without flexion[225]
2. Widening of the intervertebral disk space in excess of that observed at adjacent levels, with or without flexion–extension or traction views[48,225]
3. More than 3.5 mm of horizontal displacement of a vertebra relative to the adjacent vertebra, as measured on resting lateral or flexion–extension views (Fig. 4-3A)[255,260]
4. More than 11 degrees of angulation compared to that of either adjacent vertebra (Fig. 4-3B)[255,260]

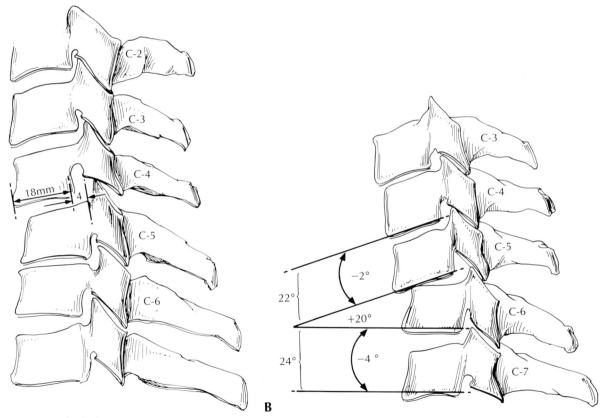

A   **B**

Figure 4-3. Method of measuring translational displacement. (A) A point at the posteroinferior angle of the lateral projection of the vertebral body above the interspace in question is marked. A point at the posterosuperior angle of the projection of the vertebral body is also marked. The distance between the two is measured (*arrows*). A distance of 3.5 mm or greater is suggestive of clinical instability. (B) The finding of abnormal angulation at a given interspace is based upon a comparison of the interspace in question with either adjacent interspace. A difference of 11 degrees or greater from that of either adjacent interspace is evidence of clinical instability. (Adapted from White AA III, Southwick WO, Panjabi MM: Clinical stability in the lower cervical spine: A review of past and current concepts. Spine 1:15–27, 1976)

Table 4-1. Diagnostic Checklist

ELEMENTS	POINT VALUE
Anterior elements destroyed or unable to function	2
Posterior elements destroyed or unable to function	2
Relative sagittal plane translation > 3.5 mm	2
Relative sagittal plane rotation > 11 degrees	2
Positive stretch test	2
Cord damage	2
Root damage	1
Abnormal disk narrowing	1
Dangerous loading anticipated	1

A total of five points or more suggests instability.

5. Disruption of the facet joints, especially with comminuted fractures that occur in and around the facet joints[255,260]

6. Evidence of severe injury, such as multiple fractures at one segment, implying disruption of one or both stabilizing complexes.[255,260]

White and associates devised a graded checklist to predict spinal instability. Two points were assigned if anterior or posterior element destruction was present, if the sagittal angulation was greater than 11 degrees, if sagittal plane translation was more than 3.5 mm, or if a positive stretch test or cord damage was present. One point was assigned if a patient demonstrated root damage or disk narrowing, or if it was anticipated that the patient would place great stress on his or her cervical spine (dangerous loading anticipated). A total of five points was regarded as evidence for instability of the spine, and treatment was assigned based on this score.[258,259,262] It should be noted that it is possible for patients with lower scores to have spinal instability[225] and for patients with higher scores to be clinically asymptomatic.[8] Repeated, rigorous examinations should be made so that potential instability is not overlooked (Table 4-1).[262]

METHODS OF TREATMENT

NONOPERATIVE METHODS

Orthotics

Cervical orthoses are used to treat a wide spectrum of clinical problems.[127,128] There are four general categories of support. The simplest and least secure is the soft collar, extending from the head to the upper part of the thorax. A more rigid category is the poster brace, which controls the head through mandibular and occipital supports. The cervicothoracic brace is essentially the same as the poster brace except that it extends further down the trunk. The most secure orthotic is the halo vest, which has a ring attached to the skull with pins and connected to the trunk by longitudinal metal uprights fixed to a cast or a vest.

The soft cervical collar is the least effective appliance in controlling any plane of motion. However, it is comfortable, affords some support, and reminds the patient to restrict motion. As such, it is useful to treat minor muscular spasm. The Philadelphia collar is more massive, and is more effective than the soft collar in controlling flexion and extension. It does not provide firm control, and is very weak in controlling rotation. Poster braces, cervicothoracic braces, and the skull occiput mandibular immobilization (SOMI) orthosis are more effective in controlling flexion, especially in the upper cervical segments. These orthoses are effective in the treatment of hangman's fractures and in the later stages of odontoid fracture treatment; however, they are especially poor at controlling lateral bending and are not indicated for the treatment of unstable fractures.[127,128,187]

The halo, basically an ambulatory form of skeletal traction, provides more rigid fixation of the head and neck. It controls rotation, lateral bending, and sagittal plane motion over the upper cervical segments, which are poorly controlled by other braces. Overall, it allows almost no motion between the occiput and the upper thoracic spine, controlling the spine in both flexion and extension.[127,128,138,154,190] There is considerable freedom of motion in the middle segments, as the halo controls the neck much as spokes on a wheel, leaving the neck in between relatively unsupported. In sagittal plane motion, more motion appears to occur at each level than over the entire spine. One segment appears to flex as the next extends, moving much as a snake does.[127,128,138,154] For this reason there are situations that are unsuitable for treatment in halo, especially lesions lower in the cervical spine and those with posterior ligamentous damage.[59,263] Application of the halo device is an invasive procedure, and care must be taken in the placement of the pins. To prevent complications, pin tracts must be cleaned, loose pins tightened, and infected pins removed and replaced.[97,99,154,174,176,190,248,263] In insensate patients, care must be taken to avoid trophic ulcers.[190,263]

Acute State Immobilization

Gardner–Wells tongs are applied easily and quickly in the emergency room. The tongs are applied to the head at its maximum diameter, just behind the external auditory meatus. Applied early, they can afford added stability in transfers and during further radiologic work-up. Crutchfield tongs are difficult to apply and occasionally loosen.[87,137,172]

The halo ring can be applied in the acute phase, allowing both early traction and later definitive care with only one invasive procedure. In most cases it is expected that a halo will be used for 3 months or longer. It must be applied with precision and care, usually with a guide. Halo size, pin length, and angulation have all been shown to be important. There is a high rate of complication with halo treatment[98,99,176] and it probably should not be initiated in the earliest phase of evaluation.[137]

Closed Reduction

The method of closed reduction is applicable for many injuries. Spinal traction is applied via halo traction with an initial weight of up to 15 lb (for lesions below C-3), increasing by increments of 5 lb until reduction is accomplished. Most reductions can be accomplished with less than 40 lb. Bilateral facet dislocations require less weight than unilateral facet dislocations.[166] If much weight is required, intravenous muscle relaxants should be considered. Reduction must be accompanied by serial neurologic examinations under radiographic control. If additional neurologic deficits occur or an increase in the height of one or more intervertebral spaces of more than 5 mm is noted, the attempt at reduction is stopped.[48,142,180]

OPERATIVE TECHNIQUES

A great controversy exists regarding the role of surgical intervention in the treatment of cervical spine injuries. Operative treatment is not essential. Many cervical fractures will undergo spontaneous fusion if treated conservatively by traction or a halo body jacket for 8 weeks and intermediate orthosis for 8 weeks.[137,263] The commonly cited reasons for surgical fusion of the cervical spine are that surgical fusions reduce pain, enhance stability, facilitate nursing care,[93,105,137] and avoid complications associated with prolonged immobilization, including recurrent dislocations, osteoporosis, pressure ulcers on the skin, thrombophlebitis, and pulmonary embolus, as well as the undesirable physiologic changes secondary to prolonged recumbency.[1,142] Some authors advocate early surgical intervention to allow for early halo-free rehabilitation of the patient.[133,178,236] Aggressive surgical intervention can decrease the duration of hospitalization and decrease the incidence of complications associated with recumbency. It is unclear, however, whether early surgical intervention leads to improved neurologic recovery. There are many instances of postoperative loss of one or more root levels, a crucial loss for future potential independence.

Fusion must be performed when the patient has undergone surgery for open reduction or decompressions. Sometimes fusions should be performed to aid in the aggressive, overall management of the multiply injured patient.[133,137,263] It should be understood that while spinal fusion is performed to provide spinal stability, immediate stability depends on the intrinsic stability of the fixation method employed. In many cases, spinal fusion should be considered an "internal splint"[64,105,265] that allows mobilization of the patient with the appropriate external support. Fusion of the traumatically unstable spine is far more difficult than in degenerative disease of the neck. In highly unstable injuries successful anterior fusion does not preclude late progressive angular deformity.[1,168]

Before considering one of the many types of treatments available for the cervical spine, a strategy for choosing the best treatment must be outlined. The mechanical and neurologic components of the injury must be considered separately. Two questions should be asked: Is the mechanical injury stable or unstable? Is the neurologic injury complete or incomplete?

Mechanically stable fractures with complete neurologic injury are uncommon; they are most often the result of penetrating trauma. Surgery is usually not indicated in this instance. Patients with mechanically unstable injuries with complete neurologic deficits usually benefit from posterior stabilization.[275] Most complete injuries occur instantaneously with impact onto the spinal cord of bone or disk.

Decompression is usually of little treatment value in patients with complete neurologic injury. A significant portion (up to one third) of patients treated conservatively experience root escape, regaining one or more levels of function.[263,275] Decompression has been advocated in those patients with complete lesions who demonstrate no root return, to allow as much chance as possible for root return to occur. Decompresssion is of greatest value in treating patients who are quadraplegic from injuries at C-5 or C-6, where one level significantly changes the abilities and rehabilitative potential for the patient.[44,187] Surgical therapy is not without its complications and potential risks. Neural deterioration can occur, with devastating effects on the patient.[158]

Patients with incomplete neurologic deficits but mechanically stable injuries do not need surgical stabilization. However, they may benefit from anterior decompression, especially if recovery is slow or has reached a plateau.[46,275] Early reduction is the best and most effective decompression of the spinal cord in many cases.[1,26] Operative decompression is reserved for incomplete lesions in which neural compression due to impingement by bone or disk persists after alignment has been restored.

In severely injured patients with both unstable injuries and demonstrable anterior compression, there are several options. Anterior decompression and fusion[25,67,152,200,247] can be performed with concomitant or staged posterior fusion, or can be stabilized with a halo.[275] An important concept in choosing an approach and a surgical construct is to create stability for the injured spine without removing structures that provide any remaining stability. It cannot be overly stressed that removal of an intact annulus fibrosus in the face of damage to the posterior elements will acutely destabilize the spine.[18,21,24,178,226,236,246,262]

In an incomplete injury, relief of compression should be accomplished by removing the offending element.[262] This is usually best achieved on the anterior aspect of the cord, using an anterior approach,[129] as this is where the majority of cord trauma occurs owing to retropulsion of the posterior aspect of the vertebral body into the cord. Subtotal vertebrectomy may be necessary to free the cord from impingement.[22,27,29,45,73,103,142,165] Similarly, a fragment of vertebral arch or articular facet that is encroaching posteriorly in a patient with an incomplete lesion must be removed. Modern neuroradiologic techniques allow localization of the offending part, and the choice of decompression can be based on an accurate definition of the anatomy.

Laminectomy without fusion in patients with complete lesions is mentioned only to be condemned. For many years, laminectomies were performed on patients without regard for their neurologic status or the anatomic location of their lesion. This effort to "do something" was made in the hopes of improving the neurologic situation. It has been shown that laminectomy without concomitant fusion decreases stability, creating possible later kyphosis, especially in cases of hyperflexion injuries where the posterior elements are the only stabilizing forces remaining intact. Laminectomy alone has never been shown to improve neurologic function where there is no posterior compression, and further neurologic injury frequently occurs as a result of instability.[30,46,121,124,169,225,262]

SPECIFIC LESIONS

SOFT-TISSUE INJURIES

Acceleration hyperextension or "whiplash" injuries of the neck have received much attention in the literature[118] and in the courts. Extension injuries of the neck were first recognized as a clinical entity with the introduction of catapult-assisted lift-offs from aircraft carriers.[80] Severy and associates were among the first to document that whiplash is an extension injury that can be sustained with impact at a relatively slow speed.[220] Of all neck injuries in the 1960s requiring medical attention, 85% resulted from motor vehicle accidents, and 85% of these were from rear-end automobile collision in which the victim sustained severe hyperextension of the neck.[182] The head and neck are subjected to acceleration forces of up to 10g at impact speeds of only 15 mph.[164] Motion of the head and neck is stopped only when the back of the head strikes the upper spine.[118,164]

Direct trauma to the head that produces sudden extension of the neck can produce injuries ranging from mild muscular strain to decapitation, depending on the location, type, and amount of force.[80] In experimentally produced extension strain of the neck, muscle tears were common, producing hemorrhage and spasm. The sternocleidomastoid process was frequently involved, being either partially torn or wholly ruptured. Occasionally, tears of the anterior longitudinal ligament or separation of the disk from the vertebral body were observed.[113,164,181,255] Front-end collisions may create posterior cervical soft-tissue injury if the flexed head strikes the dashboard or windshield. Tearing of the posterior muscles and ligaments may also occur.[118] The most severe injuries are noted with hyperextension because the potential range of motion is greater. When the neck is caused to flex anteriorly or laterally, the head strikes the shoulder or chest. The soft tissues of the neck are protected by this limitation of motion.[118]

The symptoms and signs of soft-tissue injury are variable. Often the patient experiences severe pain immediately after injury, but this may be delayed up to 24 hours. The most prominent finding immediately following injury is muscular tenderness both anteriorly and posteriorly. Injury to the strap muscles can cause difficulty in lifting the head, and especially when getting out of bed.[113,255]

Pain may radiate from the neck to one or both shoulders and down the arms, or to the interscapular area, chest, and occipital region. These patterns of referral are non-neurogenic and can be reproduced by an experimental injection at any point from C-1 to C-7.[164] The pain is probably produced by chronic irritation of musculoligamentous, joint, and intervertebral disk structures.[118] Pain radiating down the arm does not necessarily indicate nerve root compression. Frank disk herniation rarely results from soft-tissue injury. However, a frequent complaint following injury is pain or numbness along the ulnar border of the hand, and objective sensory changes may be present. This is usually due to scalenus spasm rather than true ulnar neuropathy.[119,164]

Cerebral symptoms can be present in the form of confusion, mental dullness, or mild amnesia. Patients may complain of mild headache that is intermittently manifested for months. Blurred vision, tinnitus, and vertigo are common symptoms. Dysphagia is also common, and is caused by retropharyngeal hematoma or edema.[71,164] Frankel demonstrated a significant percentage of patients who sustained temperomandibular joint injury in addition to neck injuries.[92]

Treatment of suspected soft-tissue cervical injuries should be tailored to the severity of the injury and should be directed toward mobilizing the patient as rapidly as possible. Bed rest and/or neck support in a contoured, soft cervical collar may be useful in the acute postinjury period to rest traumatized tissues. Progressive ambulation and increasing time periods spent out of the collar should be encouraged. Local heat via either a heating pad or warm showers will relieve early symptoms of stiffness and soreness. Deep heat should be reserved until several weeks after injury to prevent further irritation to damaged tissues. Analgesics and anti-inflammatory medications should be prescribed. Prolonged pain or muscle-relaxing medications should be limited or avoided in order to discourage chemical dependency. Isometric neck exercises should be prescribed carefully, and should be supervised to prevent the patient from straining his or her neck further.[14,28,71,100]

There are several signs that prognosticate against complete recovery after soft-tissue injury. Symptoms or findings referable to arm numbness or pain were positively correlated with incomplete symptomatic recovery. On the radiograph, a sharp reversal of the cervical curve carries a poor prognosis for later symptomatic degenerative changes, as does limitation of motion at one cervical level on flexion and extension films.[100] The presence of objective neurologic signs, significant neck stiffness and muscle spasm, and pre-existing degenerative changes adversely affect the outcome. Patients who needed a soft collar for more than 12 weeks or who needed home traction were also more likely to be symptomatic at follow-up. Upper back pain and interscapular pain indicate that longer therapy will be needed. Men recover more completely than women. Overall, only 57% of patients in one study obtained full, symptomatic recovery and escaped other degenerative changes.[71,94,100,107,120,179]

ATLANTO-OCCIPITAL DISLOCATIONS

Generally, this severe injury is incompatible with life. It is the most common cervical spine injury in fatal motor vehicle accidents.[5,41] The mechanism

of death seems to be transection of the medulla oblongata or the spinomedullary junction. There are, however, isolated reports of survivors with this injury.[26,55,69,79]

The mechanism of injury seems to be hyperextension of the head with a distraction force applied to the cranium. The structure that is primarily responsible for checking hyperextension and vertical translation of the occiput on the spine is the tectorial membrane, and its rupture is required for atlanto-occipital dislocation.[26,69,79] Hyperflexion is prevented by skeletal contact between the anterior margin of the foreamen magnum and the odontoid.[41]

The diagnosis is made on a lateral roentgenogram of the cervical spine. There is marked retropharyngeal swelling.[240] The anterior portion of the foramen magnum (known as the basion) nor-

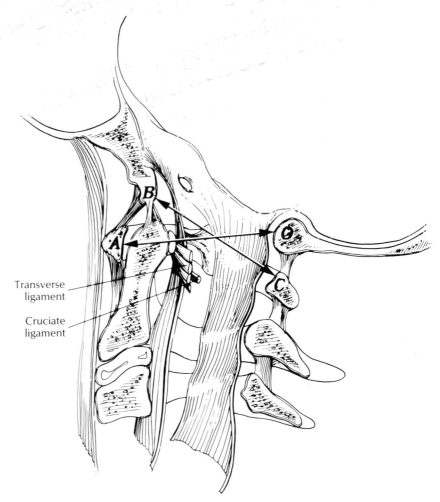

Figure 4-4. Atlanto-occipital dislocations result from disruptions of the ligaments surrounding the base of the skull. The diagnosis is made on lateral roentgenogram of the cervical spine. The basion normally should be directly over the odontoid process. The distance between the anterior foramen magnum to the tip of the posterior arch of the atlas should be the same as the distance from the anterior arch of the atlas to the opisthion. If the ratio of A to O:B to C is greater than one, then the head is forward on the spine as a result of atlanto-occipital dislocation. (A = anterior arch, O = opisthion, B = basion, C = posterior arch of C-1)

Transverse ligament

Cruciate ligament

mally should be directly over the odontoid. The distance between the anterior foramen magnum and the tip of the posterior arch of the atlas should be the same as the distance from the anterior arch of the atlas to the posterior foramen magnum (the opisthion). If the ratio of these distances is greater than one, then the head is forward on the spine as a result of atlanto-occipital dislocation (Fig. 4-4).[193] Further injury to the lower cervical spine must also be ruled out, as associated cervical spine injuries occur frequently with this dislocation.

The rare survivors with this lesion are treated with ventilatory support, gentle cervical traction (3 to 4 lb), halo stabilization,[164] and posterior spine fusion from the occiput to C-3.[41,79,140,193,277]

INJURIES TO THE C-1–C-2 COMPLEX

Injuries to this complex are related to one another by several facets of anatomy, the mechanism of injury, and methods of treatment. Damage is most commonly caused by force applied to the spine via the base of the skull.[149,257] Multiple injuries to this region are common.[149] These fractures are most often the result of combining alcohol, drugs, and motor vehicles. Falls and jumps rarely cause injury to this area.[76,87,110,153,163,187]

Serious neurologic injury occurs with relatively low incidence in patients sustaining injury to the upper cervical spine as compared with those sustaining lower cervical spine injury. Patients sustaining these lesions rarely have neurologic sequelae. In part, this is due to the relatively small proportion of the canal occupied by the cord in the upper region.[149] Here the cord and dens each occupy one third of the available space, with one third of the diameter empty. However, when neurologic injury does occur, it is frequently fatal. Lesions in the upper cervical spine are commonly found in autopsy studies of victims of fatal motor vehicle accidents.[4,5,241]

Injuries to the C-1–C-2 complex are related not only by mechanism of injury, but by the fact that treatment of injuries in this region can be concep-

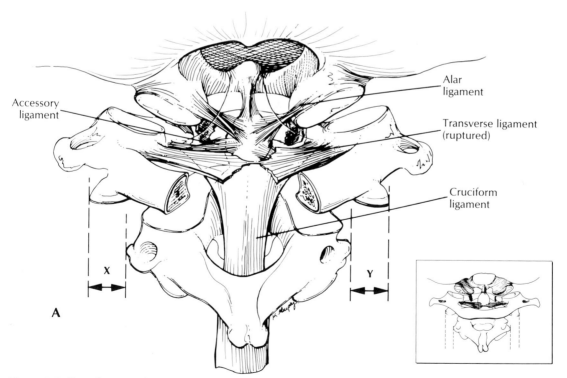

Figure 4-5. Burst fracture of C-1. (*A*) Spreading of the lateral masses of C-1 is diagnostic of a burst fracture of the ring of C-1. Rupture of the transverse ligament allows further spread of the lateral masses. In this situation, the sum of the offset (x + y) will be greater than 7 mm.

tualized together as well. With the exceptions noted below, most upper cervical injuries are best treated nonoperatively—they should heal without surgical fixation or grafting.[86,244] Posterior fusions at these levels compromise spinal motion to a larger degree than in the lower spine. The occiput–C-1 articulation supplies approximately 50% of cervical flexion and the C-1–C-2 articulation supplies approximately 50% of cervical rotation.[76,223,256] Long fusions, especially from the occiput to C-3, have high nonunion rates.[244] The decision to perform a fusion for injuries in this area is a serious one. Specific indications for each injury are outlined below.

Fracture of the Atlas

Ring of C-1. Fractures of the ring of the atlas are most frequently the result of motor vehicle accidents. The diagnosis is difficult to make on the lateral radiograph. Fractures of the posterior arch may be seen on the lateral view, and soft-tissue swelling in the retropharyngeal space may call attention to an atlantal fracture. This fracture is best demonstrated on the open-mouth view, where increased overhang of the lateral masses of C-1 is diagnostic of the fracture (Fig. 4-5). Other associated cervical spine fractures, especially type I, "hangman's fracture," and types II and III odon-

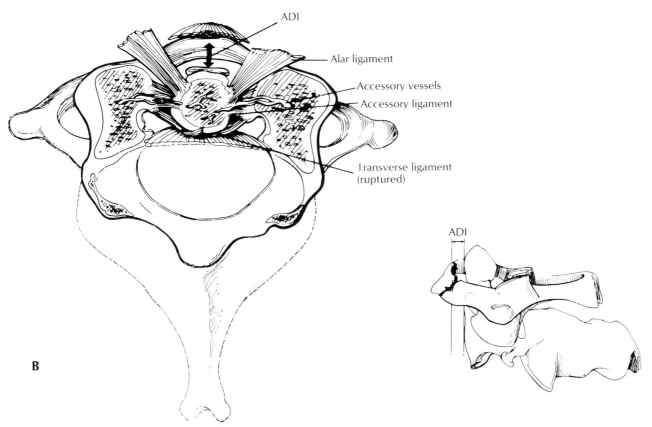

Figure 4-5. *(Continued).* *(B)* The anterior stability of the first cervical vertebra relative to the second is maintained primarily by the transverse ligaments, which run between the tubercles on the medial side of the lateral masses of the atlas in a shallow groove on the posterior surface of the dens. The strongest secondary support is provided by the alar ligaments. Transverse ligament disruption can be diagnosed on lateral roentgenogram by measurement of the antlanto–dens interval, between the posterior aspect of the anterior arch of the atlas and the anterior border of the odontoid process. Displacement of 3 to 5 mm in adults is evidence of damage to the transverse ligament, with displacements exceeding 5 mm being diagnostic of transverse ligament rupture and partial deficiency of the accessory ligaments. Displacement greater than 10 mm indicates that all the ligaments have been disrupted.

toid fractures, are noted to occur frequently in conjunction with atlantal fractures and should be specifically ruled out.[3,85]

Several major types of fracture of the ring of C-1 can be identified. Anterior arch fractures are rare, and are usually comminuted and minimally displaced. Computed tomography is necessary for documentation.[85] Posterior arch fractures account for two thirds of all atlantal fractures,[218,224] and occur at the junction of the posterior arch and lateral mass. These are the result of hyperextension, causing compression of the posterior arches of the atlas between the occiput and axial pedicles. Lateral mass fractures are uncommon.[85,218] Fracture lines pass through the articular surface anterior or posterior to the lateral mass on one side of the atlas. Displacement is asymmetric, and can be viewed on the open-mouth radiograph. Displacement of the lateral mass occurs on the same side the head was turned at the moment of impact.

Bursting fractures of the atlas were first described by Jefferson in 1920, and they still bear his name.[126] The primary force is directed vertically against the skull, with downward displacement of the occipital condyles. The occipital condyles then drive the lateral masses of C-1 apart (Fig. 4-6).[3,116,123,218,222,223] The classic Jefferson fracture, a four-part fracture of the ring of C-1 with two fractures each in the anterior and posterior arches, is uncommon. More common are those bursting fractures with less than four fractures in the ring, usually consisting of no more than one anterior and one posterior fracture.[116] A compression fracture of the lateral mass will occur if the load is asymmetric. If greater force is applied, the transverse ligament will rupture. This has important implications for the treatment of this entity.

Fractures of the ring of the atlas are being diagnosed more frequently with the advent of CT.[19,134] Unilateral fractures are undiagnosed by plain films. A new classification of C-1 ring fractures separates the less common but more severe comminuted fracture from other injuries. The comminuted fracture is more severe, and often fails to unite. Pain and stiffness result from a nonunion, preventing these patients from returning to a full level of activity.[218] Many patients report experiencing scalp dysesthesias, even with successful union.[146]

Patients present with pain in the occipital or neck region or localized stiffness. The radiographic hallmark of this fracture is the offset of the lateral masses of C-1 on the open-mouth roentgenogram. Traumatic lesions are always located in the portions of the ring adjacent to the lateral masses and are jagged in appearance. Congenital defects are more often in the midportion of the arch, and are smooth and rounded.[84,222]

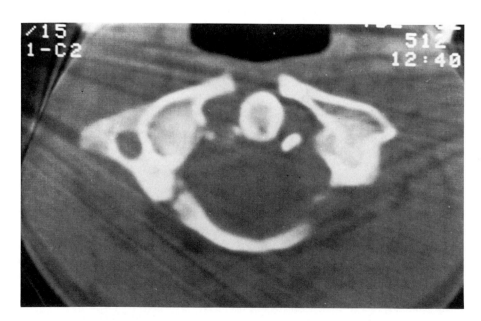

Figure 4-6. Computed tomographic scan demonstrating a three-part burst fracture of C-1 sustained in a diving accident. Note the two posterior fractures combined with the single anterior fracture.

Treatment. Fracture of the posterior arch alone does not affect the stability of the C-1–C-2 complex. Stability of the complex depends on the integrity of the transverse ligament. Therefore, treatment of these fractures depends on the status of the transverse ligament. If the combined overhang of the lateral masses on the open-mouth roentgenogram is greater than 6.9 mm, the transverse ligament has been disrupted or plastically deformed. This defines the potentially unstable Jefferson fracture (see Fig. 4-5A).[137,146,212,221,257] Rupture of the transverse ligament in this situation does not always result in significant clinical instability of C-1–C-2. Axial loading sufficient to burst C-1 may also be sufficient to rupture the transverse ligament, but the facet capsules and alar ligaments may remain intact and afford some stability. When the transverse ligament is torn by a flexion injury, the other ligaments are also damaged, diminishing the stability in this situation. Patients with bursting fractures of the atlas should have flexion–extension films performed following conservative treatment to rule out any potential instability.[86]

If the transverse ligament is intact (i.e., there is less than 6.9 mm displacement), acute surgical stabilization is not indicated. In a minimally displaced fracture, collar immobilization should be sufficient to prevent further significant displacement and allow the fracture to begin to heal.[86,146] In patients with more than 5 mm displacement, halo traction is indicated to effect reduction of the fracture. A severely displaced fracture may require 6 to 8 weeks of halo traction to prevent loss of reduction of the fracture. A halo vest may be insufficient to reverse the axial load of the cranium until the final 4 to 6 weeks.[86]

A less severely injured patient should be acutely immobilized in a cervicothoracic brace for 3 to 4 months, then reevaluated with tomography or CT for union of the fracture. If the anterior arch has healed to the lateral masses, then no further treatment is required. If there is an anterior arch nonunion, then C-1–C-2 fusion is indicated. If there is both anterior and posterior nonunion, then a fusion from the occiput to C-3 is indicated.[193,212,221] If the transverse ligament is torn and instability is present on flexion–extension films, then a primary occiput to C-2 fusion may be performed. However, if the posterior arch is allowed to heal via immobilization for 10 to 12 weeks, then it may be possible to perform a more limited C-1–C-2 fusion, thereby maximizing neck motion.[137,257]

If the posterior arch is fractured as an isolated injury, it is stable and can be treated by collar immobilization. However, it is frequently associated with other hyperextension, axial loading fractures (especially type II odontoid and type I spondylolisthesis of the axis). Failure to appreciate the posterior arch fracture can lead to suboptimal results in treatment of the other fractures. If the fracture is not appreciated and subsequent operative stabilization is based on the posterior arch of the atlas, failure of fixation and loss of position can result postoperatively. To prevent marked restriction of motion, staged reduction and stabilization may be necessary.[86]

Minimally displaced lateral mass fractures are stable, and can be immobilized in a collar. Prolonged halo traction may be necessary for displaced fractures.[86]

When a fracture occurs in conjunction with fracture of the odontoid, immobilization must be continued until the posterior arch heals. Fusion is then accomplished as necessitated by the nature of the odontoid fracture.

Transverse Ligament Disruption

The anterior stability of the first cervical vertebra relative to the second is maintained primarily by the transverse ligaments. The transverse ligament runs between the tubercles on the medial side of the lateral masses of the atlas, running into a shallow groove on the posterior surface of the dens. The strongest secondary support is provided by the alar ligaments (see Fig. 4-5B).[82,83]

Transverse ligament disruption without fracture occurs in the elderly and results from a fall with a blow to the occiput. Rupture of the transverse ligaments may occur at the midpoint, or may be associated with an avulsion fracture from the lateral mass on either side of the odontoid. These variants are functionally identical.[86,149] The average force required to experimentally rupture the transverse ligament is 84 kg. The remaining ligaments rupture secondarily when the same amount of force is applied.[83,86]

The major diagnostic criterion for this injury is instability on flexion–extension films. The diagnosis of transverse ligament disruption depends on the measurement of the atlantal–dens interval (Fig. 4-5B) on the lateral radiograh. When the odontoid is intact and shaped normally, the interval on the lateral radiograph is measured between the posterior aspect of the anterior arch of the atlas and the anterior border of the odontoid. When the odontoid is deficient, the atlantal–dens interval is measured using a line projected superiorly from the anterior body of the axis to the anterior arch of the atlas. Displacement of from 3 to 5 mm in adults is evidence of damage to the transverse ligament. If the displacement exceeds 5 mm, the transverse ligament has ruptured and the accessory ligaments are stretched and partially deficient. Displacement of greater than 10 mm indi-

cates that all the ligaments have been disrupted.[86] Spasm may make the initial flexion–extension roentgenogram falsely negative. When clinically indicated, a patient should be immobilized in a collar and follow-up studies performed.[149] Patients with transverse ligament disruption require surgical fusion. There is no effective nonoperative treatment that will predictably stabilize C-1–C-2 instability.

The purpose of any surgical construct is to reduce and prevent further anterior translation of C-1 on C-2. The upper cervical spine is most often fused posteriorly.[86,108,160] A modification of the Gallie type of fusion, advocated by Fielding, consists of a bone graft secured under wires passed between neural arch of C-1 and the spinous process of C-2. The wire is intended to hold the graft in place, not to effect reduction of the fracture

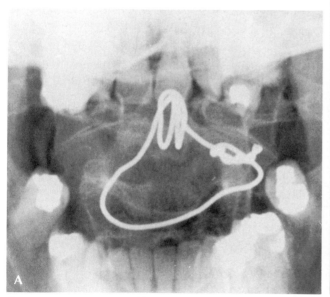
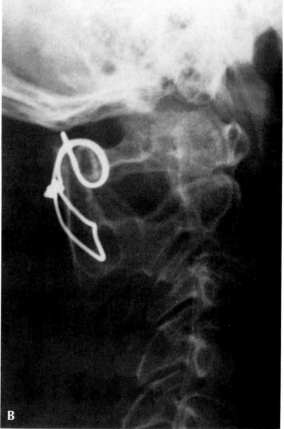

Figure 4-7. Forty-six-year-old man after a Gallie-type posterior C-1–C-2 wiring and fusion treating a type II odontoid fracture. (*A*) A/P roentgenogram. (*B*) Lateral roentgenogram.

(Fig. 4-7). This construct is very effective in stabilizing against flexion. If the fusion is continued to C-3, the wire is not necessary.[86,160,262]

The wedge compression technique, proposed by Brooks and Jenkins for posterior fusions limited to the C-1–C-2 interspace, consists of an iliac bone graft compressed under laterally placed wires between the arch of the first vertebra and the lamina of the second.[149] Postoperative stability is excellent, with good fixation against flexion, extension, lateral bending, and axial rotation. This increase in stability is offset by the increased technical risks and difficulty when compared to the Gallie fusion.[262] An intact neural arch of C-1 is a prerequisite for successful surgical stabilization, or postoperative loss of fixation will occur.[137]

Odontoid Fracture

Fractures of the odontoid are being reported with increasing frequency, though with a decreasing rate of mortality. These fractures may account for 7% to 14% of cervical spine fractures.[171] They have been disparagingly called an "unsolvable" problem.[209] Odontoid fractures are usually due to major forces. A large percentage of injuries are high energy fractures. These occur in a younger segment of the population and are correlated with alcohol ingestion and automobile accidents.[187] They occur in conjunction with other cervical spine injuries, skull fractures, mandible fractures, long bone fractures, and trunk injuries.[187] The second population of patients sustaining odontoid fractures is the elderly, who often suffer posteriorly displaced fractures after low-energy falls.[187]

Anatomic factors have profound effects on the treatment and healing of odontoid fractures. The odontoid is unique in that it is almost completely intra-articular. The ligaments that are tethered to the tip of the dens tend to distract it from its base when it is fractured. Large joint surfaces exist all around the dens: superiorly the dens is attached to the alar ligament, articulates anteriorly with the atlas, and posteriorly with the transverse ligament. Therefore, an injury at the dens, at or above the accessory ligaments, leaves the tip fragment floating entirely within synovial cavities.[206,234] The dens is left without periosteal blood supply. Fractures must heal through endosteal new bone for-

mation. In addition, the atlanto-axial apophyseal joints are horizontal and saddle-shaped, and add little if any anteroposterior stability. A fracture of the dens can therefore create a potentially unstable situation.

Odontoid fractures are usually clinically manifested by immediate, severe, high cervical pain with muscle spasm that is aggravated by the slightest motion. Pain may also radiate in the distribution of the greater occipital nerve, to the back of the head. Spasm of the neck muscles and severe limitation of motion are the most common physical findings. Neural injury, occurring in 18% to 25% of all cases, may range from high tetraplegia to minimal sensory or motor loss due to loss of one or several nerve roots.[96,188,236] The close, interlocking relationship between the atlas and the dens makes them susceptible to common injury. One third of all fractures of the atlantal ring, usually bursting fractures, occur in combination with fractures of the odontoid.[187,225]

Plain films may not adequately detect odontoid fractures.[238] If pain and spasm persist despite negative radiographs, further diagnostic measures should be pursued. The diagnosis of odontoid fracture is best made with anteroposterior and lateral tomograms.[3,238] The plane of CT slices is roughly parallel to the fracture. Nondisplaced fractures may be missed on CT. Sagittal and coronal reconstructions may be diagnostic of the fracture,[19,149] but can sometimes be misleading if original slices miss the fracture, if the patient has moved, or if there is only minimal displacement.[3,57] Flexion and extension films may be necessary to assess instability of the fragments.

The differential diagnosis of odontoid fracture must include anatomic anomalies, most specifically os odontoidium. In os odontoidium, the ossicle is smaller than the normal odontoid, usually one half its size. It is round and is separated from the hypoplastic odontoid by a wide gap. The remnant of the hypoplastic odontoid projects up like a hill, above the rest of the ring.[84,130]

An odontoid fracture is the result of the application of high velocity force to the head, but the exact mechanism is unknown. It is probably caused by complex forces, inducing lateral loading. Flexion forces the transverse ligament against the posterior aspect of the odontoid, resulting in anterior displacement. This has been reported to be the mechanism in as many as 80% of fractures.[171] Extension causes the posterior portion of the anterior ring to impinge on the anterior odontoid with posterior displacement. This pattern is seen in the remaining 20% of fractures, usually in the elderly.[171,187]

Classification of odontoid fractures is based on the level of the fracture;[10] this classification is predictive of the likelihood of nonunion (Fig. 4-8).[206] Type I fractures, or avulsion fractures of the tip, are uncommon. The blood supply to the dens is not disturbed, and the cervical spine is not rendered unstable. The transverse ligament and one alar ligament remain attached to the dens. This fracture has a good prognosis.[10]

Type II fractures occur at the junction of the odontoid and the body of C-2, and are prone to nonunion (Fig. 4-9).[206,209] This is the most common type of injury. The fracture is in the area of the attachment of the accessory ligaments. As a result of ligament damage, excessive motion of the odontoid can occur. The fracture causes a loss of blood supply to the dens. What remains is an area of hard cortical bone with a small surface area.

Nonunion is more likely to occur in patients older than 40 years of age.[10,210]

In children, type II fractures are physeal injuries at the level of the basilar epiphysis between the odontoid and the C-2 body. They will heal with gentle reduction and immobilization alone. In young children, fractures may be caused by minor falls or other trivial injuries, by forceps deliveries, and by major vehicular trauma. In children, an early roentgenogram is often negative. Persistent symptoms should around suspicion, especially if the child is reluctant to flex or extend his neck. Callus formation can been seen 2 weeks after injury. The fracture occurs at the junction of the odontoid ossification center (the subdental synchondrosis) and the body. The odontoid fragment almost always angulates anteriorly with respect to the body. Postural reduction should be followed by early rigid immobilization. Stabilization in the extended position should result in union.[9] Operative treatment seems unwarranted in younger children because the rate of union is so high.[14,19,234] After the ages of 7 to 10 years, the synchondrosis fuses, and fractures must be considered identical to their adult counterparts.[222]

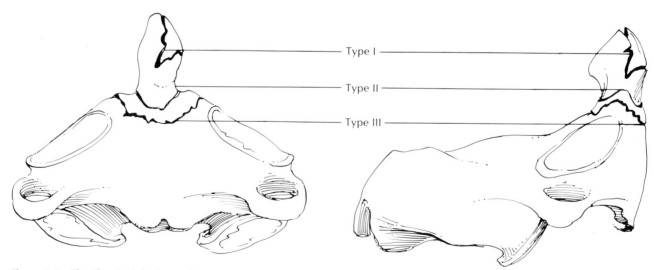

Figure 4-8. Classification of odontoid fractures is based upon level of fracture, because the level is predictive of the likelihood of nonunion. Type I fractures are avulsion fractures of the tip. Type II fractures occur at the junction of the odontoid process and the body of C-2 in the area of the attachment of the accessory ligaments, and are prone to nonunion. Type III fractures occur through the body of the axis between the junction of the dens and the axis.

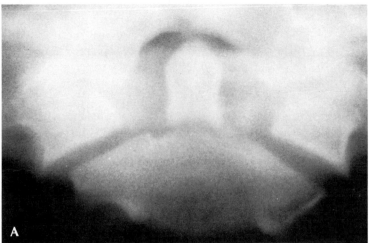

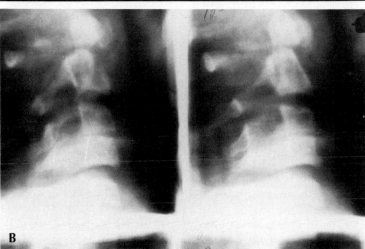

Figure 4-9. (*A*) Anteroposterior tomography of a type II odontoid fracture combined with a burst fracture of C-1. Note that the lateral masses are spread more than 7 mm, indicating concomitant injury to the ring of C-1. (*B*) Lateral tomography of a type II odontoid fracture.

There is evidence that odontoid fractures in children are the etiology of os odontoidium in later life.[130]

Type III fractures occur through the body of the axis between the junction of the dens and axis. These heal well because the fracture occurs through cancellous bone. Although displacement can occur, the injury is usually stable when reduced.[225]

Displacement plays a role in both the nature of associated injuries and in the choice of treatment modalities. Neurologic injury occurs more frequently with posteriorly displaced fractures, although nonunion is more frequent with anteriorly displaced fractures. Posteriorly displaced fractures, though less common, are associated more frequently with other cervical spine injuries and respiratory difficulties, and the mortality rate is higher.[150,187,198]

The treatment of odontoid fractures is a matter of controversy and frustration. To rationally conceptualize the treatment of these fractures one must consider each type of fracture separately. Type I fractures do not disrupt the majority of the ligamentous support or the blood supply to the dens. These fractures are thus stable and will heal well if immobilized in a collar or brace.[95,111,257]

Type III fractures are also usually stable injuries. The blood supply to the dens remains intact, and cancellous bone-to-bone contact occurs. The current initial treatment recommended is immobilization (and reduction, if necessary) in either skull tongs or halo traction. This is maintained until the symptoms of acute pain and muscle spasm have subsided. Type III fractures can be treated in a halo or brace for 3 to 4 months, with spontaneous fusion as the rule.[95,111,137,153,187,217,231,257]

The most problematic fracture to treat is the type II injury. The fracture lifts the dens off the body of C-2, and tremendous forces act at the fracture site. The blood supply is interrupted, leaving the dens avascular. Although some authors still advocate the use of halo traction for type II fractures,[153,187,217] these fractures are prone to nonunion with conservative measures, with a failure rate between 30% and 60%.[58,137,210,257]

Conservative therapy other than halo traction for this fracture can result in prolonged hospital stays, and is not without complications. These include decubitus ulcers, pin complications, and problems associated with prolonged recumbency. Prolonged immobilization may also result in a stiff neck, with loss of motion. Redisplacement of the fracture may occur.[230] Operative treatment and posterior fusion is advocated for fractures that heal slowly or not at all.[58,137,187,209,210] These include type II fractures, fractures displaced more than 4 mm, and fractures in patients older than 40 years, since these are prone to nonunion. In addition, fusion has been advocated in patients with long bone fractures because an unstable odontoid fracture complicates transfer of the patient, anesthesia for operative fixation, and rapid mobilization of the patient.[137] Many authors have reported success with posterior Gallie-type fusion[133,160,258] or the Brooks-type fusion[149,172] followed by ambulation and stabilization in a halo. Anterior stabilization for odontoid fractures has been proposed, utilizing screw fixation.[38,95,133,262]

Fracture of the Axis

Isolated fractures of the body of the axis are uncommon injuries. They are frequently associated with facial injuries and long bone fractures, along with serious thoracic injuries. Neurologic signs are usually transient, unless vertebral artery thrombosis occurs.[110,149]

Treatment of these fractures depends on the degree of displacement suffered at the time of injury. Isolated, nondisplaced fractures are stable and can be treated with a cervical collar.

Displaced fractures are unstable and require continuous traction for 4 to 14 days in extension to maintain angular reduction. The fracture may settle after removal of traction and placement into a halo vest, though almost all go on to union. This can occur without complication since translation of the segments will not decrease the size of the canal. Angular deformity, however, will alter the size of the canal.[86,206]

Traumatic Spondylolisthesis of the Axis

Traumatic spondylolisthesis is characterized by a fracture passing downward through the neural arch of the axis[187] that may result in anterior displacement of C-2 on C-3. The term "hangman's fracture" was given to this lesion because of its similarity to the lesion produced by judicial hanging. Autopsy of prisoners hung with the knot in the submental position revealed bilateral fractures of the pedicles of the axis. It was postulated that there was complete disruption of the ligaments and disk between C-2 and C-3. The mechanism of injury was hyperextension with sudden, violent distraction and complete transection of the cord.[91] The body of the axis and dens were intact.[90]

High speed automobile travel created renewed interest in this lesion. Today, the majority of patients with this lesion are injured in motor vehicle or diving accidents.[3,91,215] The large diameter of the canal at the C-2–C-3 level spares the cord from compression, thus associated neural injury is relatively uncommon. Distraction forces, which would tear the cranium away from the body, are absent, protecting the neural elements. This is different from judicial hanging, and neurologic injury is therefore less probable.[35,82,90,91,123,140] Autopsy studies of victims of fatal motor vehicle accidents demonstrate that this lesion is found commonly, second only to atlanto-occipital dislocation.[3,4,5,41]

Diagnosis of traumatic spondylolisthesis of the axis is fairly routine. Patients present with neck pain and pain with motion. Muscle spasm, especially in the sternocleidomastoid process, can be unilateral and may cause torticollis.[163] Usually the fracture is clearly evident on the lateral or oblique film (Fig. 4-10). Prevertebral swelling is common and may be associated with more unstable injuries.[187] Disk space deformities are clearly seen.[3] Extra studies are occasionally necessary to rule out associated injuries. Computed tomography is the least helpful modality to use in this entity, but scanning does alert the surgeon to the complexity of the pathology.[3,19]

There is a high incidence of head injuries and facial trauma in patients with this injury. Head trauma occurs in approximately 70% to 80% of the patients, with mandibular and other skull fractures

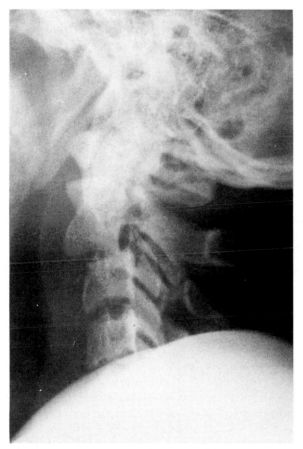

Figure 4-10. Traumatic spondylolisthesis of the axis in a neurologically intact 26-year-old man. Patient was the driver in a car involved in a collision.

being common. Frequently, there are other upper cervical lesions, such as arch fractures of C-1 or C-3 and avulsion fractures of C-2 and C-3.[74,90] Chest and extremity injuries are also present in more than one third of the patients.[187]

Traumatic spondylolisthesis is classified by both displacement and angulation of the vertebral bodies on each other.[72,223] Type I fractures are either nondisplaced or have no angulation and less than 3 mm of displacement. This is a stable injury. Neurologic injury is uncommon, but there is a high incidence of associated cervical spine fractures.[40,148,149] Type II fractures are characterized by significant angulation and translation. Anatomically, this is a bipedicular fracture, where the anterior longitudinal ligament is shortened but not disrupted. A subset of these fractures, type IIa, is characterized by an absence of translation but severe angulation. The anterior disk space is not widened, apparently owing to hinging on the anterior longitudinal ligament.[40,148,149] Type III fractures are characterized by both severe angulation and displacement and by the presence of concomitant unilateral or bilateral facet dislocations.[79,148]

Traumatic spondylolisthesis results in the separation of the cervicocranium, consisting of the skull and first two cervical vertebrae, from the remainder of the cervical spine. The junction between the axis and C-3 is a region of high stress concentration, and the neural arch of C-2 is the weakest area.[90] The fracture occurs at the narrow isthmus that separates the superior and inferior articular processes.[35] Autopsy studies have demonstrated rupture of the anterior and posterior ligaments and the disk.[60,125]

The exact mechanism of injury is unclear; it seems to be different for each type of fracture. According to Levine and Edwards, type I fractures are caused by a combined hyperextension and axial loading force that fractures the neural arch, but is not strong enough to disrupt the disk or compromise the ligaments. Type I fractures have a significant association with other axial loading fractures, such as the Jefferson fracture. Type II fractures are caused by an initial hyperextension and axial loading force, which cause the fracture of the neural arch (as in type I). A second flexion and compression force causes the anterior displacement. This needs to be reversed for reduction of these fractures. In both types IIa and III the predominant force is flexion, combined in type IIa with distraction and in type III with compression.[148] Blows to the face cause extension of the cervical spine, stretching the anterior ligamentous structures and compressing the posterior bony elements up to the pars fracture.[82] If the tension continues, the anterior longitudinal ligament and disk fail in tension. If the force continues, the disk separates from the body and the posterior longitudinal ligament ruptures, allowing the two vertebral bodies to separate. The amount of translation depends on the extent of disruption of the ligament and disk.[35,82]

Treatment. Surgical treatment is seldom necessary for this injury due to the high rate of spontaneous interbody fusion and fracture healing.[35,72,82,86,148,188,231] Specific treatment depends on the type of fracture and the extent of displacement evident on the initial lateral radiograph. The radiographic hallmark of unstable injury is the displacement of C-2 greater than half the width of C-3 or the presence of a widened anterior or posterior portion of the disk space when compared to the level below. Stability of the lesion ultimately depends on whether the interspace between C-2 and C-3 is disrupted, either at the level of the disk or at the anterior longitudinal ligament. Most injuries are stable in a halo or Philadelphia collar and do not require operative intervention.[148,231] If a patient cannot tolerate traction or bracing, posterior fusion with internal fixation can be used.[37]

In type I fractures, if there is less than 3 mm of translation on the flexion–extension roentgenogram, the patient should be treated in a cervical collar. Patients with more displacement or instability should be placed in traction with a roll under the midcervical region at approximately C-5. This will achieve reduction with approximately 10 kg of traction. Type I fractures typically go on to union in 12 weeks in a halo vest.[86,188]

The reduction of type II fractures is accomplished in the same fashion as displaced type I fractures. After reduction, the patient should be maintained in traction for 5 to 7 days, and then be reevaluated with flexion–extension films for stability. If a reduction can be maintained, the pa-

tient is placed in a halo vest for 6 weeks. If a reduction is lost, the patient should be kept in traction for 4 to 6 weeks until the fracture stabilizes, and then be placed in a halo vest for 12 weeks. In a halo vest, the reduction may "settle." If the angulation remains corrected, only the anteroposterior translation is increased. This is acceptable because the size of the spinal canal actually increases at this level as a result.[86,188]

Type IIa fractures must be treated differently from type II fractures. This subgroup of type II fractures is recognized by increased displacement at the time the patient is put into traction. Since the fractures are caused by distraction forces, the patient must be removed from traction. Treatment entails placement in a halo vest, with manual compression and slight extension of the neck. This is maintained until fracture healing is complete.[188]

Type III fractures are very unstable. Reduction of the facet dislocation is of primary importance. Therefore, halo traction should be applied immediately to attempt reduction of the dislocation component. However, it is not unusual to fail at closed reduction, since pedicular fracture may leave the facets floating. Fracture of the neural arch anterior to the facet dislocation prevents closed reduction. When the fracture is behind the facets, reduction may be obtained, but cannot be maintained. Operative intervention is necessary in order to obtain reduction of the facet dislocation. Once reduction is obtained, it can be held by a posterior fusion. The only structures with anatomic integrity are anterior and should not be disrupted. External immobilization in a halo vest is necessary to treat the bipedicular fracture postoperatively.[188]

LOWER CERVICAL FRACTURES AND DISLOCATIONS

Most fractures and dislocations in the lower cervical spine are the result of indirect forces originating on the head or trunk, causing compression or distraction forces to act on the neck. Elements of flexion, extension, or rotation may be present. Most injuries are caused by midair "flight" of the victim, either in a motor vehicle accident, diving accident, or headfirst fall. Motion is suddenly arrested by the head, while the inertial energy of the rest of the body continues. The resultant force vectors are expended in the spine, with bony or ligamentous injuries resulting.[234] Some injuries occur without blows to the head, but these are less common.[117]

The anatomy of the spine must be considered before it is possible to consider the mechanism of injury. Although some authors use a three-column system when discussing spinal anatomy[234] (see Chapter 8),[66] it is probably more useful to describe the cervical spine by two columns only: the anterior and posterior columns (Fig. 4-11).[7,114,183,262] The anterior elements consist of everything ventral to the posterior longitudinal ligament. The anterior ligamentous complex consists of the intervertebral disk, the annulus fibrosis, and the anterior and posterior longitudinal ligaments. All structures dorsal to the posterior longitudinal ligament are considered the posterior elements. The vertebral arch and the posterior interspinous ligament complex are the osseous and ligamentous elements, respectively. The anterior two thirds of the body along with the anterior longitudinal ligament and annulus fibrosis act as a tension band limiting extension, while the posterior ligamentous and bony complex acts as a tension band in flexion.[261] Flexion through the sagittal plane compresses the anterior column and distracts the posterior column. The anterior and posterior columns are thus reciprocally affected by flexion and extension forces.[114]

There are several structures that confer stability on the cervical spine. The most important anterior structure is the intact annulus fibrosis. The posterior longitudinal ligament is a well-developed structure that provides considerable stability, though the joint capsule and posterior articulations are the most important posterior elements. The ligamentum flavum, though elastic, provides stability at extremes of motion.[260]

Special consideration should be given to injuries at the extremes of the lower cervical spine. Torg and associates[242,243] believe that the lesions of C-3–C-4 react differently to the energy input at the time of injury. These injuries are rare, and the low frequency of bony injury relative to soft-tissue injuries appears to be unique. Injuries at C-3–C-4,

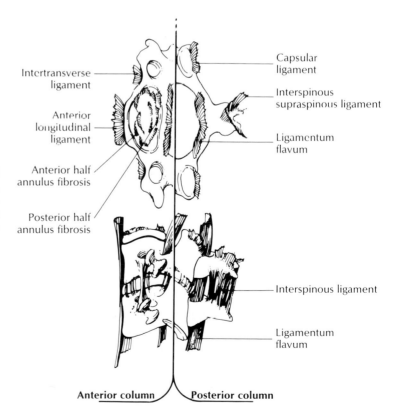

Figure 4-11. Anatomic scheme of the lower cervical spine, indicating anterior and posterior elements. (Adapted from White AA III, Southwick WO, Panjabi MM: Clinical stability in the lower cervical spine: A review of past and current concepts. Spine 1:15–27, 1976)

Intertransverse ligament

Anterior longitudinal ligament

Anterior half annulus fibrosis

Posterior half annulus fibrosis

Capsular ligament

Interspinous supraspinous ligament

Ligamentum flavum

Interspinous ligament

Ligamentum flavum

Anterior column | Posterior column

as a group, are difficult to reduce. Maintenance of reduction is also difficult. A favorable response to early and aggressive treatment can be obtained with these injuries.[242,243] In contrast, injuries at the cervicothoracic junction are not uncommon, accounting for approximately 10% of all fractures of the lower spine.[177] It is imperative that good quality radiographs be obtained in which the C-7–T-1 junction can be seen.

A single-vector force can cause different injuries in the spine, creating families of injury.[13,113,257] A direct relationship between the magnitude of force and the severity of injury exists.[113] A comprehensive classification system based on the mechanism of injury was described by Allen and associates in 1982.[7] In this classification, there are six common patterns of indirect injury to the lower cervical spine. Each pattern is divided into stages, according to the severity of musculoskeletal injury. In all families of injury, the injury described in each stage is added onto the injury incurred in the stage before. There is increasing incidence of incomplete and complete neurologic injury within each stage of the classification.[7]

The families of injuries are named accordingly to the initial, dominant force vector leading to failure and also the presumed attitude of the cervical spine at the time of failure.[7] "Compressive" indicates that compression accounts for the initial, most conspicuous damage in a motion segment, and "distractive" indicates that tension or shear is the stress that produces the initial, most evident structural failure. Ligamentous failure occurs in shear, and is inferred from abnormal relationships between vertebrae. Ligaments do not fail in compression. Rotation is not treated as a major injury vector, but rather as a localizing force.

Although we will consider individual injury patterns as described by Allen and Fergusson, it is necessary to note that few studies of cervical spine injuries follow the same classification system. The task of any system is to help one separate an injury into its components and devise a treatment plan.

Several crucial decisions must be made when contemplating the treatment of lower cervical spine fractures and dislocations. First, the nature of the lesion must be considered, along with concomitant injuries. One must determine whether the spine is stable, and whether the posterior ligamentous complex is intact. Second, consideration

to nonoperative stabilization must be given, especially to the judicious use of the cervical halo. Third, if surgical stabilization is required, a decision must be made whether an anterior approach or a posterior approach is indicated.

The anterior approach is most useful for compression injuries and bursting fractures where the posterior elements are intact, and for hyperextension injuries.[1,122,266] The most stable anterior fusion is the anterolateral trough graft.[262] Several other types of anterior arthrodeses exist and can be used in cervical spine trauma. The trough can also be placed in the anterior midline of the vertebral body and can be used to span one or more functional spinal levels.[24] Another stable variation is the keystone graft, in which the ends of the graft are cut at an angle so that it is locked into the

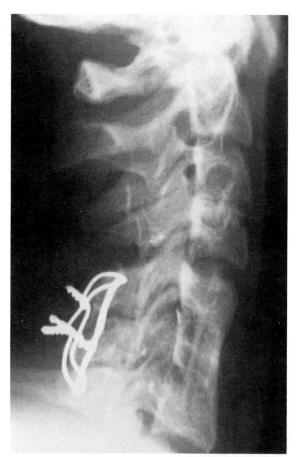

Figure 4-12. Sixteen-year-old boy following staged anterior and posterior fusions for a highly unstable C-5–C-6 fracture-dislocation.

vertebral body in which it is embedded. Supplemental stability is provided by the remaining annular fibers.[18,226,262] However, total or subtotal vertebrectomy may be necessary to free the cord from any impingement.[103,142,173] The body must then be replaced by a large cancellous graft. Such grafts cannot provide immediate postoperative stability to the spine,[262] and immobilization in a halo is usually required. The Cloward dowel graft[54,163] affords little stability and should be avoided in spinal fusions for traumatic injury.[93,103,246,262]

Posterior fusions are especially suited for unilateral and bilateral dislocations and ruptures of the posterior ligamentous complex.[1,93,122] Posterior fusions can be augmented by wiring, especially when the regional cortical bone has been only minimally injured (Fig. 4-12).[64,151,172,219,262] Iliac cancellous and corticocancellous grafts are placed over the decorticated lamina and facets. Decortication must be meticulous to prevent extension of the fusion beyond the previously intended level.[45,236] Posterior fusion may be accomplished under local anesthesia in situations where the patient's pulmonary status does not permit general endotracheal anesthesia. With patients awake and aware, further neural damage may be prevented.[276] In addition to wiring, newer surgical constructs involving plates and screws can be used to provide immediate, adjunctive stability to the grafts. Various anterior and posterior screw and plate techniques are being used with increasing frequency.[49,168,237]

The use of methyl methacrylate in spinal trauma (other than those injuries caused by pathologic fracture)[12,43] without concomitant bony fusion is not recommended. Wire and acrylic constructs are their strongest at the time of insertion, and progressive weakening occurs, with secondary loosening and loss of reduction. Deep infection is also a problem.[73,75,137]

The timing of surgical care must also be determined, whether to accomplish fusion as soon as the patient's condition permits, or to wait until clear evidence of instability is present. Clear contraindications to early, anterior surgery do exist. A patient with respiratory insufficiency is better treated conservatively until pulmonary function is stable. Early surgery on the cervical spine when cord injury is present appears to be hazardous.[158] However, if CT scanning after closed reduction shows the presence of hematoma, bone, or disk compressing the cord, immediate decompression may be warranted if the patient's condition permits.[39] In addition, tracheostomy prior to cervical fusion is a contraindication to the anterior approach.[93]

The first family of injury to be considered is *compressive flexion* injuries, which are caused by a force vector directed inferiorly and anteriorly (Fig. 4-13). This causes injury of increasing sever-

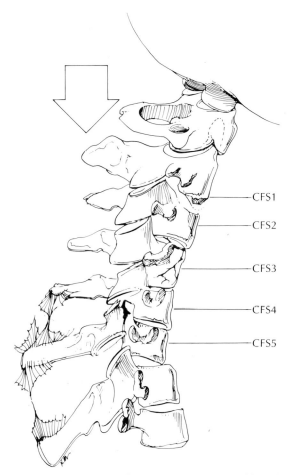

Figure 4-13. Compressive flexion injuries are caused by a force vector directed inferiorly and anteriorly. CFS1 consists of blunting at the anterior margin of the vertebral body. CFS2 adds obliquity to the anterior vertebral body and loss of some of the anterior height of the vertebral body. In CFS3 the fracture line passes obliquely from the anterior surface through the subchondral plate without displacement. In CFS4 there is less than 3 mm displacement of the inferoposterior margin of the vertebral body into the neural canal. Severe displacement of the body fragment into the canal, with separation of the articular facets and increased distance between spinous processes occurs in CFS5.

ity to the vertebral body. It occurs in approximately 20% of lower cervical injuries, and has five recognizable stages. CFS1 consists of blunting at the anterior margin of the vertebral body, changing it to a rounded contour, without failure of the posterior ligamentous elements. CFS2 adds obliquity to the anterior vertebral body, loss of some of the anterior height of the vertebral body, and "beaking" of the anteroinferior vertebral body. In CFS3 a fracture line passes obliquely from the anterior surface through the subchondral plate without displacement. Mild (less than 3 mm) displacement of the inferoposterior margin into the neural canal occurs as the next stage (CFS4). Severe displacement of the body fragment into the canal with separation of the articular facets, increased distance between spinous processes, and complete failure of both the posterior portion of the anterior ligamentous complex and the posterior longitudinal ligament is the most severe stage (CFS5) (Fig. 4-14). Compressive force, with the spine in flexion at the time of injury, creates increasing shear in the posterior elements. This links the more severe anterior compression injury with increasing posterior shear and ligamentous failure.

Compression fractures without facet fracture or subluxation are usually stable. Comminuted fractures can heal by nonoperative means (e.g., a halo

vest)[81,234] if there is no evidence of neurologic injury. Higher stages of injury (CFS3, CFS4, and CFS5) involve anterior bony injury with posterior ligamentous injury, and hence may be unstable. A frequent complication is late instability if these injuries are treated primarily with halo traction or by anterior stabilization alone.[45,46] Delayed fusion has been advocated if instability is demonstrated on flexion–extension views after 3 months in a halo vest.[234] Some authors advocate early posterior fusion, 1 to 3 weeks after injury, because they believe all patients with these injuries will need a fusion due to late reangulation.[104,276] The rate of spontaneous ankylosis is low in stages 1, 2, and 3 but rises in stages 4 and 5 due to bony comminution. These last stages are rarely unstable after conservative treatment in a halo.[99]

Patients with these injuries who are neurologically incomplete and demonstrate signs of anterior compression will need staged anterior decompression and fusion with posterior stabilization. Anterior decompression alone will destabilize a patient by means of iatrogenic rupture of an intact anterior longitudinal ligament. This is a crucial consideration and has been pointed out by many authors.[45,46,78,172,236,246,262]

Vertical compression fractures, sometimes referred to as bursting fractures, are caused by an

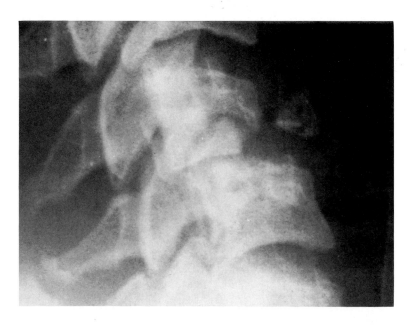

Figure 4-14. Thirty-five-year-old man rendered completely quadraplegic after an automobile accident. The patient was not restrained by a safety belt, and sustained a CFS5 fracture with retropulsion of bone into the spinal canal and involvement of the posterior elements.

axial load (Fig. 4-15). They are associated with severe incomplete and, more frequently, neurologically complete injuries.[70] Vertical compression injuries first create fracture through the center of either the inferior or superior end-plate of the vertebral body (VCS1) with a central cup-like deformity. VCS2 consists of fractures through both end-plates but minimal displacement. More force fragments the body (VCS3) and causes it to displace peripherally, with the posterior portion

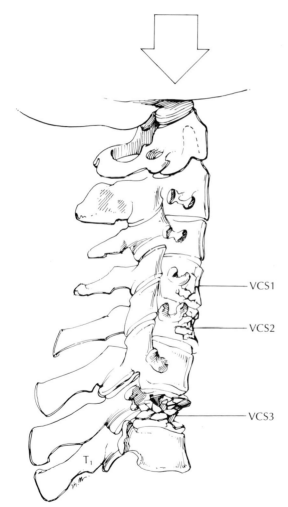

Figure 4-15. Vertical compression fractures begin with a fracture through the center of either the inferior or superior end-plate of the vertebral body (VCS1). VCS2 consists of fractures through both end-plates but minimal displacement. More force fragments the body (VCS3) and causes it to displace peripherally, abutting on or protruding into the neural canal.

abutting on or protruding into the neural canal. The neck is in a neutral position when the force is first applied. If it goes into flexion the posterior elements are placed under tension and posterior ligamentous injury occurs. If it remains in neutral or becomes slightly extended, then the vertebral arch and posterior elements are placed under compressive loads and may be fractured.

Traction is used to maintain and restore alignment, and surgical stabilization is rarely indicated.[104] Injury is primarily a compression of the vertebral body—the ligaments between the vertebrae are intact and confer continued stability. Vertical compression fractures are stable in halo treatment, and many go on to spontaneous anterior fusion.[99] However, significant posterior ligamentous injury may be present, and can lead to post-treatment kyphosis.[104,263] For this reason, all patients with this injury should undergo flexion–extension testing after 3 months in a halo, and posterior fusion should be performed if necessary.

The *distractive flexion* group is also known as the flexion dislocation injuries (Fig. 4-16). Bony integrity is usually maintained, but significant ligamentous disruption occurs with resultant dislocation of the posterior facet joints. Distractive flexion is caused by a major force vector directed away from the trunk with the neck flexed. This stresses the posterior elements in tension, with secondary anterior compression. This family of injury is the most common and is associated with significant head injuries.[202] DFS1 consists of failure of the posterior ligamentous complex, with facet subluxation in flexion and divergence of the spinous processes at injury level. This is called a "flexion sprain." Detection of this injury may be difficult, as roentgen changes are often minimal. Failure to recognize this lesion may lead to increased displacement and neurologic injury.[211,253]

Many authors have discussed "occult" injuries of the cervical spine. These are usually flexion injuries with separation of the facets, possibly with transient subluxation. Mild anterior compression may occur along with slight disk-space narrowing. Many patients have negative radiographs initially, but may demonstrate instability after 3 weeks.[191,199,259] They may be diagnosed on flexion–extension radiographs.[191,199] These purely soft-tissue injuries fail to fuse spontaneously.

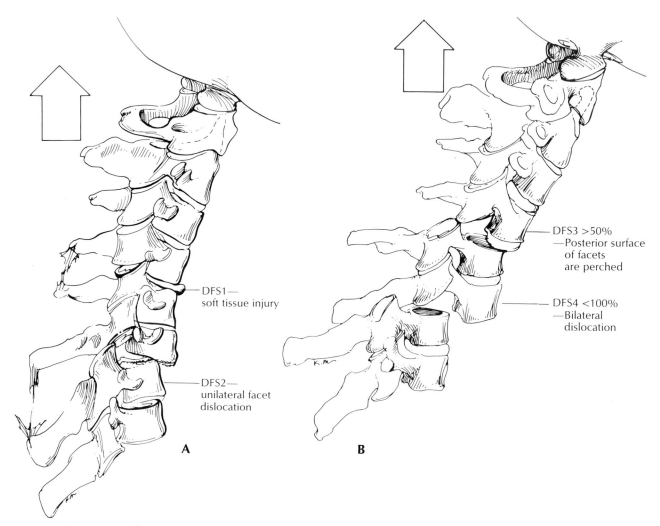

DFS1—
soft tissue injury

DFS2—
unilateral facet
dislocation

DFS3 >50%
—Posterior surface
of facets
are perched

DFS4 <100%
—Bilateral
dislocation

A

B

Figure 4-16. Distractive flexion injuries cause ligamentous injuries. DFS1 is a "flexion sprain" with failure of the posterior ligamentous complex. DFS2 is a unilateral facet dislocation and DFS3 and DFS4 are bilateral facet dislocations with increasing translation.

DFS2 is a unilateral facet dislocation (Figs. 4-17, 4-18) and DFS3 and DFS4 are bilateral facet dislocations with increasing translation. In stage 3 the anterior displacement is approximately 50%, with the posterior surface of the superior vertebral articular processes either snugly against the inferior articular processes or in a "perched" position (Figs. 4-19, 4-20) In stage 4 the vertebral body is displaced anteriorly the full width of the body, giving the appearance of a "floating" vertebral body.

When distractive flexion injury occurs, the lateral radiograph will generally be the most helpful.

In unilateral facet dislocations, the dislocation is always less than 50% of the vertebral body.[20,50,202] The facet articulations show complete loss of contact, with the lower facets of the upper segment positioned anterior to the corresponding facets of the lower segment. This lesion is characterized by the displacement of the vertebral body with a projection of the dislocated facet through the vertebral body, giving the bat wing or bow tie appearance.[50,196,202] The anteroposterior film may look deceptively normal. Close examination of the radiograph shows a tilt of the spinal column away from the lesion and rotation of the spinous pro-

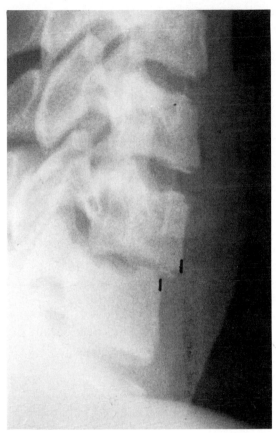

Figure 4-17. A DFS2 injury illustrating 25% offset of C-5 on C-6. Note the slightly enlarged retropharyngeal space, characteristic of lower cervical injuries.

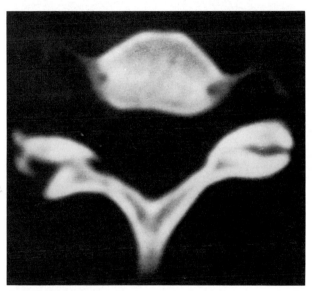

Figure 4-18. Computed tomographic scan demonstrating the empty facet sign of a DFS2 injury.

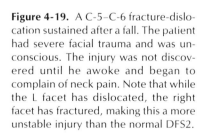
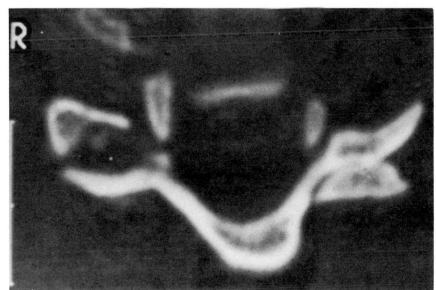

Figure 4-19. A C-5–C-6 fracture-dislocation sustained after a fall. The patient had severe facial trauma and was unconscious. The injury was not discovered until he awoke and began to complain of neck pain. Note that while the L facet has dislocated, the right facet has fractured, making this a more unstable injury than the normal DFS2.

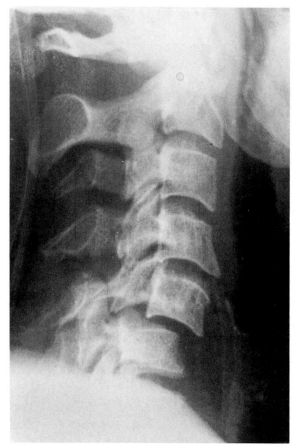

Figure 4-20. A DFS3 injury. An accident rendered this patient completely quadraplegic. He died 5 days later of a large pulmonary embolus.

cesses toward the dislocation.[50,196,202,207] A CT scan of the unilateral jumped facet includes the dislocated superior facet of the adjacent lower vertebra. It is not seen at the level of the neural arch because it has moved proximally with the dislocation.[139] Oblique views are useful if there is suspicion of this injury because this would show disruption of the facet–joint relationship.[34,202]

Unilateral facet dislocation (DFS2) covers a spectrum of injury from unilateral subluxation to unilateral perched facet to frank dislocation with or without fracture of the articular process or pedicle.[50,123] The dislocation occurs most frequently at C-6–C-7, and is often overlooked.[34,50,155,202,207] Root injury is more common than cord injury, and reduction of the dislocation is associated with re-

covery.[50,155] Neural deterioration is rare.[20,34] Alignment of the cervical spine requires skeletal traction. These injuries may be reduced closed with traction if treated in the first 2 weeks, though this may be difficult.[166,202]

The use of manipulative reduction[61] is controversial. Most authors currently agree that it is hazardous and condemn its use.[16,202] If closed reduction cannot be obtained with traction, then open reduction is called for. After 7 to 10 days have passed, an open reduction will undoubtedly be required. A locked facet left to heal in this position can lead to profound limitation of rotation, chronic pain, and possible foraminal encroachment and nerve root impingement. Another indication for open reduction is deterioration of the neurologic status in traction. If these injuries are treated after 6 weeks, the facets should be left in the locked position and foraminotomy performed for radicular pain or neurologic root impairment.[50,104,202,234] Posterior fusion should be accomplished if there is no need for anterior decompression and fusion.[50,202,275]

Bilateral facet dislocation can occur only if the posterior ligamentous structures are disrupted and the joint capsules, posterior longitudinal ligament, posterior annulus, and disks are torn. Complete neurologic injury occurs more frequently following bilateral than unilateral facet dislocations.[155,234,242] Most patients with bilateral injury will experience a reduction using traction with the appropriate weight, often with neurologic improvement.[39,166] Concomitant upper cervical injuries may make open reduction a necessity.[229] These injuries are frequently unstable after reduction and conservative treatment. There is a low incidence of spontaneous fusion, and the ligaments do not heal sufficiently.[99,142] If closed reduction is successful, then posterior fusion can be accomplished when the patient is medically stable.[104,207] Excessive distraction during treatment can worsen neurologic injury, and should be avoided.[155]

Stage 1 of *compressive extension* (Fig. 4-21) consists of a unilateral vertebral arch fracture with or without displacement. Bilateral laminar fracture without other tissue failure constitutes CES2. CES3 and CES4 are theoretical constructs of increasing severity, while CES5 consists of bilateral

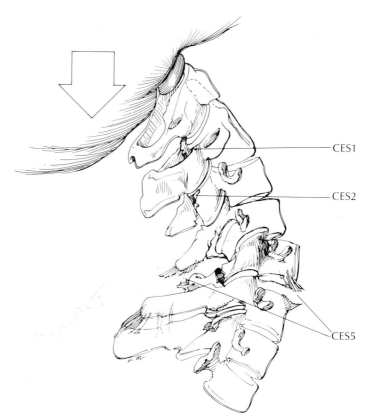

Figure 4-21. CES1 consists of a unilateral vertebral arch fracture; CES2 consists of bilateral laminar fractures. CES5 consists of bilateral vertebral arch fractures with full vertebral body width displacement anteriorly.

vertebral arch fractures with displacement of the full width of the vertebral body anteriorly. The posterior portion of the vertebral arch does not displace while the anterior portion remains with the body. Ligamentous failure occurs anteriorly between the fractured vertebra and its inferior neighbor, and posteriorly with the superior vertebra. The major injury vector is directed toward the trunk, stressing the posterior elements in compression. The frequent lateralization of the compressive stress is due to rotational forces. It is interesting to note that the severity of anatomic damage does not correlate with the severity of neural injury, with complete lesions more common in CES2 than CES5. These injuries occur approximately 20% of the time.[7]

Distractive extension injuries are caused by forces directed away from the trunk, placing the anterior elements under tension (Fig. 4-22). DES1 consists of either failure of the anterior ligamentous complex or a transverse fracture of the body. The radiographic hallmark of this stage is widening of the disk space. DES2 injuries consist of failure of the posterior ligamentous complex, which allows displacement of the superior vertebral body posteriorly into the canal. This injury is subtle and may be missed on the initial radiographic studies.[7,115,234]

Distractive extension injuries are difficult to diagnose because the injury occurs primarily through soft tissue, and roentgenograms are negative. The most frequent neurologic syndrome these patients present with is central cord syndrome, in which the hands are weak or paralyzed but there is relative sparing of the lower extremities.[7] Immobilization of the cord and immediate reduction of the inflammatory response (e.g., by steroids) are indicated to improve the neurologic situation. Recovery ultimately depends on resolution of the edema and hematomyelia that may be

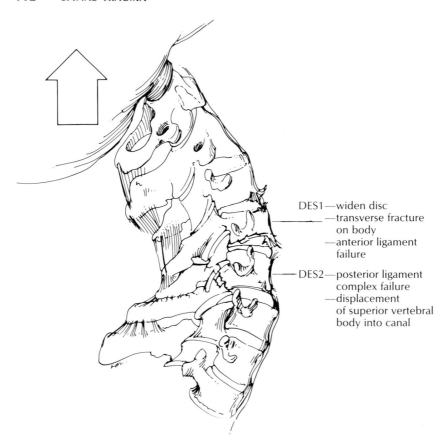

DES1—widen disc
—transverse fracture
on body
—anterior ligament
failure

DES2—posterior ligament
complex failure
—displacement
of superior vertebral
body into canal

Figure 4-22. Distractive extension injuries are caused by forces directed away from the trunk, placing the anterior elements under tension. DES1 consists of failure of either the anterior ligamentous complex or a transverse fracture of the body. DES2 is a failure of the posterior ligamentous complex.

present. Significant spontaneous recovery often occurs.[156] Decompression is indicated if diagnostic studies reveal an offending, treatable lesion. Most of the skeletal lesions are stable, and rarely go on to develop delayed deformity. Late flexion–extension testing is indicated to rule out this residual instability.[236]

Stage 1 of *lateral flexion* is an asymmetric, unilateral compression fracture of the vertebral body plus a vertebral arch fracture on the ipsilateral side, without displacement of the arch. LFS2 continues the injury, with displacement on the anteroposterior view or separation of the articular processes. Lateral flexion injuries are uncommon, and are caused by a compressive injury vector toward the side to which the spine is flexed. This is the least common family of injury.[7] Lateral flexion injuries are uncommon, and precise recommendations for their treatment have not been estab-

lished. If a patient's injury is unstable in halo vest treatment, fusion should be considered.

SUMMARY

In this chapter we have stressed the evaluation and treatment of the patient with an injured neck. Specific diagnostic criteria have been presented for each section of the cervical spine. It cannot be overstressed that treatment of these injuries begins with recognition, and that recognition of injury begins with the suspicion that injury has occurred. One must fully evaluate the patient to detect systemic and cervical spine injuries. We have also discussed the management of the patient and outlined some potential complications. Many new methods of treating cervical spine injuries are on the horizon, but the principles presented here will remain the same.

REFERENCES

1. Aebi M, Mohler J, Zack GA, Morscher E: Indication, surgical technique and results of 100 surgically treated fractures and fracture-dislocations of the cervical spine. Clin Orthop 203:244–257, 1986

2. Albin MS, White RJ: Epidemiology, physiopathology, and experimental therapeutics of acute spinal cord injury. Critical Care Clinics 3:441–452, 1987

3. Alker GJ: Radiographic evaluation of patients with cervical spine injury. In Griffen PP (ed): Instructional Course Lectures. Chicago, American Academy of Orthopedic Surgeons, 1987

4. Alker GJ, Oh YS, Leslie EV: High cervical spine and craniocervical junction injuries in fatal traffic accidents: A radiologic study. Orthop Clin North Am 9:1003–1010, 1978

5. Alker GJ, Oh YS, Leslie EV et al: Postmortem radiology of head and neck injuries in fatal traffic accidents. Radiology 114:611–617, 1975

6. Allen BL, Ferguson RL: Cervical spine trauma in children. In Bradford D, Hensinger R (eds): The Pediatric Spine. New York, Thieme, 1985

7. Allen BL, Ferguson RL, Lehman TR, O'Brien, RP: A mechanistic classification of closed, indirect fractures and dislocations of the lower cervical spine. Spine 7:1–27, 1982

8. Alpar EK, Karpinski ML: Late stability of the cervical spine. Arch Orthop Trauma Surg 104:224–226, 1985

9. American College of Surgeons: Advanced Trauma Life Support Course for Physicians, Instructor Manual. Chicago, American College of Surgeons, 1984

10. Anderson LD, D'Alonzo RT: Fractures of the odontoid process of the axis. J Bone Joint Surg [Am] 56:1663–1674, 1974

11. Aprhamian C, Thompson BM, Finger WA, Darin JC: Experimental cervical spine injury model: Evaluation of airway management and splinting techniques. Ann Emerg Med 13:584–587, 1984

12. Asnis SE, Lesniewski R, Dowling T: Anterior decompression and stabilization with methylmethacrylate and a bone bolt for treatment of pathologic fractures of the cervical spine. Clin Orthop 187:139–142, 1984

13. Babcock JL: Cervical spine injuries: Diagnosis and classification. Arch Surg 111:646–651, 1976

14. Babinski MF: Anesthetic considerations in the patient with acute spinal cord injury. Critical Care Clinics 3:619–636, 1987

15. Bachulis BL, Long WB, Hynes GD, Johnson MC: Clinical indications for cervical spine radiographs in the traumatized patient. Am J Surg 153:473–478, 1987

16. Bailey RW: Fractures and dislocations of the cervical spine. Surg Clin North Am 41:1357–1366, 1961

17. Bailey RW: "Missed" fractures of the cervical spine. Wis Med J 63:333–339, 1963

18. Bailey RW, Badgely CE: Stabilization of the cervical spine by anterior fusion. J Bone Joint Surg [Am] 42:565–594, 1960

19. Baumgarten M, Mouradian W, Boger D, Watkins R: Computed axial tomography in C1-C2 trauma. Spine 10:187–192, 1985

20. Beatson TR: Fractures and dislocations of the cervical spine. J Bone Joint Surg [Br] 45:21–35, 1963

21. Bell GD, Bailey SD: Anterior cervical fusion for trauma. Clin Orthop 128:155–158, 1980

22. Benzel EC, Larson SJ: Recovery of nerve root function after complete quadraplegia from cervical spine fractures. Neurosurgery 19:809–812, 1986

23. Berczeller PH, Bezkor MH: Deep venous thrombosis and thromboembolism, pp 117–126. In Berczeller PH, Bezkor MH (eds): Medical Complications of Quadraplegia. Chicago, Year Book Medical Publishers, 1986

23a. Blahd WH, Iserson KV, Bjelland JC: Efficacy of the posttraumatic cross table lateral view of the cervical spine. J Emerg Med 2:243–249, 1985

24. Bohler J: Anterior stabilization for acute fractures and nonunions of the dens. J Bone Joint Surg [Am] 64:18–27 1982

25. Bohler J, Gaudernat T: Anterior plate stabilization for fracture-dislocations of the lower cervical spine. J Trauma 20:203–205, 1980

26. Bohlman HH: Acute fractures and dislocations of the cervical spine: Analysis of three hundred hospitalized patients and a review of the literature. J Bone Joint Surg [Am] 61:1119–1142, 1979

27. Bohlman HH: Late anterior decompression for spinal results. Orthopaedic Transactions 4:42–43, 1980

28. Bohlman HH: Pathology and current concepts of cervical spine injuries. In American Academy of Orthopedic Surgeons (ed): Instructional Course Lectures, vol 21. St. Louis, CV Mosby, 1972

29. Bohlman HH, Bahniuk E, Raskulinecz G, Field G.: Mechanical factors affecting recovery from incomplete cervical spinal cord injury: A preliminary report. Johns Hopkins Medical Journal 145:115–125, 1979

30. Bohlman HH, Eismont FJ: Surgical techniques of anterior decompression and fusion for spinal cord injuries. Clin Orthop 154:57–67, 1981

31. Bondurant FJ, Cotler HB, Kulkarni MV, Harris JH: Magnetic resonance imaging in acute spinal cord trauma. Scientific exhibit at the 55th annual meeting of the American Academy of Orthopedic Surgeons, Atlanta, Georgia, February 1988

32. Bone L, Bucholz R: Management of fractures in the patient with multiple trauma. J Bone Joint Surg [Am] 68:945–950, 1986

33. Boynton W, Kalb R: Double lumen sign as demonstrated by computed tomography in spine dislocations. Spine 8:910–912, 1983

34. Braakman R, Vinken PJ: Unilateral facet interlocking in the lower cervical spine. J Bone Joint Surg [Br] 49:249–257, 1967

35. Brashear HR, Venters GC, Preston ET: Fractures of the neural arch of the axis: A report of 29 cases. J Bone Joint Surg [Am] 57:879–887, 1975

36. Bresler MJ, Rich GH: Occult cervical spine fracture in an ambulatory patient. Ann Emerg Med 11:440–442, 1982

37. Bridwell KH: Treatment of a markedly displaced hangman's fracture with a Luque rectangle and a posterior fusion in a 71-year-old man. Spine 11:49–52, 1986

38. Brooks AL, Jenkins EB: Atlanto-axial arthrodesis by the wedge compression method. J Bone Joint Surg [Am] 60:279–284, 1978

39. Brunette DD, Rosckswold GL: Neurologic recovery following rapid spinal realignment for complete cervical spinal cord injury. J Trauma 27:445–447, 1987

40. Bucholz R: Unstable hangman's fractures. Clin Orthop 154:119–124, 1981

41. Bucholz RW, Burkhead WZ: The pathologic anatomy of fatal atlanto-occipital dislocations. J Bone Joint Surg [Am] 61:248–250, 1979

42. Cadoux CG, White JD, Hedberg MC: High-yield roentenographic criteria for cervical spine injuries. Ann Emerg Med 16:738–742, 1987

43. Callahan RA, Johnson RM, Margolis RN et al: Cervical facet fusion for control of instability following laminectomy. J Bone Joint Surg [Am] 59:991–1002, 1977

44. Capen DA, Garland DE, Waters RL: Surgical stabilization of the cervical spine: A comparison of anterior and posterior spine fusions. Clin Orthop 196:229–237, 1985

45. Capen DA, Nelson RW, Zigler J et al: Surgical stabilization of the cervical spine: A comparative analysis of anterior and posterior spine fusions. Paraplegia 25:111–119, 1987

46. Capen DA, Zigler J, Garland DE: Surgical stabilization in cervical spine trauma. Contemporary Orthopedics 14:25–32, 1987

47. Cheshire DJ: The stability of the cervical spine following conservative treatment of fractures and fracture dislocations. Paraplegia 7:193–644, 1981

48. Cintron E, Gilua L, Murphy W, Gehweiler JA: The widened disc space: A sign of cervical hyperextension injury. Radiology 141:639–644, 1981

49. Clark CR, Keggi KJ, Panjabi MM: Methylmethacrylate stabilization of the cervical spine. J Bone Joint Surg [Am] 66:639–644, 1981

50. Clark CR, Wessels WE: Unilateral cervical facet fracture-dislocation. Surgical Rounds in Orthopedics 45:15–19, 1987

51. Clark K: Injuries to the cervical spine and spinal cord. In Youmans JR (ed): Neurological Surgery. Philadelphia, WB Saunders, 1982

52. Cline JR, Scheidel E, Bigsby EF: A comparison of methods of cervical immobilization used in patient extrication and transport. J Trauma 25:649–653, 1985

53. Cloward RB: Acute cervical spine injuries. Clin Symp 32:1–32, 1980

54. Cloward RB: Treatment of acute fractures and fracture dislocations of the cervical spine by vertebral body fusion. J Neurosurg 18:201–214, 1961

55. Collalto PM, DeMuth WW, Schwentker EP, Boal DK: Traumatic atlanto-occipital dislocation. J Bone Joint Surg [Am] 68:1106–1109, 1986

56. Cooper PR: Initial evaluation and management, pp 1–10. In Berczeller PH, Bezkor MH (eds): Medical Complications of Quadraplegia. Chicago, Year Book Medical Publishers, 1986

57. Cooper PR, Cohen W: Evaluation of cervical spinal cord injuries with metrizamide myelolgraphy CT scanning. J Neurosurg 61:281–289, 1984

58. Cooper PR, Maravilla KR, Sklar FK et al: Evaluation of cervical spinal cord injuries with metrizamide myelography CT scanning. J Neurosurg 61:281–289, 1984

59. Cooper PR, Maravilla KR, Skalr FK et al: Halo immobilization of cervical spine fractures. J Neurosurg 50:603–610, 1979

60. Cornish BL: Traumatic spondylolisthesis of the axis. J Bone Joint Surg [Br] 50:31–43, 1968

61. Cotler HB, Miller LS, DeLucia FA et al: Closed reduction of cervical spine dislocations. Clin Orthop 214:185–199, 1987

62. Daffner RH, Deeb ZL, Rothfus WE: The posterior vertebral body line: Importance in the detection of burst fractures. AJR 148:93–96, 1987

63. Dalinka MK, Kessler H, Weiss M: The radiographic evaluation of spinal trauma. Emerg Med Clin North Am 3:475–490, 1985

64. Davey JR, Roroabeck CH, Bailey SI et al: A technique of posterior cervical fusion for instability of the cervical spine. Spine 10:722–728, 1985

65. de la Torre JC: Spinal cord injury: A review of basic and applied research. Spine 6:315–335, 1981

66. Denis F: The three column spine and its significance in the classification of acute thoracolumbar spinal injuries. Spine 8:817–831, 1983

67. de Olivera JC: Anterior plate fixation of traumatic lesions of the lower cervical spine. Spine 12:324–329, 1987

68. Doris PE, Wilson RA: The next logical step in the emergency radiographic evaluation of cervical spine trauma: The five view trauma series. J Emerg Med 3:371–385, 1985

69. Dorr LD, Harvey JP: Traumatic lesions in fatal acute spinal column injuries. Clin Orthop 157:178–190, 1981

70. Ducker TB, Bellegarrigue R, Salzman M, Walleck C: Timing of operative care in cervical spinal cord injury. Spine 9:525–531, 1984

71. Dunn EJ, Blazar S: Soft tissue injuries of the lower cervical spine. In Griffen PP (ed): Instructional Course Lectures. Chicago, American Academy of Orthopedic Surgeons, 1987

72. Effendi D, Roy D, Cornish B et al: Fractures of the ring of the axis: A classification based upon the analysis of 131 cases. J Bone Joint Surg [Br] 63:319–327, 1981

73. Eismont FJ, Bohlman HH: Posterior methylmethacrylate fusion for cervical trauma. Spine 6:347–353, 1981

74. Eismont FJ, Clifford S, Goldberg M, Green B: Cervical sagittal spinal canal size in spine injury. Spine 9:663–666, 1984

75. Errico TJ, Kostiuk JP: Diagnosis and treatment of metastatic disease of the spinal column: A review. Contemporary Orthopedics 13:15–26, 1986

76. Ersmark H, Kalen R: Injuries of the atlas and axis: A follow-up study of 85 axis and 10 atlas fractures. Clin Orthop 217:257–260, 1987

77. Ersmark H, Lowenhielm P: Factors influencing the outcome of cervical spine injuries. J Trauma 28:407–410, 1988

78. Evans DK: Dislocations of the cervicothoracic junction. J Bone Joint Surg [Br] 65:124–127, 1983

79. Evarts C: Traumatic occipito-atlantal dislocation: Report of a case with survival. J Bone Joint Surg [Am] 52:1653–1660, 1970

80. Ewing CL, Thomas DJ: Human head and neck response to impact acceleration. Naval Aerospace Medical Research Laboratory Monograph, no 21, August 1971

81. Fielding JW: Cervical spine surgery: Past, present and future potential. Clin Orthop 200:284–290, 1985

82. Fielding JW: Injuries to the upper cervical spine. In Griffen PP (ed): Instructional Course Lectures. Chicago, American Academy of Orthopedic Surgeons, 1987

83. Fielding JW, Cochran GVB, Lansing JF III, Hohl M: Tears of the transverse ligament of the atlas: A clinical and biological study. J Bone Joint Surg [Am] 56:1683–1691, 1974

84. Fielding JW, Hawkins RJ: Atlanto-axial rotary fixation. J Bone Joint Surg [Am] 59:37–44, 1979

85. Fielding JW, Hawkins RJ: Roentenographic diagnosis of the injured neck. In American Academy of Orthopedic Surgeons (ed): Instructional Course Lectures. St. Louis, CV Mosby, 1976

86. Fielding JW, Hawkins RJ, Sanford RA: Spine fusion for atlanto-axial instability. J Bone Joint Surg [Am] 58:400–406, 1976

87. Fife D, Kraus J: Anatomic location of spinal cord injury: Relationship to the cause of injury. Spine 11:2–5, 1986

88. Flamm ES, Young W, Collins WF et al: Phase I trial of naloxone treatment in acute spinal cord injury. J Neurosurg 63:390–397, 1985

89. Flamm ES, Young W, Demopolous HB et al: Experimental cord injury: Treatment with naloxone. Neurosurgery 10:227–231, 1982

90. Francis WR, Fielding JW: Traumatic spondylolisthesis of the axis. Orthop Clin North Am 9:1011–1027, 1978

91. Francis WR, Fielding JW, Hawkins RJ et al: Traumatic spondylolisthesis of the axis. J Bone Joint Surg [Br] 63:313–318, 1981

92. Frankel VH: Temperomandibular joint pain syndrome following deceleration injury to the cervical spine. Bull Hosp Joint Dis Orthop Inst 26:74, 1969

93. Fried LC: Cervical spinal cord injury during skeletal traction. JAMA 229:181–183, 1974

94. Friedenberg ZB, Miller WT: Degenerative disc disease of the cervical spine: A comparative study of asymptomatic and symptomatic patients. J Bone Joint Surg [Am] 45:1171–1178, 1963

95. Fuji E, Kobayashi K, Hirabayashi K: Treatment in fractures of the odontoid process. Spine 13:604–609, 1988

96. Funk EJ, Wells RE: Injuries of the cervical spine in football. Clin Orthop 109:50–58, 1975

97. Garfin SR, Botte MJ, Centeno RS, Nickel VL: Osteology of the skull as it affects halo pin placement. Spine 10:696–698, 1985

98. Garfin SR, Botte MJ, Triggs KJ, Nickel VL: Subdural abscess associated with halo-pin traction. J Bone Joint Surg [Am] 70:1338–1340, 1988

99. Garfin SR, Botte MJ, Waters RL, Nickel VL: Complications in the use of halo fixation. J Bone Joint Surg [Am] 68:320–325, 1986

100. Gassman J, Seligson D: The anterior cervical plate. Spine 8:700–707, 1983

101. Good RP, Nickel VL: Cervical spine injuries resulting from water sports. Spine 5:502–506, 1980

102. Gopalakrishnan KC, Masri WE: Prevertebral soft tissue shadow widening: An important sign of cervical spinal injury. Injury 17:125–128, 1986

103. Gore DR: Technique of cervical interbody fusion. Clin Orthop 188:191–195, 1984

104. Grady MS, Howard MR, Jane JA, Persing JA: Use of the Philadelphia collar as an alternative to the halo vest in patients with C2-C3 fractures. Neurosurgery 18:151–156, 1985

105. Green BA, Callahan RA, Klose KJ, de la Torre J: Acute spinal cord injury: Current concepts. Clin Orthop 154:125–135, 1981

106. Green D, Lee MY, Ito VY et al: Fixed- vs adjusted-dose heparin in the prophylaxis of thromboembolism in spinal cord injury. JAMA 260:1255–1258, 1988

107. Greenfield J, Ilfeld FW: Acute cervical strain evaluation and short term prognostic factors. Clin Orthop 122:196–200, 1977

108. Griswold DM, Albright JA, Schiffman E et al: Atlanto-axial fusion for instability. J Bone Joint Surg [Am] 60:285–292, 1978

109. Grundy BL, Friedman W: Electrophysiological evaluation of the patient with acute spinal cord injury. Critical Care Clinics 3:519–548, 1987

110. Häadley MN, Sonntag VKH, Grahm TW et al: Axis fractures resulting from motor vehicle accidents: The need for occupant restraints. Spine 11:861–864, 1986

111. Hänssen A, Cabaneal ME: Fracture of the dens in adult patients. J Trauma 27:928–934, 1987

112. Härkönen M, Lepsitö P, Paakkala T et al: Spinal cord injuries associated with vertebral fractures and dislocations: Clinical and radiologic results in 30 patients. Arch Orthop Trauma Surg 94:185–190, 1979

113. Harns JH, Edeiken-Monroe P, Kopaniky DR: A practical classification of acute cervical spine injuries. Orthop Clin North Am 17:15–30, 1986

114. Harris JH: Radiographic evaluation of spinal trauma. Orthop Clin North Am 17:75–86, 1986

115. Harris WH, Hamblen DL, Ojemann RG: Traumatic disruption of cervical intervertebral disc from hyperextension injury. Clin Orthop 60:163–167, 1968

116. Hays MB, Alker GJ: Fractures of the atlas vertebra: The two part burst fracture of Jefferson. Spine 13:60–603, 1988

117. Heulke DF, O'Day J, Mendlesohn RA: Cervical injuries suffered in automobile crashes. J Neurosurg 54:316–322, 1981

118. Hohl M: Soft tissue injuries of the neck. Clin Orthop 109:42–46, 1975

119. Hohl M: Soft tissue injuries of the neck in automobile accidents: Factors influencing prognosis. J Bone Joint Surg [Am] 56:1675–1682, 1984

120. Hohl M, Hopp E.: Soft tissue injuries of the neck: II. Factors influencing prognosis. Orthopaedic Transactions 2:29, 1978

121. Holdsworth F: Fractures, dislocations and fracture-dislocations of the spine: A review paper. J Bone Joint Surg [Am] 52:1534–1551, 1970

122. Hoppenfeld S, deBoer P: Surgical Exposures in Orthopedics: The Anatomic Approach. Philadelphia, JB Lippincott, 1984

123. Jackson DW, Lohr FT: Cervical spine injuries. Clin Sports Med 5:373–386, 1986

124. Jacobs B: Cervical fractures and dislocations (C3-7). Clin Orthop 109:18–32, 1975

125. Jeanneret B, Magerl F, Stanisic M: Thrombosis of the vertebral artery: A rare complication following traumatic spondylolisthesis of the second cervical vertebra. Spine 11:179–182, 1986

126. Jefferson G: Fracture of the atlas vertebra. Br J Surg 7:407–410, 1920

127. Johnson RM, Hart DC, Simmons EF et al: Cervical orthoses: A study comparing their effectiveness and restricting cervical motion in normal subjects. J Bone Joint Surg [Am] 59:332–339, 1977

128. Johnson RM, Owens JR, Hart DC, Callahan RA: Cervical orthoses: A guide to their selection and use. Clin Orthop 154:34–45, 1981

129. Johnson RM, Southwick WO: Surgical approaches to the cervical spine, pp 93–146. In Rothman RH, Simeone FA (eds): The Spine, 2nd ed. Philadelphia, WB Saunders, 1982

130. Juhl M: Os odontodium: A cause of atlanto-axial instability. Acta Orthop Scand 54:113–116, 1983

131. Julow J, Szarvas I, Sárváry A.: Clinical study of injuries of the lower cervical spinal cord. Injury 11:38–42, 1984

132. Kamelhar DL: Respiratory care, pp 25–50. In Berczeller PH, Bezkor MF (eds): Medical Complications of Quadraplegia. Chicago, Year Book Medical Publishers, 1986

133. Karlstöm G, Olerud S: Internal fixation of fractures and dislocations in the cervical spine. Orthopedics 10:1549–1558, 1987

134. Keene GCR, Hone MR, Sage MR: Atlas fracture: Demonstration using computerized tomography. J Bone Joint Surg [Am] 60:1106–1107, 1978

135. Keene JS, Goletz TH, Lilleas F et al: Diagnosis of vertebral fractures: A comparison of conventional radiography, conventional tomography and axial tomography. J Bone Joint Surg [Am] 64:586–595, 1982

136. Kim KS, Rogers LF, Regenbogen V: Pitfalls in plain film diagnosis of cervical spine injuries: False positive interpretation. Surg Neurol 25:381–392, 1986

137. King AG: Spinal column trauma. In Anderson LD (ed): Instructional Course Lectures, vol 35. St. Louis, CV Mosby, 1986

138. Koch RA, Nickel VL: The halo vest: An evaluation of motion and forces across the neck. Spine 3:103–107, 1976

139. Kornberg M: The computed tomographic appearance of the unilateral jumped cervical facet (the "false" facet joint sign). Spine 11:1038–1040, 1986

140. Kornberg M: Upper cervical spine injuries: A review. Contemporary Orthopedics 12:61–67, 1986

141. Korres DST, Kyritsis G, Kouvaras J et al: Double level fractures of the cervical spine. Int Orthop 11:105–108, 1987

142. Kostiuk JP: Indications for the use of halo immobilization. Clin Orthop 154:46–50, 1981

143. Kraus JF: A comparison of recent studies on the extent of the head and spinal cord injury problem in the United States. J Neurosurg [suppl] 53:35–43, 1980

144. Kraus JF, Franti CE, Rigins RS et al: Incidence of traumatic spinal cord lesions. J Chronic Dis 28:471–492, 1975

145. Kulkarni MV, McArdle CB, Kopanicky D et al: Acute spinal cord injury: MR imaging at 1.5 T. Radiology 164:837–843, 1987

146. Landells CD, van Peteghem PK: Fractures of the atlas: Classification, treatment and morbidity. Spine 13:450–452, 1988

147. Leo JS, Bergeron RT, Kricheff II, Benjamin MV: Metrizamide myelography for cervical spine injuries. Radiology 129:707–711, 1978

148. Levine AM, Edwards CC: The management of traumatic spondylolisthesis of the axis. J Bone Joint Surg [Am] 67:217–226, 1985

149. Levine AM, Edwards CC: Treatment of injuries in the C1-C2 complex. Orthop Clin North Am 17:31–42, 1986

150. Lewallen RP, Morrey BF, Cabanella ME: Respiratory arrest following posteriorly displaced odontoid fractures. Clin Orthop 188:187–190, 1984

151. Light TR, Wagner FC, Southwick WO et al: Instability and recovery of neurologic loss following cervical body replacement. Spine 5:390–392, 1980

152. Lima C, deOlivea JC: Anterior fusion for fractures and dislocations of the cervical spine. Injury 2:205–210, 1971

153. Lind B, Nordwall A, Sihlbom H: Odontoid fractures treated with halo-vest. Spine 12:173–177, 1987

154. Lind B, Sihlbom H, Nordwall A: Halo-vest treatment of unstable traumatic cervical spine injuries. Spine 13:425–431, 1988

155. Maiman DJ, Barolat G, Larson SJ: Management of bilateral locked facets of the cervical spine. Neurosurgery 18:542–547, 1986

156. Marar BC: Hyperextension injuries of the cervical spine: The pathogenesis of damage to the spinal cord. J Bone Joint Surg [Am] 56:1655–1662, 1974

157. Maroon JC: "Burning hands" in football spinal cord injuries. JAMA 238:2049–2051, 1977

158. Marshall LF, Knowlton S, Garfin SR et al: Deterioration following spinal cord injury: A multicenter study. J Neurosurg 66:400–404, 1987

159. Mattox KL: The injured patient's injured neck. Emerg Med Clin North Am 16:24–48, 1984

160. Mazur JM, Stauffer ES: Unrecognized spinal instability associated with "simple" cervical compression fractures. Spine 8:687–692, 1983

161. McArdle CB, Crofford MJ, Mirfakhraee M et al: Surface coil MR of spinal trauma: Preliminary experience. AJNR 7:885–893, 1986

162. McCall IW, Park WM, McSweeney T: The radiological demonstration of acute lower cervical injury. Clin Radiol 24:235–240, 1973

163. McClelland SJ, James RL, Jarenwattanon A, Shelton ML: Traumatic spondylolisthesis of the axis in a patient presenting with torticollis. Clin Orthop 218:195–200, 1987

164. McNab I: Acceleration and extension injuries of the cervical spine, pp 647–670. In Rothman RH, Simeone FA (eds): The Spine, 2nd ed. Philadelphia, WB Saunders, 1982

165. Meyer PA Jr, Rosen JS, Hamilton BB, Hall WJ: Fracture-dislocation of the cervical spine: Transportation, assessment, and immediate management. In American Academy of Orthopedic Sur-

geons (ed): Instructional Course Lectures. St. Louis, CV Mosby, 1976

166. Miller LS, Cotler HB, de Lucia FA et al: Biomechanical analysis of cervical distraction. Spine 12:831–837, 1987

167. Miller MD, Gehweiler JA, Martinez S et al: Significant new observations on cervical spine trauma. AJR 130:659–663, 1978

168. Morgan TH, Watson GW, Austin GN: The results of laminectomy in patients with incomplete spinal cord injuries. J Bone Joint Surg [Am] 52:822, 1970

169. Morgan TH, Wharton GW, Sutin GN: The results of laminectomy in patients with incomplete spinal cord injuries. Paraplegia 9:14–23, 1971

170. Morse SD: Acute central cervical spinal cord syndrome. Ann Emerg Med 11:436–439, 1982

171. Mouradian WH, Fietti VG, Cochran GVB et al: Fractures of the odontoid: A laboratory and clinical study of mechanism. Orthop Clin North Am 985–1001, 1978

172. Murphy MJ, Ogden JA, Southwick WO: Spinal stabilization in acute spinal injuries. Surg Clin North Am 60:1035–1047, 1980

173. Murphy MJ, Southwick WO: The cervical spine. In Gossling HR, Pillsbury SL: Complications of Fracture Management. Philadelphia, JB Lippincott, 1984

174. Murphy MJ, Wu JC, Southwick WO: Complications of halo fixation. Orthopaedic Transactions 3:126, 1979

175. Myllynen D, Kammanen M, Rokkanen P et al: Deep vein thrombosis and pulmonary embolism in patients with acute spinal cord injury: A comparison with nonparalyzed patients immobilized due to spinal fractures. J Trauma 25:541–543, 1985

176. Nelson R, Capen D, Garland D, Waters R: Halo vest stabilization of cervical spine fractures and dislocations: A series review and long term follow-up. Paper presented at the annual meeting of the American Academy of Orthopedic Surgeons, Atlanta, Georgia, 1984

177. Nichols CG, Young DH, Schiller WR: Evaluation of cervicothoracic junction injury. Ann Emerg Med 16:640–642, 1987

178. Norrell H, Wilson CB: Early anterior fusion for injuries of the cervical portion of the spine. JAMA 214:525–530, 1970

179. Norris SH: The prognosis of neck injuries resulting from rear end vehicle collisions. J Bone Joint Surg [Am] 65:9–13, 1983

180. O'Brien PJ, Schweigel JF, Thompson WJ: Dislocations of the lower cervical spine. J Trauma 22:710–714, 1982

181. O'Leary P, Boiardo R: The diagnosis and treatment of injuries of the spine in athletes. In Nicholas JA, Hershman EB: The Lower Extremity and Spine in Sports Medicine. St. Louis, CV Mosby, 1986

182. O'Neill B, Haddon W, Kelly AB: Automobile head restraints: Frequency of neck injury claims in relation to the presence of head restraints. Am J Public Health 62:399–406, 1972

183. Panjabi MM, White AA III, Johnson RM: Cervical spine mechanics as a function of ligament transection. J Bone Joint Surg [Am] 57:582, 1975

184. Pennecot GF, Leonard P, Pegrot DE et al: Ligamentous instability of the cervical spine in children. J Pediatr Orthop 4:339–345, 1984

185. Penning L: Obtaining and interpreting plain films in cervical spine injury. In The Cervical Spine Research Society (ed): The Cervical Spine. Philadelphia, JB Lippincott, 1983

186. Penning L: Prevertebral hematoma in cervical spine injury: Incidence and etiologic significance. AJR 136:553–561, 1981

187. Pepin JW, Bourne RB, Hawkins RJ: Odontoid fractures, with special reference to the elderly patient. Clin Orthop 193:178–183, 1985

188. Pepin JW, Hawkins RJ: Traumatic spondylisthesis of the axis: Hangman's fracture. Clin Orthop 157:138–148, 1981

189. Perkash A, Prakash V, Perkash I: Experience with the management of thromboembolism in patients with spinal cord injury: Part I. Incidence, diagnosis and role of some risk factors. Paraplegia 16:322–331, 1978–1979

190. Pierce DS: The halo orthosis in the treatment of cervical spine injury. In Griffen PP (ed): Instructional Course Lectures. Chicago, American Academy of Orthopedic Surgeons, 1987

191. Plunkett PK, Redmond AD, Billsborough SH: Cervical subluxation: A deceptive soft tissue injury. Journal Royal Society of Medicine 80:46–47, 1987

192. Podolsky S, Baraff LJ, Simon RR et al: Efficacy of cervical spine immobilization methods. J Trauma 23:461–465, 1983

193. Powers B, Miller MD, Kramer RS et al: Traumatic anterior atlanto-occipital dislocation. Neurosurgery 4:12–17, 1979

194. Rachesky I, Boyce WT, Duncan B et al: Clinical prediction of cervical spine injuries in children. Am J Dis Child 141:199–201, 1987

195. Ravichandran G, Silver JR: Missed injuries of the spinal cord. Br Med J 284:953–956, 1982

196. Reid DC, Henderson R, Saboe L, Miller JDR: Etiology and clinical course of missed spine fractures. J Trauma 27:980–986, 1987

197. Reiss SJ, Raque GH, Shields CB, Garretson HD: Cervical spine fractures with major associated trauma. Neurosurgery 18:327–330, 1986

198. Ries MD, Ray S: Posterior displacement of an odontoid fracture in a child. Spine 11:1043–1044, 1986

199. Rifkinson-Mann S, Mormino J, Sachdev VP: Subacute cervical spine instability. Surg Neurol 26:413–416, 1986

200. Robinson RA, Riley LH: Techniques of exposure and fusion of the cervical spine. Clin Orthop 128:155–158, 1977

201. Rogers WA: Fractures and dislocations of the cervical spine: An end result study. J Bone Joint Surg [Am] 39:34–38, 1957

202. Rorabeck CH, Rock MG, Hawkins AJ, Bourne RB: Unilateral facet dislocation of the cervical spine: An analysis of the results of treatment in 26 patients. Spine 12:23–27, 1987

203. Ross SE, Schwab CW, David ET et al: Clearing the cervical spine: Initial radiologic evaluation. J Trauma 27:1055–1060, 1987

204. Rowed DW, McLean JAG, Tator CH: Somatosensory evoked potentials in acute spinal cord injury: Prognostic value. Surg Neurol 9:203–210, 1978

205. Roye WP, Dunn EL, Moody JA: Cervical spinal cord injury: A public catastrophe. AAST Abstracts. J Trauma 27:831, 1987

206. Ryan MD, Taylor THK: Odontoid fracture: A rational approach to treatment. J Bone Joint Surg [Br] 64:416–421, 1982

207. Savini R, Parsini P, Cervellati S: The surgical treatment of late instability of flexion-rotation injuries in the lower cervical spine. Spine 12:178–182, 1987

208. Schaffer MA, Doris PE: Limitation of the cross table lateral view in detecting cervical spine injuries: A retrospective analysis. Ann Emerg Med 10:508–513, 1981

209. Schatzker J, Rorabek CH, Waddell JW: Fractures of the dens. J Bone Joint Surg [Br] 53:392–405, 1971

210. Scheiss RJ, deSaussure RL, Robertson JT: Choice of treatment of odontoid fractures. J Neurosurg 51:496–499, 1982

211. Scher AT: Anterior cervical subluxation: An unstable position. AJR 133:275–280, 1979

212. Schlitke LH, Callahan RA: A rational approach to burst fractures of the atlas. Clin Orthop 154:18–21, 1981

213. Schneider RC, Cherry G, Patek H: The syndrome of acute central cervical spinal cord injury. J Neurosurg 11:546–577, 1954

214. Schneider RC, Thompson JM, Bebin J: The syndrome of acute central cervical spinal cord injury. J Neurol Neurosurg Psychiatry 21:216–227, 1958

215. Schneider RL, Livingston RE, Cave AJE, Hamilton G: "Hangman's fracture" of the cervical spine. J Neurosurg 22:141–154, 1965

216. Schrader SC, Sloan TB, Toleikis JR: Detection of sacral sparing in acute spinal cord injury. Spine 12:533–535, 1987

217. Schweigel JF: Management of the fractured odontoid with halo-thoracic bracing. Spine 12:838–839, 1987

218. Segal D, Grimm JO, Stauffer ES: Nonunion of fractures of the atlas. J Bone Joint Surg [Am] 69:1423–1434, 1987

219. Segal D, Whitlaw GP, Gumbs V, Pick RY: Tension band wiring in the cervical spine. Clin Orthop 159:211–222, 1981

220. Severy DM, Mathewson JH, Bechtol CO: Controlled automobile rear end collisions: An investigation of related engineering and medical phenomena. Canadian Services Medical Journal 11:727, 1955

221. Sherk HH: Fractures of the atlas and odontoid process. Orthop Clin North Am 9:973–984, 1978

222. Sherk HH, Shut L, Lane JM: Fractures and dislocations of the cervical spine in children. Orthop Clin North Am 7:563–604, 1976

223. Sherk HH, Snyder B: Posterior fusions of the upper cervical spine: Indications, techniques and prognosis. Orthop Clin North Am 9:1091–1099, 1978

224. Sherk MM, Nicholson JT: Fractures of the atlas. J Bone Joint Surg [Am] 52:1017–1020, 1970

225. Shields CC, Stauffer ES: Late instability in cervical spine fractures secondary to laminectomy. Clin Orthop 119:144–147, 1976

226. Simmons EH, Bhalla SH: Anterior cervical discectomy and fusion: A clinical and biomedical study with eight year follow-up. J Bone Joint Surg [Br] 51:225–237, 1969

227. Smoker WRK, Dolan KD: The "fat" C2: A sign of fracture. AJR 148:609–614, 1987

228. Soderstrum CA, Brumback RJ: Early care of the patient with cervical spine injury. Orthop Clin North Am 12:3–13, 1986

229. Sonntag VKH: Management of bilateral locked

facets of the cervical spine. Neurosurgery 8:150–152, 1981

230. Southwick WO: Current concepts review: Management of fractures dens (odontoid process). J Bone Joint Surg [Am] 62:482–486, 1980

231. Spence KF, Dedser D, Sell HW: Bursting atlantal fracture associated with rupture of the transverse ligament. J Bone Joint Surg [Am] 52:543–546, 1970

232. Spielholz NI, Benjamin NV, Ransohoff J: Somatosensory evoked potentials and clinical outcome in spinal cord injury, pp 217–222. In Popp AJ (ed): Neural Trauma. New York, Raven Press, 1979

233. Stauffer ES: Fractures and dislocations of the spine: Part I. The cervical spine, pp 987–1035. In Rockwood CA, Green DP (eds): Fractures in Adults, 2nd ed. Philadelphia, JB Lippincott, 1984

234. Stauffer ES: Management of spine fractures C3-C7. Orthop Clin North Am 17:45–53, 1986

235. Stauffer ES: Rehabilitation of the spinal cord: Injured patient. In Nichel VL (ed): Orthopedic Rehabilitation. Philadelphia, W. B. Saunders, 1983

236. Stauffer ES, Kelly EG: Fracture dislocation of the cervical spine: Instability and recurrent deformity following treatment by anterior interbody fusion. J Bone Joint Surg [Am] 59:49–48, 1977

237. Stauffer ES, Rhodes EE: Surgical stabilization of the cervical spine after trauma. Arch Surg 111:652–657, 1976

238. Streitweiser DR, Knopp R, Wales LR et al: Accuracy of standard radiographic views in detecting cervical spine fractures. Ann Emerg Med 12:538–542, 1983

239. Tearse DS, Keene JS, Drummond DS: Management of noncontiguous vertebral fractures. Paraplegia 25:100–105, 1987

240. Templeton PA, Young JWR, Mirvis SE, Buddemeyer EU: The value of retropharyngeal soft tissue measurements in trauma of the adult cervical spine: Cervical spine soft tissue measurements. Skeletal Radiol 16:98–104, 1987

241. Tolonen J, Santavirta S, Kiviluoto O, Lindqvist C: Fatal cervical spine injuries in road traffic accidents. Injury 17:154–158, 1986

242. Torg JS, Sennett B, Vegso JJ: Spinal injury at the level of the third and fourth cervical vertebrae resulting from the axial loading mechanism: An analysis and classification. Clin Sports Med 6:159–183, 1987

243. Torg JS, Truex RC, Marshall J: Spinal injury at the third and fourth cervical vertebrae from football. J Bone Joint Surg [Am] 59:1015–1019, 1977

244. van der Bout AH, Dommisse GF: Traumatic at-lanto-occipital dislocation. Spine 11:174–176, 1986

245. Van Hove E: Prevention of thrombophlebitis in spinal injury patients. Paraplegia 16:332–335, 1978–1979

246. van Peteghem PK, Schweigel JF: The fractured cervical spine rendered unstable by anterior cervical fusion. J Trauma 19:110–114, 1979

247. Verbiest H: Anterolateral operations for fractures and dislocations of the middle and lower parts of the cervical spine. J Bone Joint Surg [Am] 51:1489–1530, 1969

248. Victor DI, Keller RB: Brain abscess complicating the use of halo traction. J Bone Joint Surg [Am] 55:635–639, 1973

249. Wagner FC, Cheharzi B: Neurologic evaluation of cervical spine injuries. Spine 9:507, 1984

250. Wagner FC, Cheharzi B: Spinal cord injury: Indications for operative intervention. Surg Clin North Am 60:1048–1054, 1980

251. Walter J, Doris PE, Shaffer MA: Clinical presentation of patients with acute cervical spine injury. Ann Emerg Med 13:512–515, 1984

252. Watkins RG: Neck injuries in football players. Clin Sports Med 5:215–246, 1986

253. Webb JK, Broughton RBK, McSweeney T, Park WM: Hidden flexion injury of the cervical spine. J Bone Joint Surg [Br] 58:322–327, 1976

254. Weir DC: Roentenographic signs of cervical injury. Clin Orthop 109:11–17, 1975

255. White AA III, Johnson RM, Panjabi MM, Southwick WO: Biomechanical analysis of clinical stability in the cervical spine. Clin Orthop 109:85–96, 1975

256. White AA III, Panjabi MM: Clinical biomechanics of the occipito-atlantal complex. Orthop Clin North Am 9:867–878, 1978

257. White AA III, Panjabi MM: Clinical biomechanics of the spine. Philadelphia, JB Lippincott, 1978

258. White AA III, Panjabi MM: The role of stabilization in the treatment of cervical spine injuries. Spine 9:512–522, 1983

259. White AA III, Panjabi MM: Update on the evaluation of instability of the lower cervical spine. In Griffen PP (ed): Instructional Course Lectures. Chicago, American Academy of Orthopedic Surgeons, 1987

260. White AA III, Panjabi MM, Posner I et al: Spinal stability: Evaluation and treatment, pp 457–483. In American Academy of Orthopedic Surgeons (ed): Instructional Course Lectures, Vol 32. St. Louis, C. V. Mosby, 1983

261. White AA III, Panjabi MM, Saha S, Southwick

WO: Biomechanics of the axially loaded cervical spine: Development of a clinical test for ruptured ligaments. J Bone Joint Surg [Am] 57:582, 1975

262. White AA III, Southwick WO, Panjabi MM: Clinical stability in the lower cervical spine: A review of past and current concepts. Spine 1:15–27, 1976

263. Whitehill R, Richman JA, Glaser JA: Failure of immobilization of the cervical spine by the halo vest. J Bone Joint Surg [Am] 68:326–332, 1986

264. Whitehill R, Stowers SF, Ruch WW, Stamp WG: Cervical dislocation adjacent to a fused motion segment. Spine 12:396–398, 1987

265. Whitehill R, Wilhelm CE, Moskal JT et al: Posterior strut fusions to enhance immediate postoperative cervical stability. Spine 11:6–13, 1986

266. Whitesides TE, McDonald AP: Lateral retropharyngeal approach to the upper cervical spine. Orthop Clin North Am 9:1115–1127, 1978

267. Williams CF, Bernstein TW, Jelenko C: Essentiality of the lateral cervical spine radiograph. Ann Emerg Med 10:198–204, 1981

268. Winslow EB, Lesch M, Talano JV, Meyer PR: Spinal cord injuries associated with cardiopulmonary complications. Spine 11:809–812, 1986

269. Wojcik WG, Edeiken-Monroe BS, Harris JH: Three dimensional computed tomography in acute cervical spine trauma: A preliminary report. Skeletal Radiol 16:261–269, 1987

270. Woodring JH, Goldstein SJ: Fractures of the articular processes of the cervical spine. AJR 139: 341–344, 1982

271. Yoganandan N, Sances A, Maiman D et al: Experimental spinal injuries with vertical impact. Spine 9:855–860, 1986

272. Young W: Correlation of somatosensory evoked potentials and neurologic findings in spinal cord injury, pp 153–165. In Tator CH (ed): Early Management of Acute Spinal Injuries. New York, Raven Press, 1982

273. Young W, Flamm ES: Effect of high dose corticosteroid therapy on blood flow, evoked potential and extracellular calcium in experimental spinal injury. J Neurosurg 57:667–673, 1982

274. Young W, Flamm ES, Demopoulos HB et al: Effect of naloxone on post-traumatic ischemia in experimental cord cortesion. Neurosurg 55:209–219, 1981

275. Zigler J, Capen D, Nelson R, Nagelberg S: Management strategies for unstable cervical spine injuries. Scientific exhibit at the 55th annual meeting of the American Association of Orthopedic Surgeons. Atlanta, Georgia, February 1988

276. Zigler J, Rockowitz N, Capen D et al: Posterior cervical fusion with local anesthesia: The awake patient as the ultimate spinal cord monitor. Spine 12:206–208, 1987

277. Zigler J, Waters RL, Nelson R et al: Occipito-cervico-thoracic spine fusion in a patient with occipito-cervical dislocation and survival. Spine 11:645–646, 1987

5

CERVICAL SPINE INSTABILITY AND BIOMECHANICS OF TREATMENT

George Miz

Stability of the spine has in the past been defined in terms of clinical and radiographic parameters. Of primary concern to the clinician treating a patient with an injured spine is the concept of clinical stability. Stauffer has defined this in three parameters. First, the motion segment must not further deform or displace under physiologic loads such as gravity or active muscle contraction. Second, there must be no progressive deformity or displacement during the healing process. Third, there must be no progressive injury to the neural structures.[93] A fourth parameter used by White is the lack of incapacitating pain due to structural changes.[103] If these criteria have been met, the spine can be determined to be stable.

A differentiation must also be made between acute and chronic, or late, instability. Acute instability is that which is present at the time of injury, whereas late instability is that remaining after an appropriate time for tissue healing has elapsed.[3,78] Herkowitz[42] has additionally described the entity of subacute instability, in which, theoretically, an elastic deformation of the spinal ligaments has occurred that under physiologic loads progresses to plastic deformation. This allows for secondary displacement of the spinal motion segment.

Clinical decisions regarding treatment of the patient will hinge on the determined stability or instability of the injured spine.[8]

KINEMATICS OF THE NORMAL SPINE

Kinematics as applied to the spine is the study of motion of adjacent spinal segments without consideration of the forces involved. Prior to considering the kinematics of the individual spinal segments, several concepts require at least a brief definition.[48]

Coordinate system: The right-handed orthogonal (90-degree angle) coordinate system recommended by White and Panjabi[70] is simple

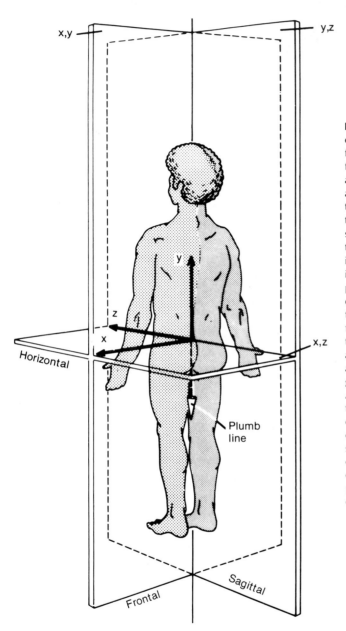

Figure 5-1. The suggested central coordinate system with its origin between the sacral cornua is shown. Its orientation is as follows. The $-y$-axis is described by the plumb line dropped from the origin, and the $+x$-axis points to the left at a 90-degree angle to the y-axis. The $+z$-axis points forward at a 90-degree angle to both the y-axis and x-axis. The human body is shown in the anatomic position. Some basic conventions are observed that make this a useful system. *The planes* are as shown: The sagittal plane is the y, z plane; the frontal plane is the y, x plane; the horizontal plane is the x, z plane. *Movements* are described in relation to the origin of the coordinate system. The arrows indicate the positive direction of each axis. The origin is the zero point, and the direction opposite to the arrows is negative. Thus, direct forward translation is $+z$; up is $+y$; to the left is $+x$, and to the right is $-x$; down is $-y$; and backwards is $-z$. The convention for rotations is determined by imagining oneself at the origin of the coordinate system looking in the positive direction of the axis. Clockwise rotations are $+\theta$ and counterclockwise rotations are $-\theta$. Thus, $+\theta x$ is roughly analogous to flexion; $+\theta z$ is analogous to right lateral bending; $+\theta y$ is axial rotation toward the left. A coordinate system may be set up at any defined point parallel to the master system described above. The location of the coordinate system should be clearly indicated for precise, accurate communications. In spinal kinematics, the motion is usually described in relation to the subjacent vertebra. The secondary coordinate system may be established in the body of the subjacent vertebra. For in vivo measurements, the tip of its spinous process may be used. (Panjabi MM, White AA, Brand RA: A note on defining body parts configurations. J Biomech 7:385, 1974)

and efficient for the description of spinal kinematics. It is detailed in Figure 5-1.

Motion segment (functional spinal unit): This consists of the two adjacent vertebrae and their connecting soft tissues.

Rotation: Rotation is defined as the angular displacement of a body about an axis, the axis being located within or without the body. This is typically measured in degrees.

Translation: This occurs when all particles of a body move in the same direction relative to a fixed point. Translation is usually measured as a distance along a straight line.

Range of motion (ROM): This is the distance or angle between two physiologic extremes of translation or rotation.

Coupled motion: Coupled motion occurs when motion about one axis consistently occurs simultaneously with motion about another axis (either translation or rotation).

Instantaneous axis of rotation (IAR): A rigid body in plane motion at any given instant has a point or extension of that point that does not move. The line passing through this point and perpendicular to the plane of motion is the IAR.

For a more comprehensive review of these topics the reader is referred to White and Panjabi's text.[103]

OCCIPITAL–ATLANTO-AXIAL COMPLEX

The upper cervical spine (occiput–C-1–C-2) is a distinct anatomic and functional unit and exhibits unique kinematics. Penning[73] postulated that motion of this complex was basically determined by movement between the occipital condyles and axis, which he likened to two rotating spheres with the atlas as a bearing between them. For the sake of simplicity we will consider the kinematics of each joint separately.

The occiput–C-1 articulation is capable of significant flexion–extension ($\pm\theta x$), minor degrees of lateral bending ($\pm\theta z$), minimal z-axis translation ($\pm z$) and negligible axial rotation ($\pm\theta y$) (Table 5-1). Werne,[101] using radiographic studies, found the occiput–C1 joint to have an average ROM in flexion–extension of approximately 13 degrees. In lateral bending he found a ROM in cadavers of an average of 11.9 degrees, and on radiographic examination 7.8 degrees. He concluded that the radiographic measurements were more accurate. His figures have been generally accepted; however, other authors have reported as much as 30 to 40 degrees of lateral bending.[23] The normal z-axis translatory motion of occiput–C-1 is generally considered to be zero to 1 mm. This is based on the cadaver studies of Werne[101] and confirmed by Weisel's[100] radiographic study of army recruits. Fielding's data[24,26] using cineradiography is also in agreement with these findings. Occipito-atlantal rotation is essentially prevented by the articulation's anatomic configuration. The opposing articular surfaces are cup-shaped and congruous, precluding rotation in the functional spinal unit with intact ligamentous structures. There is no significant coupling of motion at this articulation. The instantaneous axes of rotation of occipitoatloid motion in flexion–extension and lateral bending were estimated by Henke[40] more than 100 years

Table 5-1. Representative Values of the Range of Rotation of the Occipital–Atlanto-axial Complex

UNIT OF COMPLEX	TYPE OF MOTION	DEGREES OF MOTION
Occipital-Atlantal joint (occiput–C-1)	Flexion-extension ($\pm\theta x$)	13° (Moderate)
	Lateral bending ($\pm\theta z$)	8° (Moderate)
	Axial rotation ($\pm\theta y$)	0° (Negligible)
Atlanto-axial joint (C-1–C-2)	Flexion-extension ($\pm\theta x$)	10° (Moderate)
	Lateral bending ($\pm\theta z$)	0° (Negligible)
	Axial rotation ($\pm\theta y$)	47° (Extensive)

(Sherk HH, Dunn EJ, Eismont et al: The Cervical Spine. Philadelphia, JB Lippincott, 1987)

ago based on outlines of the articulations. Their approximate locations are shown in Figure 5-2.

The atlanto-axial joint is more complex and is more frequently involved in pathologic conditions. The articular surfaces of the joint are both convex with a horizontal orientation, permitting maximal rotation with minimal inherent stability. Its primary motion is axial rotation with smaller degrees of flexion–extension, z- and x-axis translation, and negligible lateral bending. Rotation of the C-1–C-2 joint is limited to approximately 47 degrees by the alar ligaments.[74] This accounts for nearly 50% of the rotation of the entire cervical spine. Flexion–extension was found by Werne[101] to be approximately 10 degrees, extension being limited by the tectorial membrane here as at occiput–C-1. In contrast to the occiput–C-1 articulation there is significant translatory motion at C-1–C-2. Fielding[25,27] measured z-axis translation at C-1–C-2 in cadaver specimens and concluded that the normal range was up to 3 mm. Translation exceeding this usually led to rupture of the transverse ligament. Anterior z-axis translation is restrained primarily by the transverse ligaments supplemented by the alar and other ligaments. Posterior (−z) translation is limited by abutment of the anterior atlas against the dens. Jackson's[46] radiographic study of normal subjects agreed with Fielding's data. He found a maximum anterior translation of 2.5 mm in adults and 4 mm in chil-

dren. Lateral translation (±x) at C-1–C-2 was documented by Hohl[43] in a cadaver specimen and by cineradiography. He found that translation of up to 4 mm may occur in the normal spine, but that this occurs as part of a complex coupled motion combined with lateral bending and rotation. A stronger coupling pattern occurs at this joint when axial rotation of C-1 on C-2 is associated with vertical (±y) translation. The biconvexity of the C-1–C-2 articulation results in the greatest axial separation of C-1–C-2 in neutral rotation. With an increasing degree of rotation there is a closer approximation of C-1 to C-2 (Fig. 5-3).

LOWER CERVICAL SPINE

Much of the currently accepted knowledge of kinematics of the lower cervical spine is based on the work of Lysell,[57] White,[104] and Panjabi.[69,104] Representative values of the three major motions of flexion–extension, lateral bending, and axial rotation are shown in Table 5-2. Dunsker's[20] data differs somewhat with regard to the absolute numbers, but the degree of relative motion between motion segments is in agreement. Flexion–extension is greatest in the central region, particularly at C-5–C-6.[69,76,104] The range of lateral bending and axial rotation diminishes from cephalad to caudad. Translation along the z-axis has been measured by Panjabi.[71] He found the upper limit

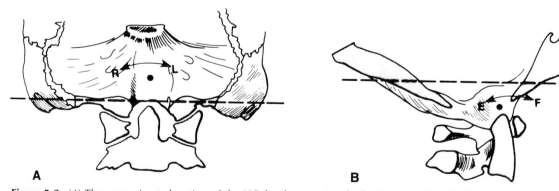

Figure 5-2. (A) The approximate location of the IAR for the occipitoatloid joint in the frontal plane. Lateral bending (R, L) of the occiput on C-1 is thought to take place around the indicated dot. The broken line indicates the approximate location of the IAR for the flexion-extension (F, E) motion in the sagittal plane. (B) The converse is shown in the sagittal plane. The broken line localizes the IAR for lateral bending and the dot shows the axes for flexion-extension. (Sherk HH, Dunn EJ, Eismont FJ, et al: The Cervical Spine. Philadelphia, JB Lippincott, 1983)

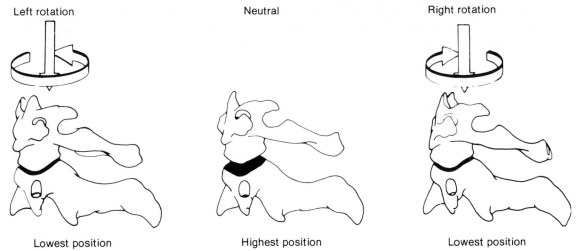

Figure 5-3. Because of the anatomic design of the lateral articulations, C-1 is highest in the middle position and lowest with the extremes of axial rotation to the right or the left. (Sherk HH, Dunn EJ, Eismont FJ et al: The Cervical Spine. Philadelphia, JB Lippincott, 1983)

of normal to be 2.7 mm. Taking radiographic magnification into account, 3.5 mm is used clinically as a guide for the upper limit of normal. Panjabi has also since shown[69] that a similar degree of lateral translation (±x) exists in a normal motion segment (3.0 mm). Y-axis translation was determined by White and associates[72] by their in vitro laboratory model for the "stretch test." They concluded that 1.7 mm was the upper limit of normal y-axis translation.[72,87] The stretch test is discussed in more detail later.

Coupling is a prominent characteristic of C-2–C-7 motion. The coupling pattern is such that with lateral bending to the left ($-\theta z$) an axial rotation to the left ($+\theta y$) occurs. An extreme example of this coupling is when this motion is carried beyond the physiologic ROM, resulting in a unilateral facet dislocation. The degree of axial rotation per degree of lateral bending can be expressed as a ratio. This ratio decreases from C-2 through C-7.[57] This is probably due to the increasingly vertical inclination of the facet joints from cephalad to

Table 5-2. Limits and Representative Values of Range of Rotation of the Lower Cervical Spine

Interspace	FLEXION–EXTENSION (X-AXIS ROTATION) Limits of Ranges (degrees)	Representative Angle (degrees)	LATERAL BENDING (Z-AXIS ROTATION) Limits of Ranges (degrees)	Representative Angle (degrees)	AXIAL ROTATION (Y-AXIS ROTATION) Limits of Ranges (degrees)	Representative Angle (degrees)
C-2–C-3	5–23	8	11–20	10	6–28	9
C-3–C-4	7–38	13	9–15	11	10–28	11
C-4–C-5	8–39	12	0–16	11	10–26	12
C-5–C-6	4–34	17	0–16	8	8–34	10
C-6–C-7	1–29	16	0–17	7	6–15	9
C-7–T-1	4–17	9	0–17	4	5–13	8

(White AA III, Panjabi MM: The basic kinematics of the human spine. Spine 3:12, 1978)

caudad. Panjabi[69] has recently detailed the coupled motion of the remaining five degrees of freedom when a force is applied along the x, y, or z axis. For more detail the reader is referred to his work.

Accurate determination of the IARs in the lower cervical spine is difficult. Most authors have concentrated on its location in the flexion–extension (z, y) plane.[18,29,33] In general, the IAR of a motion segment is found to be within the body of the subjacent vertebra. These authors have also determined geometric patterns of curvature based on radiographic studies. They hope to be able to define certain pathologic conditions because of abnormalities in the IAR of individual motion segments as well as abnormal geometric curvature patterns of the cervical spine.[47]

BIOMECHANICS OF THE SPINAL CORD

The biomechanics of the central nervous system have been well detailed by Breig.[10] He showed that the spinal cord with its investing and vascular elements exhibits good elasticity in the axial direction. Spinal extension causes the cord to shorten posteriorly and stretch anteriorly, while lateral flexion stretches the cord on the convex side and shortens it on the concave side. He also noted that the cord does not slide up and down in the spinal canal. The spinal cord is much less accommodating to translatory forces. These forces are thus more potentially injurious to the neural tissue.

CLINICAL DETERMINATION OF INSTABILITY

In the injured spine the bone–ligament complex protecting the spinal cord is disrupted. To determine the indicated course of treatment, the clinician should ask these questions: Is there unacceptable deformity? Is further deformity likely to occur? Are the neural elements endangered or injured? These questions can be answered by a systematic clinical and radiographic approach.[16,19,79]

Based on biomechanical data and pathologic observations, Louis[55, 56] proposed a three-column theory. Loss of integrity of a given column is given a score of +1. Incomplete lesions of a body or a fractured pedicle or lamina are scored +0.5. Fracture of a transverse or spinous process is scored +0.25. The lack of substance of a vertical column such as in a severe compression or bursting fracture is scored as +2. If the total injury score is +2 or greater, the lesion is considered unstable.

Louis then categorized the lesions as "temporarily unstable" or "permanently unstable." Temporarily unstable lesions are those that if appropriately protected to allow bony healing will ultimately result in a stable spine. Permanently unstable lesions are those that will yield an unstable spine even after an appropriate healing period, usually due to ligamentous or disk disruption or irreducible fracture displacement. Louis used the following criteria for the diagnosis of ligamentous instability:[55] +x-axis translation of greater than 3.0 mm above or 2.5 mm below C-4, flexion–extension range greater than 11 degrees, loss of facet contact of more than 50%, loss of facet parallelism, and interspinous widening.

White and Panjabi, based on their in vitro biomechanical studies,[72,102] developed a stretch test to determine stability. Their approach utilizes a two-column concept of the spine (Fig. 5-4). They studied cadaver specimens in flexion[102] and tension[72] with sequential transsection of supporting structures from anterior to posterior and posterior to anterior. Based on the failure patterns of their specimens they concluded that the spine could be considered clinically stable if an injured motion segment has all of its anterior elements plus one additional structure intact and, conversely, if it has all of its posterior elements plus one additional structure intact.

Flexion–extension lateral films are a clinically useful tool in determining ligamentous instability, but may be dangerous in the acutely injured spine because of the spinal cord's lack of accommodation to translatory forces. The spinal cord adapts more readily to longitudinal distraction, making stress testing in this direction neurologically safer. In their flexion testing White and Panjabi[102] concluded the spine to be unstable if +z-axis translation exceeded 3.5 mm and/or if the degree of flexion ($+\theta z$) at a motion segment exceeded the flexion at adjacent motion segments by 11 degrees. If this is apparent on initial examination no provocative tests are necessary. In doubtful cases the stretch test is a useful tool (Fig. 5-5).

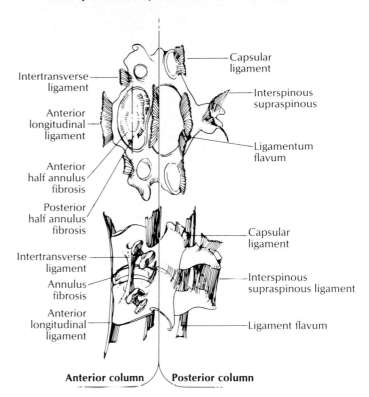

Capsular ligament

Intertransverse ligament

Interspinous supraspinous

Anterior longitudinal ligament

Ligamentum flavum

Anterior half annulus fibrosis

Posterior half annulus fibrosis

Capsular ligament

Intertransverse ligament

Interspinous supraspinous ligament

Annulus fibrosis

Anterior longitudinal ligament

Ligament flavum

Anterior column   **Posterior column**

5-4. Diagrammatic representation detailing the anatomy and separation of anterior and posterior elements.

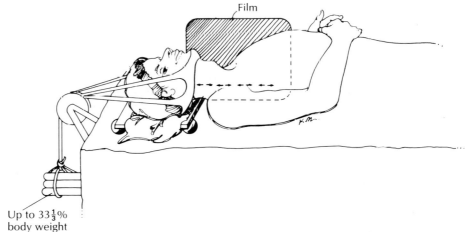

Film

Up to $33\frac{1}{3}\%$ body weight

Figure 5-5. Stretch test—this should be performed only in the presence of a physician who performs periodic neurologic examinations as the loads increase to 33% of body weight or 65 pounds. (Modified from White AA III, Panjabi MM: Clinical Biomechanics of the Spine. Philadelphia, JB Lippincott, 1978.)

Using results of the stretch test and other criteria White and Panjabi[106] developed a diagnostic checklist (Table 5-3). A score of 5 points or more determines the spine to be clinically unstable. In addition to structural damage to the spine it takes into account neural injury and the anticipation of higher-than-normal physiologic forces applied to the patient's spine in the future. Eismont and associates[22] have shown that a spinal canal that is congenitally narrow in the anteroposterior diameter increases the likelihood of neural injury in the traumatized spine. It has been suggested[106] that another point in the checklist be given for a narrow spinal canal.

BIOMECHANICS OF SPECIFIC INJURIES

Beyond the clinical history and physical examination, a major portion of useful information is obtained from radiographic examination. Using knowledge based on research data and applied in a systematic and logical fashion, the mechanism of injury can usually be deduced from the clinical picture and radiographic examination.[36,37,44,89,90,110] For the purposes of this discussion we will use the terms "major injury vector" and "minor injury vector" to describe the forces producing an injury.[2,103] Additionally, in the lower cervical spine we will use the term "transitional axis," described by Allen and associates.[2] This axis divides a motion segment into the portions exhibiting different strain patterns (different modes of tissue failure).

OCCIPITO-ATLANTAL DISLOCATION

This is a rarely encountered and usually fatal injury. Displacement can occur anteriorly, posteriorly, or rotationally. The major injury vector is along the occipital condyles in the $+z$, $-z$, or $\pm\theta y$ direction. The injury vector is presumably of fairly high magnitude, such as that seen in motor vehicle accidents. This injury may be associated with rotary subluxation or dislocation of C-1 and C-2 in the opposite direction.[75] Occiput–C1 dislocation usually causes death by injury to the spinal–medullary junction, although there are several reports of survival with varying degrees of neurologic deficit.[111] Postmortem studies have shown this to be a relatively common injury in fatal accident injuries.[1,8]

POSTERIOR ARCH FRACTURE OF C-1

This fracture occurs in a part of the ring of C-1 that is quite thin, just posterior to the lateral masses. The major injury vector is thought to be a vertical compression ($-y$) force on the posterior arch while the remainder of C-1 is fixed by the dens and facet joints. The bone then fails in the area that has the lowest sectional inertia against the

Table 5-3. Diagnostic Checklist for Spinal Stability

ELEMENTS	POINT VALUE	INDIVIDUAL CLINICAL VALUE
Anterior elements destroyed or unable to function	2	___
Posterior elements destroyed or unable to function	2	___
Relative sagittal plane translation > 3.5 mm	2	___
Relative sagittal plane rotation > 11 degrees	2	___
Positive stretch test	2	___
Cord damage	2	___
Root damage	1	___
Abnormal disk narrowing	1	___
Dangerous loading anticipated	1	___
Congenitally narrow spinal canal	1	___

Instability is defined as a total of 5 points or more, *or* a translation 20% of the anteroposterior diameter of the involved vertebra.

(White AA III, Panjabi MM: Clinical Biomechanics of the Spine. Philadelphia, JB Lippincott, 1978. Based on data from Hartman JT, Palumbo F, Hill BJ: Cineradiography of the braced normal cervical spine. Clin Orthop, 109:97, 1975)

injuring force. A minor injury vector may be a component of extension ($-\theta x$) at occiput–C-1. This injury is usually readily apparent on a good quality lateral radiograph of C-1.

JEFFERSON (BURST) FRACTURE OF C-1

The major injury vector in this injury is reasonably parallel to the y axis in a negative (caudad) direction. It is of fairly high magnitude. The geometry of the occipito-atlantal articulation is such that the axial load causes a bursting of the C-1 ring, usually into four parts: typically with two fractures anteriorly and two posteriorly. The major radiographic feature of this injury is the spread of the lateral masses of C-1 seen on the open-mouth view. Spence and associates have shown that if this spread (the combined overhang of the C-1 lateral masses) totals more than 7 mm one must assume that the transverse ligament is ruptured and the lesions must be treated accordingly.[91] In general, this is a stable injury and should heal with appropriate immobilization; however, when instability is demonstrated either early or late, surgical reconstruction should be considered.

ODONTOID FRACTURE

Odontoid fractures can be caused by a variety of flexion, extension, and rotational injuries. The precise mechanism of injury may be difficult to determine accurately because odontoid fractures have been difficult to reproduce in cadaver specimens.

Anderson and D'Alonzo[4] divided odontoid fractures into three groups. Type I is an oblique fracture through the upper portion of the dens and does not affect the stability of the motion segment. The type II fracture occurs at the junction of the dens with the vertebral body of the axis. In fractures with anterior subluxation, the major injury vector is thought to be flexion ($+\theta x$) and/or anterior translation ($+z$), whereas posteriorly displaced fractures are thought to be caused by extension ($-\theta x$) and/or posterior translation ($-z$). Undoubtedly this is oversimplified; however, no more specific data is available. Clinically, anterior displacement is much more common. Type II lesions result in an unstable C-1–C-2 motion seg-

ment and must be stabilized by the appropriate immobilization or surgical construct. Type III fractures occur through the body of the axis at the base of the dens. These usually heal with appropriate immobilization. Little is known regarding their exact mechanism of injury; however, in posteriorly displaced fractures the level (type II vs. type III), may depend on the vertical position of the ring of C-1 on the dens when the injuring force occurs.

ATLANTO-AXIAL DISLOCATION AND SUBLUXATION

Displacement of C-1 on C-2 may be anterior or posterior, or there may be rotary subluxation of C-1 on C-2. Fielding was able to consistently produce anterior subluxation of C-1 on C-2 with rupture of the transverse ligament in cadavers.[27] The major injury vector is along the $+z$ axis, although clinically the injury is probably associated with a significant degree of flexion ($+\theta x$). This is a particularly dangerous injury for two reasons. First, it is unstable. Second, anterior displacement approaching 1 cm endangers the spinal cord. This is in contrast to the anteriorly displaced odontoid fracture, in which the dens is carried forward with C-1. Posterior dislocation of C-1 on C-2 is rare. The major injury vector must combine extension ($-\theta x$) with translation directed posterosuperiorly in the y, z plane in order to carry the ring of C-1 up and over the dens. Rotary subluxation of C-1, C-2 is an unusual lesion. When caused by trauma the mechanism of injury is thought to be acute axial rotation, with the major injury vector being $\pm\theta y$. There is usually disruption of the joint capsules with subluxation or dislocation of one or both joints, resulting in varying degrees of spinal canal compromise. This lesion is usually not truly traumatic in origin. For a more detailed discussion the reader is referred to the work of Fielding.[25]

TRAUMATIC SPONDYLOLISTHESIS OF THE AXIS

This lesion is often called the "hangman's fracture." The injury caused by judicial hanging is a fracture of the axis through the pars interarticularis, separating the anterior from the posterior elements of the vertebra. The use of a submental knot causes an extension–distraction type of injury with the injury vectors in the $-\theta x$ and $+y$ directions (the major and minor injury vectors depending on which has the greater magnitude). The anterior elements (usually the annulus fibrosus) fail in tension, and bending causes failure of the pars interarticularis.

The modern counterpart of this injury is most commonly the result of a motor vehicle accident. The injury vectors here are somewhat different: the first is an axial load ($-y$) and the second is extension ($-\theta x$). Extension is usually the major injury vector. The anatomy of the neural arch helps to explain the site of failure. The pars interarticularis of the axis has a relatively low area moment of inertia to bending in the z, y (sagittal) plane. In this injury there is an extension moment on the dens and body with a balancing joint reaction force at the C-2–C-3 articulation. The force then causes failure of the pars. As continued loading occurs, disruption of the anterior longitudinal ligament takes place, followed by failure of the annulus with separation from either the superior or inferior end-plate. There is now instability between the cervix and cranium and the lower cervical spine. The next stage is anterior subluxation of C-2 on C-3, with the motion segment adopting a flexed posture. Because of an actual widening of the spinal canal, neurologic injury with this lesion is relatively rare.

FRACTURES OF THE LOWER CERVICAL SPINE

The lower cervical spine will be considered together, although certain injury patterns are more common at one level than another. Patterns and mechanisms of injury will be described using the classification of Allen and associates.[2]

Compressive Flexion

This group of injuries has a major injury vector that lies in the sagittal (z, y) plane directed obliquely caudad and posteriorly. With the spine in flexion the stress is propagated through the anterior elements. This phylogeny is divided into five stages according to the severity of the injury, ranging from blunting of the anterosuperior ver-

tebral margin in stage 1 to vertebral body disruption with canal compromise and posterior ligament disruption in stage 5. In stage 4 and 5 lesions there is a minor injury vector in tension ($+y$). The transitional axis, or the axis separating strain patterns (different modes of failure), occurs at the site where the vertebral body fracture crosses the inferior chondral plate. This marks the transition from compression to tension–shear failure.

Vertical Compression

The major injury vector in this phylogeny is along the y axis in the negative (caudad) direction. This group is divided into three stages according to the severity of the disruption. In the most severe stage (stage 3) there is compressive failure of the entire vertebral body (bursting fracture). Late in the injury there may be a minor injury vector of flexion or extension, shifting the transitional axis anteriorly or posteriorly, respectively. This may explain the presence or absence of an associated vertebral arch fracture.

Distractive Flexion

The characteristic lesion in this group is tension–shear failure of the posterior ligamentous complex. The major injury vector, therefore, is translation along the y axis in the posterior direction. If the transitional axis lies within the vertebral body there may be a minor injury vector of compression ($-y$), causing a minor vertebral body compression injury anteriorly.

The different stages of this phylogeny warrant separate discussion. The stage 1 lesion shows evidence of posterior ligamentous injury by facet subluxation in flexion, anterior displacement of the vertebral body, and kyphotic angulation of the vertebral bodies with divergence of the spinous processes, the so-called "hyperflexion sprain."[35,67,84,85,86] There may be an associated minor compression fracture of the body below. The stage 2 lesion is the unilateral facet dislocation. It is believed that, rather than being caused by a rotational force, the rotation necessary to produce this injury is an exaggeration of the normal coupled motion when lateral bending is produced by off-center distraction.[81] Stage 3 is the bilateral facet dislocation, with approximately 50% vertebral body displacement. Further loading results in stage 4, with complete anterior and posterior disruption and gross instability.

Compressive Extension

This group of injuries has a major injury vector of axial compression ($-y$) with the spine postured in extension. The posterior elements are stressed in compression. This group is divided into five stages according to the degree of injury. Stages 1 and 2 consist of unilateral and bilateral vertebral arch fractures. Stages 3 and 4 are described hypothetically, and stage 5 is essentially a traumatic spondylolisthesis-type injury with significant displacement.

Distractive Extension

The distractive extension phylogeny has a major injury vector along the $+y$ axis (axial distraction) with the spine postured in extension. This stresses the anterior elements in tension. This group has no significant minor injury vector and the transitional axis lies far posterior in the cervical spine. In stage 1 of this injury failure occurs only in the anterior column of the spine (either ligament and annulus or vertebral body), while in stage 2 the failure extends to include the posterior ligamentous complex, sometimes displacing the upper vertebral body into the spinal canal. Because of minimal residual displacement many of these injuries may go unrecognized.[13]

Lateral Flexion

This group of injuries has a major injury vector parallel to the y axis in compression ($-y$) but offset laterally ($\pm x$) to the side of lateral bending. On the side to which the lateral bend occurs there are compressive stresses, causing failure. If the transitional axis is within the spine there may be a minor injury vector of distraction, causing injury on the opposite side. This phylogeny is divided into two stages according to the severity of anatomic injury.

Which of the injuries discussed above are stable and which are unstable? Acute instability can, to a degree, be determined by applying the criteria of displacement at rest and, if necessary, employing the aid of provocative tests such as the stretch test. When making treatment decisions, however, the clinician must take into account several other factors. He or she must be aware of the natural history of a specific lesion in terms of its potential for healing and restoration of stability. This is best accomplished by determining which specific anatomic structures are injured. Other factors are the degree of neural injury present and the potential for further neural injury. Malalignment and the need for correction is a controversial topic. In general, it is accepted that if malalignment can be corrected without undue risk to the patient or his or her neurologic status, it should be.

BIOMECHANICS OF RESTORATION OF STABILITY

Once the clinician has determined the degree of injury to the patient's cervical spine, he or she must outline the specific goals to be achieved en route to a stable, pain-free spine without significant deformity. Of paramount importance is the protection of the spinal cord and nerve roots. The immediate goals may include support of the spine, immobilization, or correction of deformity. These goals may be accomplished by traction, an orthosis, surgical reconstruction, or a combination of these.

TRACTION

Traction to the cervical spine may be applied by various methods. These include a head halter, various tongs, and a halo device. It is difficult to determine how much traction should be used for a given injury.[62] When traction is used for fixation and not reduction of a deformity, White[103] has recommended a force of 8 to 18 lb. To obtain physiologic alignment he recommended 18 to 22 lb, and for correction of a deformity 22 to 62 lb. Based on clinical experience, Crutchfield recom-

Table 5-4. Cervical Traction Weights for Treatment of Fractures and Dislocations at Various Levels in the Cervical Spine

LEVEL OF INJURY	MINIMUM WEIGHT KG (LB)	MAXIMUM WEIGHT KG (LB)
C-1	2.3 (5)	4.5 (10)
C-2	2.7 (6)	5.4 (12)
C-3	3.6 (8)	6.8 (15)
C-4	4.5 (10)	9.0 (20)
C-5	5.4 (12)	11.3 (25)
C-6	6.8 (15)	13.6 (30)
C-7	8.2 (18)	15.9 (35)

(Crutchfield WG: Skeletal traction in the treatment of injuries to the cervical spine. JAMA, 155:129, 1954. Copyright © 1954, American Medical Association)

mended traction forces based on the level of injury (Table 5-4).

The use of traction for correction of deformity is common with unilateral and bilateral facet dislocation. Miller and associates[61] developed a biomechanical model likening the injured cervical spine and neck to a spring. In this model, $F_{traction}$ equals $K_{neck} \Delta X$, where F is the traction weight, K_{neck} is the calculated spring constant of the neck and X is the distraction required to achieve the perched facet position to allow reduction. Based on their clinical material they were able to calculate a consistent value for K_{neck} that differs for unilateral and bilateral facet dislocations. Using their data the

traction weight needed to reduce facet dislocations can be estimated from the formula: F = 107.1 lb/cm (X) for unilateral and F = 76.4 lb/cm (X) for bilateral dislocations.

ORTHOSES

The goal of a cervical orthosis is to control the position of the cervical spine by the application of external forces. Because of the anatomic structure of the neck these forces must be applied at the ends of the cervical spine, i.e. the thorax and skull. The degree of immobilization of any given orthosis, then, depends on how well it is attached to the skull and thorax. There are basically four categories of cervical orthoses:

1. Collars
2. Poster orthoses
3. Cervicothoracic orthoses
4. Halo devices.

The decision as to which orthosis is appropriate for a specific injury must be made on the knowledge of the degree of immobilization or corrective force that can be attained with each one.[34,49,60] Hartman and associates[39] evaluated normal motion and motion in five different orthoses using cineradiography. The results of this study are seen in Table 5-5. In another study Johnson and associates[38,50] measured cervical motion in normal

Table 5-5. Effectiveness of Cervical Spine Orthoses in Immobilization

ORTHOSIS	APPROXIMATE % RESTRICTION OF RANGE OF MOTION C-1–C-7					
	Motion Picture			Cineradiograph		
	FE	LB	AR	FE	LB	AR
Soft cervical collar	5–10	5–10	0	0	0	0
Hard plastic collar (Thomas)	75	75	50	75	75	50
Four-poster cervical	80–85	80–85	60	85	85	60
Long two-poster	95	90	90	90	90	90
Guilford two-poster	90–95	90–95	90–95	90	90–95	90
Halo device	Essentially no motion					

FE: Flexion–extension (x-axis rotation), LB: Lateral bending (z-axis rotation), AR: Axial rotation (y-axis rotation)

(White AA III, Panjabi MM: Clinical Biomechanics of the Spine. Philadelphia, JB Lippincott, 1978. Based on data from Hartman JT, Palumbo F, Hill BJ: Cineradiography of the braced normal cervical spine. Clin Orthop, 109:97, 1975)

subjects using conventional orthoses and in several patients in the halo vest. They also reported the results as the percentage of normal motion allowed by the orthosis (Table 5-6).

Using these and other data[54,109] we note that some orthoses are more effective in limiting motion at particular levels of the spine or in limiting motion in a particular plane. In our opinion, the skull occiput mandibular immobilization (SOMI) brace is most effective for limiting flexion ($+\theta x$) from C-1 to C-5, and the cervicothoracic orthosis (CTO) is more effective between C-5 and T-1 than other conventional orthoses. The CTO is effective in controlling extension ($-\theta x$) at all levels. Halo devices are most effective in controlling overall flexion and extension; however, several investigators[14,39,54,109] have noted so-called "paradoxical" motion of adjacent motion segments, where one motion segment may flex and adjacent ones simultaneously extend.

Rotational control ($\pm\theta y$) by an orthosis is less consistent. The CTO is the most effective of the conventional orthoses, but still allows 18% of normal motion.[50] Halo devices are significantly more effective when optimal rotational control is required, allowing only 1% to 2% of normal motion.[50,109] Lateral bending ($\pm\theta z$) is also difficult to control with an orthosis. The CTO and four-poster braces are the most effective of the conventional orthoses, yet limit only approximately 50% of normal motion. The halo vest is much more effec-

tive, limiting lateral bending to 4% of normal in Johnson's study.[50]

In considering individual orthoses we start with the soft collar. This device provides no significant immobilization; however, it may provide supportive treatment for minor injuries.[52] The Philadelphia collar is significantly more effective in controlling flexion–extension, but is relatively ineffective in rotation and lateral bending. Poster braces are most effective in controlling midcervical flexion and exert reasonable control in the other planes of motion nearly as well as the CTO.

The cervicothoracic orthoses are the most effective of the conventional orthoses in limiting motion. Their primary deficiency is in control of lateral bending. The SOMI brace is particularly popular because it is easy to apply and is well tolerated by patients who are not confined to bed (bedridden patients have difficulty with the posterior portions of the yoke pressing into the scapulae).

Halo devices are attached to the thorax, usually by means of either a plastic vest or plaster cast.[15] A third method, reported by Appleby,[5] is a modification using an external fixator-type framepin attached to the clavicles and scapulae. This has the advantage of greater access to the thorax and abdomen in the patient with multiple trauma. Wolf, in his study, was unable to detect a significant difference between halo–cast and halo–vest devices in efficacy of immobilization. A disturbing finding

Table 5-6. Normal Cervical Motion Allowed From the Occiput to the First Thoracic Vertebra

	NUMBER OF SUBJECTS	MEAN AGE (YRS)	MEAN % OF NORMAL MOTION		
			Flexion–Extension	Lateral Bending	Rotation
Normal	44	25.8	100	100	100
Soft collar	20	26.2	74.2	92.3	82.6
Philadelphia collar	17	25.8	28.9	66.4	43.7
SOMI brace	22	25.0	27.7	65.6	33.6
Four-poster brace	27	25.9	20.6	45.9	27.1
Rigid cervicothoracic brace	27	25.9	12.8	50.5	18.2
Halo vest	7	40.0	4	4	1

(Sherk HH, Dunn EJ, Eismont FJ et al: The Cervical Spine. Philadelphia, JB Lippincott, 1987. After Johnson RM, Hart DL, Simmons EF et al: Cervical orthoses: A study comparing their effectiveness in restricting cervical motion in normal subjects. J Bone Joint Surg (Am) 59:332, 1977)

in investigations of halo-device motion is a large degree of sum total segmental motion, as much as 51 degrees in flexion–extension.[41] Koch and Nickel[14] also found significant differences in distraction and compression forces across the spine depending on the position of the patient as well as his or her current activity, such as walking, standing, and shrugging the shoulders. They recommended the development of a constant-tension spring device to allow application of consistent forces to the injured spine.

The clinician must take all of these factors into account in selecting the orthosis that is best suited for the particular patient. The selection must be based on the specific bony–ligamentous injury and neurologic status of the patient as well as the ability of the patient to tolerate a particular appliance. Wolf and Johnson[108] have made some general recommendations for specific clinical conditions (Table 5-7).

SURGICAL RECONSTRUCTION

In reconstruction of an unstable injury of the cervical spine the goal is to restore structural integrity with minimal decrease in normal mobility and minimal disruption of the normal structure of the spine and surrounding structures. The corner-

stone of such reconstruction is the creation of an arthrodesis with or without the aid of some sort of internal fixation.[64] Spinal canal decompression is covered elsewhere in this text; however, the route and extent of a decompressive procedure obviously greatly influences both the type and the extent of reconstruction required to achieve a stable spine.[77] The indications for surgery and the description of specific procedures is well covered elsewhere in this text. We will focus here on the mechanics of surgical constructs and their respective behavior in clinical use.

An important concept in the consideration of constructs is that of immediate postoperative stability.[9,105] This is the stability present at the completion of the surgical procedure prior to any healing. This is dependent on the composition, shape, and placement of the graft material as well as the preoperative degree of instability. It may be augmented by both internal and external fixation. Autogenous bone, especially in children,[92] is usually preferable, although there is some data showing that the bone source makes little difference.[88] The graft is most commonly harvested from the ilium and less frequently from the fibula, ribs, or tibia. Figure 5-6 shows a representative selection of grafts for various constructs. A common misconception in the use of bone grafts is that

Table 5-7. Wolf and Johnson's Recommendations for Orthoses for Use in Selected Clinical Conditions and Injuries

CLINICAL CONDITION	PLANE OF INSTABILITY	RECOMMENDED ORTHOSIS
"Cervical Strain"	None	Philadelphia collar
Ring of C-1 (Jefferson fracture)		
Stable	None	Cervicothoracic
Unstable	All	Halo
Odontoid fracture		
Type I	None	Cervicothoracic
Types II and III	All	Halo
C-2 neural arch fracture (hangman's fracture)		
Stable	Flexion	SOMI
Unstable	All	Halo
Flexion injuries		
Midcervical C-3–C-5	Flexion	SOMI, cervicothoracic
Low cervical C-5–T-1	Flexion	Cervicothoracic
Extension Injuries		
Midcervical C-3–C-5	Extension	Halo, Cervicothoracic
Low cervical C-5–T-1	Extension	Halo

(Wolf JW, Johnson RM: Physiology and biomechanics. In Cervical Spine Research Society (ed): The Cervical Spine, Philadelphia, JB Lippincott, 1983)

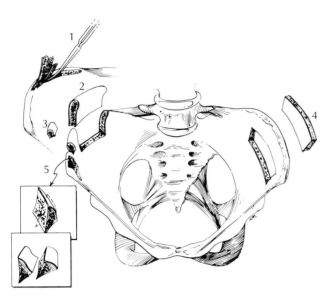

5. Fashioned for
Brooks C-1 to C-2

Figure 5-6. Diagrammatic representation of some of the various combinations and configurations of bone grafts available from the ilium. (1) Cancellous bone may be curetted from any portion of the iliac crest. (2) Various lengths of horseshoe-shaped tricortical cancellous graft may be taken for trough grafts and vertebral body replacements. (3) The smaller horseshoe configuration used in the Smith–Robinson fusion. (4) A bicortical piece of iliac crest may be harvested. This will preserve the natural contour of the iliac crest, but at the expense of weakening the graft compared to a tricortical piece. (5) A part of the ilium of variable sizes may be taken and fashioned for the Brooks C-1–C-2 fusion. (Adapted from White AA III, Panjabi MM: Clinical Biomechanics of the Spine. Philadelphia, JB Lippincott, 1978)

bone grafts loaded under tension will be resorbed. According to Wolff's law, bone is laid down according to the stress applied; the bone laid down under tensile stress, of course, will have a different structure and different biomechanical properties than the bone laid down in a compression. According to White and Panjabi,[105] any resorption of a fusion mass is more likely to be related to a level of strain that exceeds the strength of the differentiating tissue.

Stabilization of the Upper Cervical Spine (Occiput–C-1–C-2)

Anterior Constructs. Anterior constructs for fusion of the occiput–atlanto-axial complex utilize diffi-
cult surgical approaches such as that of Henry[41] or the proximal extension of the anterolateral Smith–Robinson approach described by DeAndrade and MacNab.[17] DeAndrade and MacNab described their approach for performance of anterior occipitoatloid fusion when a posterior approach or construct is not feasible. The fusion construct is an onlay bone graft and adds no immediate postoperative stability. It is recommended that postoperative immobilization be achieved with a halo device. Another anterior construct is that described by Barbour for atlanto-axial fusion.[6] This construct involves an anterior facet fusion at C-1–C-2 with bilateral screw fixation. This construct is very technically demanding to achieve; however, it provides good immediate postoperative stability. The transoral route is another approach to this region of the spine; however, it is difficult to achieve a construct that lends any immediate stability with this route.

Posterior Constructs. Indications for fusion to the occiput are rare. When there is little concern for immediate postoperative stability, a simple onlay bone graft with postoperative halo fixation will suffice. For the acutely unstable situation Robinson and Southwick have described a construct using two large cortical cancellous grafts wired segmentally from the occiput caudad as far as the fusion is required to extend.[80] Such a fusion should only extend as far caudad as absolutely necessary because of the great loss of motion already caused by the fusion of occiput to C1 and C1 to C2. Murphy[65] has used Harrington instrumentation in a modified manner as an anchor for the segmental wires following a laminectomy.

Three fusion constructs are most commonly used for C-1–C-2 fusions: the Gallie,[31] Fielding's modification of the Gallie,[28] and Brooks'[11] fusion and its modifications. With each specific injury one must consider the plane or planes of instability involved. The Gallie, or midline wiring technique with an onlay bone graft, provides little protection against axial rotation ($\pm\theta y$), which is a major component of normal C-1–C-2 motion. Additionally, when the wire is tightened, C-1–C-2 is drawn into extension ($-\theta x$) as the laminae are approximated. This may result in further displacement or redisplacement of a posteriorly displaced odontoid fracture. A mechanically sounder construct for C-1–C-2 fusion is Fielding's modification.[28] Fixation is provided by a cortical cancellous H-shaped graft tailored to fit the arch of C-1 and notched for the spinous process of C-2. It is fixed with a wire passed around the arch of C-1 and through the base of the C-2 spinous process. The graft provides a block in extension, the wire blocks flexion, and the apposition of the graft to the arch of C-1 and the lamina of C-2 provides some degree of rotational control. The best rotational control is probably provided by the Brooks type of construct, in which a cortical cancellous wedge is fixed to either side of the midline by either one or a pair of sublaminar wires passed around the arch of C-1 and the lamina of C-2. The wires, being some distance from the midline, provide improved control of axial rotation. Paired wires on each side improve the degree of control, but with greater risk of neural injury.

Stabilization of the Lower Cervical Spine (C-2–C-7)

The decision as to whether an anterior or posterior construct would best stabilize the spine in a given situation is often complicated by a simultaneously contemplated spinal canal decompression. Capen and associates[12] reported on the results of anterior compared to posterior fusions with regard to perioperative morbidity, late complications, and efficacy of stabilization. The complication rates were similar but the anterior group had more serious complications, such as visceral injury and transient neurologic loss. There were also six cases of graft dislodgment (6%). On late follow-up, 36% of the anterior fusion group developed a kyphosis averaging 22 degrees between the time of surgery and complete healing of the fusion. The posterior fusion group, in contrast, had no late changes in alignment. Nearly 75%, however, had significant extension of their fusion mass beyond the originally intended levels. They concluded that posterior fusion is the treatment of choice for cervical spine instability and that when anterior spinal canal decompression is necessary, simultaneous posterior fusion or halo immobilization should be considered to maintain alignment.

Capen and associates also noted that posterior ligamentous disruption is not always evident on radiographic examination. This is particularly true in those lesions most often treated by anterior decompression and in fusions such as compressive flexion stages 4 and 5 and vertical compression stage 3 injuries. Many other authors have also warned against relying on an anterior fusion construct to provide stability in the face of posterior ligamentous disruption.[30,53,58,94,97,98]

Ulrich and associates,[95,96] using cadaver specimens, compared the stability of several anterior and posterior constructs both in the intact spine and after severance of all the discoligamentous structures at a particular motion segment. They compared an anteriorly applied H-plate affixed to the vertebral bodies above and below the lesion; a posteriorly applied "hook" plate affixed with screws to the lateral masses of the superior vertebra, with a hook extending around the base of the spinous process below (creating a tension band effect); interspinous wiring; and anterior–posterior combinations. The constructs were tested by applying a distractive (+y) force to the base of the superior spinous process, creating a flexion (+θx) moment in the motion segment. With posterior disruption alone, both posterior constructs were superior to the anterior plate and little was gained by adding the anterior plate to the posterior constructs. In combined anterior–posterior instability, the combined anterior–posterior constructs provided superior stability; however, the authors felt that based on their data the hook plate alone may be sufficient. Posterior wiring alone provided much less stability. Anterior plating alone was grossly inadequate in this situation, again confirming the need for a posterior column stabilizer, either internal or external.

Anterior Constructs. Several grafting techniques have been described for anterior cervical spine fusions. Simmons[103] has described a keystone bone graft for a single-level fusion and has shown it to be clinically efficacious as well as biomechanically sound. White and associates[101] compared the immediate load-bearing capacities of three other commonly used constructs: Cloward's dowel graft, Smith and Robinson's tricortical iliac crest graft, and Bailey and Badgley's graft. The Smith–Robinson type of graft provided superior resistance to vertical loading, to a degree because the vertebral end-plates are left intact. Vertebrectomy requires the use of a larger graft, which may be a modified Bailey and Badgley-type graft or another variation using tricortical iliac crest or fibula. The fibular graft is the strongest of these, but takes much longer to become completely incorporated.

Adjunctive internal fixation with anteriorly applied plates has been described by several authors.[7,32,51,66,98] Some have used AO (Arbeitsgemeinschaft für Osteosynthese) "small-fragment" plates, while others have designed plates specifically to fit the anterior cervical spine. These authors document the successful clinical use of anterior cervical plates; however, there is little experimental evidence in the literature documenting the degree of enhanced stability provided.[95,96] This information is necessary before one can decide whether the potential benefits justify the additional risks of the procedure.

Posterior Constructs. The simplest posterior fusion construct is onlay bone graft, which obviously provides no immediate postoperative stability. Posterior fusions, therefore, are usually augmented by some form of internal fixation. Posterior wiring techniques offer a degree of immediate postoperative stability. The wire is passed through the base of the spinous process at the superior level and around the base of the spinous process below. If multiple levels are to be fixed, the process is repeated so that the entire length of the fusion is encircled with an additional wire. Ulrich found the "hook" plate to provide somewhat better stability than simple wiring techniques.[95,96]

For multiple-level fusions in which the spinous processes and lamina are incompetent or missing, Robinson and Southwick[80] have described a posterolateral facet fusion. Here a strong cortical cancellous graft is wired to the respective facet joints on either side of the spine. Stability is enhanced by segmental fixation as well as the strength of the particular graft chosen. Murphy[63] has augmented fixation in this situation with segmental wiring to a U-shaped rod or with modified Harrington instrumentation, which offers the versatility of using compression or distraction as necessary to help achieve or maintain reduction of a particular deformity.

Roy-Camille[82] uses a construct of his own design featuring small metal plates anchored by screws to the articular masses of the adjacent vertebrae. Savini[83] has found this method particularly useful in a staged approach for correction of late post-traumatic deformities. Successful use of all these techniques is reported regularly; however, there is little experimental biomechanical data to support the selection of a particular technique in a given clinical situation.

Methyl Methacrylate

Polymethyl methacrylate (PMMA) is well accepted as an adjunct to cervical spine reconstruction in tumor cases. Its role in traumatic instability remains to be clarified. In general, spinal reconstruction for trauma will be subjected to greater forces for a longer period of time than that for tumor, thus longevity of the construct is a primary consideration. The weak point of any construct using bone and PMMA is, of course, the bone–PMMA interface. It is also well known that the bone–PMMA interface and PMMA itself resist compressive loading much better than they resist tensile loading.[105]

Polymethyl methacrylate may be used clinically as a spacer or for internal fixation. Used as a spacer anteriorly, it provides adequate stability against flexion and, to a degree, lateral bending and rotation.[103] Wang and associates have tested several such anterior constructs to determine their stability in extension.[99] None of the many constructs tested were able to regain the normal structural strength in extension. An additional finding was that combined anterior and posterior fixation did not provide further strength, although it did increase the rigidity of the fixation.

Panjabi and associates tested the spine of a patient 7 years after anterior and posterior reconstruction for a tumor using PMMA.[68] They found the PMMA to be essentially intact, and also noted the formation of a bony arthrodesis. The spine exhibited reduced motion in flexion–extension with little change in rotation and lateral bending. It also displayed good strength when loaded to failure. It appears that the formation of a bony arthrodesis had a protective effect on the PMMA. The authors concluded on the basis of this that the clinical use of PMMA in stabilization of the cervical spine is biomechanically sound, especially if some provision can be made for the formation of a bony arthrodesis. The use of PMMA posteriorly in the cervical spine places the cement under a tensile load, however. In this biomechanically disadvantaged situation the PMMA has a high incidence of loosening at the bone–PMMA interface.[21]

SUMMARY

As is apparent from this review, there is much work to be done to elucidate the biomechanical behavior of the cervical spine in its normal and abnormal states. Several mathematical models[45,59,107] have been developed that show promise in helping toward this end. Using these models we should be able to both test existing surgical constructs and develop new and improved fixation methods. We should then be able to predict the in vivo behavior of the new constructs even prior to their first clinical use.

REFERENCES

1. Alker GJ, Oh YS, Leslie EV: Post mortem radiology of head and neck injuries in fatal traffic accidents. J Neuroradiol 114:611–616, 1975
2. Allen BL, Ferguson RL, Lehmann TR et al: A mechanistic classification of closed indirect fractures and dislocations of the lower cervical spine. Spine 7:1–27, 1982
3. Alpar EK, Karpinski M: Late stability of the cervical spine. Arch Orthop Trauma Surg 104:224–226, 1985
4. Anderson LD, D'Alonzo RT: Fractures of the odontoid process of the axis, J Bone Joint Surg [Am] 56:60–64, 1974
5. Appleby DM, Fu FH, Mears DC: Halo-clavicle traction. J Trauma 24:452–455, 1984
6. Barbour JR: Screw fixation in fracture of the odontoid process. South Australian Clinics 5:20–24, 1971
7. Bohler J, Gaudernak T: Anterior plate stabilization for fracture dislocations of the lower cervical spine. J Trauma 20:203–205, 1980
8. Bohlman HH: Acute fractures and dislocations of the cervical spine. J Bone Joint Surg [Am] 61:1119–1142, 1979
9. Boni M, Denaro V: Surgical treatment of traumatic lesions of the middle and lower cervical spine. Ital J Orthop Traumatol 6:305–320, 1980
10. Breig A: Biomechanics of the Nervous System: Some Basic Normal and Pathologic Phenomena. Stockholm, Almquist & Wiksell, 1960
11. Brooks AL, Jenkins EG: Atlanto-axial arthrodesis by the wedge compression methods. J Bone Joint Surg [Am] 60:279–284, 1978
12. Capen DA, Garland DE, Waters RL: Surgical stabilization of the cervical spine: A comparative analysis of anterior and posterior spine fusion. Clin Orthop 196:229–237, 1985
13. Carter DR, Frankel VH: Biomechanics of hyperextension injuries to the cervical spine in football. Am J Sports Med 8:302–309, 1980
14. Coch PR, Nickel VL: The halo vest and evaluation of motion and forces across the neck. Spine 3:103–107, 1978
15. Cooper PR, Maravilla KR, Sklar FH et al: Halo immobilization of cervical spine fractures. J Neurosurg 50:603–610, 1979
16. Daffner RH, Deeb ZL, Rothfus WE: Fingerprints of vertebral trauma: A unifying concept based on mechanisms. Skeletal Radiol 15:518–525, 1986
17. DeAndrade JR, MacNab I: Anterior occipital cervical fusion using an extrapharyngeal exposure. J Bone Joint Surg [Am] 51:1621–1626, 1969
18. Dimnet J, Pasquet AL, Krag MH: Cervical spine motion in the sagittal plane: Kinematic and geometric parameters. J Biomech 15:959–969, 1982
19. Dolan KD: Radiological determination of cervical spine fracture and stability. Clin Neurosurg 27:368–384, 1980
20. Dunsker SB, Colley DP, Mayfield FH: Kinematics of the spine. Clin Neurosurg 25:174–183, 1977
21. Eismont FJ, Bohlman HH: Posterior methyl methacrylate fixation for cervical trauma. Spine 6:347–353, 1981
22. Eismont FJ, Cliffort S, Goldberg M et al: Cervical sagittal spinal canal size in spine injury. Spine 9:663–666, 1984
23. Fick R: Handbuch der Anatomie und Mechanik der Gelenke. Jena, S Fischer, 1904
24. Fielding JW: Cineroentgenography of the normal cervical spine. J Bone Joint Surg [Am] 39:1280–1285, 1957
25. Fielding JW: Injuries to the upper cervical spine. In Griffin PP (ed): Instructional Course Lectures, Vol 36. Chicago, AAOS, 1987
26. Fielding JW: Normal and selected abnormal motion of the cervical spine from the second cervical vertebra to the seventh cervical vertebra based on cineroentgenography. J Bone Joint Surg [Am] 46:1779–1784, 1964
27. Fielding JW, Cochran GVB, Lansing JF III et al: Tears of the transverse ligament of the atlas: A

clinical and biomechanical study. J Bone Joint Surg [Am] 56:1683–1687, 1974

28. Fielding JW, Hawkins RJ, Sanford AR: Spine fusion for atlanto-axial instability. J Bone Joint Surg [Am] 58:400–407, 1976

29. Fineschi GF, Logroscino CA, Leali PT: Lower cervical spine: Biomechanical and clinical combined approach. In Cervical Spine I. New York, Springer-Verlag, 1987

30. Foley MJ, Lee C, Calenoff L et al: Radiologic evaluation of surgical cervical spine fusion. AJR 138:79–89, 1982

31. Gallie WE: Fractures and dislocations of the cervical spine. Am J Surg 46:495–501, 1939

32. Glynn MK, Sheehan JM: Fusion of the cervical spine for instability. Clin Orthop 179:97–101, 1983

33. Gonon JP, Deschamps G, Dimnet J et al: Kinematic study of the inferior cervical spine and sagittal plane. In Cervical Spine I. Chicago, Springer-Verlag, 1987

34. Grady MS, Howard MA, Jane JA et al: Use of the Philadelphia collar as an alternative to the halo vest in patients with C2, C3 fractures. Neurosurgery 18:151–156, 1986

35. Green JD, Harle TS, Harris JH: Anterior subluxation of the cervical spine: Hyperflexion sprain. AJNR 2:243–250, 1981

36. Gui L, Savini R, Martucci E et al: Diagnosis and treatment of cervical instability. Ital J Orthop Traumatol 8:131–144, 1982

37. Harris JA, Edeiken-Monroe B, Kopaniky DR: A practical classification of acute cervical spine injuries. Orthop Clin North Am 17:15–30, 1986

38. Hart DL, Johnson RM, Simmons EF et al: Review of cervical orthoses. Phys Ther 58:857–860, 1978

39. Hartmann JT, Palumbo F, Hill BJ: Cineradiography of the braced normal cervical spine. Clin Orthop 109:97–112, 1975

40. Henke W: Handbuch der Anatomie und Mechanik der Gelenke. Leipzig & Heidelberg, 1863

41. Henry AK: Extensile Exposure. Baltimore, Williams & Wilkens, 1963

42. Herkowitz HN, Rothman RH: Subacute instability of the cervical spine. Spine 9:348–357, 1984

43. Hohl M, Baker HR: The atlanto-axial joint radiographic and anatomical study of normal and abnormal motion. J Bone Joint Surg [Am] 46:1739–1752, 1964

44. Huelke DF, Mendelsohn RA, States JD et al: Cervical fractures and fracture dislocation sustained without head impact. J Trauma 18:533–538, 1978

45. Huelke DF, Nusholtz GS: Cervical spine biomechanics: A review of the literature. Journal of Orthopedic Research 4:232–245, 1986

46. Jackson H: Diagnosis of minimal atlanto-axial subluxation. Br J Radiol 23:672–676, 1950

47. Jirout J: Persistence of the synkinetic patterns of the cervical spine. Neuroradiology 18:167–171, 1979

48. Jofe MH, White AA III, Panjabi MM: Physiology and biomechanics. In Cervical Spine Research Society (ed): The Cervical Spine. Philadelphia, JB Lippincott, 1983

49. Johnson JL, Cannon D: Nonoperative treatment of the acute teardrop fracture of the cervical spine. Clin Orthop 168:108–112, 1982

50. Johnson RM, Hart DL, Simmons EF et al: Cervical orthoses: A study comparing their effectiveness in restricting cervical motion in normal subjects. J Bone Joint Surg [Am] 59:332–339, 1977

51. Korkala O, Kytomaa J: Reduction and fixation of late diagnosed lower cervical spine dislocations using the Daab plate. Arch Orthop Trauma Surg 103:353–355, 1984

52. LaRocca H: Acceleration injuries of the neck. Clin Neurosurg 25:209–217, 1978

53. Light TR, Wagner FC et al: Correction of spinal instability and recovery of neurologic loss following cervical vertebral body replacement. Spine 5:392–394, 1980

54. Lind B, Sihlbom H, Nordwall A: Forces in motions across the neck in patients treated with halo vests for unstable cervical spine fractures. In Cervical Spine I. Chicago, Springer-Verlag, 1987

55. Louis R: Stability and instability of the cervical spine. In Cervical Spine I. Chicago, Springer-Verlag, 1987

56. Louis R, Bonsignour JP, Ouiminga R: Reduction orthopedique controlee des fractures du rachis. Rev Chir Orthop 61:323–328, 1975

57. Lysell E: Motion of the cervical spine. Acta Orthop Scand [Suppl] 123:5–58, 1969

58. Mazur JM, Stauffer ES: Unrecognized spinal instability associated with seemingly simple cervical compression fractures. Spine 8:687–692, 1983

59. Merrill T, Goldsmith W, Dang YC: Three dimensional response of a lumped parameter head–neck model due to impact and impulse of loading. J Biomech 17:81–95, 1984

60. Milington PJ, Ellingsen JM, Hauswirth BE et al: Thermoplastic minerva body jacket: A practical alternative to current methods of cervical spine stabilization. Phys Ther 67:223–225, 1987

61. Miller LS, Cotler HB, Delucia FA et al: Biome-

chanical analysis of cervical distraction. Spine 12:831–837, 1987

62. Misasi N, Milano C, Cotugno GF et al: Closed treatment of cervical fractures and dislocations. Ital J Orthop Traumatol [Suppl] 9:57–81, 1983

63. Murphy MJ, Daniaux H, Southwick WO: Posterior cervical fusion with rigid internal fixation. Orthop Clin North Am 17:55–65, 1986

64. Murphy MJ, Ogden JA, Southwick WO: Spinal stabilization in acute spinal injuries. Surg Clin North Am 60:1035–1047, 1980

65. Murphy MJ, Southwick WO: Surgical approaches and techniques. In Cervical Spine Research Society (ed): The Cervical Spine, Philadelphia, JB Lippincott, 1983

66. Oliveira JC: Anterior plate fixation of traumatic lesions of the lower cervical spine. Spine 12:324–329, 1987

67. Paley D, Gillespie R: Chronic repetitive unrecognized flexion injury of the cervical spine (high jumpers neck). Am J Sports Med 14:92–95, 1986

68. Panjabi MM, Goel VK et al: Biomechanical study of cervical spine stabilization with methyl methacrylate. Spine 10:198–203, 1985

69. Panjabi MM, Summers DJ, Pelker RR et al: Three dimensional load displacement curves due to forces on the cervical spine. J Orthop 4:152–161, 1986

70. Panjabi MM, White AA III, Brand RA: A note on defining body parts configurations. J Biomech 7:385–394, 1974

71. Panjabi MM, White AA III, Johnson R: Cervical spine mechanics as a function of transsection of components. J Biomech 8:327–334, 1975

72. Panjabi MM, White AA, Keller D et al: Stability of the cervical spine under tension. J Biomech 11:189–197, 1978

73. Penning L: Functional Pathology of the Cervical Spine. Baltimore, Williams & Wilkins, 1968

74. Penning L: Normal movements of the cervical spine. AJR 130:317–326, 1978

75. Pierce DS, Barr JS: Fractures and dislocations. In Cervical Spine Research Society (ed): The Cervical Spine, Philadelphia, JB Lippincott, 1983

76. Pipino F, Bancale R: Biodynamics of the lower cervical spine. In Cervical Spine I. Chicago, Springer-Verlag, 1987

77. Raynor RB, Pugh J, Shapiro I: Cervical facetectomy and its effect on stability. In Cervical Spine I. Chicago, Springer-Verlag, 1987

78. Rifkinson-Mann S, Mormino J, Sachdev VP: Subacute cervical spine instability. Surg Neurol 26:413–416, 1986

79. Roaf R: A study of the mechanics of spinal injuries. J Bone Joint Surg [Br] 42:810–823, 1960

80. Robinson RA, Southwick WO: Surgical approaches to the cervical spine. In American Academy of Orthopedic Surgeons: Instructional Course Lectures, Vol 17. St. Louis, CV Mosby, 1960

81. Rorabeck CH, Rock MG, Hawkins RJ et al: Unilateral facet dislocation of the cervical spine. Spine 12:23–27, 1987

82. Roy-Camille R, Judet TA, Saillant G et al: Tumeurs du rachis. Encycl Med Chir Techniques Chirurgicales Orthopedic 44165, 4.6.04

83. Savini R, Parasini P, Cervellati S: The surgical treatment of late instability of flexion-rotation injuries in the lower cervical spine. Spine 12:178–182, 1987

84. Scher AT: Anterior cervical subluxation: An unstable position. AJR 133:275–280, 1979

85. Scher AT: Ligamentous injury of the cervical spine: Two radiological signs. S Afr Med J 53:802–804, 1978

86. Scher AT: Radiographic indicators of traumatic cervical spine instability. S Afr Med J 62:562–565, 1982

87. Schlicke LH, White AA III, Panjabi MM et al: A quantitative study of vertebral displacement in angulation in the normal cervical spine under axial load. Clin Orthop 140:47–49, 1979

88. Schneider JR, Bright RW: Anterior cervical fusion using preserved bone allografts. Transplant Proc 8[Suppl 1]:73–76, 1976

89. Shapiro R, Youngberg A, Rothman S.: The differential diagnosis of traumatic lesions of the occipitoatlanto-axial segment. Radiol Clin North Am 11:505–526, 1973

90. Sherk HH: Stability of the lower cervical spine. In The Cervical Spine I. Chicago, Springer-Verlag, 1987

91. Spence KF Jr, Decker J, Sell KW: Bursting atlantal fracture associated with rupture of the transverse ligament. J Bone Joint Surg [Am] 52:543–548, 1970

92. Stabler CL, Eismont FJ, Brown MD: Failure of posterior cervical fusions using cadaveric bone graft in children. J Bone Joint Surg [Am] 67:371–375, 1985

93. Stauffer ES: Management of spine fractures C3 to C7. Orthop Clin North Am 17:45–53, 1986

94. Stauffer ES, Kelly EG: Fracture dislocations of the cervical spine: Instability and recurrent deformity following treatment by anterior interbody fusion. J Bone Joint Surg [Am] 59:45–48, 1977

95. Ulrich C, Worsdorfer O, Claes L et al: Comparative stability of anterior and posterior cervical spine fixation. In vitro investigation. In Cervical Spine I. Chicago, Springer-Verlag, 1987

96. Ulrich C, Worsdorfer O, Claes L et al: Comparative study of the stability of anterior and posterior cervical spine fixation procedures. Arch Orthop Trauma Surg 106:226–231, 1987

97. Van Peteghem PK, Schweigel JF: The fractured cervical spine rendered unstable by anterior cervical fusion. J Trauma 19:110–114, 1979

98. Waisbrod H: Anterior cervical spine fusion for unstable fractures. J Injury 12:389–392, 1981

99. Wang GJ, Lewish GD, Reger SI et al: Comparative strengths of various anterior cement fixations of the cervical spine. Spine 8:717–721, 1983

100. Weisel SW, Rothman RH: Occipitoatlanto hypermobility. Spine 4:187–191, 1979

101. Werne S: Studies in spontaneous atlas dislocation. Acta Orthop Scand [Suppl] 23:1–28, 1957

102. White AA III, Johnson RM, Panjabi MM et al: Biomechanical analysis of clinical stability in the cervical spine. Clin Orthop 109:85–96, 1975

103. White AA III, Panjabi MM: Clinical Biomechanics of the Spine. Philadelphia, JB Lippincott, 1978

104. White AA III, Panjabi MM: The basic kinametics of the human spine. Spine 3:12–20, 1978

105. White AA III, Panjabi MM: The role of stabilization in the treatment of cervical spine injuries. Spine 9:512–522, 1984

106. White AA III, Panjabi MM: Update on the evaluation of instability of the lower cervical spine. In Griffen PP (ed): Instructional Course Lectures, Vol 36. Chicago, AAOS, 1987

107. Williams JL, Belytschko TB: A three dimensional model of the human cervical spine for impact simulation. J Biomech Eng 105:321–331, 1983

108. Wolf JW, Johnson RM: Physiology and biomechanics. In Cervical Spine Research Society (ed): The Cervical Spine, Philadelphia, JB Lippincott, 1983

109. Wolf JW, Jones HC: Comparison of immobilization in halo casts and halo-plastic jackets. Orthopaedic Transaction 5:118–119, 1981

110. Yoganandan N, Sances A, Maiman DJ et al: Experimental spinal injuries with vertical impact. Spine 11:855–860, 1986

111. Zigler JE, Waters RL, Nelson RW et al: Occipito-cervical-thoracic spine fusion in a patient with occipito-cervical dislocation and survival. Spine 11:645–646, 1986

6

SURGICAL TECHNIQUES IN CERVICAL SPINE SURGERY

R. Geoffrey Wilber

John G. Peters

Matt J. Likavec

Many injuries to the cervical column are appropriately treated by nonoperative means. There are, however, some conditions in which we feel that clear indications for surgical management exist. This chapter deals with the surgical approach in the management of cervical spinal column and cord injuries.

Initial management at the scene of the accident and in the emergency room is concerned with maintaining the alignment and immobilization of the cervical spine. Attention to the ABCs of trauma management is essential to more predictable patient outcomes. The initial triage assessment includes a lateral radiograph of the cervical spine.

Prevention of further damage to both neural and structural elements is essential in the management of these injuries.[56] Injury patterns must be recognized and appropriate treatment applied.[1,8,12,23,55,69] Assessment of neurologic function to determine whether it is normal, incomplete, or complete will guide in planning treatment.[34,39,67] After obtaining diagnostic cervical spine films, unstable or displaced spinal column injuries are safely treated initially in cervical traction, usually applied through a device such as Gardner–Wells tongs.[20,32,45] For mid- to lower cervical spine lesions 10 lb of traction can be safely applied. This can act as a temporary measure until definitive management can be instituted. In most upper cervical lesions, a hard cervical collar is applied until an accurate diagnosis is made, as inappropriate traction can potentially harm the patient.

Once cervical traction is applied, immediate follow-up lateral radiographs are essential to judge the overall effect and alignment.[74] Further weight increments are applied by a pulley to the cervical tongs, or realignment of the vector of traction is made on the basis of these follow-up radiographs[20] coupled with serial neurologic assessments. Cervical traction is most often applied to facet dislocation injury patterns or fracture–

dislocations. It is generally safer and easier to place tong traction early in the course of patient care. If, in the final assessment, cervical traction is not needed, the tongs can be removed with little risk of morbidity to the patient.

Once the spinal column is aligned and/or stabilized, the injury needs to be further defined.[28,52] Supplemental cervical radiographs, including oblique views, tomography, computerized axial tomograms, myelography, and magnetic resonance imaging, can be applied as indicated.[5] Dynamic studies such as flexion and extension radiographs, although potentially hazardous, can have a place in assessing ligamentous injury.

An accurate diagnostic assessment allows definition of the underlying injury pattern. General classification schemes based on the mechanism and level have been devised to permit a prediction of outcome and guide in the choice of a treatment modality.[2,5,8,12,14,23,40,44,55] Most helpful in our experience is the grading system outlined by White, Johnson, Panjabi, and Southwick.[77,79]

Surgical management can address stabilization of the spine,[78] decompression of compromised neural elements, or a combination of the two. At times decompression of neural elements should be accomplished whether or not there is neurologic deficit. Neurologic compression is often released as a benefit of simple spinal realignment and stabilization. Surgical options include reduction, reduction and internal stabilization, decompression, and decompression and internal stabilization.

In general, an operative approach is rarely the treatment of choice for the patient in the very early phases of care.[29] There are, however, indications for immediate surgical intervention for a patient in whom a fluctuating or degrading neurologic picture is seen.[34] Many cervical injuries are by nature so complex that it is justified to allot time for adequate evaluation by all modalities at hand in order to delineate the entire injury pattern before proceeding with surgery. In addition, a brief delay in operative intervention due to other surgical or medical problems may allow for a better-directed operation in a medically-improved operative candidate.

In the patient with instability as the primary injury, a posterior approach is most likely to be chosen as the definitive treatment for the patient.

However, if a patient has neurologic compromise, anterior compression, or anterior or middle column injury, there is a greater emphasis on the anterior approach and decompression of the spinal canal.[6,14,15,24,53,58,70]

The remainder of this chapter will deal with operative approaches to the injured cervical spine using the more traditional fixation techniques and bone grafting. Other fixation or hardware techniques will be discussed in other chapters of this book.

OCCIPITO-ATLANTAL DISLOCATIONS

There are increasing numbers of case reports of survival of occiput—C-1 dissociation.[87] This probably reflects better on-site care and transportation of patients with multiple injuries. This lesion occurs fairly frequently in those who die in motor vehicle accidents.[12] Surgical intervention must address stabilization and permanent fixation of the occipital–cervical junction.

Immobilization is best accomplished in the halo vest preoperatively. This allows for maintenance of alignment in either the supine or prone position and permits safe positioning of the patient in surgery. Usually, the surgery can be accomplished around the halo and vest with appropriate draping. If necessary, the posterior vest can be removed to facilitate the procedure.

Surgically, a midline posterior approach is made from the inion to the midcervical region. The dissection is performed in the midline. Deep self-retaining retractors are advanced during dissection for both visualization and tamponade. The occiput and upper cervical posterior elements are identified and subperiosteally stripped. Dissection on the posterior atlas must remain within 2.5 cm of the midline to obviate injury to the vertebral artery laterally. Dissection is carried inferiorly onto the posterior elements of C-2. Care should be taken to avoid damage to the C-2–C-3 interspinous ligament. Occipital fixation is facilitated either by drill holes through the occiput to the dura or through the outer table of the skull with undermining of the inion, allowing wires to be passed between the outer and inner tables.

A three-wire technique is used (Fig. 6-1). Double 20-gauge wires are passed through these occipital fixation sites. One is used for stabilization of the bone graft. The other is passed inferiorly through a drill hole in the spinous process of C-2 to secure spinal fixation. A third wire is passed through the C-2 spinous process to stabilize the inferior end of the bone graft. A wire can also be passed under the ring of C-1 to further stabilize the cervical spine to the overlying bone graft. Usually a cortical cancellous iliac crest strip, approximately 1.5 cm in width, is used for bone grafting. This can be supplemented with additional autogenous cancellous bone. If there are problems with inadequate wire fixation, a simple onlay technique can be used for bone grafting.

We recommend maintaining the patient in a halo vest for 3 to 4 months postoperatively. This supplements the internal fixation used and increases the likelihood of fusion. At the time of halo removal, flexion–extension radiographs or tomography can be used to assess fusion healing.

FRACTURES OF THE ATLAS

Vertical compression forces to the ring of the atlas result in a burst injury termed a Jefferson fracture.[46] This fracture can be deemed stable or unstable depending on the preservation of the transverse ligament (Fig. 6-2). Stability is best judged on the open-mouth anteroposterior radiographic

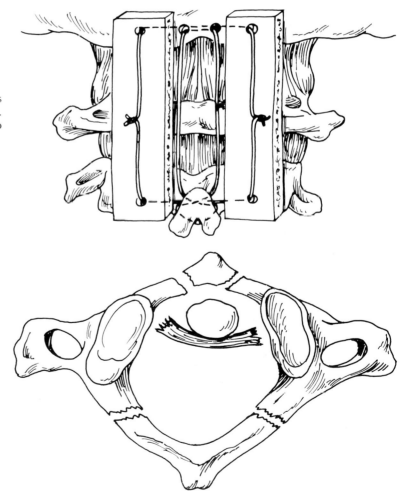

Figure 6-1. Occiput–C-2 fusion employing wires placed through the outer occipital cortex only. This technique utilizes three 20-gauge wires to firmly affix the two corticocancellous grafts.

Figure 6-2. An "unstable" Jefferson fracture with transverse ligament disruption.

view. The sine qua non of a transverse ligament injury is the spread of greater than 7 mm of the C-1 lateral masses on C-2 (Fig. 6-3). Ligamentous damage may also be indicated if there is comminution of the ipsilateral C-1 ring with a floating C-1 articular process. This is best seen on computed tomography.[10]

Jefferson fractures that are stable are best treated with halo immobilization. Unstable C-1 injuries are best initially treated in a halo vest for 6 to 8 weeks to allow for ring healing, which should be confirmed radiographically. This is followed by a C-1–C-2 posterior fusion to stabilize the ligamentous component. Techniques for this will be discussed in a later section. The surgical approach to the management of this fracture pattern is an occiput–C-2 fusion. This, however, compromises a significant amount of cervical motion and should be avoided if possible. The indication for an occiput–C-2 fusion is damage to the occiput–C1 facet joint associated with a comminuted Jefferson fracture. Fortunately, this is rare.

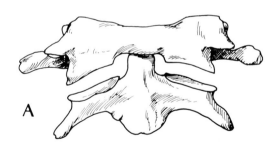

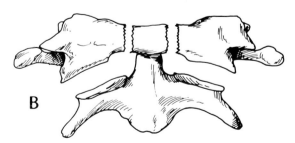

Figure 6-3. (*A*) The normal lateral mass relationship is seen. (*B*) When the combined bilateral spread of the C-1 lateral mass on C-2 is greater than 7 mm, then "instability" is likely.

ODONTOID FRACTURES

Fractures involving the odontoid process have been classified into three distinct types according to the location of the fracture.[3] Types 1 and 3 are have a high likelihood of union when treated with immobilization.[60] Type 2 fractures, or fractures to the waist of the odontoid process, represent the most common type of odontoid fracture. They may be nondisplaced or displaced. Displaced odontoid waist fractures have a higher incidence of nonunion (Fig. 6-4). There is, however, a significant incidence of poor healing in both groups.[61]

Halo immobilization can be expected to give the greatest chance for healing by nonoperative means.[76] Most surgical approaches deal with instability between the C-1 and C-2 vertebrae.[47] The usual approach is through a posterior fusion, with wire fixation by the standard Gallie or Brooks fusion techniques. Anterior approaches at the fusion of C-1 to C-2 have also been described.[64] Lateral mass fusion has been described by Barbour[7] and Simmons and du Toit[64] and may have a place when a deficient posterior arch of C-1 or C-2 is present.[49] This procedure is quite difficult in both exposure and fixation techniques. An anterior screw fixation technique has been described by Bohler using small-fragment cancellous screws directed superiorly from the body of C-2 into the odontoid process (Figs. 6-5, 6-6).[11] This provides interfragmentary fixation of this fracture and has been reported in Europe with good results.[7]

There are two basic techniques of posterior C-1–C-2 wiring and fusion. The Gallie technique is older and has a long track record of success.[36,40] It uses a block-shaped single bone graft over the posterior ring of C-1 and the lamina and surrounding the spinous process of C-2 (Fig. 6-7). It is held in place with a single wire, which is placed around the posterior ring of C-1 and through the spinous process of C-2. This technique requires the use of a halo vest or Minerva jacket for immobilization postoperatively. Using this technique, a high incidence of fusion can be expected. Theoretical disadvantages of this technique include loosening of the fixation due to bone graft resorption, and potential pivoting and translation of C-1 on C-2 because the spinous process of C-2 is slightly posterior to the articular facet.

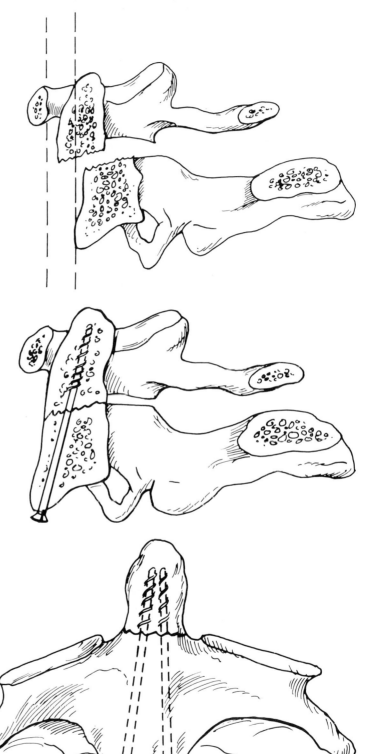

Figure 6-4. Displaced odontoid waist fracture (type II).

Figure 6-5. Lateral view of transodontoid screw fixation in a type II odontoid fracture.

Figure 6-6. Frontal view of transodontoid screw fixation.

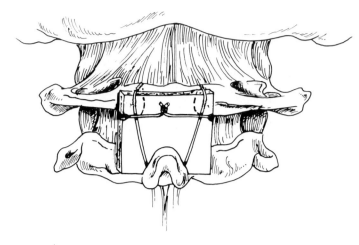

Figure 6-7. Gallie type of posterior wiring and grafting of C-1–C-2 used by authors.

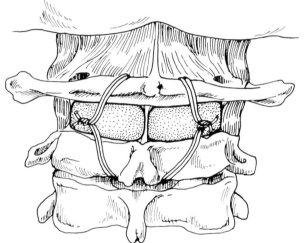

Figure 6-8. Posterior view of Brooks and Jenkins' technique with trapezoidal corticocancellous bone grafts lying between the posterior elements of C-1 and C-2.

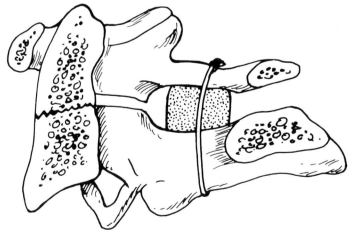

Figure 6-9. Lateral view of Brooks and Jenkins' technique.

The technique of Brooks and Jenkins[18] uses two to four wires passed sublaminarly under C-1 and C-2, holding the interlaminar bone graft in place (Fig. 6-8). The wires do not hold the bone graft over the lamina of C-1 (Fig. 6-9). There is probably more stability in the Brooks construct, and this may in fact obviate halo vest immobilization in the postoperative period.[42] Its disadvantages are the intrusion of wire into the spinal canal and the potential for neurologic compromise.[84]

Supplementation of posterior fixation with methyl methacrylate probably has no place in the injured spine. It is, however, advocated by some authors.[30] It carries with it a higher incidence of infection and does not give long-term biologic (bony) stability.[50]

After reduction and posterior stabilization of odontoid fractures, there is occasionally continued compression anteriorly by a nonunion or a malunion of the dens. Anterior débridement of the odontoid process may have an application in this situation. This can be accomplished either by a high anterior approach or through transoral resection.[33,43]

HANGMAN'S FRACTURES

Traumatic spondylolisthesis of the axis is a spinal fracture that can usually be treated nonoperatively.[48] Management involves application of halo traction for a 2-week period to achieve reduction. The patient is then immobilized in a halo vest for 3 months. The outcome from this is usually satisfactory.

In the uncommon instance in which surgical management is indicated,[17] the options are an anterior or posterior approach. Each approach has its advantages and disadvantages. The posterior approach provides better stability, but adds an additional level of fusion. The anterior arthrodesis technique fuses only the C-2–C-3 level (i.e., the anteriorly involved level). The major disadvantage of this approach is that the anterior longitudinal ligament, which can be the last competent structural element in this fracture pattern, is compromised.

In the posterior approach, a standard midline incision is made to the posterior elements from the base of the occiput to C-3. The posterior elements are subperiosteally dissected of soft tissues over the posterior elements of C-1, C-2, and C-3. Wires are placed in the base of the spinous processes of C-2 and C-3, and a sublaminar wire is placed under the posterior ring of C-1. This is a modification of the Gallie technique. Some authors recommend placing sublaminar wires from C-1 to C-3 in a modified Brooks technique. In either technique of wiring, the use of a halo vest in the postoperative period is suggested.

Anterior arthrodesis for a hangman's fracture is probably indicated when there has been a severe disruption of the C-2–C-3 disk space by the fracture. Initial treatment is immobilization in a halo vest for 6 weeks. After this period, a modified Smith–Robinson[26,51,66,84] approach is used with a C-2–C-3 diskectomy and interbody fusion. Interbody fusion allows for bony stabilization of the fracture with preservation of the C-1–C-2 articulation. This is indicated if the patient is involved in an occupation in which cervical mobility is essential. Patients with marked degenerative disease of the cervical spine should also be considered. This fusion technique requires halo vest immobilization postoperatively.

An anterior approach that parallels the anterior board of the sternocleidomastoid muscle may also be used. The carotid pulse is retracted laterally and the strap muscles are retracted medially. The dissection is blunt and usually no traversing vessels need ligation. The pretracheal and prevertebral fascia are entered sharply, and the anterior longitudinal ligament and longus colli muscles are visualized. The anterior longitudinal ligament and the annulus of the disk are excised at the disk level with a #15 scalpel blade and the disk material is removed with curettes and pituitary rongeurs. Exposure can be facilitated with the use of a small laminar spreader in the disk space. The hard subchondral bone is left intact except for small puncture holes made with a 3-0 angled cervical curette. This allows for vascular ingress and may increase graft incorporation. A tricortical graft from the iliac crest is then placed into the interbody space and recessed 1 mm from the anterior vertebral border. Close follow-up with serial radiographs with the patient in a halo vest is essential to detect potential problems with the bone graft or alignment of the spine. The anterior approach is made safer and easier with the use of magnification and illumination (microscope vs. loops and headlight).

FACET DISLOCATIONS

Unilateral (Figs. 6-10, 6-11)[16] and bilateral (Fig. 6-12)39 facet dislocations with or without fractures represent a major subgroup of cervical injuries. The mode of injury is usually flexion. Typically there is damage to the posterior ligaments and facet capsules with preservation of the anterior longitudinal ligament. There may be damage

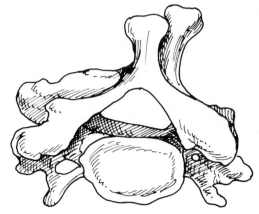

Figure 6-10. Superior view of a unilateral facet dislocation.

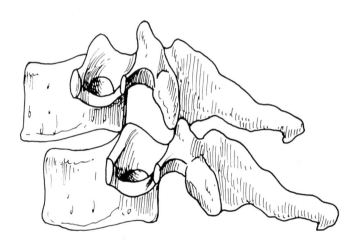

Figure 6-11. In unilateral dislocations, the cephalad body is displaced anteriorly approximately 25% on the body below.

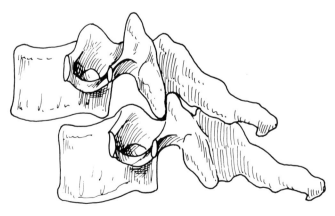

Figure 6-12. Bilateral facet dislocations have at least 50% anterior displacement.

to the disk itself with or without retropulsion of fragments into the canal. Computed tomography and myelography following reduction are important in determining canal compromise with disk material. Anterior disk removal must be considered if there is significant disk damage or spinal impingement.

The possibility of early surgical intervention should be raised if there are locked facets that cannot be reduced by closed means.[54,57] In this case, it is essential to monitor the patient's neurologic function with intraoperative evoked potentials (spinal or cortical) or by a postreduction wake-up test. Disk prolapse into the canal can occur, with resultant quadriplegia postoperatively.[53] Therefore, consideration for intraoperative myelography or ultrasound to determine canal patency should be made.

The operative technique for open reduction of a facet dislocation requires a posterior approach with the patient in tong or halo traction. The anterior approach is dangerous and rarely employed.[27,31,48,68,72] The superior facet of the caudal

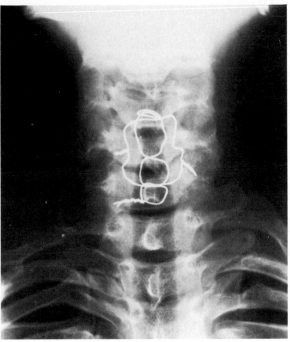

Figure 6-13. Anteroposterior radiograph of three-wire technique of stabilization.

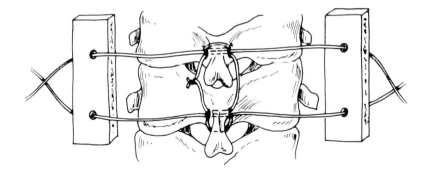

Figure 6-14. Three-wire fixation technique.

vertebra is visualized. The superior aspect of this is then removed with a burr. This will result in a controlled, intraoperative reduction. If there is an associated facet fracture with radiculopathy, a laminotomy or foraminotomy is a consideration.

Stabilization techniques include posterior spinous process wire fixation,[13] wire and spinous process Steinmann's pins,[25] sublaminar wire fixation,[83] Luque rods, spinal plates, and methyl methacrylate fixation.[4,65,75] We favor the posterior three-wire technique described by Bohlman for fixation of these injuries (Fig. 6-13).[13] This utilizes three 20-gauge stainless steel wires with fixation to the vertebral spinous processes through small drill holes in their bases. The technique is seen in Figure 6-14. This has shown to be mechanically stronger than other constructs. Sublaminar wires, while strong, have the potential for increased neurologic injury and should be avoided in the cervical spine[84] if possible. In the face of associated spinous process fractures, there may be an indication for this, however.

Threaded Steinmann's pins (Fig. 6-15) percutaneously placed into the base of the spinous processes offer strong fixation; incorporating the adjacent iliac crest graft into the pins will further enhance graft fixation. An interlocking 16- or 18-

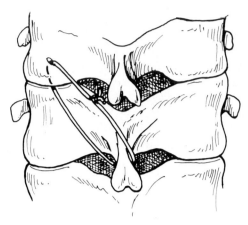

Figure 6-16. In unilateral facet dislocations, single-sided facet to spinous process wiring can be performed.

gauge wire provides increased rigidity. This technique is probably comparable to the three-wire technique, although good mechanical testing has not been done.

Facet wiring may offer increased rotational stability to facet dislocations, and can be placed unilaterally (Fig. 6-16) or bilaterally (Fig. 6-17). The Southwick facet wiring technique (Fig. 6-18) has the disadvantage of potential damage to the inferior nonfused mobile segment articulation. Facet wiring from facet to inferior spinous process has the potential for better rotational control. Plate fixation techniques will be discussed elsewhere.

The purpose of posterior fixation is the allowance of bony healing and bone graft incorporation. This provides a long-term stable construct that is not expected to deteriorate over time. Methyl methacrylate provides nonbiologic fixation that may, in fact, deteriorate with time.[30,81] There is also a higher incidence of infection with increasing amounts of implanted foreign material.[50] We feel that the use of methyl methacrylate in young patients is controversial and prefer the biologic approach with traditional bone grafting techniques.

Bone grafting can be accomplished from autografted, allografted,[19] or xenografted sources. The gold standard, however, is autogenous iliac crest bone. Cortical cancellous bone graft is preferable for posterior cervical fusion. Other autogenous bone sites are available, including the rib and fibula. Allograft bone is also a viable alternative,

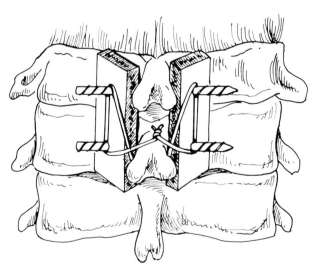

Figure 6-15. Percutaneously placed Steinmann's pins directed through corticocancellous grafts and the spinous processes above and below the injury. These are then interconnected with heavy stainless steel wire.

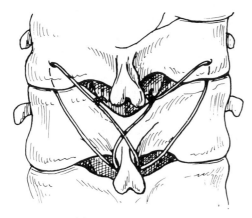

Figure 6-17. Bilateral facet to spinous process wiring.

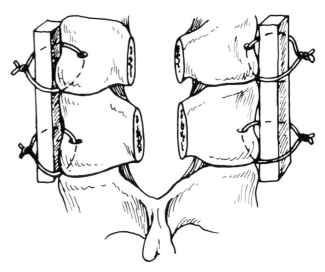

Figure 6-18. Southwick-type facet wiring with fixation to corti-cocancellous bone graft in the spine following laminectomy.

especially if autogenous bone is not readily available. The potential for nonunion is probably higher, and depending on the processing of the graft, there is a potential for viral transmission to the patient and its resultant sequelae. Xenograft bone has a high rejection potential and in general should represent a last choice or not be considered at all.

Luque-type rod fixation (Fig. 6-19) with either sublaminar or spinous process wires requires the inclusion of additional vertebrae for a strong mechanical construct. This has an adverse effect on spinal motion. Luque-type rod fixation with closed rings on shorter segments provides much weaker constructs. The potential for subluxation and/or redislocation is probably higher. Posterior sub-

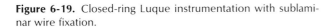

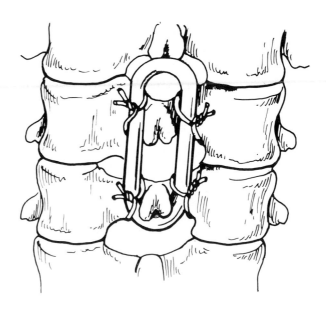

Figure 6-19. Closed-ring Luque instrumentation with sublaminar wire fixation.

laminar wiring techniques have a higher potential for neurologic injury and should be avoided when possible.[85]

BURST FRACTURES

Burst fractures can involve two or three spinal columns (Fig. 6-20). In two-column burst injuries, there is bony disruption anteriorly with varying degrees of canal compromise by bone and disk material.[53] The pathology involves mainly the anterior spinal elements.[73] Operative approaches should be directed at the anterior pathology.[15,53,70]

In three-column injuries, there is additional damage to the posterior elements. Posterior stabilization followed by anterior decompression offers a reasonable therapeutic approach.[9,22,71,82] These can be done as a combined procedure or separately in the medically unstable patient. Posterior stabilization can be performed under local anes-

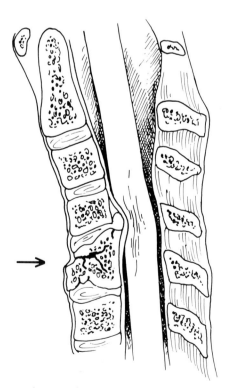

Figure 6-20. A bursting fracture with anterior and middle column involvement (*arrow*).

thesia with the patient on a turning frame if necessary. The senior author has had experience with this technique and has had few problems in the cooperative patient.

After posterior stabilization is accomplished, the burst fracture can be managed as a two-column injury. In the case of complete quadriplegia, the posterior procedure alone may suffice. Some authors recommend consideration of anterior decompression, however, to gain additional root levels.[12,67] In incomplete spinal cord lesions in which significant bony or disk encroachment is suspected, appropriate studies, including a myelogram, computed tomographic scan, or magnetic resonance imaging, are used to determine the degree of canal involvement. Significant canal intrusion of bone and/or disk provides a rationale for anterior decompression of the involved spinal cord and nerve roots followed by a strut graft.[15,37]

The anterior approach described by Smith and Robinson[66] is used with the adaptation of making a transverse incision and carrying the dissection medial to the sternocleidomastoid muscle and lateral to the strap muscles. The cricothyroid membrane is used as a point of reference and usually allows excellent exploration of the C-5–C-6 level. The omohyoid muscle and superior thyroidal artery can often be retracted but may be ligated if exposure is limited. The carotid pulse is kept laterally, and dissection is carried through the pretracheal and prevertebral fascia. A needle is placed into the disk space and an roentgenogram taken to document the appropriate level. The disk spaces immediately above and below the involved level are excised using scalpel, curette, and pituitary rongeur. This dissection should be carried to the posterior longitudinal ligament and the joints of Luschka laterally. The vertebrectomy is then started by creating a bony trough 14 mm wide centered on the midline. This usually allows for adequate decompression without endangering the vertebral arteries laterally. An air-powered bur system usually works best for this débridement. The regular notched bur tip is changed to a diamond bur as the dissection approaches the canal. This allows for removal of bone safely, even over the ligament and dural sac.[15] Final resection of bone is accomplished with a 3-0 cervical curette or fine Kerrison rongeur (1 to 2 mm) (Fig. 6-21). This allows for safe, atraumatic decompression of

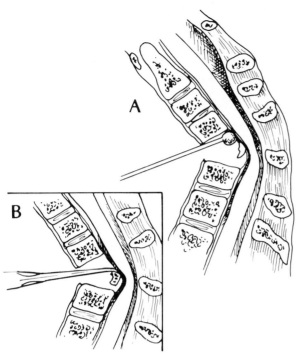

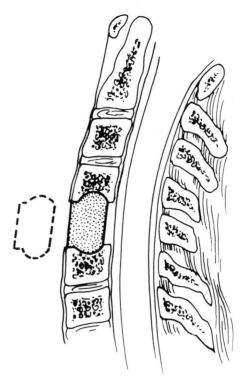

Figure 6-21. (*A*) A diamond burr tip is used as the posterior longitudinal ligament is approached. (*B*) A 3-0 curved curette is used to "pick" remaining osseous fragments away from the dura or posterior longitudinal ligament.

Figure 6-22. Notched graft (iliac crest) S/P anterior corpectomy.

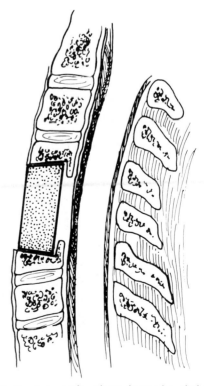

the spinal canal. Lateral decompression of the cord as well as nerve roots is carried out at this time with angled curettes and Kerrison rongeurs.

After decompression of appropriate segments, the vertebral bodies above and below are contoured to accept a bony interposition graft. There are two basic grafting techniques. In the notched graft,[6,41] the end-plates above and below the injured level are channeled with both an anterior and posterior bony lip (Fig. 6-22) to prevent anterior or posterior migration of the graft. In the keystone technique,[63] a 10-degree beveled shaping of the vertebral bodies above and below the defect is made (Fig. 6-23). The posterior lip of bone prevents the migration of the keystone-shaped graft posteriorly.

A tricortical iliac crest bone graft is usually of sufficient size for defects of one to two levels of decompression. Because the natural curvature of iliac bone precludes straight grafts of longer than 5 cm, when more than two levels of vertebral

Figure 6-23. Keystone graft with 10-degree beveled graft ends. Note iliac crest grafting material.

bodies require decompression, fibula is a better grafting material (Fig. 6-24).[58,80] The disadvantage of fibular bone graft, however, is its slower incorporation as compared to the iliac crest. The fibula, fortunately, does have a lower incidence of long-term graft failure.

The Cloward technique[24] of interbody fusion does not usually allow for enough bone removal for adequate decompression. The Cloward dowel graft may be unstable in lateral bending and the graft itself is not as strong as iliac tricortical material.[38,86]

Lateral tomograms and/or computed tomography provide good postoperative assessment of spinal decompression.[59] Orthotic management postoperatively can be achieved either with a two-poster style brace or a halo vest, depending on the surgeon's assessment of the underlying stability. If there is a question as to the stability of the operated construct, the safer approach is to use the halo system. Externally, immobilization can usually be removed in 2 to 3 months.

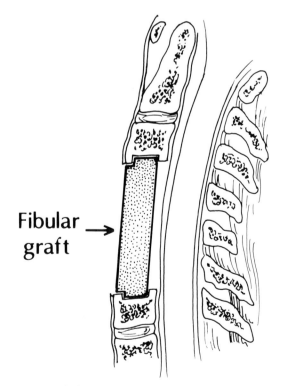

Figure 6-24. Fibular graft is used for an anterior strut following corpectomy.

SUMMARY

This chapter represents an overview of the management of cervical spine injuries. Certainly, the majority of injuries can be treated appropriately on a conservative, nonoperative basis. We advocate realignment of the spine with stabilization of the posterior elements and posterior decompression of neural impingement when the injury pattern and neurologic picture warrant posterior procedures or posterior stabilization. Laminectomies without fusion, however, are potentially destabilizing procedures.[21] Central canal compromise by bone usually represents anterior pathology, and this route should be employed for safe, rational decompression. Occasionally, combined anterior and posterior approaches are appropriate in the management of three-column injuries. These can be performed as a combined procedure or at separate times.

An adequate evaluation of the injury and identification of the underlying pathology are essential. It is certainly better to approach a spine nonoperatively than to perform an unwarranted or poorly advised procedure. Usually, surgical techniques are best done in the controlled environment of a spinal cord injury center by experienced surgeons who have adequate resources available to them.

REFERENCES

1. Aebi M, Mohler J, Zach GA, Morscher E: Indication, surgical technique, and results of 100 surgically treated fractures and fracture-dislocations of the cervical spine. Clin Orthop 203:244–251, 1986
2. Allen BL, Ferguson RL, Lehmann TR, O'Brien RP: A mechanistic classification of closed indirect fractures and dislocations of the lower cervical spine. Spine 7:1–27, 1982
3. Anderson LD, D'Alonzo RT: Fractures of the odontoid process of the axis. J Bone Joint Surg [Am] 56:1663–1674, 1974
4. Asnis SE, Lesniewski P, Dowling T: Anterior decompression and stabilization with methylmethacrylate in a bone bolt for treatment of pathologic fractures of the cervical spine: A report of two cases. Clin Orthop 187:139–143, 1984

5. Babcock JL: Cervical spine injuries: Diagnosis and classification. Arch Surg 111:646–651, 1976

6. Bailey RW, Badgley CE: Stabilization of the cervical spine by anterior fusion. J Bone Joint Surg [Am] 41:565–594, 1960

7. Barbour JR: Screw fixation in fracture of the odontoid process. South Australian Clinics 5:20–24, 1971

8. Beatson TR: Fractures and dislocations of the cervical spine. J Bone Joint Surg [Br] 45:21–35, 1963

9. Bell GD, Bailey SI: Anterior cervical fusion for trauma. Clin Orthop 128:155–158, 1977

10. Bernhang AM, Fielding JW: Combined atlas and axis fractures visualized by computerized tomography. Clin Orthop 212:255–259, 1986

11. Bohler J: Anterior stabilization for acute fractures and non-unions of the dens. J Bone Joint Surg [Am] 64:18–27, 1982

12. Bohlman HH: Acute fractures and dislocations of the cervical spine: An analysis of 300 hospitalized patients and review of the literature. J Bone Joint Surg [Am] 61:1119–1142, 1979

13. Bohlman HH: The management of cervical spine fractures and dislocations. In American Academy of Orthopedic Surgeons (ed): Instructional Course Lectures, Vol 34, pp 163–187. St. Louis, CV Mosby, 1985

14. Bohlman HH: Pathology and current treatment concepts of cervical spine injuries. In American Academy of Orthopedic Surgeons (ed): Instructional Course Lectures, Vol 21, pp 108–115. St. Louis, CV Mosby, 1972

15. Bohlman HH, Eismont FJ: Surgical techniques of anterior decompression and fusion for spinal cord injuries. Clin Orthop 154:57–67, 1981

16. Braakman R, Vinken PJ: Unilateral facet interlocking in the lower cervical spine. J Bone Joint Surg [Br] 49:249–257, 1967

17. Bridwell KH: Treatment of a markedly displaced hangman's fracture with a Luque rectangle and a posterior fusion in a 71-year-old man: Case report. Spine 11:49–52, 1986

18. Brooks AL, Jenkins EB: Atlanto-axial arthrodesis by the wedge compression method. J Bone Joint Surg [Am] 60:279–284, 1978

19. Brown MD, Malinin TI, Davis PB: A roentgenographic evaluation of frozen allografts vs. autografts in anterior cervical spine fusions. Clin Orthop 119:231–236, 1976

20. Burke DC, Berryman D: The place of closed manipulation in the management of flexion-rotation dislocations of the cervical spine. J Bone Joint Surg [Br] 53:165–182, 1971

21. Callahan RA, Johnson RM, Margolis RN et al: Cervical facet fusion for control of instability following laminectomy. J Bone Joint Surg [Am] 59:991–1002, 1977

22. Capen DA, Garland DE, Waters RL: Surgical stabilization of the cervical spine: A comparative analysis of anterior and posterior spine fusions. Clin Orthop 196:229–237, 1985

23. Cheshire DJE: The stability of the cervical spine following the conservative treatment of fractures and fracture-dislocations. Paraplegia 7:193–203, 1969–1970

24. Cloward RB: Treatment of acute fractures and fracture-dislocations of the cervical spine by vertebral-body fusion: A report of 11 cases. J Neurosurg 18:201–209, 1961

25. Davey JR, Rorabeck CH, Bailey SI et al: A technique of posterior cervical fusion for instability of the cervical spine. Spine 10:722–728, 1985

26. De Andrade JR, MacNab I: Anterior occipito-cervical fusion using an extra-pharyngeal exposure. J Bone Joint Surg [Am] 51:1621–1626, 1969

27. De Oliveira JC: Anterior reduction of interlocking facets in the lower cervical spine. Spine 4:195–202, 1979

28. Dorr LD, Harvey JP, Nickel VL: Clinical review of the early stability of spine injuries. Spine 7:545–550, 1982

29. Ducker TB, Bellegarrigue R, Salcman M, Walleck C: Timing of operative care in cervical spinal cord injury. Spine 9:525–531, 1984

30. Eismont FJ, Bohlman HH: Posterior methylmethacrylate fixation for cervical trauma. Spine 6:347–353, 1981

31. Eismont FJ, Borja F, Bohlman HH: Complete dislocations at two adjacent levels of the cervical spine. Spine 9:319–322, 1984

32. Evans DK: Reduction of cervical dislocations. J Bone Joint Surg [Br] 43:552–555, 1961

33. Fang HSY, Ong GB: Direct anterior approach to the upper cervical spine. J Bone Joint Surg [Am] 44:1588–1604, 1962

34. Feuer H: Management of acute spine and spinal cord injuries: Old and new concepts. Arch Surg 111:638–645, 1976

35. Fielding JW, Cochran GVB, Lawsing JF, Hohl M: Tears of the transverse ligament of the atlas: A clinical and biomechanical study. J Bone Joint Surg [Am] 56:1683–1691, 1974

36. Fielding JW, Hawkins RJ, Ratzan SA: Spine fusion for atlanto-axial instability. J Bone Joint Surg [Am] 58:400–407, 1976

37. Fielding JW, Pyle RN, Fietti VG: Anterior cervical

vertebral body resection and bone grafting for benign and malignant tumors. J Bone Joint Surg [Am] 61:251–253, 1979

38. Flynn TB: Neurologic complications of anterior cervical interbody fusion. Spine 7:536–539, 1982

39. Forsyth HF, Alexander E, Davis C, Underdal R: The advantages of early spine fusion in the treatment of fracture-dislocation of the cervical spine. J Bone Joint Surg [Am] 41:17–36, 1959

40. Gallie WE: Fractures and dislocations of the cervical spine. Am J Surg 46:495–499, 1939

41. Gore DR: Technique of cervical interbody fusion. Clin Orthop 188:191–195, 1984

42. Griswold DM, Albright JA, Schiffman E et al: Atlanto-axial fusion for instability. J Bone Joint Surg [Am] 60:285–292, 1978

43. Hall JE, Denis F, Murray J: Exposure of the upper cervical spine for spinal decompression by mandible and tongue splitting approach. J Bone Joint [Am] 59:121–123, 1977

44. Holdsworth FW: Fractures, dislocations, and fracture-dislocations of the spine. J Bone Joint Surg [Br] 45:6–20, 1963

45. Horlyck E, Rahbek M: Cervical spine injuries: A clinical and radiologic follow-up study, in particular with a view to local complaints and radiological sequelae. Acta Orthop Scand 45:845–853, 1974

46. Jefferson G: Remarks on fractures of the first cervical vertebra. Br Med J 2:153–157, 1927

47. Lee PC, Chun SY, Leong JCY: Experience of posterior surgery in atlanto-axial instability. Spine 9:231–239, 1984

48. Levine AM, Edwards CC: The management of traumatic spondylolisthesis of the axis. J Bone Joint Surg [Am] 67:217–226, 1985

49. Lipson SJ, Hammerschlag SB: Atlanto-axial arthrodesis in the presence of posterior spondyloschisis (bifid arch of the atlas): A report of three cases and an evaluation of alternative wiring techniques by computerized tomography. Spine 9:65–69, 1984

50. McAfee PC, Bohlman HH, Ducker T, Eismont FJ: Failure of stabilization of the spine with methylmethacrylate: A retrospective analysis of 24 cases. J Bone Joint Surg [Am] 68:1145–1157, 1986

51. McAfee PC, Bohlman HH, Riley LH et al: The anterior retropharyngeal approach to the upper part of the cervical spine. J Bone Joint Surg [Am] 69:1371–1383, 1987

52. Nash CL: Acute cervical soft-tissue injury and late deformity: A case report. J Bone Joint Surg [Am] 61:305–307, 1979

53. Norrell H, Wilson CB: Early anterior fusion for injuries of the cervical portion of the spine. JAMA 214:515–530, 1970

54. O'Brien PJ, Schweigel JF, Thompson WJ: Dislocations of the lower cervical spine. J Trauma 232:710–714, 1982

55. Rogers WA: Fractures and dislocations of the cervical spine: An end-result study. J Bone Joint Surg [Am] 39:341–376, 1957

56. Rogers WA: Treatment of fracture-dislocation of the cervical spine. J Bone Joint Surg [Am] 24:245–258, 1942

57. Rorabeck CH, Rock MG, Hawkins RJ, Bourne RB: Unilateral facet dislocation in the cervical spine: An analysis of the results of treatment in 26 patients. Spine 12:23–27, 1987

58. Rossier AB, Hussey RW, Kenzora JE: Anterior fibular interbody fusion in the treatment of the cervical spinal cord injuries. Surg Neurol 7:55–60, 1977

59. Rothman SLG, Glenn WV: CT evaluation of interbody fusion. Clin Orthop 193:47–56, 1985

60. Schatzker J, Rorabeck CH, Waddell JP: Fractures of the dens (odontoid process): An analysis of 37 cases. J Bone Joint Surg [Br] 53:392–405, 1971

61. Segal LS, Grimm JO, Stauffer ES: Non-union of fractures of the atlas. J Bone Joint Surg [Am] 69:1423–1434, 1987

62. Sherk HH, Nicholson JT: Fractures of the atlas. J Bone Joint Surg [Am] 52:1017–1024, 1970

63. Simmons EH, Bhalla SK, Butt WP: Keystone graft in cervical spine surgery. J Bone Joint Surg [Br] 51:225–228, 1969

64. Simmons EH, du Toit G: Lateral atlanto-axial arthrodesis. Orthop Clin N Am 9:1101–1115, 1978

65. Six E, Kelly DL: Technique for C1, C2, and C3 fixation in cases of odontoid fracture. Neurosurgery 8:374–377, 1981

66. Smith GW, Robinson RA: The treatment of certain cervical-spine disorders by anterior removal of the anterior vertebral disc and interbody fusion. J Bone Joint Surg [Am] 40:607–623, 1958

67. Stauffer ES: Neurologic recovery following injuries to the cervical spinal cord and nerve roots. Spine 9:532–534, 1984

68. Stauffer ES, Kelly EG: Fracture-dislocations of the cervical spine: Instability and recurrent deformity following treatment by anterior interbody fusion. J Bone Joint Surg [Am] 59:45–48, 1977

69. Stauffer ES, Rhoades ME: Surgical stabilization of the cervical spine after trauma. Arch Surg 111:652–657, 1976

70. Svendgaard NA, Cronqvist S, Delgado T, Salford

LG: Treatment of severe cervical spine injuries by anterior interbody fusion with early mobilization. Acta Neurochir 60:91–105, 1982

71. Tew JM, Mayfield FH: Complications of surgery of the anterior cervical spine. Clin Neurosurg 23:424–434, 1976

72. Van Peteghem PK, Schweigel JF: The fractured cervical spine rendered unstable by anterior cervical fusion. J Trauma 19:110–114, 1979

73. Verbiest H: Anterolateral operations for fractures and dislocations in the middle and lower parts of the cervical spine: Report of a series of 47 cases. J Bone Joint Surg [Am] 51:1489–1530, 1969

74. Wagner FC, Chehrazi B: Surgical results in the treatment of cervical spinal cord injury. Spine 9:523–524, 1984

75. Wang G, Lewish GD, Reger SI et al: Comparative strengths of various anterior cement fixations of the cervical Spine. Spine 8:1717–1721, 1983

76. Wang G, Mabie KN, Whitehill R, Stamp WG: The Non-surgical management of odontoid fractures in adults. Spine 9:229–230, 1984

77. White AA III, Johnson RM, Panjabi MM, Southwick WO: Biomechanical analysis of clinical stability in the cervical spine. Clin Orthop 109:85–96, 1975

78. White AA, Panjabi MM: The role of stabilization in the treatment of cervical spine injuries. Spine 9:512–522, 1984

79. White AA, Southwick WO, Panjabi MM: Clinical instability in the lower cervical spine: A review of past and current concepts. Spine 1:15–27, 1976

80. Whitecloud TS, LaRocca H: Fibula strut graft in reconstructive surgery of the cervical spine. Spine 1:33–43, 1976

81. Whitehill R, Reger SI, Fox E et al: The use of methylmethacrylate cement as an instantaneous fusion mass in posterior cervical fusions: A canine in-vivo experimental model. Spine 9:246–252, 1984

82. Whitehill R, Reger SI, Kett RL et al: Reconstruction of the cervical spine following anterior vertebral body resection: Mechanical analysis of a canine experimental model. Spine 9:240–245, 1984

83. Whitehill R, Wilhelm CE, Moskal JT et al: Posterior strut fusions to enhance immediate postoperative cervical stability. Spine 11:613, 1986

84. Whitesides TE, McDonald AP: Lateral retropharyngeal approach to the upper cervical spine. Orthop Clin North Am 9:1115–1127, 1978

85. Wilber RG, Thompson GH, Shaffer JW et al: Postoperative neurologic deficits in segmental spinal instrumentation: A study using spinal cord monitoring. J Bone Joint Surg [Am] 66:1178–1187, 1984

86. Williams JL, Allen MB, Harkess JW: Late results of cervical discectomy and interbody fusion: Some factors influencing the results. J Bone Joint Surg [Am] 50:277–286, 1968

87. Zigler JE, Waters RL, Nelson RW et al: Occipital-cervical-thoracic spine fusion in a patient with occipital-cervical dislocation and survival. Spine 11:645–646, 1986

7

RATIONALE AND TECHNIQUES OF INTERNAL FIXATION IN TRAUMA OF THE CERVICAL SPINE

Raymond Roy-Camille
Christian Mazel
Gerard Saillant
Jean Pierre Benazet

When analyzing the pathology of traumatic lesions of the cervical spine, it can be seen that the majority of lesions evidence posterior column disruption. Fractures of the vertebral body are, in fact, rare. In our own research consisting of a continuous series of 274 cases of cervical spine injuries, only 30 cases, or 11%, were vertebral body fractures. Most lesions were seen in the region of the posterior arch. These consisted of:

Unilateral or bilateral articular dislocations (56/274 cases = 20%).

Fracture-dislocations of the facets (97/274 cases = 35%), fractures of the superior facets of underlying vertebrae being the most common.

Separation fractures of the articular mass (24/274 cases = 9%).

Finally, we found severe sprains (38/274 cases = 14%) and teardrop fractures, which are similar in nature (29/275 cases = 11%), to be not uncommon.

A simple rule in surgery is that when one has the choice among several operative approaches, it is advisable to choose the path that leads directly to the most serious lesions. It is for this reason that in the injured cervical spine we primarily perform the posterior approach, which leads directly to correcting the posterior column disruption. When the lesions are situated predominantly on the anterior vertebral body, we of course use the anterior approach in the cervical spine.

With the posterior approach, we routinely carry out internal fixation of the cervical spine with screw plates implanted into the articular masses. Internal fixation of the cervical spine is simple and provides a rigid fixation. The technical simplicity of implanting screws into the articular masses of the cervical spine is the basis for our technique.

It must be pointed out that in the cervical region as opposed to the thoracic and lumbar spine, screws are *not* transpedicular but rather are implanted into the articular masses. Anatomically, the pedicles of the cervical spine are very small in diameter and are oblique in a direction that is difficult to define when using the posterior approach. In addition, from C-3 to C-6 they lie too close to the vertebral artery to allow safe implantation. To implant a screw into the vertebral pedicle between C-3 and C-6 would be to take an unacceptable risk. At C-7 the vertebral artery does not cross the transverse process and the pedicle is very similar to the one in the dorsal spine. Thus, at C-7 a screw can be implanted into the vertebral pedicle. At C-2, the relationship of the vertebral artery to the articular mass and the pedicle changes. We will discuss at a later point the technical feasibility of implanting a screw into the pedicle of the axis, taking very precise technical precautions.

From C-6 to C-3 the vertebral artery extends vertically across the foramina, which perforate the transverse processes and are situated lateral to the vertebral bodies. The vertebral artery is adjacent to the uncus, which limits laterally the superior vertebral end-plate, and anterior to the nerve roots, which exit transversally from each foramen. In a posterior and lateral position in relation to the vertebral artery is the articular mass, which forms a bony block, the posterior aspect of which is convex. Toward the apex it supports the superior articular process, which faces backward and toward the base; it also supports the inferior articular process, which faces forward (Fig. 7-1).

A screw implanted into the middle of the posterior aspect of the articular mass and directed obliquely toward the exterior will have a solid purchase within the dense cancellous bone between the posterior and anterior cortices. By angling outward, the screw avoids the vertebral artery, which is more medial and is situated in the center of the articular mass; it also avoids the two nerve roots, which are situated above and below at the level of the foramina.

The technique of implanting screws into the cervical spine is based on clear and precise ana-

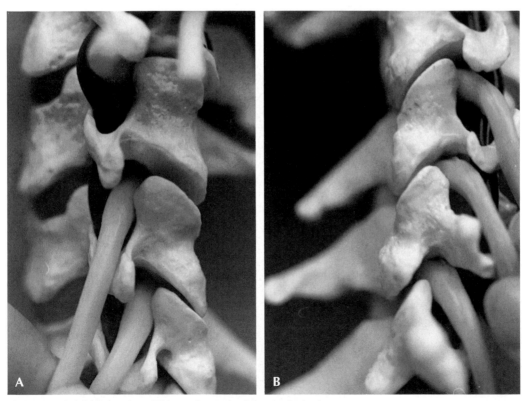

Figure 7-1. (*A*) Oblique view. (*B*) Lateral aspect of the cervical spine.

tomic landmarks, making this a technique that is both simple and reliable. It is simpler than the technique using wire passed through the articular masses and brought out in the articular space. It is more solid than the technique using wire passed through the spinous processes, and safer than passing wire under the laminae, which, in the cervical spine, can cause injury to the spinal cord.

At first, in the 1950s, we used this implantation of cervical screws to perform cortical cancellous iliac grafts, achieving simultaneously both internal fixation and fusion. We then began to use this technique with the introduction of heterologous grafts such as Kiehl grafts. Later, on reviewing the files of patients who had undergone operations, we noted that in many cases the heterologous graft disappeared after 1 or 2 years, leaving just the screws in place. The dislocated articular masses that had been reduced remained stable and fused. We concluded that when a traumatic dislocation was reduced and the articular masses were immobilized, the modification of the articular cartilage

led to its fusion. With our fixation, grafts were unnecessary. So we replaced heterologous grafts by specially designed plates. These are 1 cm wide and 2 mm thick and have a slight posterior concavity that follows or reproduces the normal lordosis of the cervical spine. The holes are spaced at intervals of 13 mm, which is the average normal distance between two articular masses in the cervical spine from C-3 to C-7.

LOWER CERVICAL SPINE

ANATOMY

The anatomy of the lower cervical spine is not generally well known. When a posterior fixation is carried out, only the dorsal aspect of the posterior arches is visible. The position of the anterior elements are thus determined by their relationship to the posterior vertebral arch.

The posterior vertebral arch (Fig. 7-2) comprises the spinous process, situated in the center

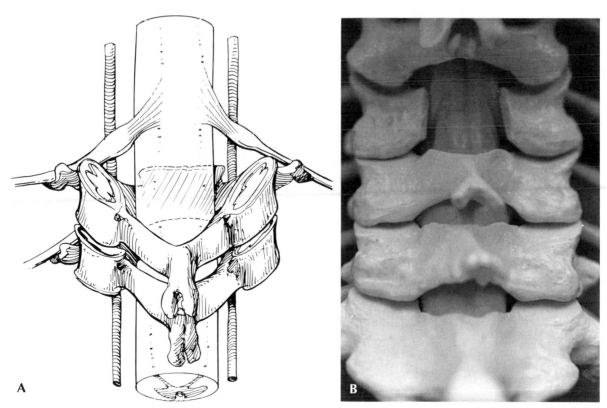

Figure 7-2. (*A, B*) Posterior aspect of C-4 and C-5.

with the laminae on either side, and the articular masses, which are more lateral. A valleylike groove is located at the border between the lamina and articular mass, which protrudes like a small hill, called a hillock. The spinal cord is in front of the spinous process and the laminae. The vertebral artery is situated to the front of the valleylike groove, which serves as an excellent landmark (Fig. 7-3). The roots exit from the canal through the foramina and lie at the level of the articular joints, which are their posterior borders.

In internal fixation of the cervical spine, the plates are placed over the articular masses and the screws are implanted into these masses. When the anatomy is thoroughly understood and the landmarks are located, implantation of the screws into the articular masses is relatively easy.

EXPERIMENTAL STUDY

With Rollin Johnson in New Haven, Connecticut, we investigated the mechanical properties of internal fixation of the cervical spine in flexion and extension stress.

Two cervical vertebrae were removed from a fresh cadaver and, after removal of all the ligaments and interbody disk material, were fixed together posteriorly with a symmetrical pair of two-hole plates. The lower vertebra was fixed firmly in place, while stress was applied to the upper vertebra. The entire experiment was performed in a large glass box in order to maintain a constant hygrometric level and remain as close as possible to in vivo conditions. Displacements during stress

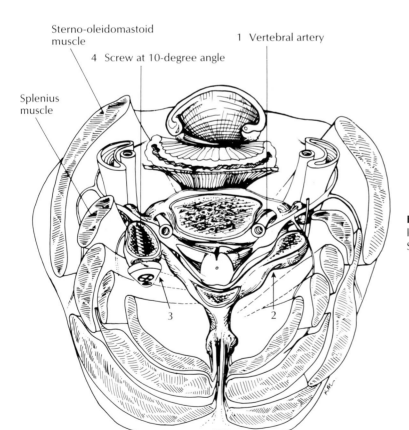

Sterno-oleidomastoid muscle

4 Screw at 10-degree angle

1 Vertebral artery

Splenius muscle

Figure 7-3. Cross section of the neck at the C-4 level. (1) Vertebral artery. (2) Valley. (3) Plate. (4) Screw orientation.

were analyzed with displacement gauges and were radiographed. All results were computerized.

The average breaking load in extension stress was found to 52.5 kg (515 N). This represents 60% of the load necessary to dislocate two normal cervical vertebrae. These results were compared with those obtained using other methods of posterior fixation. In extension stress, posterior wiring of the spinous processes or in the articular masses was found not to be sufficient to stabilize the spine. The fixation with posterior plates increased normal stability by 60%, and a methyl methacrylate fixation on the spinous processes increased stability by 99%.

In flexion stress, posterior wiring between the spinous processes increased stability by 33%. The same system of wiring around a complementary bone graft provided a 55% increase in stability. This reached 88% when the wiring went through the articular masses. Plate fixation increased stability by 92%.

SURGICAL PROCEDURE

In our technique of internal fixation of the lower cervical spine, surgery is performed through a midposterior approach. The patient lies in a prone position with his or her head fixed firmly in a head holder that permits a flexion–extension range of motion. If necessary, a traction device can be attached to the operating table. A local infiltration of lidocaine (Xylocaine) and epinephrine (Adrenalin) makes it easier to separate the muscles on the midline and diminishes bleeding. The posterior approach is generally performed by electrocautery down to the lateral side of the articular masses in order to locate the reference marks exactly.

The precise point for drilling and implantation of screws is at the tip of the articular mass hillock, exactly in its center (Fig. 7-4). For a 3.6 mm screw, a 2.8 mm drill is used. A specially adapted drill with a depth gauge block at 19 mm prevents drilling too deeply. The power on the drill should be lowered to allow for a slow drilling speed. The drilling direction is perpendicular to the spinal

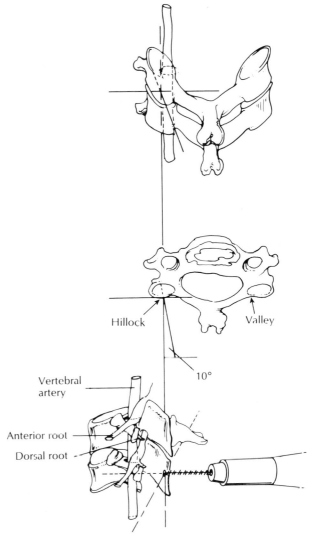

Figure 7-4. Drilling at the tip of the hillock, exactly in its center and 10 degrees oblique laterally.

plane and 10 degrees oblique laterally, never medially. This lateral obliquity increases safety and ensures that the vertebral artery, situated medially in front of the valley, is avoided.

When performed with such precision, this surgical procedure has not led to any vascular complications. The screws are 3.6 mm in diameter and 16 or 19 mm in length. Usually two plates are implanted symmetrically. These have two to five holes, depending on the number of vertebrae to be fixed (Fig. 7-5).

POSTERIOR PLATE FIXATION IN SPECIFIC LOWER CERVICAL SPINE INJURIES

Predominant posterior disrupted lesions are best treated by performing the posterior technique, and anterior lesions by the anterior technique.[11,12] Horizontal lesions of the mobile vertebral segment can be treated either posteriorly or anteriorly. As we are very confident in our technique, if there is any question as to whether to use the posterior or anterior technique, we usually choose posterior plate fixation. Thus our surgical technique, by which screw plates are implanted into the articular masses, is used to stabilize all cervical spine injuries with predominant posterior lesions, as well as severe sprains.

Cervical Dislocation

Cervical dislocations can be unilateral or bilateral. In the case of unilateral dislocations, reduction is achieved operatively with spatulae introduced be-

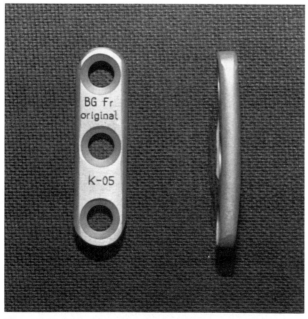

Figure 7-5. Three-hole cervical plate.

tween the laminae at the dislocated level. The first spatula is introduced near the midline, close to the spinous process. While the first spatula is kept in position, a second one is introduced laterally. The first one is then placed further on, between the dislocated articular facets. With a tire-lever maneuver it is then possible to spring the lower articular facet backward over the upper one. The reduction is stabilized by positioning the table head holder in extension. A first posterior two-hole plate is implanted into the dislocated side, then the fixation is completed by a second plate implanted into the opposite side (Fig. 7-6).

For bilateral dislocations the same maneuver is carried out on both sides symmetrically. Again the stabilization is achieved by implanting two posterior two-hole plates.

Single-level dislocations fixed with two-hole plates are strong enough that any secondary displacement is prevented. After the operation the patient will wear a simple collar for 5 weeks.

We prefer to perform this surgical procedure on an emergency basis without previous traction. A precise, smooth reduction is made possible by the direct visual control obtained with open reduction. The posterior fixation, performed simultaneously, shortens the length of postoperative care. Patients without neurologic involvement ambulate on the first postoperative day and are usually discharged from the hospital on the fifth postoperative day.

Facet Fracture and Dislocation

A facet fracture combined with a dislocation is usually situated in the upper articular facet. The displacement of this facet follows the upper vertebral one, and the broken fragment, pushed into the foramen, can compress the cervical nerve root. This creates two problems: possible cervicobrachialgia induced by the compression of the nerve root, and lack of stabilization following reduction, this stabilization normally being provided by the articular facet.

The displaced compressive fragment must be removed from the foramen before carrying out the fixation (Fig. 7-7). This can only be performed by a posterior approach through the articular facet.

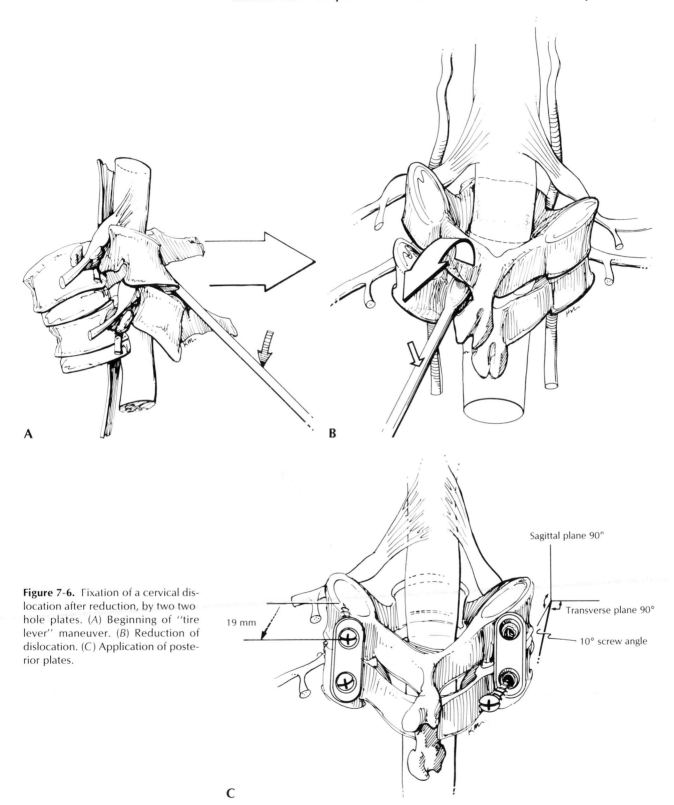

Figure 7-6. Fixation of a cervical dislocation after reduction, by two two hole plates. (*A*) Beginning of ''tire lever'' maneuver. (*B*) Reduction of dislocation. (*C*) Application of posterior plates.

19 mm

Sagittal plane 90°

Transverse plane 90°

10° screw angle

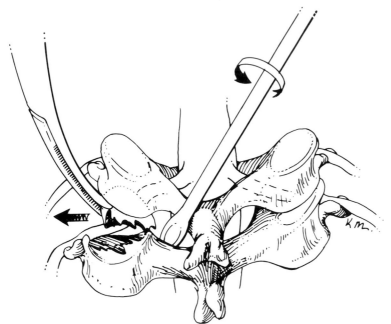

Figure 7-7. Removal of a fractured upper articular facet compressing a nerve root.

The fixation is performed by reconstructing the removed articular facet using a special tile-shaped plate (Fig. 7-8). This is a very precise technique of joint replacement. The upper part of the plate is oblique and is slipped beneath the facet of the upper rotated vertebra (Fig. 7-9). The lower part of the plate is fixed onto the articular mass with screws. In the earlier stages of our study just one plate was used; however, we now prefer to use both a tile plate and a standard two-hole plate. The normal plate is placed over the tile plate like a portemanteau. The fixation is performed by driving a screw through the lower holes of the two plates, and implanting a screw upward into the articular mass of the vertebra above (Fig. 7-10). To increase the stability a normal plate is then implanted on the opposite side. If there is significant instability, it is possible to use the same portemanteau fixation with a long tile plate, bridging three vertebrae.

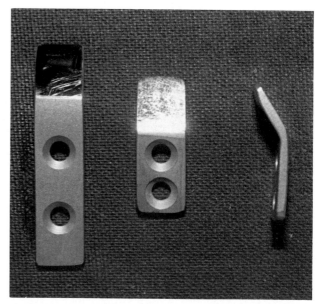

Figure 7-8. Long and short tile-shaped plates.

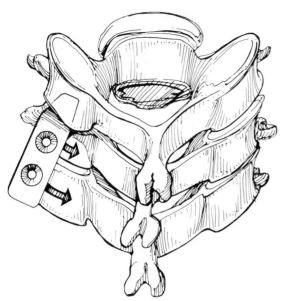

Figure 7-9. The oblique segment of the tile-shaped plate replaces the broken upper facet.

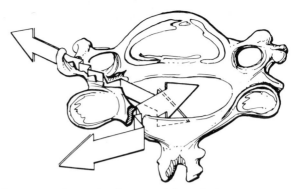

Figure 7-11. Separation fracture of the articular mass.

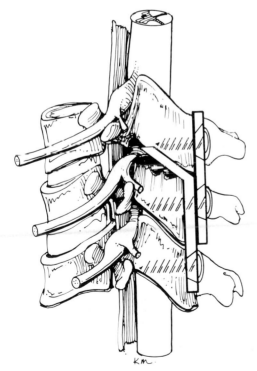

Figure 7-10. Cross section of a "porte manteau" fixation.

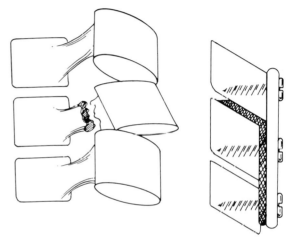

Figure 7-12. (*A*) The separated articular mass (C-4) has a pathognomonic horizontal displacement. (*B*) Reduction and fixation with a long "porte manteau" procedure.

Separation Fracture of the Articular Mass

This is a particularly difficult fracture to stabilize. Two fracture lines separate the articular mass from the rest of the vertebra. Both fracture lines are on the same side, the first on the pedicle and the second on the lamina (Fig. 7-11). In this way the articular mass, completely liberated from the vertebra, will rotate with either the upper or lower adjacent vertebra. Visualized on a lateral radiograph, it is in a horizontal position and is no longer parallel to the adjacent facets (Fig. 7-12A): this is pathognomonic. The fracture lines can be seen on the lamina via the anteroposterior view, and on the pedicle via the oblique view. The correct method of reduction and fixation for such fractures is a long portemanteau fixation on the side of the articular mass fracture. Pushing the lower part of the tile plate against the articular mass of the vertebra below, reduction of the fractured articular mass and of the cervical spine above is achieved. The fixation is performed by placing the normal plate over the tile plate (Fig. 7-12*B*). A simple three-hole plate is implanted on the other side.

Teardrop Fracture

The teardrop fracture is more like a severe sprain than a fracture. Lesions occur principally on the disk and ligaments. The small broken bony fragment of the vertebral body is not significant (Fig. 7-13). Instability is due to the severity of the sprain. When the injury is mainly posterior with

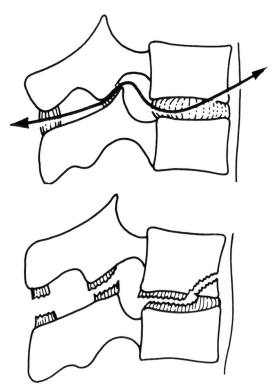

Figure 7-13. Teardrop fracture with the line of the lesions, similar to a severe sprain.

demonstrative interspinous widening and articular facet posterior opening, surgical treatment can be performed posteriorly with posterior plates in the same way as for severe sprains (Fig. 7-14).

Severe Sprains

Sprains are often misdiagnosed. The entire mobile vertebral segment is involved by the trauma but there is no bony lesion. The severe sprain is the stage just prior to the complete tear of a dislocation. Displacement may occur a few weeks or months after the initial sprain injury, induced by the continuous mobilization of the neck. Severe sprains involve interspinous widening, facet subluxation, disk posterior opening, and anterior listhesis of the upper vertebra. Fixation with posterior plates and screws is a simple and ideal technique for the stabilization of these lesions.

RATIONALE OF POSTERIOR PLATE FIXATION

There are a number of advantages of this fixation technique in the lower cervical spine. Posterior fixation with plates and screws is a very simple and effective method of achieving a fusion following an unsuccessful attempt using an anterior technique. A stable posterior fixation induces an anterior fusion.

The posterior approach and the use of posterior plates and screws implanted into the articular masses make it possible to perform further associated procedures. Because the plates are placed laterally to the laminae on the articular masses, it is simple to perform a laminectomy if necessary. It has already been pointed out that grafting is not necessary in cases of pure dislocation; however, when associated fractures are present a Hibbs' operation on the laminae is possible if desired.

Postoperative care in many cases is simplified. Straightforward injuries such as unilateral dislocations are immobilized for 5 weeks by a simple collar. More unstable lesions with associated fractures are immobilized for 2 to 3 months by a light Minerva jacket. In cases of spinal cord injury with quadriplegia, the stable fixation induced by the plates facilitates nursing care.

The mechanical stability of this fixation was demonstrated in a continuous series of 221 cases

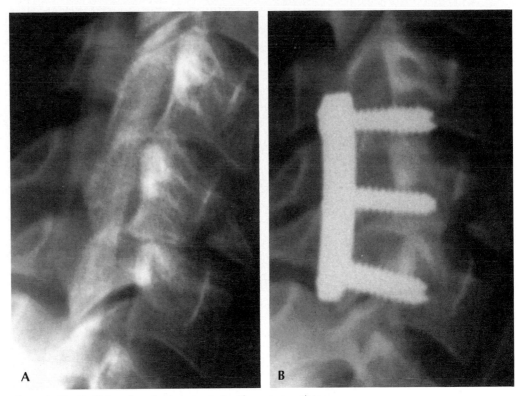

Figure 7-14. (*A, B*) Teardrop fracture treated with posterior plates.

of lower cervical spine injuries treated by this technique. In 85.2% of the cases there was no secondary displacement, in 8.8% there was a displacement of less than 5 degrees, in 3% the displacement was 5 to 10 degrees, and in 3% displacement was more than 10 degrees. No breakage of plates or screws was observed.[3]

The only contraindication for posterior plate fixation is in severe cases of osteoporosis.

UPPER CERVICAL SPINE

ANATOMY

The normal occipitocervical angulation is 105 degrees, giving the eyes their normal horizontal direction. Internal fixation with plates must maintain this angulation.

The longitudinal posterior venous sinus is situated on the midline of the occipital bone. To the lateral side of this sinus the bone is approximately 10 to 12 mm thick with two cortices. Because of these two cortices, a short but nevertheless strong screw purchase can be obtained.

If it is necessary to implant a screw into a C-2 pedicle, it is important to know its direction as well as its relationship to the spinal cord and vertebral artery. A C-2 pedicle has an oblique upward and inward direction of 10 to 15 degrees (Fig. 7-15). A screw implanted into this pedicle must have the same direction.

The C-1 ring is normally divided into three equal surfaces: one for the odontoid process, one for the cord, and one that is free. At C-2 the ring is still large and there is no intimate contact between the spinal cord and the pedicles.

The vertebral artery makes a loop similar to a horizontal "S" within the C-2 articular mass. The posterior aspect of the articular mass, reached through a posterior approach, can be divided into four quadrants. The vertebral artery occupies the

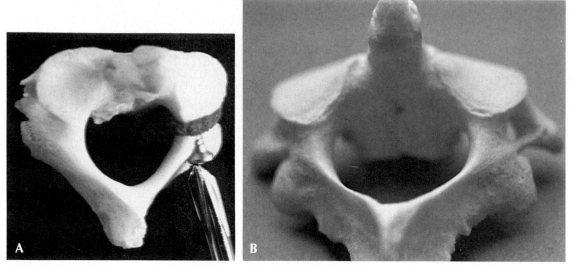

Figure 7-15. (*A, B*) C-2 pedicle has 15 degrees of upward and inward obliquity.

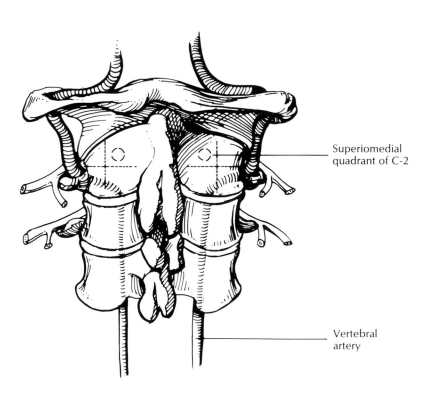

Superiomedial
quadrant of C-2

Vertebral
artery

Figure 7-16. A screw can be implanted safely into the upper medial quadrant of the C-2 articular mass.

upper lateral and two inferior quadrants. A screw can be implanted into the upper medial quadrant, which is free (Fig. 7-16).

ARTHRODESIS FOR OCCIPITOCERVICAL PATHOLOGY

The classical method of occiput–C-2 grafting has several elements that can lead to failure, including:

The fragility of the fitting
Delays in taking of the graft caused by compulsory micromotion in the absence of internal fixation
The difficulty in setting the position of the head in relation to the neck.

In order to avoid these problems, we perform this fusion by screwing two plates laterally onto the occipital bone and the cervical articular masses. These plates provide immediate support, which in turn favors successful graft incorporation. Since the plates are premolded to fit the normal 105-degree curvature of the occipitocervical joint (Fig. 7-17), a perfect and automatic positioning of the skull over the cervical spine is assured.[7]

The vertical portion of the plate is made with reinforced holes, 13 mm apart, for the application of screws into the articular masses. The horizontal portion is slightly curved and perfectly adaptable to the skull. This portion is made thinner by the absence of any embossing around the holes, and does not therefore stick under the skin. There are two sizes of occipitocervical plates. The small plate has three cervical holes, making it possible to reach the articular masses at C-3 and C-4. The larger one has four cervical holes, allowing one to reach the level of C-5. If it is necessary to extend the arthrodesis further down, we use dorsolumbar plates that are molded prior to surgery.

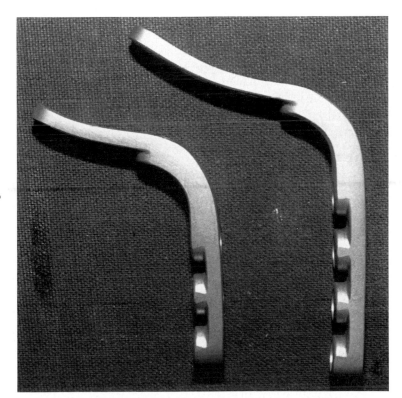

Figure 7-17. Special occipitocervical plates, two sizes.

The patient is operated on in a prone position. The table is equipped with a head holder, which can easily be adjusted during the operation. This makes it possible for the skull to support traction if necessary.

In order to control bleeding during the operation, the head of the table should be placed high enough to assure that the operative field is reasonably bloodless. Controlled hypotension should be established.

A preoperative radiograph should be available for checking the best positioning of the occiput and cervical spine.

The skin incision starts from the occipital protuberance and follows the line of the spinal processes. The two paravertebral grooves are retracted in order to obtain a perfect exposure of the cervical vertebral articular masses. Care is needed when exposing the posterior arch of C-1. To avoid bleeding from the venous plexuses that follow the vertebral artery, one must not exceed 1 cm on either side of the medial line. The occipital sheath is exposed subperiosteally.

For the implantation of the screws, which are 3.5 mm in diameter, drilling is first performed in the articular masses. The same technique as that used for the lower cervical spine should be followed, aiming in a perpendicular direction and 10 degrees oblique laterally at the top of the hillock formed by each articular mass. The plates are then applied, the inferior holes corresponding to the holes drilled in the articular masses.

The head is gently mobilized so that the upper part of the plates fits neatly against the occipital sheath. Here the drilling is done carefully with a slow drill speed, through the two cortices of the occipital bone. It is very helpful to use a protected drill depth of 13 mm in order to avoid any penetration that could injure the dura mater, although this was never observed. If the posterior thoracic wall makes it difficult to hold the motor in the correct direction, one may use a flexible drill or bend the head carefully a few degrees in flexion.

Screws 13 mm in length are first implanted into the occipital bone, then screws 16 or 19 mm in length are implanted into the articular masses. The occipital bone is then decorticated with a gouge or bur. The spinal processes and vertebral laminae are also decorticated. Cortical cancellous scrapings are cut off the posterior iliac crest and applied directly over the decorticated areas. A large cortical cancellous graft from the posterior iliac crest is placed between the two plates. It is fixed with a screw in the medial occipital line by contouring a midline notch around the spinal process of the inferior involved vertebra.

During the postoperative period, the patient becomes ambulatory within 48 hours. He or she must wear a molded cervicothoracic orthosis for 3 months.

Certain procedures can be associated with the occipitocervical arthrodesis. A laminectomy can be carried out with extreme caution at the level of C-1 without interposing any instrument between the bone and the neural axis. An enlargement of the occipital bone to the back may also be performed.[5] The bony sheath behind the hole is perforated. The occipital bone is then chipped with a rongeur or bur, working from back to front.

The occipitocervical arthrodesis technique is simple and reliable. The stability obtained following the application of the plates assures a good take of the graft and light postoperative retention. We use this method in cases of dislocation of the occipitocervical junction (Fig. 7-18).

LATERAL ARTHRODESIS OF C-1–C-2 ARTICULAR PROCESSES (DU TOIT)[2]

If a fusion is necessary on the upper cervical spine it must be as short as possible. If the classical posterior C-1–C-2 fusion is not possible, the internal fixation technique is very helpful. This approach should give direct access to the lateral masses of C-1 and C-2 down to the vertebral bodies.

Positioning of the patient is normal, with the head in a frontal position for the bilateral approach. The ear lobe is stitched above and to the front of the pretragal region in order to free the tip of the mastoid.

The approach to the articular processes of C-1–C-2 is posterior to the sternomastoid muscle and above the hyoid.[6] The approach is left and right. The incision, 5 to 6 cm long, is retromastoidal and starts at the tip on the mastoid apo-

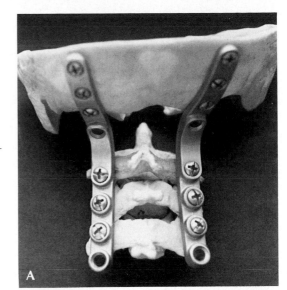

Figure 7-18. (*A, B*) Occipitocervical fixation for a complex fracture-dislocation of C-2. (C) Lateral view with the graft.

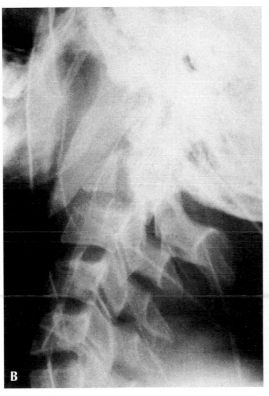

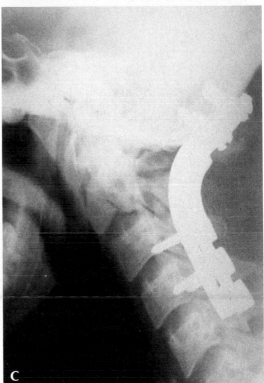

physis (Fig. 7-19). The upper part of the incision can be convex frontward.

The sternomastoid muscle can be partially retracted from the mastoid toward the front. The carotid vessels and the spinal nerve are protected, at the front, by the muscle. Two approaches are possible: through the muscle or from behind it (Fig. 7-20).

The essential landmark here is the transverse apophysis of C-1. This is the most external bony structure; prominent and easily located with palpation, it is situated 1 cm below the mastoid. The anterior aspect of the transverse apophysis is freed until the anterior aspect of the lateral mass of C-1 is reached. The transverse apophysis of C-2 can be detected below that of C-1 and slightly deeper.

The intertransverse muscles are left intact because they protect the vertebral artery in the transverse canal. The anterior aspect of the C-2 transverse apophysis is in turn freed in order to reach the anterior aspect of the articular line and the two lateral masses of C-1 and C-2. The long muscles of the neck are retracted from the anterior aspects of the C-1 and C-2 bodies and pulled toward the front. From this point on, it is possible to free the anterior tubercle of C-1 and reach the retropharyngeal space. The C-1–C-2 joint is opened by excising the capsule. It is well exposed by a narrow Homan's retractor resting on the base of the odontoid.

The joint is cleared from the front with a small osteotome and a motor-powered bur. Cortical

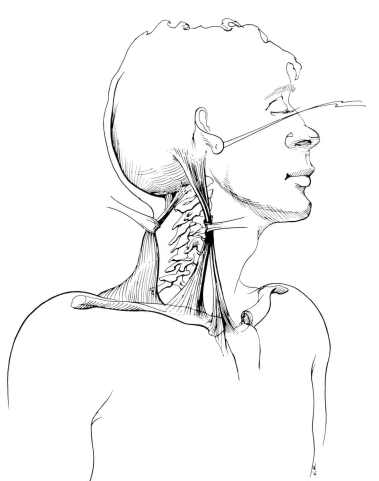

Figure 7-19. Incision for C-1–C-2 lateral approach.

Sternocleido
mastoid muscle

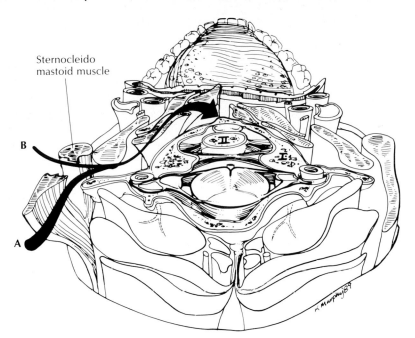

Figure 7-20. Cross section with arrows indicating the approach through (*A*) or behind (*B*) the muscle.

cancellous grafts are taken from the iliac crest or from the transverse process of C-1 and packed into the joint. Fixation of the fusion is achieved by an oblique screw. Its point of entry is just at the anterior border of the base of the transverse process of C-1; it passes obliquely downward at an angle of 25 degrees to the horizontal in the frontal plane (Fig. 7-21). The length of the screw varies from 25 to 35 mm.

The prominence of the mastoid process may impede the drilling by making the drill hole too horizontal or too anterior. In this case, the fixation can be made with a small staple across the joint or by screwing an anterior short plate into the C-1 and C-2 articular processes.

The operation can be done bilaterally by two teams working simultaneously, or successively by one surgeon. Following the operation the patient is ambulatory and will need to wear a Minerva jacket for an average of 3 months.

This technique can be used in case of failure of a posterior C-1–C-2 arthrodesis, or in cases of a Jefferson fracture or a dens fracture with an associated posterior arch fracture of C-1.

C-1–C-2 POSTERIOR ARTHRODESIS BY DIRECT IMPLANTATION OF SCREWS IN THE ARTICULAR FACETS

There are three radiographic landmarks that it is important to study prior to the operation (Fig. 7-22):

> The superior end-plate of C-3 and the inferior end-plate of C-2
> The anterior arch of C-1
> The facet of C-2.

These landmarks can be detected on the image taken in profile.

The relationship between the lateral masses of C-1 and C-2 and the vertebral arteries is intimate. Thus at C-2 the implantation of screws will first be in the isthmus of the pedicles and then in the facet joint. It is advisable to avoid the superolateral face of the pedicle, which is the point at which the vertebral artery passes. The screw emerges in the center of the C-2 articular surface before penetrating the lateral mass of C-1. At this level there is

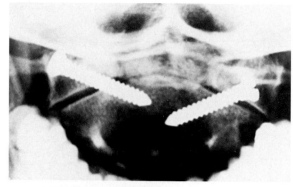

Figure 7-21. (A, B, C) Lateral fixation of C-1–C-2 articular masses by an oblique screw at 25 degrees to the horizontal in the frontal plane.

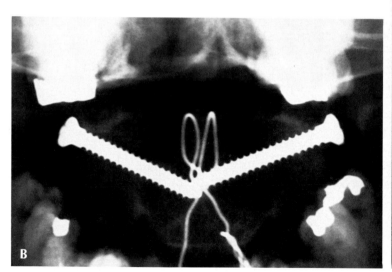

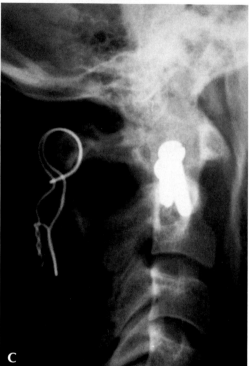

no longer any risk to the vessels because the vertebral artery forms a posterior loop and rests against the upper part of the posterior C-1 arch.

At the point at which the extremity of the screw emerges at the anterior cortex of C-1, there are no other elements in front of C-1 apart from the suprahyoid portion of the pharynx. The mucous membrane is separated from C-1 and C-2 by the common anterior vertebral ligament and the long muscles of the neck.

Two screws are needed to stabilize the lateral masses of C-2 and C-1. The alignment of each screw must be strictly straight ahead in the sagittal plane and directed obliquely upward and forward at an angle of 60 degrees in relation to the lower portion of the C-2 body.[4]

If the orientation of this screw is not strictly straight ahead, it is better for it to be slightly medial rather than lateral; we have noted that the medial intracanal margin of security is greater

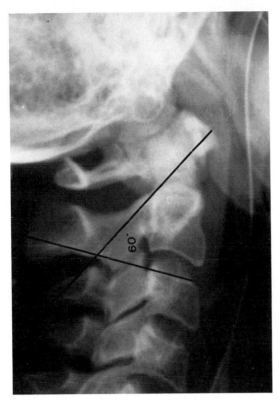

Figure 7-22. Radiographic landmarks.

than the lateral margin of security, which is limited by the passage of the vertebral artery.

In the cranial caudal plane, drilling should be directed obliquely upward at an angle of 60 degrees with a possible variation of 5 degrees. If the drilling is any lower, it will tend to come out between the lateral masses of C-2 and C-1. Furthermore, if the drilling is too lateral or too inferior, it may injure the vertebral artery.

This technique necessitates a perfect exposure of the posterior arches of C-1 and C-2 and positioning to diminish the inconvenient contour of the cervicodorsal junction. The patient is put in a ventral decubitus position with a thick block under each shoulder. The head is fixed in a head holder. The upper part of the cervical spine is put in kyphosis to free C-1 and C-2.

An image intensifier is fundamental to this technique because it reduces the time spent in operation that is due to frequent radiographic filming of the progression of the drill and screws. Through a posterior medial incision, the paravertebral grooves and then the C-2 laminae are freed laterally to the lateral border of the facets. It is not necessary to open up the atlanto-axial membrane as one does when locating the pedicle if implantation of the screws is monitored by an image intensifier.

If no image intensifier is available, the internal and superior borders of the pedicle are located with a spatula while keeping a distance from the medullary axis. Progression with a spatula is carried out on the first centimeter of the pedicle, making it possible to define its direction in the two planes.

The point of entry is situated at the junction of the lamella and facet on the posterior arch of C-2, as near as possible to the C-2–C-3 joint line. Drilling must remain strictly straight ahead in the sagittal plane and be directed obliquely upward at an angle of 60 degrees in relation to the tangent line in the inferior plateau of C-2. The direction is perfect when, on the lateral image, the extremity of the drill is directed toward the anterior tubercle of C-1 (Fig. 7-22).

After penetrating the resistance of the first cortex of C-2, the drill encounters resistance when it passes into the anterior portion of the pedicle and then strikes the cortex of the superior facet of C-2. The third area of resistance is due to the perforation of the cortex of the inferior aspect of the lateral C-1 mass, and finally a fourth resistance is encountered, indicating that the drill has reached the anterior aspect of the atlas.

A flexible drill holder is very helpful. This makes control of direction and access much easier in relation to the spinous processes of C-7–D-1. The drilling is achieved with a 2.8 mm drill, but the first part of the drilling, in C-2, can be carried out with a 3.5 mm drill in order to obtain a better compression. Philipp's 3.5 mm screws are 36, 38, and 41 mm in length, making it possible to reach the anterior cortex of the atlas.

For ease of drilling into C-2 and then C-1, traction must be applied to the spinous process of C-2 using a forceps. Furthermore, it must be known that one never has too much of an upward direction; therefore, the drill must lie as flat against the spinous process of C-7 as possible. The two screws

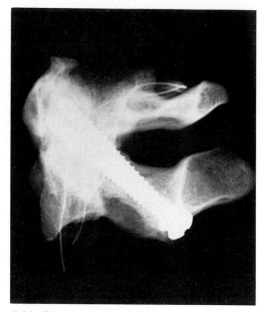

Figure 7-23. Direct posterior implantation of screws in the articular masses for C-1–C-2 arthrodesis.

are implanted successively. Perfect stabilization of C-1–C-2 is observed (Fig. 7–23).

The difficulties that may arise in use of this technique often lie in the morphology of the subject, including a short or thick neck or a prominent cervicodorsal articulation. As far as complications are concerned, the main problem is perforation of the vertebral artery.

This type of fixation can be used in cases of pseudarthrosis of the odontoid, but can also be performed in cases of odontoid fractures associated with a congenital or acquired abnormality of the posterior arch of C-1 or C-2, with a Jefferson fracture, or with a severe C-1–C-2 sprain. It is competitive with the Du Toit technique.

POSTERIOR C-1–C-2 FIXATION WITH AN IMPLANT

Fusion of the upper cervical spine must be avoided as often as possible. In some cases a tem-

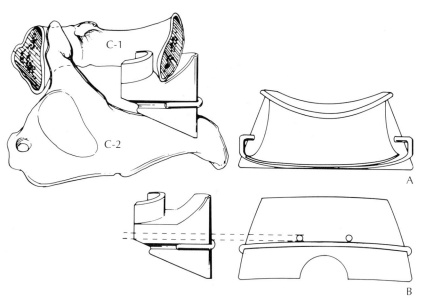

Figure 7-24. The C-1–C-2 polyethylene implant. (A) Superior view. (B) Anteroposterior and lateral view.

porary C-1–C-2 fixation may induce consolidation of a dens fracture.

We use a polyethylene implant with the shape and size of a usual C-1–C-2 graft. It is anteriorly concave with a groove in its upper border and a notch in the lower one[9] (Fig. 7-24). There are two different sizes, which can be adapted to the patients.

The polyethylene implant is placed between the posterior arches of C-1 and C-2 to maintain their normal separation and to ensure a correct reduction in the sagittal plane of an odontoid fracture. It is used in the same way as a classical bone graft. The posterior arch of C-1 is placed in the upper groove and the lower notch is placed astride the spine of C-2. Fixation is achieved by either a thick nylon suture or a wire. The nylon is easier to tighten, but the wire is safer. The suture first passes from behind, forward through the two holes in the middle of the implant. The two sutures are passed round the posterior arch of C-1 from below, upward, and then behind the implant under the loop of the wire. One of the ends is passed through the interspinous ligament between C-2 and C-3 before being tied tightly to the opposite end (Fig. 7-25). In this way, the fixation is very stable and in anatomic alignment.

This technique is recommended for odontoid

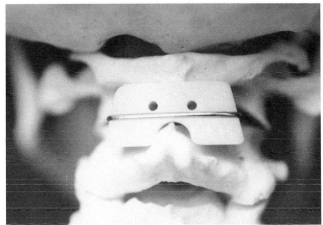

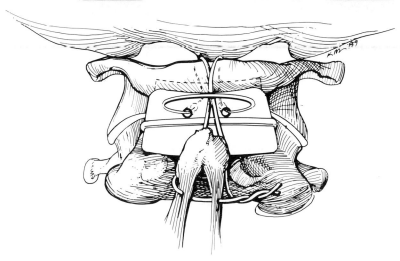

Figure 7-25. C-1–C-2 fixation with the polyethylene implant. (*A*) Posterior view. (*B*) Lacing in place.

fractures with an oblique line descending anteriorly because anterior displacement is easy to reduce with the wire positioning.

ANTERIOR SCREW FIXATION OF THE ODONTOID PROCESS

Originally described by Jorg Bohler in 1975,[1] anterior screw fixation of the odontoid is difficult to perform; however, it preserves the function of the C-1–C-2 joint, which is very important.

The patient is placed in a supine position on a radiolucent table. Nasal intubation using a flexible tube avoids superimposition on radiographs. The shoulders are pushed forward by a small transverse sandbag. The head is positioned in flexion or extension for better reduction of the displacement. The head is positioned almost straight but is turned slightly to the left.[8]

It is advisable to use two image intensifiers simultaneously. The lateral view is easily obtained, but the anteroposterior view is more problematic. The beam is centered on the maxilla or mouth, depending on the position of the head. It is inclined slightly obliquely in an upward or downward direction (Fig. 7-26).

The approach is in front of the sternomastoid muscle and below the hyoid on the right side, working from below upward.

The fixation should only be made after the fracture has been reduced. This is usually done after

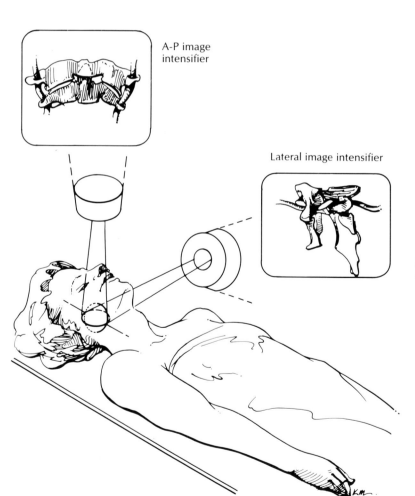

A-P image intensifier

Lateral image intensifier

Figure 7-26. The anteroposterior control of a dens fracture with the image intensifier.

the patient has been positioned and only exceptionally by direct manipulation of the fracture. The point of entry of the drill is determined in the frontal and sagittal planes. In the frontal plane, the screw enters into the inferior surface of the body of C-2 through the C-2–C-3 disk (Fig. 7-27). The anterosuperior corner of C-3 sometimes needs to be trimmed. In the frontal plane, because access is from the lateral side, the screws are slightly oblique from right to left.

The point of entry of the drill is made with an awl. In the sagittal plane, the line of drilling is the most vertical possible in the axis of the cervical spine. Drilling is impeded by the prominence of the thoracic cage, against which the motor of the drill rests. This problem can be helped by using a flexible cable for drilling.

The drilling is controlled by using the two image intensifiers simultaneously. Care must be taken not to be too anterior or posterior. The drill must pass from the anteroinferior corner of the C-2 body to the most superior and posterior part of the tip of the odontoid in order to obtain a solid fixation. The screw is normally between 32 and 38 mm long and is 3.5 mm in diameter.

The second screw is inserted in the same way, but the point of entry is more lateral. The method is the same (Fig. 7-28).

Postoperative immobilization in a Minerva jacket is preferable, with the purchase on the occiput and chin to control rotation as well as flexion and extension of the cervical spine. In certain cases, a simple rigid collar is sufficient. Bony union is monitored by anteroposterior and lateral tomographs.

This technique is excellent in cases of odontoid fractures with an oblique line descending posteriorly. However, if the line descends in an oblique anterior direction, the screw is almost parallel to this line and one may have a loss of reduction.

INTERNAL FIXATION OF C-2 PEDICLES WITH SCREWS AND PLATES BETWEEN C-2 AND C-3

The direct fixation of C-2 pedicles in a hangman's fracture is the most logical method of osteosynthesis of this lesion. The implanted screws must avoid the vertebral arteries, the anatomy must be

well known, and the technique must be very precise (see the previous section).[10]

The posterior approach facilitates reduction in cases of C-2–C-3 dislocation. Once reduction has been achieved, the lesion is stabilized using pedicular screw fixation and two plates bridging the dislocated C-2–C-3 joint. The difficulty lies in the C-2 pedicular screws. A drill is first introduced in the upper and medial quadrant of the inferior articular facet of C-2 (see Fig. 7-16). It should be placed very high, in a medial position close to the medial border of the C-2 pedicle. This pedicle must be probed with a spatula placed in the spinal canal while the hole is being drilled. Starting from the point of entry in the superomedial quadrant of the articular process, the hole should be drilled in a 15-degree upward direction and a 15-degree medial direction (Fig. 7-29). As the drill hole is being made, one can feel the passage of the drill across the fracture to the cancellous bone of the C-2 body as far as its anterior cortex. The drill hole normally measures 30 mm in length. A screw is applied through the upper hole of a two-hole plate and tightened. Another screw is then applied to the articular process of C-3 through the second hole in the plate. An identical plate with two screws is applied on the opposite side. Stabilization of the fracture of the pedicles and the dislocation of the C-2–C-3 joint is thus achieved (Fig. 7-30).

This technique may be used in cases of unstable hangman's fractures with dislocation of the C-2–C-3 facets. The direct long screws stabilize the pedicles and the plates stabilize the C-2–C-3 dislocation.

ANTERIOR INTERNAL FIXATION OF THE CERVICAL SPINE WITH STAPLES

Specially designed for the spine, these staples are safe and simple to implant. There is no risk of penetrating the spinal canal. They are used to improve stability after the insertion of an anterior bone graft.

The staples are 1 cm wide and of different lengths. They have four feet with serrated edges

(Text continues on p. 186)

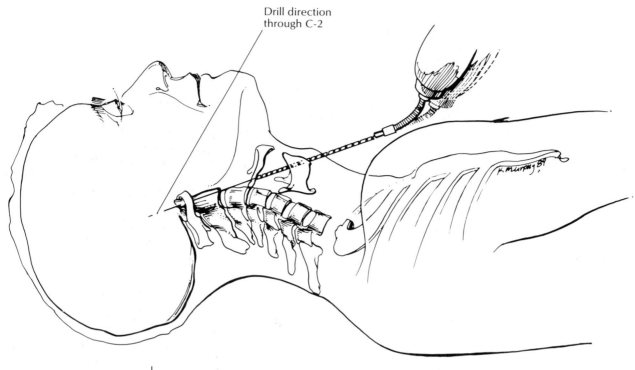

Drill direction
through C-2

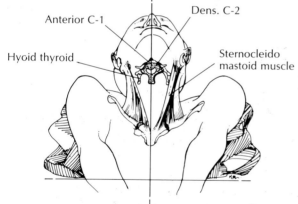

Anterior C-1

Hyoid thyroid

Dens. C-2

Sternocleido
mastoid muscle

Figure 7-27. The drill enters into the inferior surface of the body of C-2. The use of a flexible cable is helpful to avoid the prominence of the thoracic cage.

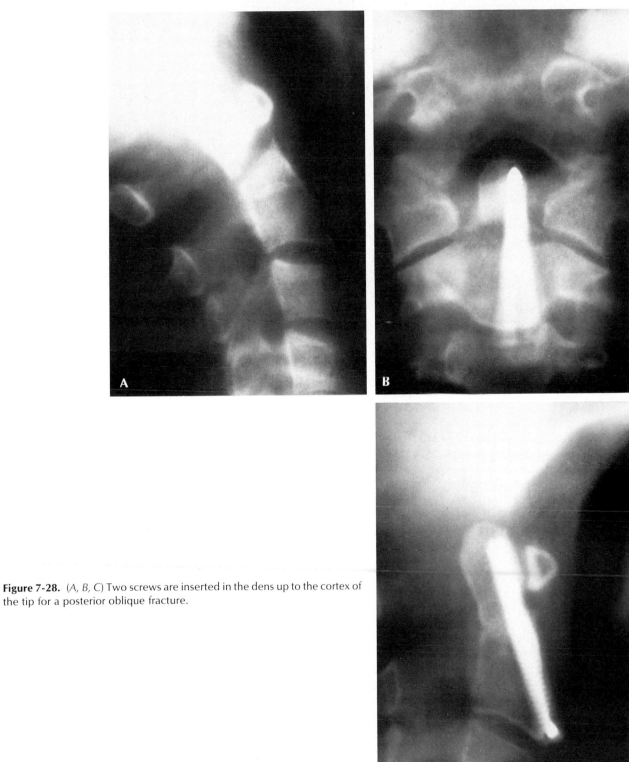

Figure 7-28. (*A, B, C*) Two screws are inserted in the dens up to the cortex of the tip for a posterior oblique fracture.

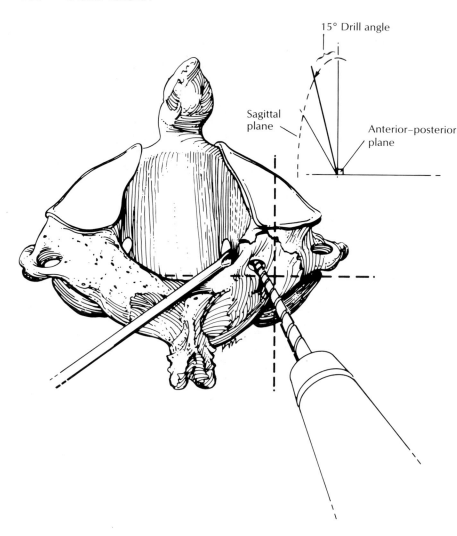

15° Drill angle

Sagittal plane

Anterior–posterior plane

Figure 7-29. Drilling of the C-2 pedicle 15 degrees obliquely upward and inward with the control of a spatula into the vertebral canal.

that will support the underlying and overlying vertebrae (Fig. 7-31). Templates are used for positioning the staples.

The length of the staple is selected with an adequate template placed over the graft. The template has a hole in each corner corresponding to the 4 feet of the staple. The positions of the holes are determined to give, if possible, a purchase on the end-plates of the vertebrae without bridging any normal disk. The template, which is attached to a handle, is placed on the midline of the cervical spine. The vertebrae are drilled to a depth of 1 cm through the four holes corresponding to the four feet of the adequate staple. The staple is then placed in the same position with its oblique carrier, and the four feet are introduced into the four holes by hammering on the carrier with a punch (Fig. 7-32). The feet are short enough to prevent penetration of the vertebral canal (Fig. 7-33).

The staples are used in cases where it is necessary to improve stability after the insertion of an anterior or bone graft.

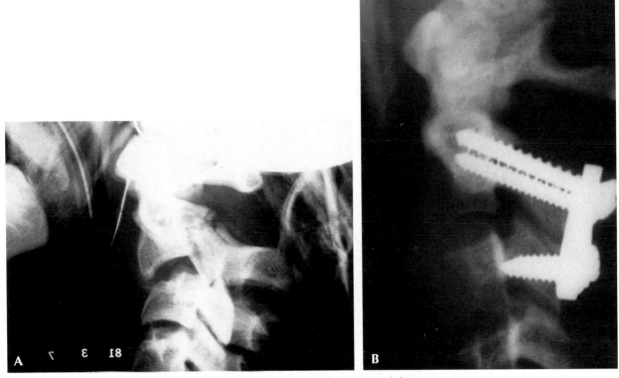

Figure 7-30. (*A, B*) Stabilization of the C-2 pedicle fracture and of the C-2–C-3 dislocation.

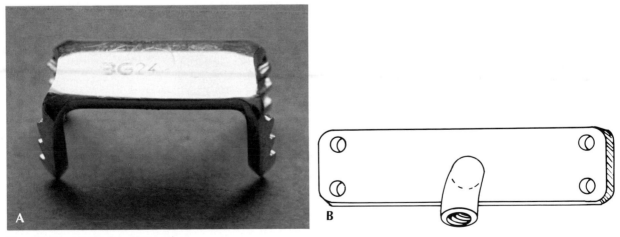

Figure 7-31. (*A*) Staples. (*B*) Template.

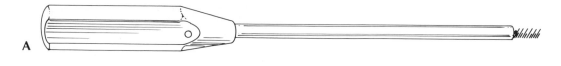

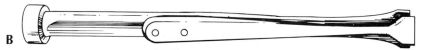

Figure 7-32. (*A*) Template handle. (*B*) Staple carrier.

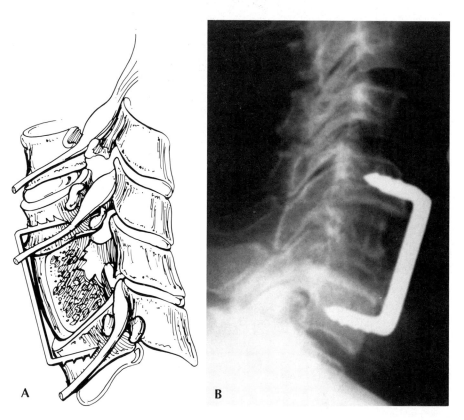

Figure 7-33. (*A*) Anterior graft. (*B*) Staple.

REFERENCES

1. Bohler J: Anterior stabilisation for acute fractures and nonunions of the dens. J Bone Joint Surg [Am] 64:18–27, 1982
2. Du Toit G: Lateral atlanto-axial arthrodesis: A screw fixation technique. S Afr J Surg 14:9–12, 1976
3. Roy-Camille R, Saillant G, Mazel C et al: Rachis cervical traumatique non neurologique. In Roy-Camille R (ed): Lères Journées d'Orthopédie de la Pitié. Paris, Masson Publisher, 1979
4. Roy-Camille R, Benazet JP, Leonard PH, Lazennec JY: L'arthrodese C1-C2 par vissage articulaire posterieur, pp 44–48. In Roy-Camille R (ed): 5èmes Journées d'Orthopédie de la Pitié: Rachis Cervical Supérieur. Paris, Masson Publisher, 1986
5. Roy-Camille R, Bouchet TH, Saillant G: Decompression posterieure occipito-atloidienne par elargissement du trou occipital et laminectomie de C1, pp 32–35. In Roy-Camille R (ed): 5èmes Journées d'Orthopédie de la Pitié: Rachis Cervical Supérieur. Paris, Masson Publisher, 1986
6. Roy-Camille R, Bouchet TH, Saillant G, Ferron JM: Technique de l'abord lateral de C1-C2, pp 62–65. In Roy-Camille R (ed): 5èmes Journées d'Orthopé-die de la Pitié: Rachis Cervical Supérieur. Masson Publisher, 1986
7. Roy-Camille R, Gagna G, Lazennec JY: L'arthrodese occipito-cervicale, pp 49–51. In Roy-Camille R (ed): 5èmes Journées d'Orthopédie de la Pitié: Rachis Cervical Supérieur. Masson Publisher, 1986
8. Roy-Camille R, Mazel CH, Benazet JP, Cavagna R: Vissage anterieur de l'odontoide, pp 58–61. In Roy-Camille R (ed): 5èmes Journées d'Orthopédie de la Pitié: Rachis Cervical Supérieur. Masson Publisher, 1986
9. Roy-Camille R, Morin O, LaPresle PH: La prothese en polyethylene C1-C2, pp 39–41. In Roy-Camille R (ed): 5èmes Journées d'Orthopédie de la Pitié: Rachis Cervical Supérieur. Masson Publisher, 1986
10. Roy-Camille R, Saillant G, Bouchet TH: Technique du vissage des pedicules de C2, pp 41–43. In Roy-Camille R (ed): 5èmes Journées d'Orthopédie de la Pitié: Rachis Cervical Supérieur. Masson Publisher, 1986
11. Roy-Camille R, Saillant G, Lazennec JY: Chirurgie par abord posterieur du rachis cervical. In Encyclopédie médico-chirurgicale, Paris, Techniques chirurgicales (Orthopédie), 3-22-09, 44176, 1987
12. Roy-Camille R, Saillant G, Sagnet P: Luxation-fracture du rachis, pp 750–766. In Detrie PH (ed): Chirurgie d'Urgence. Masson Publisher, 1985

THORACIC AND
LUMBAR SPINE

8

THORACOLUMBAR SPINE INJURIES

R. David Bauer
Thomas J. Errico

Interest in the treatment of thoracolumbar spinal fractures has intensified within the last 10 years. Dissatisfaction with the results of conservative treatment of fractures has led to the redefinition of the role for and the increased utilization of surgical techniques. In the 1980s a greater understanding of the abnormal anatomy of the area of a spinal fracture has been achieved by the use of computed tomography and metrizamide myelography. Detection of spinal injury and bone in the canal has been enhanced by these techniques. The conservative approach stressed by Guttman and Bedbrook[12,13,104,105] has yielded to a more aggressive operative approach as convincing evidence that secure and adequate stabilization of unstable thoracic and lumbar spine fractures promotes faster rehabilitation, easier nursing care, and fewer complications is presented.

In this chapter, we will discuss the detection of thoracolumbar injuries and the associated injuries that accompany them. We will review the classification of injuries and the role of both conservative and operative care for these injuries. Specific types of injuries will be discussed in detail.

CLINICAL FEATURES

Thoracolumbar fractures tend to affect a younger segment of the population. They are most often due to motor vehicle accidents, winter sports accidents,[137,244] airplane crashes,[114,209,254] industrial accidents, falls, jumps, and suicide attempts, and less frequently due to direct violence.

A thorough evaluation of all patients suspected of having a thoracolumbar spine fracture is mandatory. Suspicion that a fracture has occurred is the first step in the detection of injury. Screening radiographs should be obtained of the thoracolumbar spine in patients involved in a fall from a height and in patients involved in motor vehicle accidents who complain of pain or have an altered neurologic status.[159]

A careful physical and neurologic exam is essential. The patient's awareness of pain or the level of the patient's apparent neurologic injury is the most important clinical factor. Examination of the back reveals tenderness at the site of fracture. A palpable gap between spinous processes at the level of the dislocation may be present and is the most reliable physical sign of dislocation and damage to the posterior elements.[109,118,119,135,141,228] Any retained muscular function or sensation below the injury must be sought, as this has tremendous prognostic significance for eventual recovery. Preserved sensation is occasionally limited to the perianal area, and should not be overlooked. The degree of anal sphincter tone should also be assessed, and the bulbocavernous reflex checked.

Blunt trauma to the chest or abdomen severe enough to cause a thoracolumbar fracture will also have adverse effects on other organ systems.[4,28,45,63,96,145,222,251] Life-threatening emergencies are often present, especially in the cardiovascular or pulmonary systems, and severe head trauma may be present. Approximately 50% of patients with thoracolumbar fractures have multisystem trauma: Almost 30% have injuries to one organ system other than the spine, 10% to 20% have injuries to two, and approximately 5% have injuries to three or more other organ systems. There are concomitant injuries to the skull and head in approximately one third of patients with thoracolumbar fractures, and significant injuries to the chest and abdomen occur in almost one quarter. Facial, head, and neck injuries, including cervical spine fractures, occur in the majority of patients.[14,235] Displaced thoracic fractures are always accompanied by painful rib fractures and often by underlying lung contusions,[45,83,145,180] hemothorax or hemopneumothorax.[14,45,96,180,251] Aortic arch arteriograms may be necessary to rule out trauma to the great vessels.[14] Splenic injury and other intra-abdominal injury is not uncommon. Scapular fractures also occur, especially in conjunction with upper thoracic fractures.[180] The care of life-threatening emergencies takes precedence over injuries to the spine and spinal cord.[4,48,63,180,181,235]

Considerable violence is necessary to produce a fracture or dislocation of the upper part of the thoracic spine. It is more rigid than other parts of the spine, and is stabilized by the contiguous rib cage. This markedly resists lateral bending and extension. The facets and laminae are oriented so as to restrict motion in the rotatory plane. At each level, there are 4 degrees of flexion and extension motion in the upper thoracic spine (T-1–T-6) and 6 degrees in the lower thoracic region (T-6–T-10). There are 8 degrees of rotation present at each level.[14,22,25,100,243] The narrower spinal canal in the upper thoracic spine, along with its critical vascular supply, makes it almost inevitable that patients with injuries at this level also sustain a severe concomitant neurologic injury.[22,66,145,237]

The lumbar spine is the second most mobile region of the spine. It is relatively free to move in flexion, extension, lateral bending, and rotation; this freedom of motion increases with caudal progression toward L-5. Flexion–extension motion increases gradually from 12 degrees at L-1–L-2 to 20 degrees at L-5–S-1. Lateral bending is similar at all levels, with approximately 6 degrees. Long interlaminar distances and the sagittal orientation of the facet joints contribute to lateral bending, but tend to restrict rotation. The overall configuration of the lumbar spine may be changed from normal lordosis to neutral or slight flexion by the position of the pelvis. At the time of impact, this may influence the area of injury. The lumbar spine is susceptible to injury only when the physiologic range of motion is exceeded. As flexion–extension mobility increases caudally, force can be dissipated at each segment.[145,243]

The thoracolumbar junction is the region at greatest risk of sustaining a fracture; the majority of fractures occur here. The thoracolumbar junction is the first mobile area distal to the stabilizing influence of the ribs, and acts as the fulcrum of motion for the thorax. It is situated between the distal end of the relatively long lever arm of the thoracic complex and the highly mobile lumbar spine. It sits in an area of transition from the kyphotic thoracic spine to the lordotic lumbar spine.[9,22] The thoracolumbar junction is also the point at which the facets are in the process of changing their orientation from the coronal plane to the sagittal plane.[9]

Approximately 80% of fractures of the upper part of the thoracic spine with cord injury result in complete paraplegia.[14,22,145] Flexion injuries without posterior disruption result in complete injuries 50% of the time. If there is evidence of subluxation, 95% of the patients sustain complete neurologic injury (Fig. 8-1). Rotational injuries result in complete injuries 60% of the time, and two thirds of patients with burst fractures sustain complete injuries.[22] Gunshot wounds may produce a complete or incomplete spinal cord injury in the upper thoracic region, but are usually quite stable from an osseous standpoint.[22] The most common type of incomplete cord lesion sustained after thoracic fracture is the anterior cord syndrome, accompanied by sacral sensory sparing.[22,145] Less common is the central cord syndrome. The Brown–Séquard syndrome with hemiparesis and sensory dissociation may occur, either in association with stab wounds of the back or, less commonly, unilateral protrusion of bone into the spinal canal (Fig. 8-2).[22]

The majority of thoracolumbar neural injuries are incomplete injuries with a good prognosis. The neural injury that occurs most commonly is combined conus and root injuries. This is because the majority of lesions are at the thoracolumbar junction, at the location of the major functioning roots to the lower extremities and bladder.[30,37,83,135] Other injuries include complete division of the sacral spinal cord and lumbar nerve roots, complete division of the sacral spinal cord with escape of the lumbar nerve roots on one or both sides, and incomplete division of the sacral spinal cord with escape of lumbar nerve roots to varying degrees. Lower motor neuron injury to the cauda equina does occur, but isolated injury of this type is the least frequent type of injury.[83,119]

Fractures of the thoracolumbar junction are most often associated with injuries to the conus medullaris.[30,37,48,84,136,139,176,181,235] In the thoracolumbar region the conus broadens, and the reserve

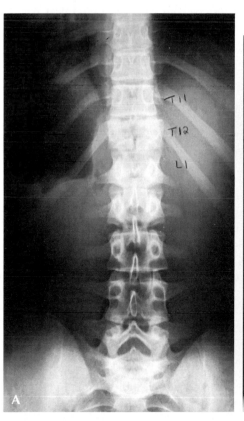
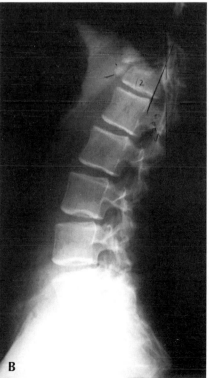

Figure 8-1. Twenty-one year-old man injured in a motor vehicle accident. Complete paraplegia was noted on admission. (*A*) Anteroposterior and (*B*) lateral views.

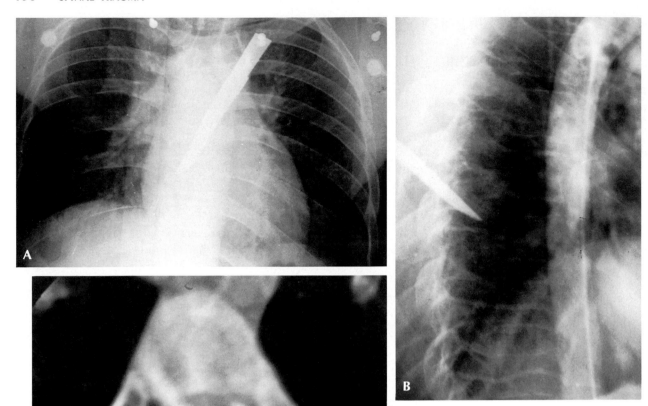

Figure 8-2. *(A, B, C)* Sixteen-year-old boy involved in street drug dealings stabbed during a territorial dispute. He presented to the emergency room with Brown–Séquard syndrome. Computed tomographic scan reveals the tip of the knife blade occupying the right side of the spinal canal.

space between the neurologic structures and spinal elements is minimal at the thoracolumbar junction. Injuries to the conus can be detected by noting decreased or absent anal sphincter tone, anal sensation, and bladder function and the continued absence of the bulbocavernous reflex after distal sensation has returned.[240]

Reserve space available for the neural structures increases significantly at levels caudal to the thoracolumbar junction. For a given degree of displacement, neural injury in this region is often less significant and has a greater potential for recovery than at other levels. The lumbar spine has a large canal area and the roots of the cauda equina are the only contents. There is poor correlation between the degree of canal compromise as measured by CT scanning and the resulting neurologic deficit (Fig. 8-3).[55,70,95,124,143,219] Neural injuries in this area are root rather than cord lesions, and thus have a greater potential for recovery.[145] Injuries occurring in the lower lumbar area are associated with a lower incidence of related injuries to other organ systems. The exception to this is the frequent involvement of the genitourinary system.[135]

Injury to the thoracolumbar area is missed less often than injuries in the cervical region. Retrospective review revealed that only 5% of all fractures in the thoracolumbar region are missed, but that these delays in diagnosis often led to an increase in or the emergence of new neural deficits.

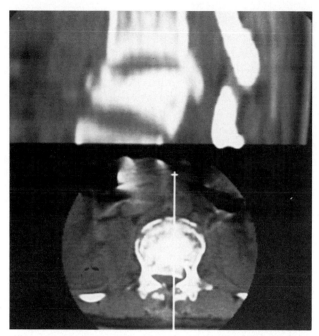

Figure 8-3. Twenty-one year-old woman involved in a motor vehicle accident. She was noted to have a burst fracture of L 1. She was neurologically completely intact. Computed tomography and saggital reconstruction reveal significant canal compromise.

The two most frequent reasons that lesions are missed are the failure to appreciate the severity of an injury and omission of the appropriate radiograph, and the overlooking of injuries at initial evaluation. Factors that confound correct diagnosis include intoxication of the patient, multiple levels of spinal injury, multi-system injuries, or an altered state of consciousness.[205]

A major error in early patient evaluation is failure to demonstrate other concurrent spinal injury.[159] Four to seventeen percent of individuals with spinal fractures have noncontiguous fractures, approximately 20% of which are potentially unstable fracture-dislocations.[39,137,142,218,229] The majority of noncontiguous injuries are at the extremes of the spine, especially at C-1–C-2 and L-4–L-5.[16,39] Forty percent occur above the primary lesion, and 60% occur below it. There are three main patterns of noncontiguous injuries: low cervical fractures (from C-4 to C-7) are combined most often with low thoracic and lumbar (T-12–L-5) fractures; high thoracic fractures (from T-2 to T-4) are often combined with cervical fractures (C-1 to C-7); and thoracolumbar fractures (T-12–L-2) are associated with low lumbar (L-4–L-5) fractures. Most frequently, a compression fracture occurs either above or below a severe burst fracture in the thoracolumbar spine. Thoracolumbar injuries below cervical spine fractures that are associated with significant neurologic injuries are frequently missed. As soon as a fracture at any level has been identified, screening radiographs of the entire spine should be taken, and special attention should be paid to the craniocervical and lumbosacral junctions.[9,16,39,136]

The severity of neurologic injury can be classified using Frankel's functional classification scheme.[137] The letters A to E are used, A representing no motor or sensory function, B preserved sensation only, C preserved motor (nonfunctional), D preserved motor (functional), and E complete recovery. Group D, with preservation of functional motor power, is a large and heterogeneous group. In an attempt to make the system more sensitive, Bradford suggested subdividing this group with respect to muscular power and bladder function. D_1 represents patients with preserved motor function at the lowest functional grade (3+/5+) or with bowel or bladder paralysis. D_2 represents patients with preserved motor function at the midfunctional grade (3 to 4+/5+) or neurogenic bowel or bladder dysfunction. D_3 is reserved for patients with preserved motor function at a high functional grade (4+/5+) and normal voluntary bowel and bladder function.[29,30]

Genitourinary dysfunction may represent a subtle neurologic deficit undetectable by conventional physical examination.[137] Patients with fractures at the thoracolumbar junction who have normal sacral sensation and anal sphincter tone may have poorly functional bladders. Urodynamic evaluation of patients with fractures of the lower thoracic and upper lumbar vertebrae begins with a determination of the postvoiding residual urine volume. If this volume is greater than 60 ml, a thorough urologic evaluation, including a cystometrogram and an intravenous pyelogram, should be considered to rule out injuries to the upper collecting system.[138,201]

Somatosensory evoked potentials (SEPs) should be obtained on patients with neurologic injury and intraoperatively on all patients who demonstrated repetitive waveforms preoperatively. Somatosensory evoked potentials have some prognostic value and provide an objective supplement to the clinical examination.[154,223]

Pediatric patients may sustain significant neurologic injury without evidence of skeletal injury. Up to one quarter of all patients under the age of 18 sustain complete injuries without fracture.[106,134,198,249] The incidence of this phenomenon rises as age drops, and is especially true of patients under 10 to 12 years of age.[106,215] Significant neurologic recovery may occur in pediatric patients without surgical intervention.[106] A large percentage of patients with complete neurologic injuries develop progressive spinal deformities even in the absence of bony injury. Younger children experience a greater degree of spinal deformity and a greater chance for progression of curvature than do older patients after total neurologic injury.[249]

RADIOLOGY

Radiographic assessment provides objective evidence to document the level of injury, demonstrates bony and soft-tissue injuries, and provides the information necessary to determine the stability of the injury.[136,137] The adage that "one view is no view" underscores that the minimum evaluation of any patient is two views, preferably in perpendicular planes.[111] At a minimum, lateral radiographs should be obtained before the patient is moved off the back board. The patient should be logrolled, with as little movement as possible, to obtain the remainder of the radiographs.[9,107,111,200] A physician should accompany the patient into the radiology suite for all special studies.[9]

Plain films are critical to proper radiologic work-up. Standard anteroposterior and lateral radiographs are obtained to determine if and where a thoracic or lumbar fracture has occurred.[137,139,181,200,202] The presence of soft-tissue damage may be inferred by the malalignment or disharmonious arrangement of the vertebral elements.[220] Increased radiodensity of a segment may be due to superimposed vertebral bodies.[121] A paraspinal hematoma, demonstrated by the widening of the paraspinal line in the thoracic spine or by a change in the contour of the margins of the

psoas shadows in the lumbar area, usually points to the area of maximum injury to the spine.[9,51] Pneumothorax or hemothorax must be specifically excluded. Associated fractures of the transverse processes and the ribs imply severe trauma to the spine.[9] The posterior intercostal spaces may be distorted or narrowed, and there may be disproportion between the number of rib pairs and the thoracic vertebral bodies.[121]

Compression of the vertebral body can be measured on the lateral radiograph (Fig. 8-4).[9] Disruption of the posterior vertebral margin is as-

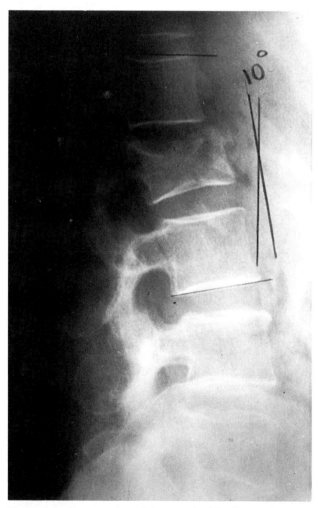

Figure 8-4. Compression of the vertebral body may be measured on the lateral radiograph by the percentage of lost height or the degree of kyphosis. Measurement is from the superior end-plate of the vertebra above to the inferior end-plate of the vertebra below.

sociated with protrusion of a fragment of the vertebral body into the neural canal (Fig. 8-5).[50] The alignment of the posterior margins of the vertebral body should be assessed for anterior or posterior displacement, which would indicate a dislocation.[9] Exaggerated lordosis in the lumbar spine may be evidence of a fracture-dislocation.[121] Increased vertical separation of adjacent spinous processes gives indirect evidence of ligamentous damage.[220] The spinous processes should be midline in a patient without scoliosis, and displacement indicates damage to the neural arch or the posterior ligamentous complex.[9]

Computed tomography (CT) is ideal for assessment of the spine and is the optimal adjunct to plain radiographs.[9] It should be mandatory in all major thoracolumbar spinal column injuries.[111,145,229] The CT scan gives much more information about the status of the middle column than does conventional radiography, and reveals obscure fractures of the posterior elements (Fig. 8-6). Computed tomography clearly demonstrates impingement of the neural canal (Fig. 8-7)[9,26,32,33,70,115,124,136,137,139,145,176,193,202,244] and best demonstrates small fragments within the canal.[32,44,108,202] Plain radiographs underestimate encroachment on the spinal canal.[9] Nondisplaced fractures are best demonstrated by CT, as are soft-tissue abnormalities in the paraspinal space or intraspinal blood.[202] Computed tomography gives an accurate display of the cross-sectional anatomy and can detect concomitant chest and abdominal injuries, especially fractures of solid organs.[9,136,137,139]

The patient remains supine throughout CT evaluation, rather than transferring to the lateral decubitus position required for lateral tomograms, decreasing the risk of neural compromise.* The average radiation exposure for CT is 10 times less

* Reference numbers 9, 32, 33, 108, 111, 136, 137, 139, 194.

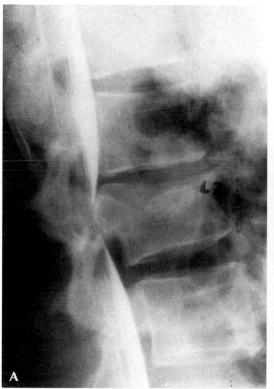
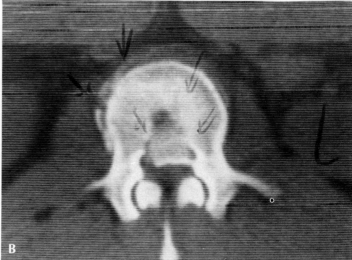

Figure 8-5. Burst fracture of L-2. (*A*) Disruption of the posterior vertebral margin may be apparent on the lateral radiograph or may be "hidden" behind a pedicle. Note the myelographic defect at the posterior margin of the pedicles. (*B*) The CT scan reveals the bony aspects of the canal defect.

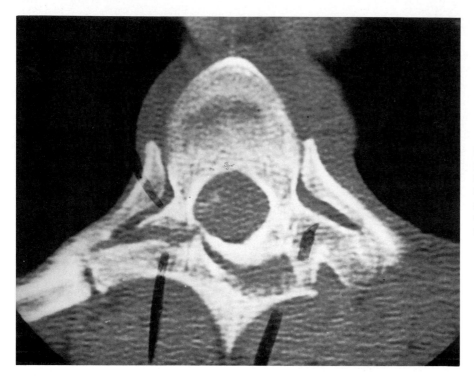

Figure 8-6. This fracture of the posterior elements in the thoracic spine was not well seen on a plain radiograph. Computed tomographic scanning, however, delineated the fracture in exquisite detail.

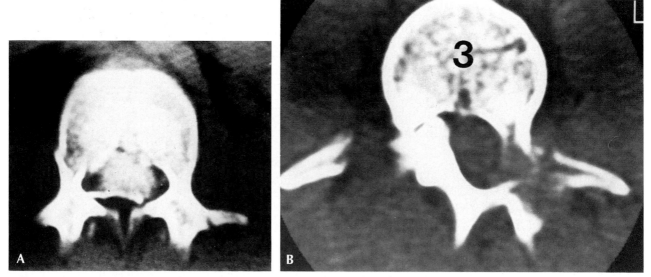

Figure 8-7. (A) Computed tomographic scan shows a large fragment of bone retropulsed into the spinal canal. (B) Computed tomographic scan reveals the dislocation of posterior elements into the spinal canal.

than that required for conventional tomography.[32,33,108,111,136,137,139,194]

Computed tomographic scanning is not wholly accurate, nor should it be used to the exclusion of other modalities. Computed tomography cannot localize lesions, and the amount of vertebral compression cannot be easily determined.[136,137,139,202] Computed tomographic scans can miss an increase in the intervertebral space unless reformatting and reconstructions are performed.[172] Alignment in the anteroposterior or lateral dimension is difficult to correlate and may also be missed without reformatting of images. Optimal reformatting requires overlapping scans[9] and an extra expenditure of time, and the result lacks sufficient clarity.[33,124,143,172] Rotational deformities or kyphotic deformities can produce pseudofractures that can be seen on CT.[19,107] Computed tomography should be used only as the next step after conventional radiography, not as a screening tool.[107,108,136,172,194]

One must pay special attention to the anatomy of and spatial relationships between facets. The superior facet is oriented medially and posteriorly toward the vertebral body. The articular surface of the superior facet is concave. The inferior facet is either flat or slightly convex at its articular surface, and is oriented in an anterolateral direction with respect to the vertebral body.[172] The relationship of the superior to the inferior facet remains constant over several successive scans.

Water-soluble myelography (metrizamide or iopamidol) demonstrates by direct visualization the spinal cord, cauda equina, and nerve roots, and localizes compression (Fig. 8-8).[9,111,176] Myelography can distinguish between intramedullary and extramedullary cord or root injury and can demonstrate root avulsion or dural tears.[111] It is best performed with the patient supine, via C-1–C-2 puncture.[9,200] The indications for myelography are changing,[197] and it should probably be reserved for situations in which the bony injury demonstrated on the CT scan or plain radiograph is inconsistent with neurologic findings, or when the neurologic lesion is rapidly progressive or is inconsistent with SEP findings.[3,48,85,137,140,181] Combined CT and myelography has the advantage of demonstrating three-dimensional anatomy. It thus affords better evaluation of spinal contents than plain myelography, and can define the cause

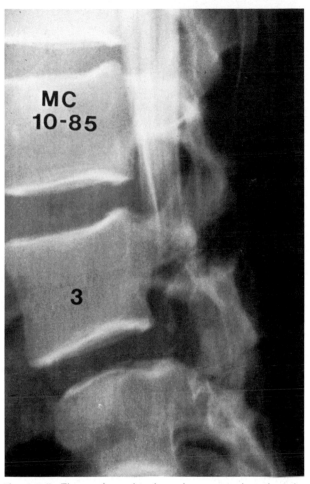

Figure 8-8. The myelographic dye column stops abruptly at the level of posterior element disruption in this distractive flexion injury.

of myelographic block.[9,176] Intraspinal hematoma can be optimally demonstrated, as can transection of the cord.[9] A dural tear can be detected by identifying leakage of dye more easily with combined CT and myelography than with myelography alone.[9,32,176]

Intraoperative spinal sonography[48,179,204] has been used to evaluate reduction of intraspinal fragments, to detect residual fragments or indentation of the cord, and to demonstrate the free flow of the cerebrospinal fluid and the configuration of the canal while the patient remains in the operating room.[9,16,39,136,234]

CLASSIFICATION OF INJURIES

Nicoll was the first to attempt to differentiate between stable and unstable injuries in his classic study of injuries sustained by coal miners.[191] He classified isolated anterior and lateral vertebral body wedge fractures and all laminar fractures above L-4 as stable injuries, and any fracture-dislocation with rupture of the interspinous ligament and all laminar fractures below L-4 as unstable.

Holdsworth and Hardy modified the Nicoll classification in 1953,[119] and Holdsworth later modified and expanded this in his classic 1970 review paper.[118] His classification led to better understanding of the mechanisms of injury and began to clarify when operative treatment was indicated. His scheme recognized that the thoracolumbar spine may be subjected to many types of forces, including flexion forces, which cause injuries in which the posterior ligaments do not rupture; flexion forces with a rotatory component, which may cause rupture of the posterior ligamentous complex; hyperextension of the spine, which causes injury to the posterior elements with the potential for dislocation; and axial compression forces. Each individual or coupled force could result in specific fracture patterns identifiable on radiographs.

Holdsworth insisted that rupture of the posterior column alone was sufficient to create instability of the spine. Wedge compression fractures and burst compression fractures were considered stable fractures, while all dislocations, extension fracture-dislocations, and rotational fracture-dislocations were considered unstable. Holdsworth treated stable fractures with bed rest and rehabilitation after osseous healing, while advocating operative intervention for fractures he considered unstable. Although the Holdsworth classification has remained the cornerstone of all subsequent classification schemes, this classification is no longer considered wholly accurate. Many burst compression fractures that Holdsworth considered stable are now classified as unstable.

The two-column concept of spinal anatomy was first introduced by Kelly and Whitesides, ushering in the second generation of classifications.[141] They differentiated the hollow column of the neural canal from the solid column of the vertebral bodies. According to their classification, if only one column is destroyed, collapse is incomplete and surgical treatment can be directed at that column responsible for the neurologic deficit. Destruction of both columns permits pronounced collapse. Burst fractures with retropulsion of the posterior wall of the vertebral body into the vertebral canal were identified as a distinct pattern and treated with direct anterior decompression. Most unstable flexion patterns were managed by posterior interspinous wiring, plating, or, eventually, by utilization of Harrington rods.

The descriptive two-column classifications rapidly yielded to a three-column theory with the advent of CT.[22,55] Denis introduced the concept of the middle column, an osteoligamentous column whose integrity is critical to the stability of the spine (Fig. 8-9). The basic premise is that spinal stability is also dependent on the status of the middle spinal column, and not solely on the posterior ligamentous complex.

The middle column mode of failure correlates with the type of spinal fracture and also with the neurologic injury the patient sustains. Denis avoided any radical departure from traditional mechanistic approaches by noting that one or more of the three columns predictably fail in axial compression, axial distraction, or translation from combinations of forces in different planes.[55] With compression alone the middle column can remain intact and will act as a hinge, resulting in anterior or lateral wedge fractures. For example, "Chance" fractures involve failure of the posterior and middle columns due to flexion and distraction. Burst fractures represent disruptions of the anterior and middle columns via axial load.

Denis further subdivided burst injuries according to whether there is failure of superior, inferior, or both end-plates, and whether there is a rotational component or evidence of lateral flexion.[55,56] Denis was the first to postulate that spinal fracture-dislocations are a heterogenous group of injuries secondary to various combinations of compression, tension, rotation, and shear forces that can result in failure of all three columns. He identified three major classes of fracture-dislocations: flexion–rotation, shear, and flexion–distraction. Although Denis ushered in the age of mechanistic classifications, his is an unwieldy system that has too many subdivisions to be clinically useful.[176]

McAfee and associates similarly described injury patterns based on mechanism of injury to the middle column in patients examined by CT.[176] They described three modes of failure: axial compression, axial distraction, and translation in the transverse plane. With minimal overlap, six fracture patterns can be described. Injuries were categorized as wedge compression, stable burst, unstable burst, Chance type, flexion-distraction, and translational. McAfee and associates were also the first to differentiate between stable and unstable burst fractures. This division hinges on the presence or absence of posterior column disruption in addition to the characteristic anterior and middle column injuries. The middle column fails in compression while the posterior column can fail in compression, lateral flexion, or rotation.[176]

Ferguson and Allen[76,77] expanded on the work of Denis and evolved a mechanistic classification system based on the forces that cause the injury. They realized that the majority of fractures are not caused by a single force but rather by a dominant force and minor components. Each fracture group is labelled according to the presumed mechanism of injury. This is deduced from the patterns of injury: compression is inferred if an element of the vertebral body has been shortened. If an element of the vertebral body has been lengthened, tension is the predominant force. Torsional forces are assumed to cause rotational failure, while translational failure causes anterior, posterior, or lateral displacement of the loaded segment. Each injury can be classified by observing what occurs in each of the three anatomic regions.

Ferguson and Allen describe seven major groups of injuries: compressive flexion, distractive flexion, lateral flexion, translational, torsional flexion, vertical compression, and distractive extension injuries (Table 8-1). Descriptions of these injuries will be expanded on below.

CONSERVATIVE TREATMENT

PATIENT MANAGEMENT

The mainstays of nonoperative treatment in the past were postural reduction and prolonged recumbency.[9,12,13,86] Bed rest was utilized to remove the force of axial compression, i.e. gravity, from the spine. If a patient were kept on bed rest long enough, osseous stability could be achieved. The limitation of bed rest is that it does not provide rotational stability, an axial distraction force, or hyperextension, and cannot fully reduce many fractures.[160]

Historically, "conservative treatment" meant postural reduction for 6 to 12 weeks. Pillows were used in the lumbar region to maintain lordosis, and this posture had to be maintained continually for 2 to 3 weeks to prevent redisplacement. The patient was turned frequently to prevent decubitus.[13,37,160] Injudicious handling during the early postinjury period could result in redisplacement of unstable fractures, losing reduction and potentially allow further injury to nerve roots that would otherwise have the capacity to recover.[252] Recollapse of crushed vertebrae was common.[37] Bed rest was followed by mobilization in a cast or orthosis[13,21,37,77] for a prolonged period. Nonoperative care of unstable fractures required a heavy investment in skilled staff and prolonged hospitalization.

Operative reduction allows earlier ambulation, anatomic fracture reduction, and, at times, improvement in neurologic function in those patients with neurologic compromise. The advantages of operative treatment are less clear in the neurologically intact patient with a stable fracture or a fracture that will be stable once healing has occurred. The neurologically intact patient does not present the same formidable rehabilitation problems as patients with cord injuries. The nonoperative management of selected patients with intact neurologic function can yield long-term results similar to those obtained with operative management.[51,151,239]

(*Text continued on p. 208*)

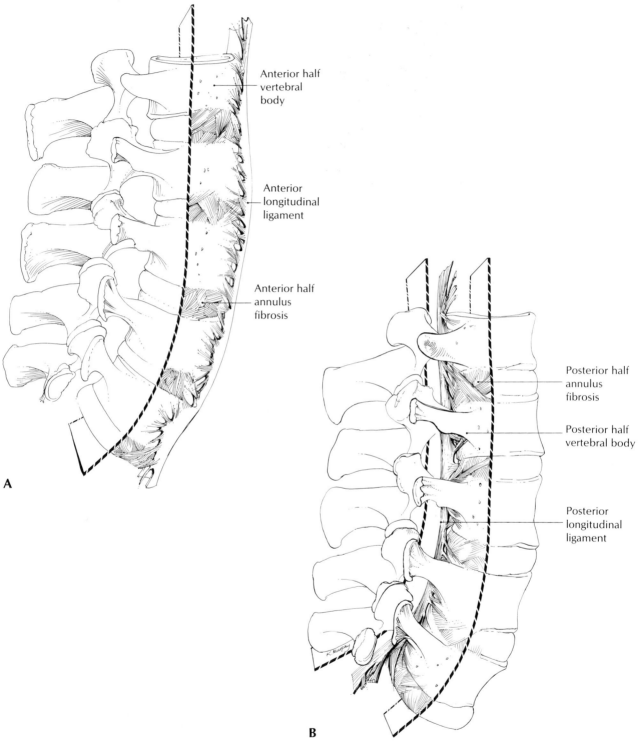

Figure 8-9. (*A, B, C, D*) The anterior, middle, and posterior elements of the spine. (Adapted from Denis F: The three-column spine and its significance in the classification of acute thoracolumbar spinal injuries. Spine 8:817–831, 1983)

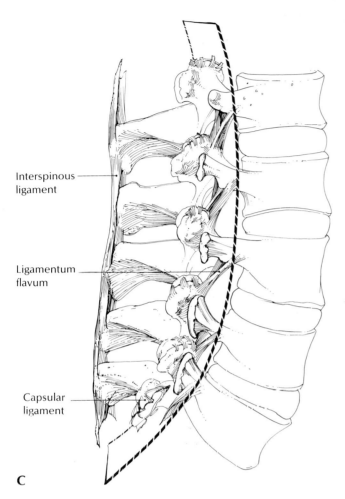

Interspinous ligament

Ligamentum flavum

Capsular ligament

C

Figure 8-9. (*continued*).

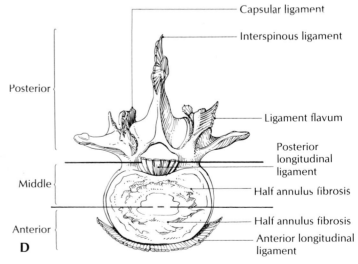

Capsular ligament

Interspinous ligament

Posterior

Ligament flavum

Posterior longitudinal ligament

Middle

Half annulus fibrosis

Half annulus fibrosis

Anterior

Anterior longitudinal ligament

D

Table 8-1. Mechanistic Classification of Thoracolumbar Spine Fractures

	COLUMNS		
	Anterior	Middle	Posterior
Compressive flexion	comp		
stage 1	</= 50%	—	—
stage 2	>/= 50%	—	tens
stage 3	>/= 50%	burst*	+/− tens
Distractive flexion	+/− tens	tens	tens
Vertical compression	comp	comp**	comp
Lateral flexion	uni comp	+/− comp	+/− tens
Torsional flexion	comp + tors	tens + trans	tens + trans
Translation	shear	shear	shear
Distractive extension	tens	—	comp

key:	comp:	compressive loading
	tens:	failure in tension
	uni comp:	unilateral compression
	tors:	torsion
	trans:	translation
	shear:	failure in shear

* The portion in between the pedicles rotates into the canal. This subgroup of fractures has a very high incidence of kyphosis.

** Low incidence of kyphosis.

The choice between surgical and conservative treatment is made on the basis of serial neurologic examinations and after examination of fracture morphology on plain radiographs and CT scans. An assessment of initial fracture instability, kyphosis, age at the time of injury, and degree of canal compromise is necessary to choose the best possible candidates for conservative management.[151] Considerations in this decision include the patient's neurologic status and medical condition, the fracture morphology, presence of associated injuries, and desires of the patient. *No patient with both progressive neurologic involvement and documented neural compression is suitable for nonoperative treatment.* Other contraindications include evidence of motor weakness, bowel or bladder paralysis, and painful paresthesias. Minor motor loss such as loss of one reflex, the loss of strength of one grade, or subjective changes in the distribution of a single root should not automatically disqualify a patient from nonoperative care.[151]

Certain fracture patterns are not suitable for conservative therapy. All translational and flexion–rotation fracture-dislocations and the major-ity of three-column fractures require operative intervention. Distraction injuries with posterior ligamentous disruption and kyphotic deformities of greater than 30 degrees should be surgically reduced and stabilized. Computed tomographic scans must be carefully examined for evidence of occult posterior element injury and bony canal compromise that would disqualify a patient from conservative management.[151] The presence of canal compromise secondary to retropulsed bony fragments is not in itself an adequate indication for surgical decompression. Patients with canal compromise of up to 60% who are neurologically intact have been managed nonoperatively without further compromise.[151,239]

Krompinger and associates[151] have described an excellent protocol for the conservative treatment of thoracic and lumbar fractures. Nonoperative treatment begins with logrolling immediately after admission, with use of appropriate measures to prevent pressure sores. Serial neurologic examinations, including assessment of motor power, sensation, and reflexes, are essential in patient management. Bed rest is maintained for 72 to 96 hours or until all medical complications are assessed and resolved, including the usual ileus.[151,160,241] Stryker frames may be used, as may regular beds with observance of proper turning procedures. Many centers are now using the Roto-rest kinetic bed.[151,160] Patients with fractures above T-8 are maintained on bed rest for 6 to 8 weeks. Mobilization earlier than this has resulted in progressive kyphosis and neurologic loss in some patients.[151]

The advantage of the Roto-rest frame is that it allows for rapid and safe transfer from the prone to the supine position, facilitating skin management. These frames are relatively effective for immobilization of thoracic injuries due to the intrinsic stability of the rib cage, which offers protection against rotatory instability.[160] In the lumbar spine, rolling from the supine to the prone position significantly increases the lordosis of the spine and therefore the degree of flexion or extension of individual segments. The position of the pelvis influences the relative flexion or extension of the lumbar spine. With continued changes in position, significant changes in the relative degree of kyphosis may cause movement of fracture fragments, increasing the potential for further neural damage.[160] The Roto-rest frames are therefore not as useful in patients with lumbar injuries.

Patients with fractures at the thoracolumbar junction or below are managed with an underarm cast or a total contact thoracolumbar sacral orthosis. A cast can be applied with the patient on a Risser table, achieving three-point fixation by careful contouring over the symphysis pubis, sternum, and fracture. According to the protocol of Krompinger and associates, patients with more than 50% canal compromise are not allowed to ambulate immediately. Patients with canal compromise between 50% and 60% are kept on bed rest for an additional 4 to 6 weeks before ambulation is allowed.[151] Upright radiographs are taken as soon as possible and at 6-week intervals for 4 months, and all forms of immobilization are discontinued at 4 months.[151]

Neurologically intact patients treated conservatively occasionally suffer from residual kyphosis, spinal stenosis, late instability, or radiculopathy, which interfere with a good functional result. Back pain seen in these patients may be caused by either instability, kyphosis, retained fragments, or

foraminal stenosis, which might have been corrected at the time of injury with anatomic reduction and rigid fixation.[151,160] Approximately 20% of neurologically intact patients with burst fractures developed either frank neurologic symptoms[56] or severe leg pain[151] when treated nonoperatively. The presence of canal occlusion at the time of injury does not guarantee that it will remain occluded. Bony resorption of canal compromise does occur, especially in those patients with less than 50% canal occlusion.[79,151] Krompinger and associates demonstrated that canal occlusion of greater than 25% decreased in more than 75% of the patients and canal compromise of 25% or less resolved completely in 50%.[151]

Conservative care can lead to progressive kyphotic deformity of 10 degrees or more in at least 20% of patients. Progression occurs most frequently at the thoracolumbar junction in patients with initial kyphosis of greater than 15 degrees or greater than 50% canal occlusion. Patients with initial kyphosis of 10 degrees or less do not progress more than 10 degrees.[151,247] Residual kyphosis must be compensated for by hyperlordosis in the adjacent, uninjured segments in order for the patient to regain a vertical posture.[71] Late back pain is not uncommon in patients with more than 20 degrees of residual post-traumatic kyphosis.[96] Correction of this late post-traumatic kyphosis may require combined anterior and posterior fusion or anterior osteotomy, instrumentation, and fusion.[149,171,178]

Degenerative changes, including facet hypertrophy and foraminal stenosis, are noted in more than 20% of patients treated without surgery. The majority of patients experiencing degenerative changes were older than 40 years of age. Residual pain was noted in patients with either foraminal stenosis or canal occlusion greater than 15%.[151]

Conservative nonoperative care is not without other general medical complications. The incidence of thrombophlebitis and pulmonary embolism increases in recumbent patients. The incidence of urinary tract infections is significant, but decreases with intermittent catheterization.[12,159] Chest therapy diminishes the occurrence of pulmonary complications; it is easier in mobile patients dressed in removable orthotics.[13] Bed sores are more frequent after conservative care, though the incidence has decreased with impeccable nursing care and the advent of removable orthotics, enabling daily hygiene.[159]

SPINAL ORTHOSES

Orthoses, though used extensively in the care of thoracolumbar fractures, do not fully immobilize the thoracolumbar spine (Fig. 8-10). There is no direct pressure on the elements of the spine and no dramatic reduction in load.[153] Orthoses act to decrease patient discomfort, in part by raising intra-abdominal pressure and converting the abdomen into a semi-rigid cylinder allowing it, rather than the spinal column, to transmit some force.[160,186,233,237] No orthosis decreases the myoelectric activity in the erector spinae in standing tasks,[153,237] and there were many instances in which the signal levels increased after an orthosis was applied.[152]

Orthoses can achieve good fixation on the lower thorax but fail to control the pelvis.[186] A pantaloon spica cast can consistently control L-4–L-5 and L5–S-1 movement in all planes of motion because it also controls the pelvis.[80,160] The standard body jacket may be effective at the L-2–L-3 and L-3–L-4 area. A thoracolumbosacral orthosis is more effective in restricting gross body motion than a lumbosacral corset or chairback brace. However, all orthoses are relatively ineffective in restricting flexion, and are not significantly effec-

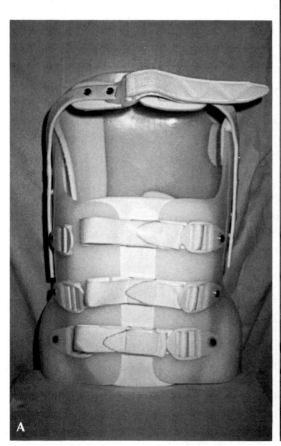
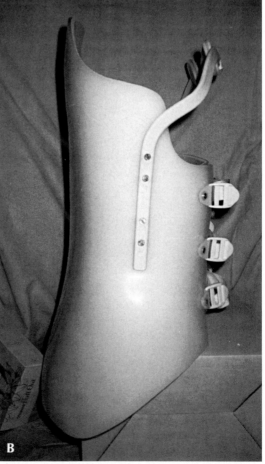

Figure 8-10. (*A, B*) Custom-molded thoracolumbosacral orthosis with clavicular bars.

tive in restricting twisting, lateral bending, and extension.[152]

There are limitations to the application of orthoses in the care of fractures in the lumbar spine. Certain orthotics, such as the Jewett brace, act to increase motion at the level of injury, rather than immobilize it, if applied to lesions below L-1. The brace causes a concentration of forces at or near the thoracolumbar junction.[160,192] No brace significantly decreases the axial compression of gravity in the upright position.[160,186] No brace effectively controls rotation or flexion–extension in the low lumbar or lumbosacral area.[160] A thoracolumbar orthosis used to treat a fracture must not be expected to do more than it is biomechanically able to do.

OPERATIVE TREATMENT

HISTORICAL TRENDS

Conservative therapy was stressed by Guttman[104,105] and Bedbrook,[12,13] both of whom recommended postural reduction of spinal fractures by keeping the patient recumbent until physiologic stabilization of the fracture had occurred. Holdsworth, among others, attempted to distinguish stable fractures from unstable ones. He suggested that the stabilization of unstable fractures by internal fixation would speed overall patient recovery and prevent greater damage to neural elements.[118,119]

This approach has subsequently been stressed by many authors. There is convincing evidence that secure and adequate stabilization of unstable thoracic and lumbar spine fractures promotes faster mobilization and rehabilitation, increased ambulation and wheelchair use, and easier nursing care with fewer complications. Operative therapy is associated with less residual deformity and prevents further deformity. Back pain due to altered spinal mechanics and abnormal motion at the fracture site can be avoided with successful surgical fusion. Residual displacement of thoracic fractures is correlated with pain after healing; however, the incidence of pain is lessened after fusion and anatomic reduction. Rapid mobilization is the current aim of operative treatment. As with all other trau-

matic injuries, emphasis has been placed on rapid mobilization and early rehabilitation via the use of rigid internal fixation.[22,123] Operative therapy prevents the high expense and complications that are associated with recumbent management and decreases hospitalization in minimally injured patients with mobilization in the space of days rather than months.*

Although spinal fractures or fracture-dislocations almost always occur at a single motion segment, early attempts at surgical stabilization by single-level wiring were largely unsuccessful.[135] Plates fixed to the spinous processes were then introduced, attached one or two levels above and below the level of fracture.[161] Surgical stabilization based on the strength of the spinous processes frequently was inadequate and fixation was frequently lost. There was a substantial rate of infection and the rate of continued deformity remained constant,[89,161] with approximately one third of the plates removed for pain associated with displacement. With these poor results, those early advocates of conservative management that vehemently opposed surgical intervention seemed justified.

Introduction of the Harrington double distraction system revolutionized the surgical treatment of spinal fractures, affording the ability to achieve an anatomic reduction with excellent stabilization yet with an acceptable complication rate (Fig. 8-11). The rule became instrumentation and fusion stretching two levels above and two levels below the fracture site.[4,28,59] Since the advent of this system there has been continued uncertainty over and development toward the most appropriate instrumentation and the timing for and length of instrumentation and fusion.

INDICATIONS

There are no universally accepted guidelines for the treatment of thoracolumbar fractures.[145] Spinal fracture healing will occur in most situations; nonunion is rare.[11,13] The exceptions occur when there is excessive distraction and separation of

* Reference numbers 4, 21, 27, 31, 34, 45, 62, 63, 77, 83, 89, 96, 123, 124, 135, 161, 162, 197, 222, 224, 228, 238, 247, 248, 250, 251.

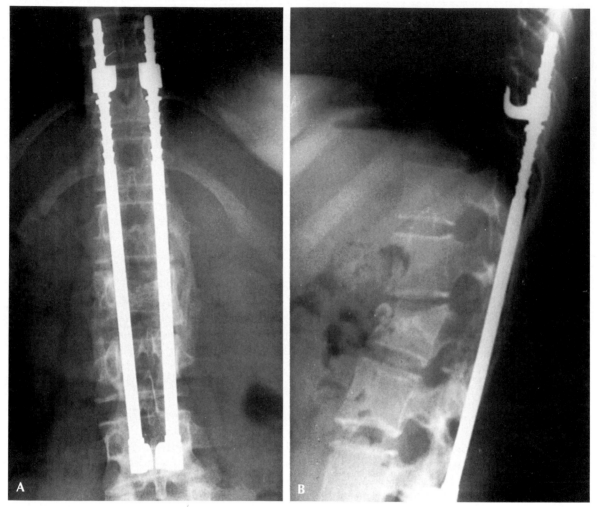

Figure 8-11. (*A, B*) Dual Harrington instrumentation and fusion.

fragments,[180] when the fracture is grossly translated and the fragments are not in apposition,[12,13,53] or when a patient without stabilization is ambulated too soon, which causes additional compression and displacement of fragments to occur.[83]

Patient-related factors may influence the decision to operate. Poor patient compliance with recumbent therapy (e.g., due to head injury, irritability, or another neurologic defect),[53,89] injury in an organ system whose management would be simplified by mobilization of the patient,[89] and changes in the patient's neurologic status may influence the decision.[4,76]

The strongest indication for surgical stabilization is an injury that can be considered unstable on a mechanical basis.[48] The determination of whether or not a patient's injury is stable is not an easy one. Stability is a relative term that depends on the degree of injury, the anatomy of the injury, and the potential stresses that will be applied to a spinal motion segment both prior to and after successful healing.[28,89] Different authors have attempted to define stability.

Denis defines stable injuries as those that can be ambulated with or without external immobilization. First-degree instability occurs in those cases in which the spinal column may buckle or angulate. Severe compression fractures and seat belt type fractures are categorized as first-degree unstable due to their tendency to buckle around the stable anterior (seat belt) or middle (compression) columns. These patients must be treated with either external immobilization in extension or open reduction and internal fixation. Second-degree instability occurs in those patients with neurologic instability, where acute or chronic neurologic damage has been done or may continue. Burst fractures are unstable in this fashion, since the middle column has ruptured and there will be continued impingement of the neural elements with bony fragments. The spine will continue to sag with immediate ambulation, demonstrated by continued widening of the interpedicular distance as the middle column fails to hold its load. Third-degree instability is demonstrated in those cases in which structural integrity is absent and neurologic damage has been done. Fracture-dislocations of all types and burst fractures are unstable in this manner. Major secondary displacements and progression of the deficit may occur in both types of fractures.[55]

Jacobs defines any spine that is sufficiently displaced to allow neurologic symptoms or signs as unstable. Any injury to the thoracolumbar spine severe enough to be associated with neurologic deficit is assumed to be mechanically unsound for early ambulation. Patients with "chronic instability" are those in whom neural damage is not demonstrated initially nor is likely to develop in the peri-injury period, but in whom it can appear late due to progressive deformity (specifically, the compression fracture with greater than 50% loss of height).[123,124]

The following definitions are suggested as an integration of current knowledge. A "stable fracture" is a fracture in which only a few days of bed rest are required to ameliorate the acute effects of the fracture. The patients may then be mobilized upright, walking either with or without immobilization. An "unstable fracture" can then be defined as one in which early mobilization in a cast or brace leads to an unacceptable risk of fracture fragment mobilization, subluxation, or frank dislocation that may lead to a long-term deleterious effect. This deleterious effect may be manifested by pain, loss of neurologic function, or spinal deformity. Conservative management of an unstable

fracture is possible: a period of bed rest or postural reduction allows enough healing to occur over 6 to 12 weeks to then permit mobilization in a cast or brace. Some late deleterious effects may occur, but they are thought by proponents to be acceptable.

"Highly unstable" fractures represent a subcategory of unstable fractures. These are fractures in which it is hard to obtain or maintain reduction of the spine even with prolonged bed rest followed by immobilization. These fractures include fracture-dislocations, especially those with translation, and burst fractures with posterior element damage. Highly unstable fractures almost demand to be treated surgically (Fig. 8-12).

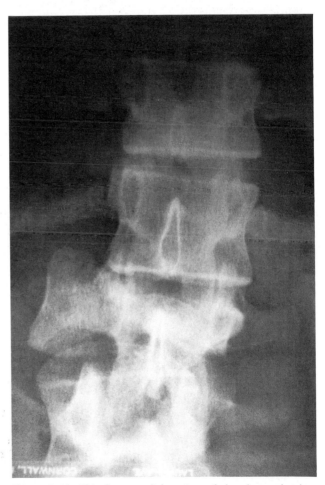

Figure 8-12. This fracture-dislocation of the thoracolumbar junction is highly unstable and almost "demands" a surgical attempt at reduction and stabilization.

SURGICAL INTERVENTION

An issue that is as yet unsettled is at what juncture postinjury surgical fusion should be performed. Immediate intervention may salvage neural tissue that is in jeopardy of ischemic necrosis by lessening ischemic time. Early mobilization decreases pulmonary and other complications. Early surgery is less complex, and less force is required to achieve an anatomic spine reduction than surgery performed several days or weeks after injury. There is no increase in postoperative complications in those patients treated on the day of injury than those treated later, although there is a slight increase in blood loss. Patients with multiple trauma are often better operative candidates on admission than several days later. In patients without multi-system trauma and without salvageable neurologic deficits the advantages are less clear-cut.[63,71] In a retrospective study, a short delay to stabilize patients was correlated with better results.[225] The quality of reduction depends on when it is obtained, with little improvement seen in the canal area of patients treated with posterior rod–sleeve stabilization if treatment was delayed more than 2 weeks. Best results were obtained if reduction was obtained within 48 hours.[71] Surgery performed more than 3 to 4 weeks after injury compromises correction of angulation and displacement.[28,71,83,137,140]

The optimal length of fusion has not yet been established. Harrington's original work specified that two intact vertebrae above and below the fracture were necessary to produce a lever arm long enough to reduce the fracture and maintain the reduction.[63] Subsequent work has confirmed these findings. Distraction hooks placed at least three levels above and two or three levels below the injured vertebral segment have a significantly higher success rate for correction of the angle of deformity, and increase the stability of instrumentation in flexion.[123,137,140,203] In patients with instrumentation spanning five levels or more, ambulation occurred earlier, the patient was discharged earlier, and a better correction was obtained.[128]

Scoliosis literature demonstrates that after a five- to seven-level fusion there are some modest functional limitations, inherent in the loss of mo-

tion segments.[1,8,41,43,89] Fusions extending to L-3 and below limit flexibility significantly, and fusions for scoliosis that extend down into the lower lumbar spine increase the incidence of low back symptoms and degenerative changes.[76,89] Long spinal fusion after fracture decreases spinal extensor power in paraplegics and decreases the range of extension and flexion.[110] Paraplegics with minimal fusions are able to reach their feet and dress without assistance. They are able to reach the ground from the sitting position and can perform walking exercises without difficulty.[175] Clearly, techniques should be employed that allow minimal interference with spinal mechanics yet are consistent with stable fixation.

With these considerations in mind, the maxim "rod long and fuse short" was advocated to minimize the number of permanently stabilized spinal segments and to provide more spinal mobility across the thoracolumbar junction. Jacobs proposed instrumenting three levels above or below the fracture site with one-level fusion, and removing the instrumentation 1 year after injury.[123]

The work of developers following this maxim has not been proven with long-term follow-up study.[89] Some authors have noted that in a significant number of patients with localized fusion, kyphosis increased to close to admission levels, a progression not seen in patients with longer fusions.[247] Jacobs and associates state that normal flexibility returns to the nonfused, immobilized segments and reported that patients experienced no increased incidence of back pain after removal of the rods.[123,125] Microscopic studies, however, have demonstrated that immobilized facet joints show areas of fibrillation, fissures, and thinning of the normal cartilaginous surfaces—changes typical of osteoarthritis.[132] These degenerative facet changes have been demonstrated in animal models and in humans at the time of rod removal. The changes occur as early as 2 months after instrumentation, so early removal of the rod (i.e. at 6 months) is not beneficial in reducing the osteoarthritis. Segments that have been instrumented for 9 to 12 months have not been shown to return to mobility, nor is there any improvement in the degenerative changes already present.[131,132] The mechanics of the back remain abnormal even 6 months after rod removal, with less mobility in flexion, lateral bending, and axial rotation than in normal subjects.[64] Only long-term follow-up of the initial patient population will determine whether these theoretical considerations will lead to clinical symptoms.

Both the proponents and opponents of surgical treatment of thoracolumbar injuries have noted that surgical therapy is not without its risks. Pressure sores remain a difficulty in the operative patient,[28,83] but their incidence has decreased with the improved physical hygiene permitted by the advent of removable orthoses.[71,228] Thrombophle-

bitis remains a major complication, although the incidence after operative treatment and early mobilization is lower than that in conservatively treated patients.[4,28,71,83,222,228] Urinary tract infection, hematoma, and pneumonia are other possible complications.[6,71,83,128,222,228]

Complications specifically related to the surgical treatment of the fractures include a 2% to 10% incidence of pseudarthrosis, rod loosening or breakage (Fig. 8-13),[6,28,48,63,77,83] or painful hardware.[4,28,83] Rod migration or dislodgement is one of the most frequent complications. The incidence

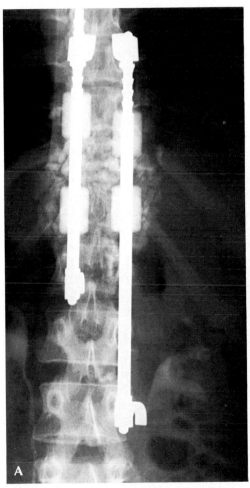
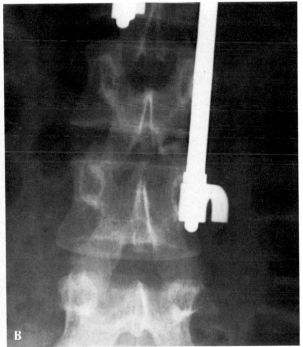

Figure 8-13. (*A, B*) Patient with T-11–T-12 injury who was rendered a complete paraplegic. Her treatment followed the "rod long fuse short" methodology. Bilateral Harrington rods and rod sleeves were employed. Prior to transfer to a rehabilitation facility her lower hook site dislodged. The shorter fusion site, however, fused solidly, as determined by exploration at the time of complete rod removal 1 year after the date of injury.

of hook dislodgement is between 2% and 23%, and is especially prevalent in those fusions that cross the lower lumbar spine. The junction of the upper hook and the lamina was the most common site of failure.[6,63,72,83,96,170,173,228]

Neurologic damage can also occur after surgical treatment. Besides direct risk from surgical intervention, there is additional risk from anesthesia, positioning on the operating table, hypotension, hypothermia, and changes in alignment.[181] Hematoma may cause neurologic loss,[96] and spinal cord vascularity may be impeded by distraction.[181] The neurologic status of 2.4% of patients degraded after posterior stabilization (vs. 0.3% in conservatively treated patients), while 15.5% improved one Frankel grade (vs. 6.6% in conservatively treated patients), suggesting a strongly positive risk to benefit ratio.[181]

DECOMPRESSIVE PROCEDURES

The indications for decompression of the spinal cord in the thoracolumbar spine are similar to those outlined for the cervical spine. Decompression is carried out only in the presence of significant *partial* neurologic deficits with evidence of canal compromise by bony or disk material. Single nerve root lesions are probably not an indication for decompression, as this problem usually improves spontaneously. Complete paraplegia after 48 hours and the termination of spinal shock does not require any decompressive procedure.[22,145] In the past, decompression had a poor reputation; many authors were unable to document any neurologic improvement after surgical procedures.[4,28,53,63,135,197] Because incomplete lesions tend to improve with time and nonoperative therapy, it has been difficult to demonstrate that surgical decompression had any positive effects.[23,28,86,135]

Restoration of normal spinal alignment may lead to adequate decompression if the canal is restored to normal dimensions early, if there are no comminuted fragments in the canal, and if the posterior longitudinal ligament is intact.[4,28,70,83,89,175] Restoration of foraminal and canal areas is maximized by the correction of vertebral height, alignment, and displacement, which indirectly relieves the pressure.[71] However, even a technically

acceptable Harrington rod reduction and stabilization of a thoracolumbar fracture does not necessarily alleviate continued compression from displaced fragments of bone or disk within the canal.[51,92,169,174] Dickson[62,63] and Flesch[83] both described iatrogenic progressive neurologic deficit and transient paresthesias in several patients after Harrington rod instrumentation without anterior decompression. Fountain used intraoperative myelography to demonstrate that dual Harrington distraction rods frequently do not decompress the spinal canal.[85] Dual posterior Harrington instrumentation with or without posterolateral decompression often leaves persistent anterior impingement (Fig. 8-14).[29,30,51]

The debate as to what the correct decompressive operation should be continues today. Holdsworth and Hardy were the first to demonstrate that laminectomy adversely affects spinal stability and can cause increased neurologic damage.[22,83,104,105,109,119,224,237] Laminectomy is not synonymous with decompression. Laminectomy does not improve the neurologic situation[4,25,83,128] nor does it relieve the myelographic block.[135,201] Laminectomy unnecessarily increases operative time. Patients with laminectomy experience a higher incidence of blood loss, postoperative pain, and subsequent instrument failure.[128,197,226] As in the cervical spine, laminectomy leads to increased instability and a potential worsening of the neurologic situation. Patients lose function after laminectomy and take longer to ambulate.[31,83,135,141,154,184,197] The most significant postinjury kyphosis occurs in patients in whom laminectomy has been performed. Laminectomies spanning more than 1.5 segments will complicate stabilization by necessitating fusion over a greater length than the injury would otherwise dictate.[48,62,63,73,83,128,137,140,159,174,176]

The presence of a dural tear on CT–myelography is not an indication for laminectomy and repair because traumatic dural tears are frequently located on the anterior surface of the dura and these cannot be repaired by a laminectomy.[159] Laminectomy cannot reduce the pressure exerted on the dura and neural elements by an anterior mass.[7,201] Great penetration of the anterior dura can occur with almost negligible displacement of the posterior dura.[230]

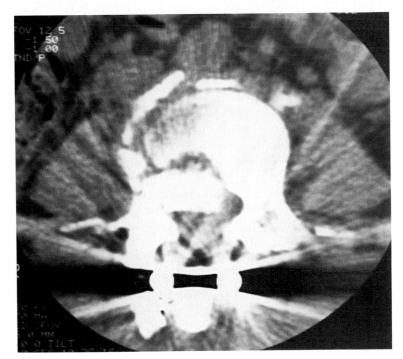

Figure 8-14. Computed tomographic scan obtained following Harrington instrumentation. Despite the artifact scatter from the metallic rod, incomplete canal decompression is seen.

It has been demonstrated that laminectomy has no decompressive effect with up to 35% occlusion of the canal. No surgical manipulation other than removal of the anterior mass is beneficial when there is anterior compression of the cord. Laminectomy and release of all nerve roots has no effect if the anterior ligaments are intact.[231] Although routine laminectomy has been condemned frequently in the past, these points deserve to be reemphasized here. Thirty percent of fractures recently reported to a regional spinal cord injury center are still being treated with routine laminectomies.[7] The only (rare) indication for laminectomy is significant posterior impingement by fragments of the neural arch.[71,159]

Unilateral or bilateral posterolateral decompression has been proposed as a method of decompressing the anterior surface of the spinal canal (Fig 8-15). This process attempts to excise bony or soft-tissue fragments compressing the dura anteriorly via partial or complete removal of the pedicle through a costotransverse approach.[73,83,92,123,154,169] An advantage of this approach is that concomitant posterior stabilization

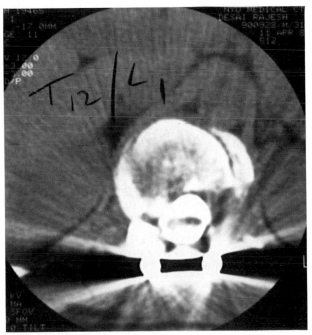

Figure 8-15. L-1 burst fracture treated with a posterior dual Harrington distraction rod and posterolateral decompression. Note the residual bone in the canal on the opposite side from the decompression.

can be performed without changing the patient's position on the table.[73,83,92,169,177,226] Intraoperative sonography can be used to confirm the adequacy of decompression of the spinal canal when posterior reduction and posterolateral decompression of fragments in the canal are attempted.[124,179,234]

Posterolateral decompression adds considerable risk to the stabilization procedure. It requires retraction of the dura, conus, and adjacent nerve roots, with the potential for cord retraction injury.[46,68,124,127,129] Retraction may be made difficult by the presence of tethering and scarring at the fracture site.[127] Too often the posterolateral approach does not offer adequate visualization across the entire length of the canal.[46,68,129,144,174] It can lead to excessive hemorrhage.[124] Pneumothorax occurs frequently.[169] Removal of a pedicle can add significant instability to the already injured spine.[30,83]

The results of posterolateral decompression are extremely dependent on the skill of the surgeon, and are not uniformly good. Although this approach has been shown to lead to some improvements in SEP,[154] improvements are not universal. One proponent of the procedure noted that posterolateral decompression does not "necessarily improve neurologic function." Recovery was no different in patients treated with posterolateral decompression than in patients treated conservatively.[92] Computed tomography frequently demonstrates inadequate decompression after posterior procedures.[92,98,176]

The failure of posterior Harrington instrumentation to adequately decompress the neural canal occurs more commonly than failure to restore normal alignment. Anterior decompression is the most common secondary surgical procedure after posterior stabilization in patients with incomplete neurologic injury and radiographically demonstrable residual neural compression by bony or disk fragments.[29,30,129,169,173,174]

Anterior decompression allows direct visualization and relief of the compression with less forceful reduction, allowing the optimum environment for the recovery of incomplete neural deficits (Fig. 8-16).[4,17,22-25,46,68,93,145,174,199,209,245,252] Anterior decompression can lead to complete recovery in most patients who improve at least one Frankel class.[69,148,174,195] Progressive deficits are halted after anterior decompression.[129] Bradford and McBride demonstrated greater neurologic improvement in patients after anterior spinal decompression than after either posterior or posterolateral decompression procedures. The return of bowel and bladder function were more frequent after anterior decompression than after either posterior procedure. Only 17% of those approached anteriorly failed to improve, compared with 69% of those approached posteriorly. The inferior results following the posterior procedures were correlated with residual bony stenosis on CT. Following posterior procedures the average area found to still be occupied by bony fragments was approximately 25% of the canal area. After anterior procedures, less than 1% stenosis remained (Fig. 8-17).[29,30]

Bradford and McBride have advocated anterior decompression as a second-stage procedure in the patient with incomplete neurologic injury if residual canal narrowing greater than 25% is still present after posterior procedures and if the patient shows no recovery or plateaus with disabling symptomatic residual deficits.[30] Other research has shown that fragments do not contact the spinal cord at T-11 until about 30% of the neural canal is occluded. These authors concluded that it may be reasonable to accept residual canal occlusions in that range (Fig. 8-18).[231]

Unless proper stabilization is provided as part of the procedure, the anterior approach provides improved exposure at the risk of increasing spinal instability. The anterior approach should not be used alone in the presence of significant posterior ligamentous disruption because the anterior ligaments may be all that remains in an unstable burst fracture. Anterior treatment does not provide any real stability until fusion occurs.[124,174] Decompression and anterior iliac strut grafting do not alter the usual indications for posterior surgical instrumentation.[24,174,210] The anterior approach can be performed at the same time as a posterior procedure, to add protection. Whitesides and Shah[245] advocated the two-stage approach with

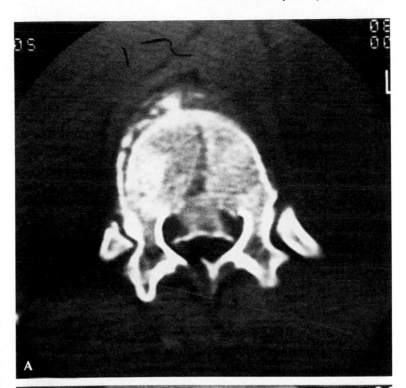

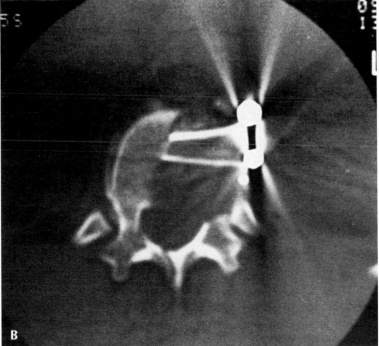

Figure 8-16. (*A*) A bone fragment from a T-12 burst fracture is compressing the spinal cord, causing Frankel class B incomplete paraplegia. (*B*) With prompt recognition of the offending fragment and single-stage anterior decompression, Kostvik–Harrington instrumentation, and fusion the patient improved to Frankel class E. A CT scan reveals the complete canal clearance afforded by the anterior decompression.

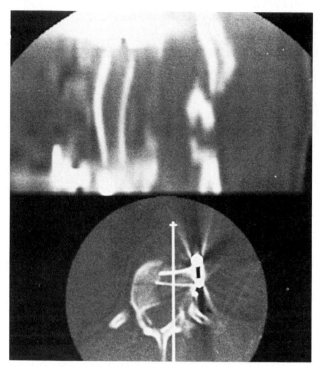

Figure 8-17. Less than 1% stenosis can routinely be achieved with anterior decompression.

The two-step approach for incomplete injuries may not be the optimum approach, however. In treating an unstable burst fracture two issues must be addressed. The first is the issue of decompression, followed by the restoration of spinal stability. Posterior instrumentation will provide stability if fusion is achieved, but can only achieve indirect and probably incomplete spinal canal decompression. Early posterior instrumentation without iatrogenic neural injury may preclude the necessity of a second-stage decompression. If residual compression exists, the definitive anterior procedure to alleviate neural compression is often delayed 7 to 10 days. Many centers have moved to solve the dilemma by advocating simultaneous anterior decompression with posterior instrumentation, and others have suggested single-stage anterior de-

posterior spinal fusion for stability, followed by anterior decompression. Several authors have endorsed this strategy.[85,93,174,177,245]

There are several complications specific to anterior surgery. These include retrograde ejaculation,[30] failure to obtain primary union,[69] blood loss averaging 1800 ml,[69,210] chest tube insertion, atelectasis, and prolonged intubation,[71] ileus, and a high degree of postoperative pain.[71]

Classically, a surgeon has the option of performing an initial posterior reduction and stabilization with Harrington distraction rods, and assessing whether protruding fragments of bony or disk material are compressing the neural structures to any significant degree. If there is significant compression and no evidence of neural recovery, an anterior decompression via a separate anterior approach can be performed.[95] Translational fractures, flexion–rotation fractures, fractures with angular displacement, and complete injuries are treated with posterior procedures alone.[30,95]

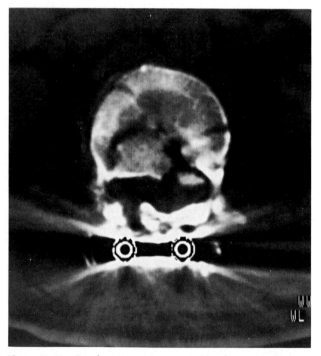

Figure 8-18. Canal compromise remaining after posterior Harrington instrumentation of an L-1 bursting fracture. Some authors feel this amount of residual canal compromise is acceptable. In this particular patient, 3 months of slow improvement in a rehabilitation facility was observed. A delayed anterior decompression and iliac crest strut grafting was performed. Immediately postoperatively the patient noted subjective sensory improvement and new quadriceps function. Subsequent progress in rehabilitation was significantly speeded.

compression and instrumentation to obtain stabilization.[68,133,147,148]

Obviously, there is great variation in different surgeons' approaches to decompression. The basic premise of decompression is that neural tissue loses function when compressed by bony and disk fragments.[65] Depending on the seriousness of the injury to the underlying neural tissue, one of three scenarios is possible:

1. Neural function will improve partially or totally without surgical intervention.
2. Neural function will not improve despite any and all types of surgical intervention (e.g., complete spinal cord injuries).
3. Neural function will improve to a higher degree, either partially or totally, if the pressure is removed from the underlying tissue.

Each damaged neural element has an unquantified innate ability to heal itself. To date our only objective means of measuring this ability is to decompress partial lesions and observe case by case what the result is. Certainly the cumulative knowledge leads authors to predict outcomes based on different treatment protocols. Unfortunately, the common flaw in all studies will be the varied traumatic forces applied to the neural elements despite comparable levels and lesions, as well as the unknown innate ability of each neural lesion to heal itself either with or without decompression. In comparing different treatment methods, even with extensive experiences obtained with similar lesions at similar spine levels, the answers we seek may remain elusive.

SPECIFIC INJURIES

The mechanistic classification of thoracolumbar fractures as described by Ferguson and Allen is an instructive classification, although it is sometimes difficult to use. One must be cognizant of the fact that on many occasions the injuries seen are not pure injuries. A judgment must be made on the maximum deformity and the predominant mechanism of injury. This classification is helpful in the determination of most variables necessary for trauma assessment and the type of stabilization needed.[48]

COMPRESSIVE FLEXION

Axial loading of the spine in the flexed position causes compressive stress to pass through and damage the anterior elements. The three patterns of injury in this group (Fig. 8-19)[54,55,124] depend on whether the posterior and middle elements fail in tension.[22,55,77]

The first pattern (Fig. 8-20A) is the simple anterior wedge compression fracture. The anterior elements fail in compression and the posterior and middle elements remain intact.[36,54,55,77,160] Due to the stabilizing effect of the rib cage, simple wedge compression fractures are most commonly seen in the thoracic spine.[36] Typically, less than 50% of the body vertebral height is lost. If anterior compression is limited to less than 50%, sufficient posterior ligamentous integrity remains and the fracture is stable.[54,55,77,113,241] The radiographic hallmark of this fracture is decreased anterior vertebral height with unchanged posterior height. The posterior vertebral cortex is intact, so the middle column is not been disturbed. Computed tomography demonstrates an irregular arc of anterior bony density displaced circumferentially from the vertebral body, confirming that the neural elements are not disrupted and that the canal has not been transgressed.[54,55,143]

In stage 1 of this fracture pattern neurologic injury is uncommon, unless multiple adjacent vertebrae are involved.[55,77] Complete neurologic lesions are rare. When there is neurologic involvement, 80% of the injuries are incomplete; most of these improve dramatically without intervention.[48] Patients with multiple adjacent compression fractures with kyphosis of 60 to 70 degrees are predisposed to continued kyphosis and serious neurologic injury, with a high incidence of late pain.[176] These injuries should be treated with surgical stabilization even if less than 50% anterior compression is demonstrated at each level.[76]

Posterior element disruption in conjunction with an anterior wedge fracture is the second stage of injury (Fig. 8-20B). There is greater than 50% compression of the anterior vertebral body, usually combined with tension failure and severe

(*Text continued on p. 224*)

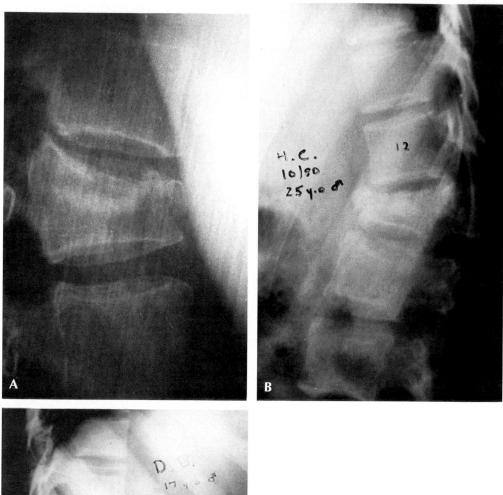

Figure 8-19. Compressive flexion injury. (*A*) Stage 1. (*B*) Stage 2. (*C*) Stage 3.

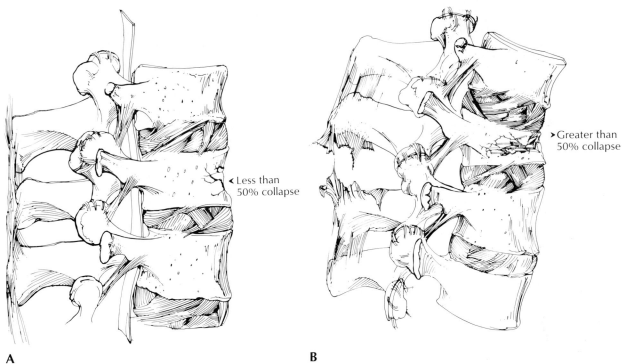

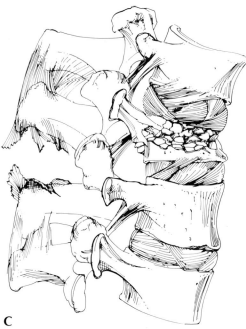

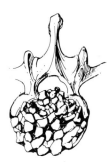

A

B

C

Figure 8-20. Compressive flexion injury. (*A*) Stage 1 is a simple anterior wedge compression fracture in which the anterior elements fail in compression and the posterior and middle elements remain intact. If anterior compression is limited to less than 50%, sufficient posterior ligamentous integrity remains and the fracture is stable. (*B*) Posterior element disruption in conjunction with an anterior wedge fracture is the second stage of injury. There is greater than 50% compression of the anterior vertebral body. This is usually combined with tension failure and severe disruption of the posterior ligamentous complex. (*C*) The third stage is failure of the middle element along with the other two columns. The lateral radiograph shows that the posterior vertebral wall height is equal to or greater than the adjacent inferior vertebral body. The pedicles remain in continuity with the vertebral body and are not splayed.

Less than 50% collapse

Greater than 50% collapse

disruption of the posterior ligamentous complex.[22,76,77,137,160] Progression of deformity is more likely in stage 2, due to tension failure of the posterior elements. Concomitant neurologic injury is also more likely. The middle column remains intact and acts as a hinge around which the vertebral body rotates. The middle column prevents the fracture from subluxation and protects the neural elements.[54,55] The posterior injury is demonstrated on the lateral radiograph with widening of the spinous processes and adjacent pedicles.[54,124] The articular processes are usually subluxated or dislocated.[54,55,77,189,241] This is the most common dislocation in the lumbar spine.[135] An unacceptable late, painful deformity may result from the vertebral body collapse.[145]

The third pattern is the most severe (Fig. 8-20C). It is a combined injury, with middle element failure along with failure of the other two columns. Because failure of the middle column to bear load creates a high probability of progression and neurologic injury, this injury must be recognized and properly treated.[77] The lateral radiograph shows that the posterior vertebral wall is the same height as or taller than the adjacent, inferior vertebral body. This is not as easily measured on CT as it is on plain films. In contradistinction to burst fractures, the pedicles remain in continuity with the vertebral body and are not splayed apart.[160] The middle column fails in tension and the posterior wall of the vertebral body is not shortened.[76,77] This pattern has a marked propensity for neurologic injury and progressive deformity.

Computed tomography should be performed for patients with compressive flexion injuries in several instances. The first is in fractures that demonstrate 50% or greater anterior vertebral collapse on plain films, in which case posterior and potential middle element injury need to be defined. The second instance in which CT should be performed is in patients with multiple adjacent wedge compression fractures.[176] Computed tomography probably will not be beneficial, however, if anterior compression is less than 50% and there is no plain film evidence of posterior ligamentous damage.

Treatment

Wedge compression fractures with anterior failure alone have no propensity for further progression of spinal deformity or progression of neurologic injury. If there are no other spinal injuries, these fractures remain unchanged even with early ambulation.[64,113,241] This stable injury is treatable in a Jewett or other hyperextension brace.[113,141,160,176,187,233,245]

When the anterior and posterior elements have failed and the middle column is intact, surgical stabilization is required to prevent further deformity.[145] Either Luque or Harrington instrumentation might be used.[76,77] Luque instrumentation requires no postoperative immobilization and places no tension over the posterior elements. Harrington instrumentation, countering axial compression forces via three-point fixation, places tension over the posterior elements that have already failed in tension. For this reason, some authors prefer L-rod segmental spinal instrumentation for this injury.[77] Most authors prefer Harrington instrumentation, and many variations on this instrumentation have been used for this injury. Harrington instrumentation with bilateral distraction has been shown to effect restoration of vertebral body height.[15,71,109,176,181,228] Combined distraction and compression instrumentation with an additional midline compression rod acts to preserve lumbar lordosis.[140,228] An interspinous compressive wire has also been used with Harrington instrumentation to preserve lordosis.[84] Locking hook and spinal rod devices,[125,126] segmental interspinous process wiring,[67] and sublaminar wires[35,91,166,227] have been used to increase the stability of the construct and in an attempt to preserve lordosis. Sublaminar wires decrease the incidence of pseudarthrosis and lessen the need for external immobilization, speeding rehabilitation (Fig. 8-21).[91,227]

When all three elements have failed and the middle element has protruded into the neural canal, axial compression must be prevented. A distraction apparatus should be used when the posterior approach has been chosen.[77,83,236,251] Partial indirect decompression of the retropulsed

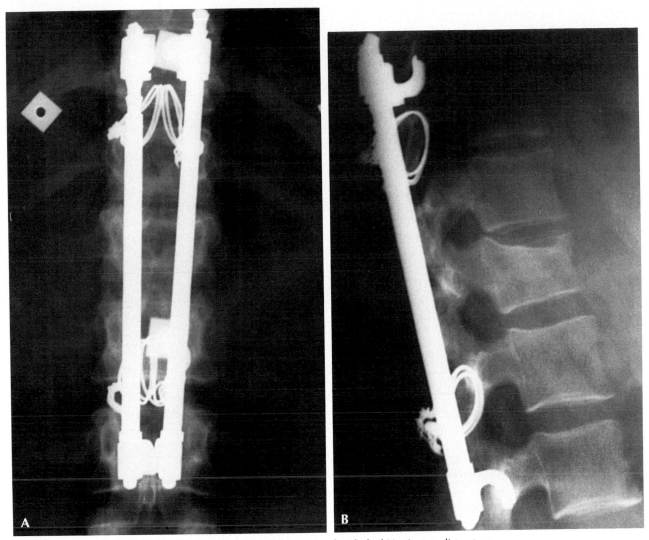

Figure 8-21. (*A, B*) Compressive flexion stage 2 injury of L-1 treated with dual Harrington distraction rods and sublaminar wires adjacent to the hooks only.

fragment is sometimes possible when the posterior longitudinal ligament remains attached to this fragment. When sufficient lordosis is restored to the spinal segment, the fragment is reduced back into position by ligamentaxis.[160] Although several authors advocate the use of L-rods,[167,168] Luque rod instrumentation is not appropriate for compression fractures of the thoracolumbar spine. Segmental instrumentation does not produce the

distracting forces necessary to reduce compression fractures.

DISTRACTIVE FLEXION

This injury occurs by tension failure of all three columns. The original fracture that Chance described in 1948[42] is a purely bony injury with horizontal splitting of the spinous process and neural arch. Currently, three types of distractive flexion injuries are recognized. The first is the chance-type fracture, in which the fracture occurs through the bony spine. The second is the pure dislocation in which tension failure occurs through the ligamentous structures alone, predominantly leading to unilateral or bilateral facet dislocation. This is an uncommon lesion caused by a high-energy injury, often resulting from motor vehicle accidents or falls. The pure dislocation fracture differs prognostically and therapeutically from the remainder of the thoracolumbar fractures because it is an ominous, unstable fracture.[158,172,245] The third type, a variation of the first two patterns, is more common. This type includes partial bony and ligamentous tension failure (Fig. 8-22).

Concomitant intra-abdominal injury is common with the distractive flexion fracture, and may be difficult to diagnose in patients with complete cord lesions. This fact stresses the importance of performing minilaparotomy and paracentesis on patients with spinal injury.[40,94,102,158,207,221] Cecal perforation is common after this injury, probably due to traction on the fixed cecum.[207] Other intra-abdominal injuries include traumatic pancreatitis and pancreatic laceration, along with other ruptured viscera. These skeletal injuries are also associated with rib fractures, sternal fractures, and other long bone fractures.[47,101,102,120,158,207,221] Craniofacial trauma is also common, because distractive flexion fractures are associated with motor vehicle accidents in which the victim's face and head strike the dashboard or seat in front of him as he is thrown forward, constrained by a lap seat belt. This fracture has been associated with nerve root avulsions in the thoracic cord.[130]

When flexion with an element of distraction is applied to the spine in a high energy mode, the result is a complete disruption of the posterior ligamentous complex and ligamentum flavum, and disruption of the intervertebral disk.[22,54,55,157,158,160] The posterior wall of both vertebral bodies remains intact, although there may be mild anterior compression.[157,158] The majority of patients with facet dislocations have extreme kyphosis, especially if the injury is in the midthoracic spine. The spinal cord and roots bowstring anteriorly and are injured in tension.[176]

Howland and associates[101] suggested that the mechanism of this injury was similar to breaking a stick across one's knee, creating tension failure of all elements. The axis of rotation generated by the flexion force, rather than being within the intervertebral disk, is displaced anteriorly to the anterior longitudinal ligament and lies at the level of the abdominal wall.[22,47,77] This is why the injury is so frequently associated with lap seat belt wear.[18,47,94,102,176,207,221] The seat belt acts as a fulcrum around which hyperflexion occurs (Fig. 8-23).

Distraction is an important component of the disruptive force.[55,102,176,207] Distractive flexion injuries are especially likely to occur if the victim is wearing a high-riding or otherwise malpositioned seat belt[101,221] or has submarined under the belt after impact.[102] The injury is rare in individuals not wearing belts, and the victim usually is not the driver.[221] A distractive flexion injury can also occur in a lateral direction if the axis of rotation is placed over the patient's flank rather than abdomen.[116] Distractive flexion injuries are located in the upper lumbar spine, occasionally as high as T-12[47] and rarely below L-3.[55,94,102,135,161,221] Dislocation of the facets is less common than a fracture.[158,172] Although the majority of distractive flexion injuries occur at T-12–L-1,[135,158,161] purely ligamentous disruptions can be located higher in the thoracic spine. This same mechanism is responsible for facet dislocations in the cervical spine.

Classically, the distractive flexion injury is acutely stable, and rarely is associated with neural injury.[55,137] Neurologic injury in this lesion is proportional to the amount of translation of the injured segment either anteriorly or laterally. When facet dislocation occurs, complete neurologic injury is more common due to stretching and shearing of the dural sac combined with the direct trauma of the intact neural arch on the cord.[157,158] Pure dislocations are "highly unstable" injuries, with a high propensity for progression of deformity and neurologic injury, whether or not translation is present. Lesions with partial bony or ligamentous injuries that have translation of one segment on another may also have a propensity for progression of neurologic injury or progression of deformity.[77,120,221]

Injuries sustained by this same mechanism are more frequently associated with significant neurologic injuries in children than in adults. There is

(Text continued on p. 229)

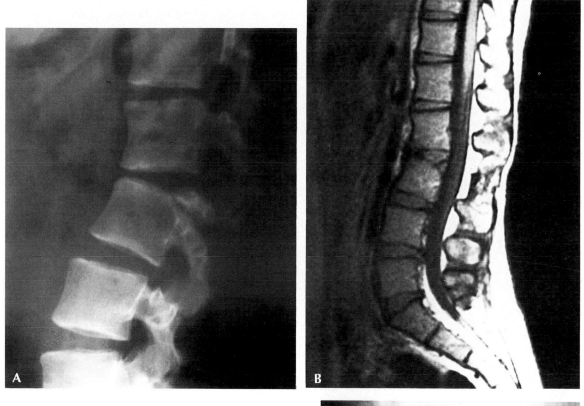

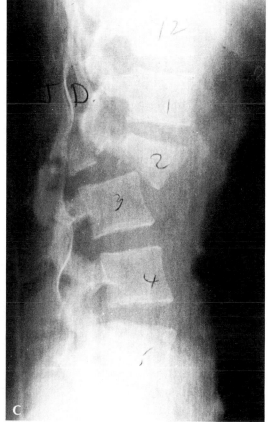

Figure 8-22. (*A*) Distractive flexion injury at L-2–L-3. (*B*) Magnetic resonance imaging of distractive flexion injury L-2–L-3. (*C*) Severe distractive flexion injury with dislocation of L-2 on L-3.

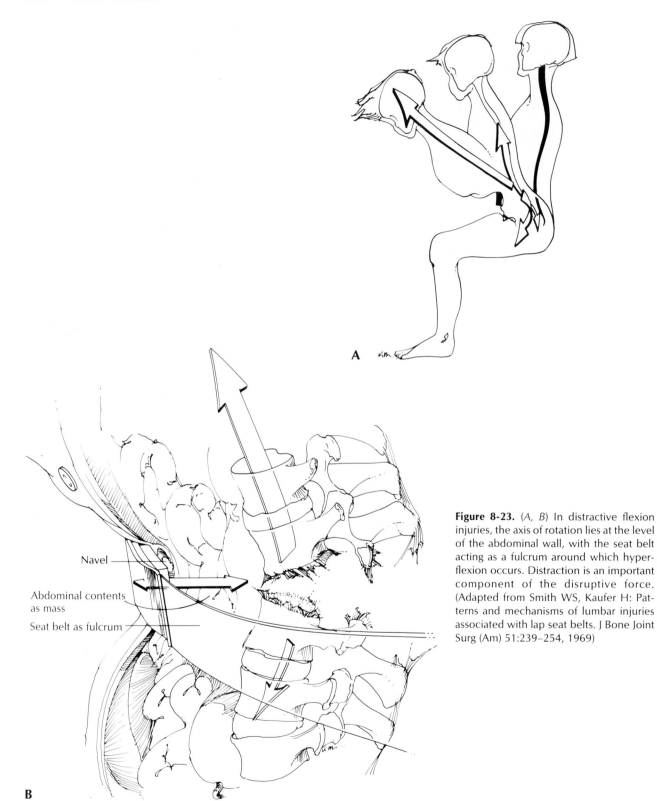

A

B

Navel

Abdominal contents
as mass

Seat belt as fulcrum

Figure 8-23. (*A, B*) In distractive flexion injuries, the axis of rotation lies at the level of the abdominal wall, with the seat belt acting as a fulcrum around which hyperflexion occurs. Distraction is an important component of the disruptive force. (Adapted from Smith WS, Kaufer H: Patterns and mechanisms of lumbar injuries associated with lap seat belts. J Bone Joint Surg (Am) 51:239–254, 1969)

considerable instantaneous stretching due to disruption of the posterior elements and hinging of the posterior portion of the vertebral body off the anterior longitudinal ligament. The disk is relatively elastic and tolerates this distraction. The spinal cord does not tolerate this stretching. Complete paraplegia results, often several levels above the bony injury.[156,160]

The distractive flexion injuries have been subclassified by Denis, using the direction and the type of tissue through which the injury progressed, from posterior to anterior, to distinguish four types of injuries.[55] Type A fractures are one-level fractures that pass through bone. This is the classic Chance fracture. Type B fractures are a one-level injury that is purely ligamentous in nature, called a distractive flexion dislocation. Type C fractures are two-level injuries, passing through bone at the level of the middle column. Type D is a two-level injury, passing through ligamentous tissue at the level of the middle column (Fig. 8-24). Gumley and associates[102] demonstrated that injury to the posterior elements may enter through the middle or base of the spinous processes, or there may be an asymmetrical injury of the posterior elements due to rotatory forces.

Radiographically, this injury will demonstrate a lengthening disruption through the body, pedicle, lamina, and spinous processes, or through the disk space. The flexion force on the spine causes a horizontal split of the transverse processes and pedicles. It may also cause fractures of the spinous processes or pars, or avulsion of part of the spinous process. Disruption of the joint capsules, ligamentum flavum, and posterior longitudinal ligament occurs.[221] Widening of the distance between spinous processes gives evidence of disruption of the posterior elements.[47,54,55,221] Although there is usually minimal or no decrease in the anterior vertebral height of the involved vertebral body and minimal or no forward or lateral displacement,[120,221] there may be associated compression or bursting of the anterior vertebral body.[94] The fracture line in the "true Chance fracture," the type A injury, passes in the transverse plane, through the cancellous portion of the body, out through the pedicles and extends posteriorly through the spinous process. Partial lesions reveal disruptions through portions of the bony structure and ligamentous structure.[137,160]

Lateral tomograms are diagnostic, demonstrating the separation of the neural elements. Although computed tomography confirms the disruption of the bony neural arch with normal articulating facets,[194] these fractures are difficult to detect by CT.[176] Sagittal reconstructions are diagnostic only if the original cuts pick up the fracture. Computed tomography is the least helpful modality in evaluation of this injury.[140]

Radiographs of a distractive flexion dislocation demonstrate either no anterior bony compression fracture or a minimal one.[55,140] The separation of the vertebral bodies occurs through the ligamentous structures with a widening of the interspinous distance, dissociation of the articular processes, widening of the disk space,[77] and, frequently, translation of the vertebral bodies.[77,157,158] All patients with abnormal separation of the posterior spinous processes have varying degrees of partially dislocated, "perched," or completely dislocated facets.[220] Upper thoracic lesions may be difficult to diagnose on the emergency portable radiographs obtained in trauma situations. Overpenetrated radiographs should be obtained if clinical suspicion is aroused.[51,158]

Computed tomographic scanning demonstrates that the inferior facets of the superior vertebral body have dislocated superiorly. They can come to rest in any one of four positions.[172] The facets can return to the normal position, resulting in an apparently normal CT scan. The medially oriented concave superior facets can be identified posterior to the flatter forward-facing inferior facets if they are jumped anteriorly. The facets may also appear translated laterally or may appear "naked" due to superior dislocation without significant anterior subluxation. Naked facets are diagnostic of a dislocation.[107,157,158,172,194] The presence of two vertebral bodies within the same axial slice suggests fracture-dislocation.[9,244] Sagittal reconstructions of the CT scan demonstrate the degree of canal compromise through anterior translation of the spinal elements.[158]

Treatment

The true Chance fracture, Denis's type A, is fairly uncommon. Union of the vertebral cancellous surfaces occurs with regularity if the fracture is re-

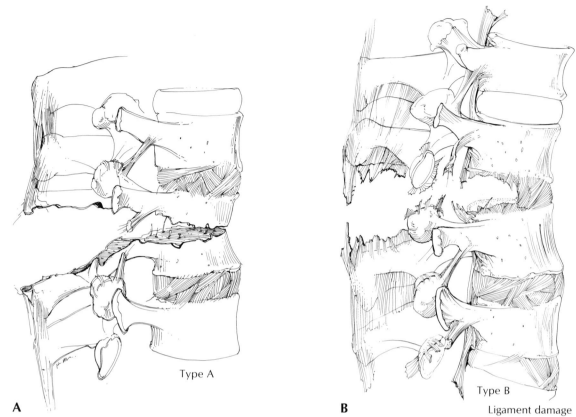

Figure 8-24. (*A, B, C, D*) Types of distractive flexion injuries. (*A*) Classic chance fracture completely through bone. (*B*) One level injury, purely ligamentous in nature.

duced and there is coaptation of the cancellous surfaces.[102] This requires reduction and immobilization, which can be accomplished with hyperextension casting or bracing. Surgical reduction and bracing is also an acceptable option for more immediate mobilization.[176,187,226]

Operative treatment is necessary for the majority of distractive flexion injuries, which occur through ligamentous tissue. Although they are stable initially, there can be late instability.[102,145] Since the posterior anatomic hinge has been disrupted, the instrumentation of choice is bilateral compression instrumentation to counter the tension failure of the posterior elements (Fig. 8-25).[28,71,77,123,124,137,176,181,251] If there is moderate to severe anterior compression of the vertebral body, distraction rods[94] or the combination of distraction and compression instrumentation may be

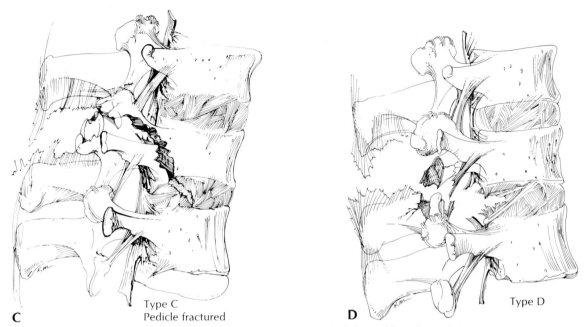

C
Type C
Pedicle fractured

D
Type D

Figure 8-24. (*continued*). (*C*) Two level injury through bone at the level of the middle column. (*D*) Two level injury passing through ligamentous tissue at the level of the middle column. (Adapted from Denis F: The three-column spine and its significance in the classification of acute thoracolumbar spinal injuries. Spine 8:817–831, 1983)

necessary.[137] If the patient has sustained a complete neurologic lesion, segmental spinal instrumentation with L-rods might be used so that the patient does not require postoperative immobilization.[77]

When a facet dislocation has occurred, reduction of the facets may be difficult due to the intact bony buttress of the vertically oriented facets, which block repeated translation. Surgical intervention is mandatory:[37,53,160] even Bedbrook noted that irreducible facet dislocation requires surgical intervention.[11,13] The goal of treatment is to achieve bony fusion, using a tension band construct to prevent further flexion and translation.[22,135,160]

Harrington compression instrumentation acts as a hinge, creating a posterior tension banding system (Fig. 8-26).[71,76,124,140,181,251] Compression

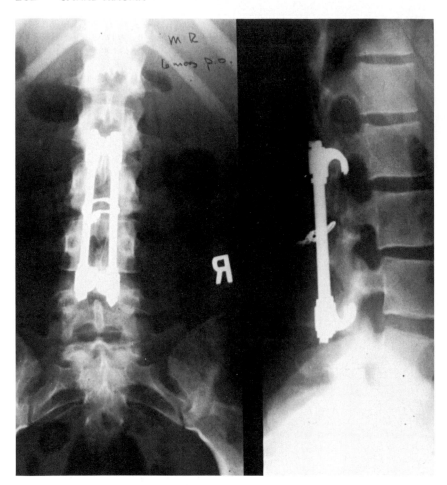

Figure 8-25. Anteroposterior and lateral radiographs of dual Harrington compression rods used to reduce and stabilize a distractive flexion injury. The injury passed through the posterior bony elements of L-2 and then through the L-2–L-3 disk space. Notice the loss of disk height at the injured L-2–L-3 disk in this 17-year-old girl.

instrumentation gives the best restoration of anatomy compared with other types of instrumentation, and is more stable.[140,158] Distraction instrumentation prevents disk compression but requires fusion over a longer distance, requiring an average of 5.5 segments, compared to the two segments compression instrumentation requires.[71,76,90,157,158] In the lower lumbar spine compression instrumentation with a concomitant discectomy may be required.[158] Roy-Camille plates [146,212-214] and Dick's internal fixator[60,61,175] have been used for this injury.

LATERAL FLEXION

Lateral flexion injuries are secondary to eccentric axial loading forces, which cause lateral bending of the spine.[77] There are two stages of lateral compression fracture. The anterior and middle elements may fail unilaterally in the first stage, while the posterior elements remain intact. Radiologically this is manifested by an acute lateral bending deformity of the spine with unilateral shortening of the vertebral body height. This is the more common pattern, according to Denis (Fig. 8-27).[55]

The second stage in this family of injuries is reached when sufficient force causes the posterior elements also to be disrupted.[77] Compression failure occurs on the concave side of the spine, while tension failure of the bony and ligamentous structures occurs on the convex side, with the fulcrum being located within the vertebral body. An acute lateral bending deformity is present on the radiograph with a unilateral articular process dislocation. Computed tomography demonstrates a vacant facet unilaterally.[77]

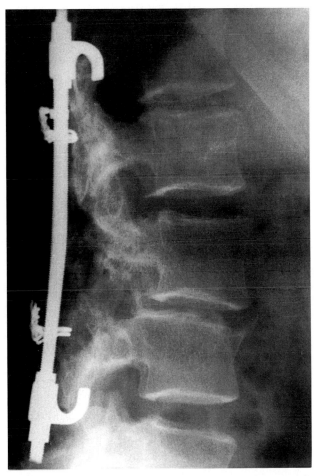

Figure 8-26. The posterior dual Harrington compression rods act as a posterior tension band. This fracture healed and fused in a position of slight subluxation of L-3 on L-4.

If only the middle and anterior elements are involved, this lesion is unlikely to progress. If the posterior elements also fail, the incidence of late pain due to continued deformity increases. Neurologic injury may occur if the middle element encroaches on the neural canal.[77,141] Patients with neural injuries resulting from this fracture showed the best overall improvement with the least profound deficits when compared to patients whose neural injuries resulted from other types of fractures.[48]

Several treatment modalities can be employed for this fracture pattern. Harrington distraction instrumentation or segmental spinal instrumentation have been successfully used.[76,77] Harrington distraction rods can be used on the concave side of the deformity combined with compression rods on the convex side (Fig. 8-28).[48] If middle element failure has caused neural canal impingement, then Harrington distraction instrumentation is the instrumentation of choice to prevent axial loading and possible further encroachment on the neural canal by the middle element. Anterior decompression is not usually necessary.[77]

TRANSLATIONAL OR SHEAR TYPE FRACTURE-DISLOCATION

Fracture-dislocations secondary to shear are caused by forces that displace the vertebral body anteriorly, posteriorly, or laterally.[22,54,55,77] Shearing forces are most commonly the result of massive blows to the back.[9,57] Gross displacement of the vertebral bodies is associated with fractures of the articular processes and ligamentous rupture. Significant neurologic damage is common (Fig. 8-29).[9]

Shear predominantly occurs in the sagittal plane. Posteroanterior shear, when the segment above shears forward off the segment below, occurs with the patient in the extended position. There is no loss of vertebral height.[55] The posterior arch of the vertebral segment is fractured as it rides forward through the posterior elements of the level below, leading to free-floating laminae,

(*Text continued on p. 236*)

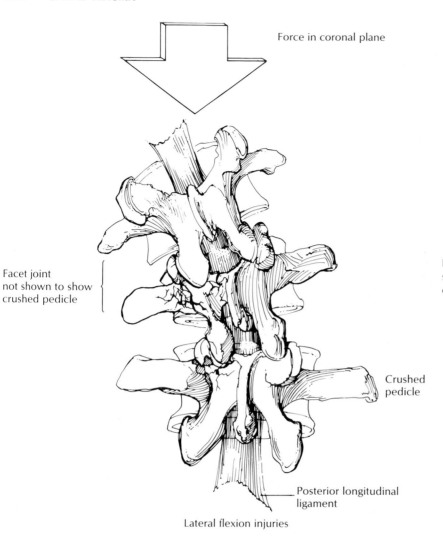

Force in coronal plane

Facet joint
not shown to show
crushed pedicle

Crushed
pedicle

Posterior longitudinal
ligament

Lateral flexion injuries

Figure 8-27. Lateral flexion injuries result from unilateral forces compressing one portion of the vertebral body.

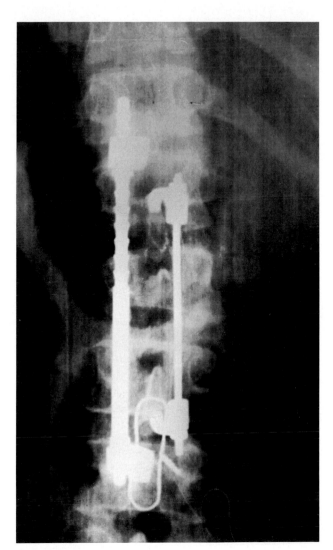

Figure 8-28. This lateral flexion injury was treated with a Harrington distraction rod on the concave side of the deformity and a compression rod on the convex side. The spinous process of L-3 was wired to the spinous process of L-4 in an attempt to maintain lordosis.

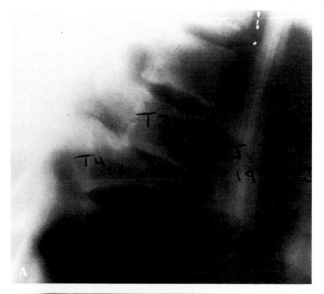

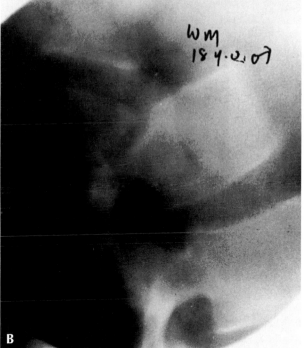

Figure 8-29. (*A*) Fifty-percent anterior translation of T-3 on T-4 resulted in paraplegia in this 19-year-old man. (*B*) Posterior translation of T-12 on L-1.

fractures of several spinous processes, fracture of the superior facet of the inferior vertebra, and disruption of the anterior longitudinal ligament (Fig. 8-30).[9,55,238]

Anteroposterior shear causes the cranial segment to be displaced in a posterior direction.[55] Posterior arch fractures do not occur because there is no interference to the posterior elements as they travel posteriorly. The articular processes disengage and displace, rupturing the articular joint capsules, without producing free-floating

laminae. There may be spinous process fractures, though usually at one level alone.[55,57] There may be fractures at the junction of the pedicle with the body (permitting more severe retrolisthesis) or a fracture of the anteroinferior margin of the superior vertebral body.[57] The anterior aspect of the upper segment may be locked on the superior facet of the body below (Fig. 8-31).

With displacements of 25% or more, the articular processes and all ligamentous structures, including the anterior longitudinal ligaments, are

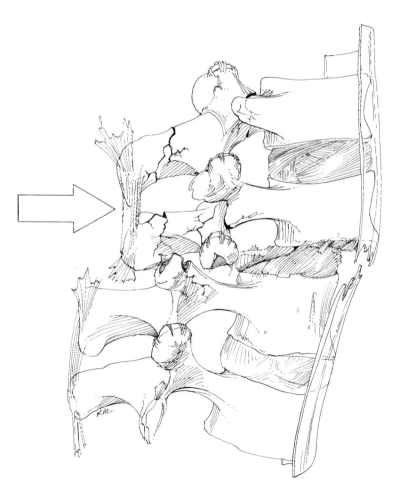

Figure 8-30. Lateral diagram of a posteroanterior shear injury. (Adapted from Denis F: The three-column spine and its significance in the classification of acute thoracolumbar spinal injuries. Spine 8:817–831, 1983)

ruptured. If the articular processes are also fractured, there are few or no remaining stabilizing structures in the spine. Acute and chronic deformities may result. These are highly unstable lesions that require operative stabilization.[9,22,54,55,145,238] Shear is frequently associated with other injury mechanisms and rarely occurs in the pure form. Associated injuries usually include rib fractures, lung contusions, sternal fractures, and most frequently, pneumothorax, hemothorax, or both.[83,180,238]

Serious neurologic injury occurs in a high percentage of patients.[9,77,160] Due to the extreme degree of canal compromise, 80% or more of patients with injuries at the thoracolumbar junction and above sustain complete paraplegia. Spinal discontinuity is nearly complete.[55,160,176] There are isolated reports of patients who sustained significant bony injuries without neurologic compromise. Such injury can occur when multiple pedicular fractures dissociate the anterior elements from the posterior elements. This traumatic spon-

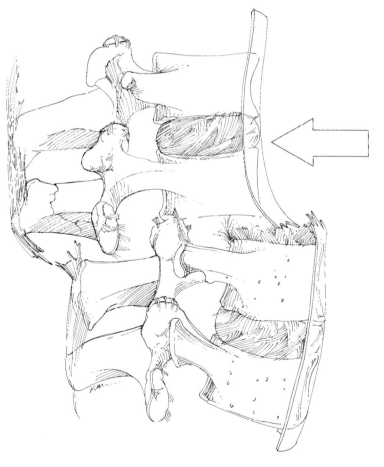

Figure 8-31. Anteroposterior shear injury. (Adapted from Denis F: The three-column spine and its significance in the classification of acute thoracolumbar spinal injuries. Spine 8:817–831, 1983)

dylolysis causes widening of the spinal canal, leaving the spinal cord untouched.[97,112,122,217,232,238] In the lumbar spine, there is a large area for the spinal cord, thus few patients sustain significant neural injury after lumbar fracture.[57,160]

Shear injuries are usually not difficult to detect on plain films. The vertebral body can be seen to be translated a variable distance directly anteriorly, laterally, or posteriorly. More subtle signs include increased radiodensity of an involved segment due to superimposition of vertebral bodies, exaggerated lordosis of the lumbar spine due to dislocation,[121] and distortion of the posterior intercostal spaces in the thoracic spine.[220] Computed tomography demonstrates the double body sign at the level of the dislocation, and confirms the injury to the posterior elements.[112,124]

Reduction of shear type dislocations can be difficult,[57] especially when there is dissociation of the body from the spinous process. Surgical treatment in the past has revolved around the use of Harrington distraction rods.[62,109,228] The posterior longitudinal ligament is usually completely transected. If the body is displaced more than 25%, the anterior longitudinal ligament may also be ruptured, allowing overdistraction to occur.[77,173] To minimize overdistraction, the posterior elements of the injured vertebra may be wired together before distraction.[84] A short midline compression rod placed across the injured vertebral segments may counteract the distraction.[140,188] Segmental fixation with either Harrington distraction rods supplemented by sublaminar[35,88,91,166,227] or interspinous wires[67] or L-rods may be used.[77] Since L-rods require no stability from the anterior longitudinal ligament, overdistraction cannot occur. These rods afford an excellent means of stabilizing translational injuries.[77]

Use of Harrington rods to treat this injury is associated with a significant failure rate. Pseudarthrosis is most likely to occur following distraction instrumentation of translational injuries, and is associated with hook dislodgement.[48,173,197] The use of Harrington distraction rods supplemented by sublaminar wires improves resistance to axial loads, lateral bending, and forward flexion, but the greatest improvement is in resistance to rotatory stresses. Sublaminar wires also cause a decrease in the pseudarthrosis rate and in the incidence of

hook cutout.[35,91,187,227] L-rod fixation with sublaminar wiring is the most rigid type of fixation, especially with respect to rotation.[78,181] This form of fixation is best reserved for complete neural injuries[6,35,88,168,181,226] because external immobilization is no longer necessary when segmental fixation is employed.[166] Roy-Camille plates[146,212,213,214] and Dick's internal fixator[60,61,175] have been used for this injury.

TORSIONAL FLEXION OR ROTATION–FLEXION DISLOCATION

The most unstable fracture of the thoracolumbar spine is the rotatory fracture-dislocation.[9,55,77,141,245] These unstable rotation–flexion dislocations are frequently located at the thoracolumbar junction.

This injury occurs when there is torsion and compression in the anterior elements, and tension and torsion about the posterior elements.[36,54,55,77] The articular processes are usually fractured and dislocated, providing physical evidence of the rotatory nature of the injury.[9,36,55] The middle elements are likely to be involved as well. Middle column injuries occur either through the vertebral body or purely through the disk. Disk injuries are associated with wedging through the inferior vertebral body.[55] Usually, a slice of the inferior vertebral body attached to the annulus is fractured in the sagittal plane and translated anteriorly or laterally.[9,22,36,55,127] Ligamentous structures are very susceptible to rotation. The anterior longitudinal ligament is usually stripped from the anterior border of the involved vertebra (Fig. 8-32).[22,55,77]

Rotation–flexion fractures are due to significant trauma. Associated injuries, especially to the chest, are common. Hemothorax is the most common associated injury,[83,180,238] along with rib fractures, sternal fractures, and extremity fractures.[83]

On the anteroposterior radiograph, the cephalad vertebral body is usually displaced to the side of the shear fracture (Fig. 8-33). The anteroposterior film may appear innocuous, although careful inspection reveals the articular process fractures[55] or a subtle increase in the disk height.[54] Rotation between segments is recognized by the orientation of the pedicles and spinous processes.[55] The fracture is associated with multiple

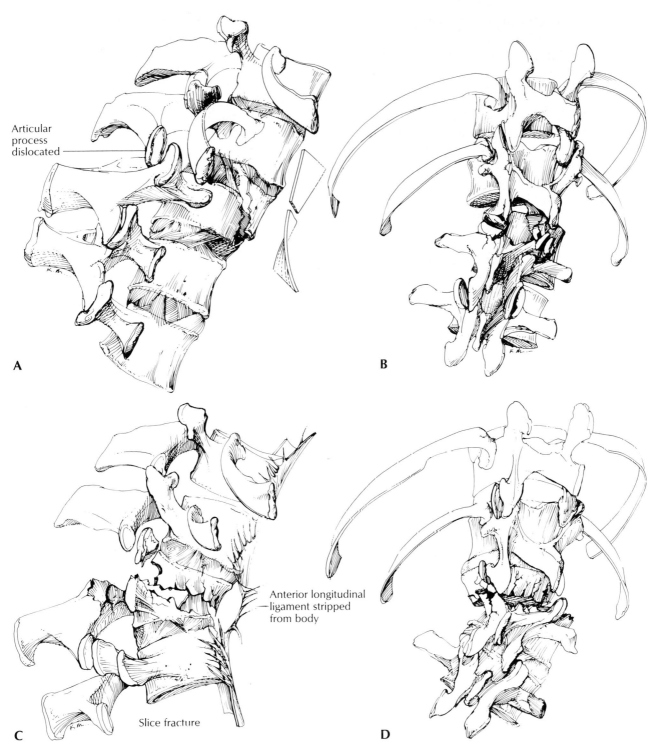

Articular process dislocated

A

B

Slice fracture

Anterior longitudinal ligament stripped from body

C

D

Figure 8-32. Rotatory fracture-dislocation of the thoracolumbar spine. Injury can occur through the disk (*A* and *B*) or totally through bone (*C* and *D*). Rotation between segments is recognized by the orientation of the pedicles. (Adapted from Denis F: The three-column spine and its significance in the classification of acute thoracolumbar spinal injuries. Spine 8:817–831, 1983)

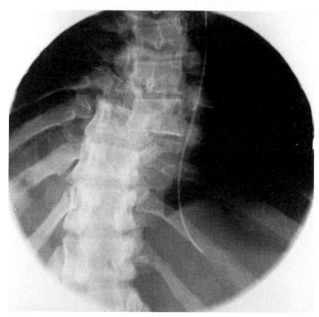

Figure 8-33. The cephalad vertebral body is displaced to the side of the inferior vertebral body.

transverse process fractures and rib fractures, and its presence should be suspected if these injuries are evident.[54,55] On the lateral radiograph the spine appears telescoped, with one vertebra overlapping the other. The lateral film usually clearly demonstrates the subluxation or dislocation; however, the fracture may be obscured by overlying shoulders, hips, or soft tissues.[55,121] One can clearly see conservation of the posterior wall of the vertebral body.[55]

Computed tomography demonstrates the offset of the vertebra above on the one below. Constriction or occlusion of the canal at that level is due to the offset.[54,55] Jumped facets are best demonstrated on CT, along with fractures at the base of the articular processes or at the base of the pedicles.[55] The retropulsed fragment of posterior vertebral body that is seen in the vertebral canal is associated with a torn posterior longitudinal ligament. This is in contradistinction to the burst fracture, in which this is intact and ligamentaxis might work to reduce the fragment from the canal.[54] For this reason, the rotation–flexion fracture is less stable than a burst fracture.

Because of the extensive ligamentous and bony injury, this fracture type is thought to have both acute and chronic propensity to deform the spinal column and cause progression of the neurologic injury.[37,77,145] Holdsworth[119] stated that rotational fracture-dislocations are the most unstable of all spinal fractures and that they are invariably associated with paraplegia. He also pointed out that injudicious handling of the patients could lead to further neurologic injury.

This lesion is most common in the thoracic spine, with the majority of patients sustaining complete neurologic injury. The most unstable patients are those with anterior subluxation. Roberts and Curtiss[211] were able to demonstrate only a very low incidence of spontaneous fusion, with progressive deformity in most patients. Although Denis noted no neurologic injury in 25% of his fracture-dislocations, in more than 50% of his patients there was a complete neurologic injury.[55] Other authors have documented profound neurologic injuries from this lesion, 60% to 70% of these being complete injury, and the remainder significant, though incomplete injury.[48,83] Neural recovery after decompression of rotation–flexion injuries is not as complete as that obtained after decompression of burst fractures.[210]

Patients with complete cord injury and grossly unstable rotatory fracture-dislocation require posterior open reduction and internal fixation with posterior arthrodesis. These torsional flexion injuries may be treated with Harrington instrumentation[22,28,48,62,77,83,109,228] because bilateral Harrington rod instrumentation acts like a beam lying between the spinous processes and facets, preventing rotation (Fig. 8-34).[123,163] Since Harrington rods are relatively weak in preventing rotation,[175] supplementation with either a short compression rod to resist tensile forces or with sublaminar wires is recommended.[88,188,226] L-rods with sublaminar wires have been recommended for this injury.[35,77,88] L-rods are best for preventing rotation.[175] Roy-Camille describes his experience with pedicular screw plating for this fracture.[146,212,213,214] Patients who have sustained complete neurologic injury may be better treated by compression instrumentation because a shorter length of spine needs to be instrumented and fixation is stronger.[123]

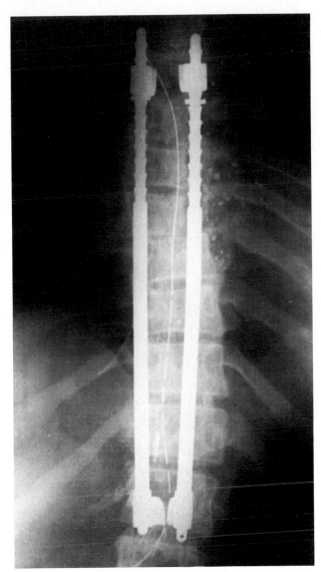

Figure 8-34. Dual Harrington distraction rods used to reduce a fracture-dislocation.

BURST FRACTURE

The burst compression fracture of the thoracolumbar spine is the most common major spinal injury presenting to an orthopedic service. This fracture has received considerable recent interest, with new information becoming available on its classification, and new concepts being developed regarding its stability. Indications for surgery and

selection of the most appropriate surgical implant are also matters of intense debate.[58,144]

Holdsworth[119] believed that this injury occurs when the thoracic spine is placed into a linear relationship with the cervical and lumbar spine. Axial loading forces are applied to either the foot or the buttock,[9] allowing compressive force to be delivered to the injured vertebral body by the intact cephalic disk. Axial compression applied to the body in a relatively symmetrical fashion causes the vertebral body to explode. The height of the vertebral body diminishes as the anterior, posterior, and lateral walls of the vertebral body are disrupted. The longitudinally running anterior and posterior longitudinal ligaments are vertically shortened and bowed out around the expanded bone. As the cephalic half of the vertebral body is crushed, the rim of cortical bone is broken into a number of fragments, which displace circumferentially outward.[9,22,54,55,58,77,144,160]

The majority of injuries occur between T-10 and L-2.[10,55,56,63,172,177,210,239,245] There is a significant association of burst fractures with calcaneal fractures, long bone fractures, ligamentous injuries to the knee, and intra-abdominal injuries.[56] Severe burst fractures are frequently accompanied by compression fractures above or below the fractured level.[9,10] Burst fractures may be associated with posterior dural tears, allowing posterior interlaminar herniation of the cauda equina and possible entrapment or amputation of nerve roots.[182]

Burst fractures as a group are associated with less kyphotic deformity than compressive flexion fractures. The incidence of progressive kyphosis after burst fractures depends on the location of the injury.[55] The injury is rare in the thoracic spine. Burst fractures occur most often at the thoracolumbar junction or in the upper lumbar spine (L-1–L-3), and most often involve the superior end-plate alone.[55,127] Burst fracture in the upper lumbar spine is associated with a moderate tendency toward kyphotic deformity, owing to the natural tendency of an axial load to cause flexion at the thoracolumbar junction, which in turn leads to greater involvement of the anterior portion of the vertebral body. In addition, the posterior third of the vertebral body is somewhat stabilized by the pedicular attachments, leaving the anterior third

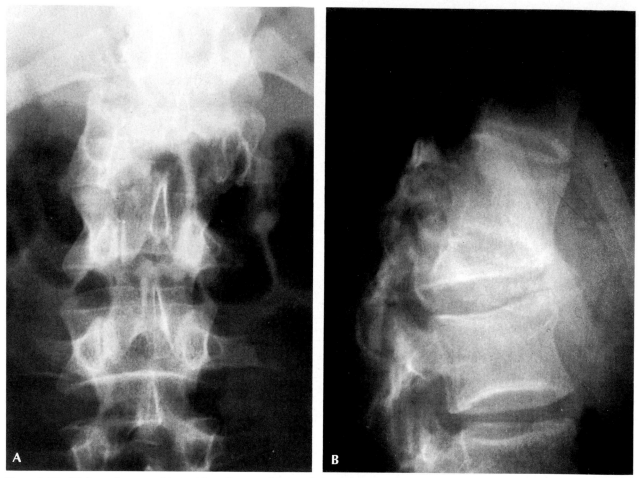

Figure 8-35. (*A*) Burst fracture of L-1 with widening of the pedicle and overall appearance of the body. (*B*) Lateral x-ray shows severe destruction of the vertebral body with widening of the body.

more vulnerable to the axial force. At the lower lumbar levels, an axial load more commonly leads to spinal extension, creating a symmetrical injury with little tendency toward kyphosis.[54,55]

Axial compression can lead to lateral flexion, with lateral compression of the vertebral body. Burst fracture differs from lateral compression fracture in that the interpedicular distance is widened and there is a retropulsed fragment in the canal.[54,55] If the predominant force vector is anteriorly directed, a minor component of lateral bend or rotation may be applied. The vertebral body will be compressed to a greater degree on that side, resulting in an asymmetrical burst.[55]

There may be a significant change of the rotational alignment in the cross-sectional plane, amounting to 5 to 10 degrees through the vertebral body. This can be easily evaluated on plain films by assessing the alignment of the spinous processes above and below the fracture.[144] This rotation is unchanged following Harrington instrumentation, and should be considered before use of pedicular instrumentation is contemplated if pedicular instrumentation is used.[144]

The radiographic hallmark of burst fractures on plain films is widening of both the anteroposterior and mediolateral diameters of the vertebral body (Fig. 8-35). On the anteroposterior film there is widening of the interpedicular distance.[10,55,77,145] On the lateral, radiograph posterior height is lost with spreading of the vertebral body, representing failure of the middle column.[54,55,124,145] Disruptive abnormalities of the posterior vertebral line are reliable signs on plane films that a burst fracture has occurred and that compromise of the vertebral canal and subarachnoid space is present (Fig. 8-36).[50] The integrity of the middle column is sometimes difficult to ascertain by standard anteroposterior and lateral radiographs.[145] Failure to appreciate, evaluate, and appropriately treat significant involvement of the middle column can lead to rapid neurologic deterioration.[9]

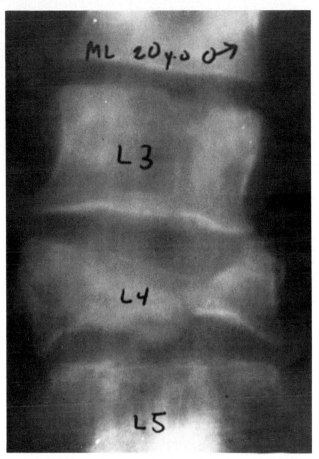

Figure 8-37. Lateral tomography shows the retropulsion of fragments into the spinal canal.

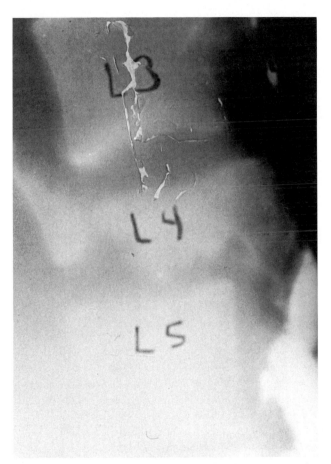

Figure 8-36. Anteroposterior tomography demonstrates the "explosion" of fragment in this burst fracture of the L-4 vertebral body.

Computed tomography is very helpful in evaluation of burst fractures, especially with regard to neural impingement* and the detection of small fragments in the canal (Fig. 8-37).[56,115,176,177] Computed tomography offers the best assessment of facet congruity[176] and the degree of foraminal and spinal canal compromise.[172] Disruption of the anterior and posterior borders of the vertebral body and comminution of the vertebral bodies are easily demonstrated.[55,99,176] Sagittally oriented fractures of the vertebral body are usually noted in the lower third of the vertebral body.[143,164] Vertebral body fragments are distributed in a centripe-

* Reference numbers 9, 10, 26, 32, 33, 70, 115, 124, 133, 136, 137, 139, 143, 145, 176, 193, 202, 244.

tally oriented array, indicating that the longitudinal ligaments are intact,[10,144,164] which is the usual case.[173,242] The fragments, however, do not always remain attached to the longitudinal ligaments.[147]

The optimal method for assessing the posterior elements is the CT scan.[82,176] It shows that the pedicles, which are attached to the bone of the centrum in the cephalic third of the vertebral body, are radially displaced with the bone or, if the posterior ring remains intact, sheared off from the bone at the pedicular base. The cortical bone between the pedicles is usually thin and concave posteriorly, and displaced posteriorly into the canal.[144] A fracture of the facet or at the base of the pedicle is often demonstrated.[127] The bone that is driven into the canal is often at the level of the pedicle and can be difficult to visualize on the lateral radiograph (Fig. 8-38).[99,127,133]

Vertical laminar fractures, usually located on the anterior portion of the lamina, are always noted on the CT scan.[10,55,99,143] At the time of impact the pedicles are forced apart with the expanded vertebral body. The structures that are attached to them cannot remain intact. The posterior bony ring must be damaged, or the cephalic facet joints disrupted, in at least two places.[55,143,144] Longitudinal fractures of the laminar arch, adjacent to the spinous process, are usually seen on the side of maximum compression.[127]

The hallmark of axial compression is retropulsion of bone from the middle element into the canal. The fragment may pivot so that the cortical surface normally facing the spinal canal no longer is vertical but projects into the canal. The fragment is displaced 2 to 4 mm posteriorly so that it is posterior to, rather than directly below, the lower corner of the adjacent vertebral body.[14,127,143]

Examination of the posterior wall of the vertebral body by CT can differentiate between compression fractures and burst fractures. In burst fractures, fractures of the posterior wall of the vertebral body and laminae are present, with disruption of the posterior joints.[55] This is not true of compression fractures.

Denis has subdivided burst fractures into five types (Fig. 8-39). Type A burst fractures, seen in the lower lumbar spine, rupture both end-plates.

Due to pure axial compression, type A fractures do not seem to lead to progressive kyphosis. The most frequent subtype, type B, is seen at the thoracolumbar junction. Rupture of the superior end-plate is frequently accompanied by a sagittal split of the lower body. Fracture of the inferior endplate, type C, is rare. Types A, B, and C best diagnosed on the lateral radiograph.[54-56]

Type D is the highly unstable burst rotation fracture, occurring most frequently in the midlumbar spine. Translation of the spine follows the devastating injury to the posterior elements. This fracture resembles the rotation–flexion dislocation, but can be differentiated from it due to the increased interpedicular distance and comminution of the vertebral body. Type E fractures are burst fractures due to lateral flexion. They differ from the lateral flexion injury in that they have an increased incidence of neurologic injury due to fracture of the posterior vertebral wall and extrusion of bony contents into the canal. Types D and E are best diagnosed on the anteroposterior radiograph.[54-56]

Burst fractures have been considered stable if the posterior column remains intact. A burst fracture becomes unstable in the presence of subluxation of one or more facet joints, displaced fracture of the neural arch, posterior ligamentous injuries, or gross displacement of neural elements.[10,76,176,177,189,245] Posterior element failure can occur in tension, rotation, or lateral flexion.[176,177] The criteria for instability of burst fractures also include progressive neurologic deficit, progressive kyphosis in the presence of a neural deficit, and greater than 50% loss of vertebral body height with facet subluxation.[177]

Neurologic injuries sustained after burst fractures are usually incomplete lesions.[30,55] Unstable burst fractures have the most severe neural deficits, although there are instances in which the canal can be occluded up to 90% in "stable" burst fractures.[174,176] Although Denis found few neurologic injuries in which the canal was compromised 50% or less and few injuries of Frankel grade B or C with canal occlusions 75% or greater,[55] most authors have found no simple direct correlation or reliable predictor between the amount of canal encroachment and concomitant neurologic in-

(*Text continued on p. 248*)

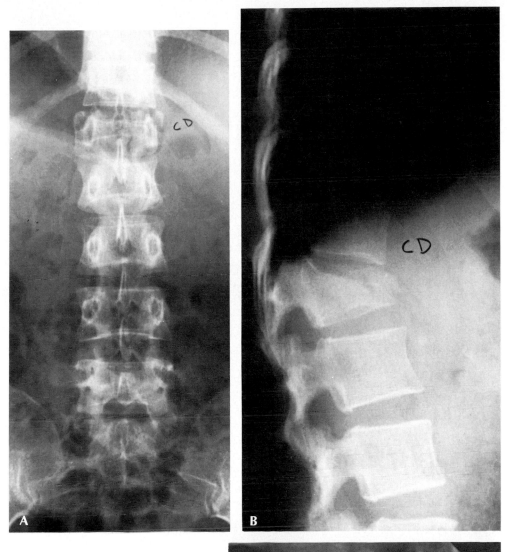

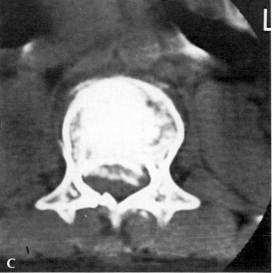

Figure 8-38. Fracture of L-1. (*A*) Subtle widening of the pedicles is seen on the anteroposterior view. (*B*) There is no evidence on the lateral view that bone fragments from the posterior vertebral wall are out of alignment. (*C*) Computed tomographic scan shows bony fragments "hidden" behind the pedicles and impinging on the spinal canal.

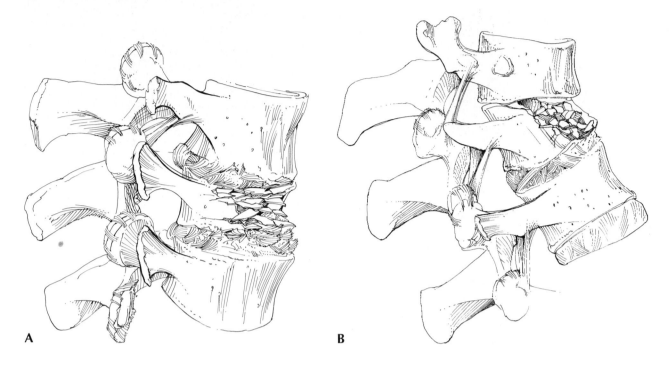

A

B

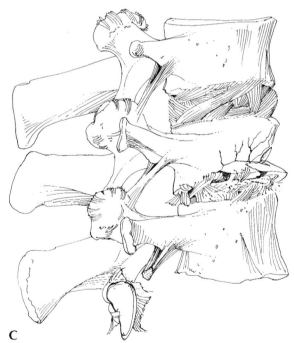

C

Figure 8-39. (*A–E*) Denis' classification of burst fractures. Types A, B, and C are primarily diagnosed on the lateral radiograph. Type A is usually in the lower lumbar spine with rupture of both end-plates. Type B is a rupture of the superior end-plate with a sagittal split of the lower body. Type C is a fracture of the inferior end-plate.

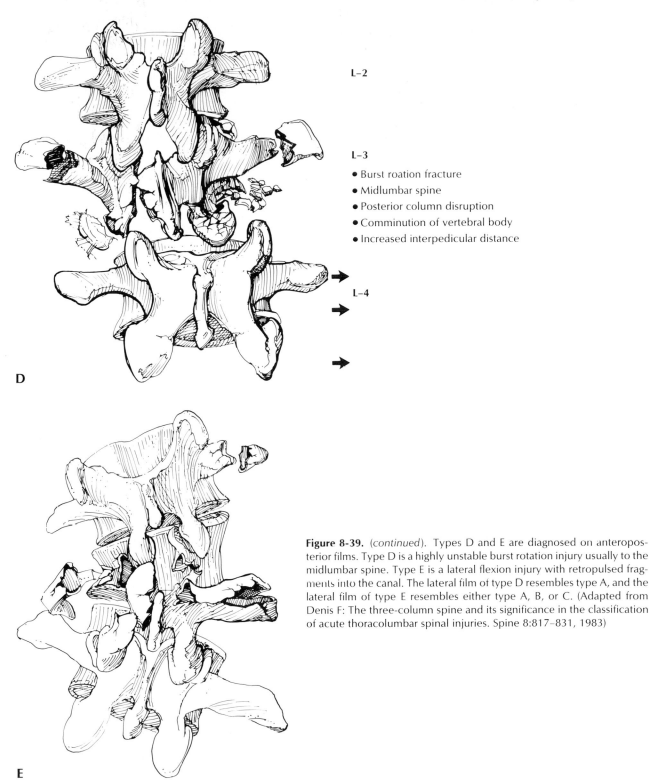

L–2

L–3

- Burst roation fracture
- Midlumbar spine
- Posterior column disruption
- Comminution of vertebral body
- Increased interpedicular distance

L–4

D

E

Figure 8-39. (*continued*). Types D and E are diagnosed on anteroposterior films. Type D is a highly unstable burst rotation injury usually to the midlumbar spine. Type E is a lateral flexion injury with retropulsed fragments into the canal. The lateral film of type D resembles type A, and the lateral film of type E resembles either type A, B, or C. (Adapted from Denis F: The three-column spine and its significance in the classification of acute thoracolumbar spinal injuries. Spine 8:817–831, 1983)

jury.[48,55,70,95,143,176,177,219] This may be because the final resting place of the fragments may reflect less impingement than what occurred at the time of injury. Significant canal narrowing may be present without encroaching on the cord or cauda equina, due to incomplete filling of the spinal canal by neural material in the lumbar region. A greater degree of canal compromise can be tolerated without major neural element compression.[70,219] Burst fractures may also result in central or lateral canal stenosis rather than just midaxial compression. This can be demonstrated on CT.[177,219]

Treatment

The issue of the stability of burst fractures is controversial. Classically, Holdsworth considered all burst fractures to be stable, treating them with a body cast or an orthosis.[176,226] Experience has shown that ambulation of a patient with a disrupted middle column may cause further axial loading of the spine, with progression of the neural deficit.[76,133] Conservative treatment of burst fractures may be associated with progressive neural deficits and post-traumatic spinal stenosis. Paraparesis and radicular symptoms were demonstrated in 17% of patients treated nonoperatively in one study,[56] although deterioration is not an absolute in patients with canal compromise.[151,239] Resolution of small bony fragments and adaptive changes in canal morphology by bony remodeling may occur. These changes are age-related, present more frequently in younger patients.[151] Post-traumatic kyphosis increased by at least 20 degrees with conservative treatment.[56,239]

Many authors feel that there is an unacceptable percentage of unsatisfactory results after conservative treatment of burst fractures. Computed tomography, since its advent, has led us to better understand the pathologic anatomy of these fractures, and many of these fractures have been redefined into the unstable category. Within this subgroup of unstable fractures, there are fractures with relative inherent stability ("stable" burst fractures) and those that are *highly* unstable (therefore, "unstable" burst fractures). This point has great importance in the choice of treatment and will be returned to later.

Prophylactic fixation of stable burst fractures, with stabilization and fixation of acute burst fractures in the absence of neurologic deficits, prevents neurologic deficits from occurring and allows early, safe mobilization. At the same time it prevents late kyphosis and decreases postoperative pain and the incidence of late degenerative changes.[56,135,165] However, by choosing this route one runs the risk of iatrogenic complications, including failure of fixation, pseudarthrosis, neurologic damage, and failure to decompress the neural elements adequately.[151]

Distraction performed in the first 2 weeks after injury may lead to significant reduction of the middle element from the canal. The best results are obtained when distraction is performed within 48 hours after injury.[76,98] Overdistraction can occur in unstable burst fractures during attempts to correct retrodisplacement.[173] The overdistraction is usually of only a minor degree, due to plastic deformation of the longitudinal ligaments.[144]

Bilateral Harrington distraction instrumentation has been used most frequently when posterior surgical repair is performed. It has been the most effective instrumentation in restoring vertebral height. Harrington instrumentation lengthens the middle element and may reduce the retropulsed posterior wall of the vertebral body (Fig. 8-40). It will prevent axial compression forces from shortening the vertebral body.

Harrington instrumentation has many weaknesses that limit its effectiveness in treating burst fractures. Angulation is resisted by the beam effect on the intact lamina.* While distraction does tend to lengthen the middle element, Harrington instrumentation depends on distraction to keep the hooks under the lamina. Harrington rods have very limited firm skeletal purchase.[144,187]

A burst fracture may settle even after Harrington instrumentation. There is a tendency for the angular deformity to recur if straight Harrington rods are used.[96] This is due to viscoelastic relaxation and creep in the anterior structures, leading to 10 to 15 degrees more kyphosis than was obtained at surgery.[4,96,127,144] A more anteriorly directed force is required to restore the anatomy of the vertebral body.

Several adaptations of posterior instrumentation attempt to correct these shortcomings. Harrington

---

* Reference numbers 22, 69, 71, 77, 98, 109, 124, 137, 140, 176, 181, 228, 236.

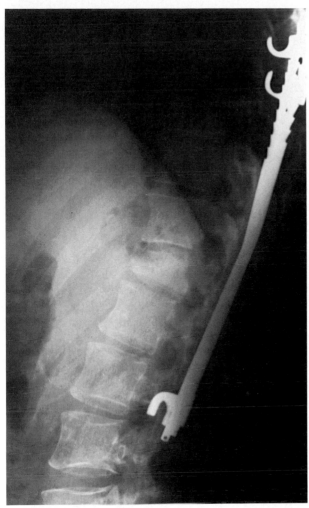

Figure 8-40. Lateral radiograph of a Harrington rod used to reduce L-1 burst injury.

and "universal" rods have been supplemented by the application of variously sized rod sleeves. These allow shorter fusions and application of an anteriorly directed force while preserving lordosis. If the posterior elements are not intact, rod sleeves can be used in a bridging construct. Rod sleeves allow the use of noncontoured rods and make it easier to insert hooks.[71,144] The locking rods of Jacobs can also be used, with contouring of the rods to preserve the lordosis and maintain the tension on the anterior structures.[125,126]

Wired Harrington rods provide improved axial stability and are best at resisting compressive loads. Many authors consider them the best posterior method to treat unstable burst fractures.[35,76,166,175,187,226,242] The addition of sublaminar wires prevents increasing kyphosis,[144] decreases the need for external immobilization,[6,35,88,226] and, if applied two to four lamina above the fracture, provides strength equal to the original spine in flexion.[183] While sublaminar wires add stability, they do not increase the ability of posterior instrumentation to reduce bony fragments that protruded into the canal.[5] The use of segmental spinal fixation with sublaminar wires must be carefully considered in light of its risk in intact patients.[181]

Cotrell–Dubousset instrumentation is now being used more frequently in the treatment of burst fractures (Fig. 8-41). Like the classic Harrington system, it accomplishes three point-bending. It is rigidly attached to the uppermost vertebra so that overdistraction is not necessary to maintain the superior hook in position. Segmental fixation is accomplished without the need for sublaminar wires. Rotational stability can be improved by the use of the device for transverse traction (DTT) between the two rods.[74,103,144]

The pedicle is considered by some to be ideal for fixation in burst fractures.[3] Pedicle screw plates have been used.[213,214] The internal spinal skeletal fixator was designed by Dick and Magerl for use in fixation[60,61] (Fig. 8-42). The major advantage of this posterior instrumentation is that it need be applied to only the vertebrae immediately adjacent to the fracture, decreasing the limits of surgical fusion and preserving lordosis. Strong fixation allows rapid mobilization with or without an orthosis, with good restoration of vertebral anatomy and decompression of the neural canal without the need for further anterior decompression.[2,3,61,134,175,196] There are situations in which the use of this instrumentation still requires anterior bone grafting through the pedicle or via an anterior approach to reduce the incidence of fatigue failure of the internal fixator.[61,134,175,196] The internal fixator can be used in any type of lesion; it does not require the presence of intact longitudinal ligaments, nor does it depend on the condition of the posterior elements or the posterior wall of the vertebral body.[61,175]

There is no role for the use of Luque instrumentation in the treatment of burst fractures because there is no built-in axial distraction mecha-

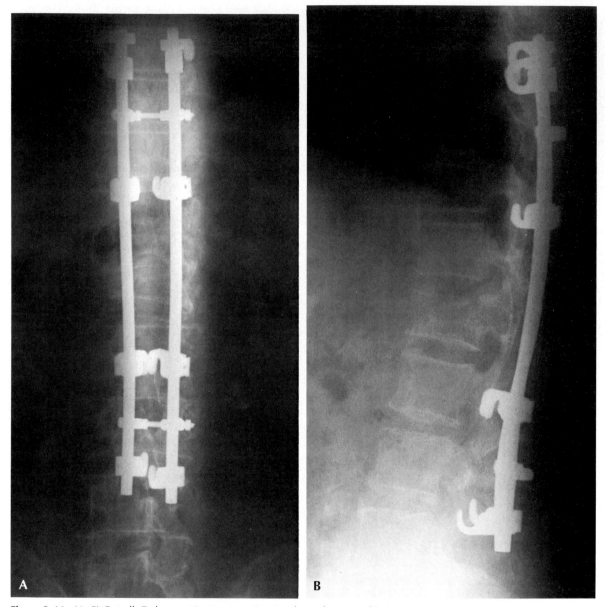

Figure 8-41. (*A, B*) Cotrell–Dubousset instrumentation in a burst fracture of L-1.

nism.[168] Patients in whom L-rods had been used to treat burst fractures required the highest percentage of reoperation of any form of instrumentation.[4] Although favored in the past, Harrington rods have not been a panacea in the treatment of burst fractures, and should not be the primary treatment in patients with incomplete neurologic injuries.[23,147] Although vertebral body fragments within the canal are usually attached to the inferior portion of the vertebral body, and in some cases can be successfully reduced with distraction, ligamentaxis may not always be successful in reducing the fragment.[51,70,115,124] Many authors have found that better results can be obtained from removal of the anterior vertebral body.[22,51,63,70,77,98,144,147,148,160] Dickson[63] and

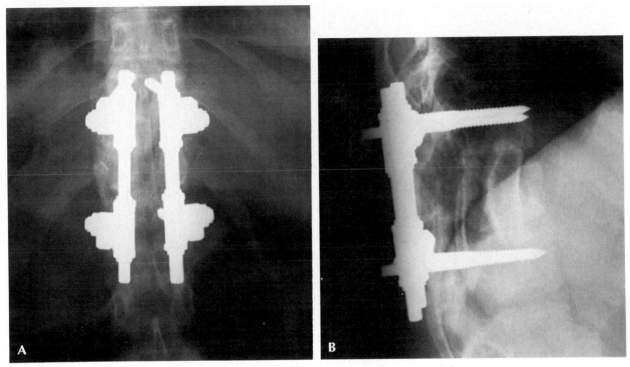

Figure 8-42. (*A, B*) Internal fixator used to stabilize a T-12 burst fracture with complete paraplegia. In this case the surgeon decided to do a second-stage anterior decompression and strut graft.

Flesch[83] both demonstrated that there could be progressive neurologic deficit and transient paresthesias after Harrington rod instrumentation without anterior decompression.

When anterior decompression should be performed, and whether anterior or posterior instrumentation should be employed are controversial issues. Some authors believe that it is not necessary to perform anterior surgery immediately. They prefer to treat developing neurologic compromise or a plateau in recovery with later anterior surgical decompression.[24,25,89] Whitesides and Shah were the first to advocate the two-stage approach: posterior spinal fusion followed by anterior decompression.[93,174,177,245] Many authors believe that the posterolateral approach used with posterior instrumentation affords sufficient decompression.[73,83,177,226]

There have been varied attempts at anterior decompression and instrumentation. Anterior fusion without instrumentation was associated with progressive kyphosis, though this was no greater than

that allowed by posterior Harrington instrumentation.[252] Zilke instrumentation was used, but was found to be not biomechanically suited for fracture management.[93] AO broad plates were used for anterior fixation after Harrington instrumentation was used for distraction,[238] but these plates were associated with nonunion.[147] Dunn instrumentation[68] was also associated with nonunion and has been withdrawn from the market.[144]

Kostuik reported on anterior decompression along with anterior fixation for burst fractures in patients with and without incomplete neurologic injuries (Fig. 8-43).[147,148] There is no need for posterior fusion and instrumentation when using the Kostuik–Harrington distraction rods supplemented by a heavy compression rod. This combination is sufficiently rigid to allow early rehabilitation and ambulation with an orthosis. The anterior third of the vertebral body is preserved as viable graft, and is supplemented by iliac crest grafting.[147] The indications for this approach include acute burst fractures with neurologic injury in-

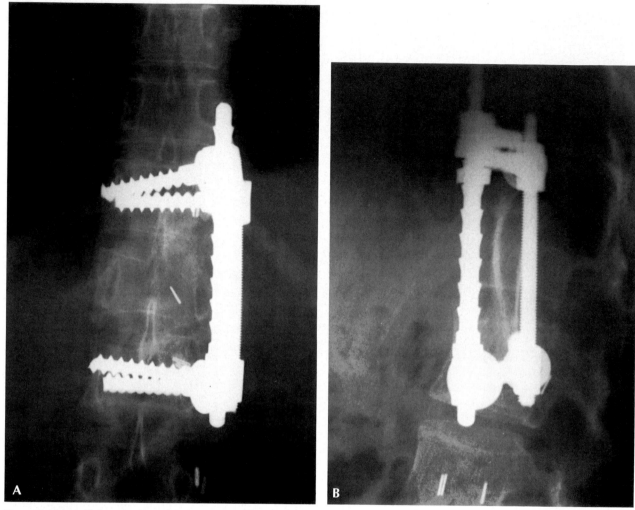

Figure 8-43. (A, B) Anterior Kostuik–Harrington instrumentation and fusion of an L-1 burst fracture. There is an anterior distraction rod and a posterior heavy-threaded rod.

volving the anterior and middle column with retropulsion into the canal, late burst injuries (those that are treated 10 or more days after injury) that are difficult to reduce posteriorly, and painful or progressive kyphosis with or without neurologic changes.

There are a number of advantages to the anterior approach. Anterior surgery serves to preserve motion segments if there is injury at the lower lumbar spine.[68,133,145] There is frequently a void left anteriorly after posterior reduction that needs to be filled in with graft; this void can be filled by anterior surgery.[144] Stabilization is limited to one vertebral body above and below the fracture.[133,144] Lordosis can be preserved with this approach, and kyphosis is directly eliminated (Fig. 8-44).[133]

It is clear that the consensus of opinion regarding the treatment of burst fractures remains as fragmented as the fractures themselves.[68,93,174,177,245] Recommended therapy for this lesion has run the gamut from prolonged bed rest with postural reduction to combined anterior decompression with concomitant posterior stabili-

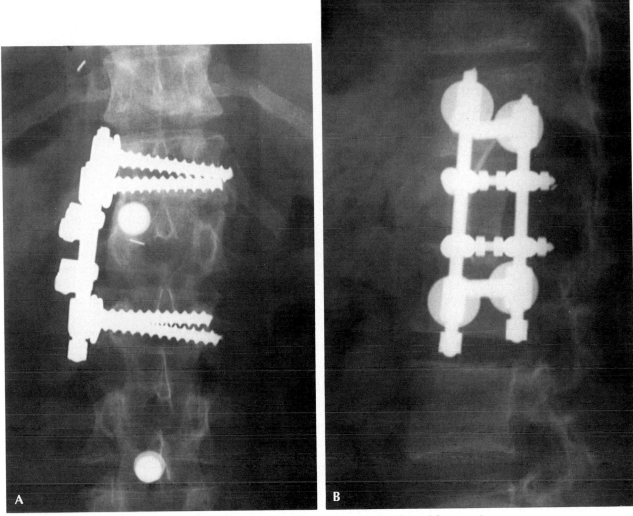

Figure 8-44. (*A, B*) Modification of anterior Kostuik–Harrington instrumentation allowed for use of two heavy compression rods connected by two devices for transverse traction.

zation. To better understand the various options available, it is necessary to better define the goals of treatment of burst fractures.

Modern goals of fracture treatment include early mobilization and ambulation, reduction of the localized area of kyphosis to minimize postoperative deformity, restoration of normal canal dimensions (especially in the neurologically impaired), and long-term stabilization to prevent the late onset of deformity or neurologic deficit. All of these should be accomplished while sacrificing as few levels of lumbar mobility as possible. Furthermore, these goals must be accomplished without creating an iatrogenic neurologic problem.

In order to best select the treatment that achieves these goals, it is necessary to delineate between upper burst fractures (T-12–L-1), middle burst fractures (L-2–L-3), and lower burst fractures (L-4–L-5). Each of these areas demands special consideration because of unique anatomic considerations. In each category the differentiation between a stable and an unstable burst injury should be made.

Upper Burst Fracture.   The upper burst fracture is anatomically unique from the other two because the canal still contains cord or conus medullaris. This segment represents the transitional zone of facet morphology from the coronally oriented thoracic facets to the sagittally oriented lumbar facets. Of considerable importance as well is the availability of at least four to five open interspaces below the fracture, depending on the exact level of injury and the presence or absence of lumbosacral anomalies. Each of these factors will weigh in treatment decisions.

The presence or absence of neural deficits is the single most important priority in the decision-making procedure. The presence of profound neural deficit in association with canal compromise is an urgent indication for surgical decompression. There are three methods of decompression available: two direct and one indirect. Indirect decompression is accomplished by a variety of posterior instrumentation, relying on correction of kyphosis and ligamentaxis to achieve canal clearance. This is not without risk of iatrogenic neural injury and at best produces incomplete canal decompression. This technique is the most dangerous at the upper level, where both the cord and the conus are present.

Direct decompression techniques include posterolateral and anterior decompression. Posterolateral decompression often follows partial indirect decompression via the posterior instrumentation, in an attempt to overcome the recognized inadequacies of the posterior instrumentation. Resection of the pedicle is usually limited to one side in order to minimize iatrogenic instability. It is difficult to decompress the far side of the canal with unilateral posterolateral decompression, even in highly experienced hands, and there is the risk of iatrogenic neural injury or incomplete decompression. Therefore, bilateral posterolateral decompression has been performed. This increases iatrogenic instability but provides increased canal clearance.

The remaining option is direct anterior decompression, either combined with anterior stabilization or following a posterior instrumentation and decompression. The risk of iatrogenic neurologic injury is lowest with this procedure, given the proximity of the cord and conus, and this procedure is the most effective in establishing a wide canal clearance.

In the neurologically intact patient no firm criteria have yet been established concerning the need for canal decompression and the extent to which it must be performed. Appropriate treatment can only be determined after long-term follow-up. A partial decompression in the neurologically intact patient combined with reduction of the kyphus and a stable fusion may well suffice.

No one particular instrumentation system is suggested to the reader. The surgeon has great latitude in selecting a surgical technique for treatment of patients with a burst fracture in the upper region. Each surgeon should select a procedure he is familiar with and is within his surgical capabilities. The availability of multiple open segments below the level of the injury allows a surgeon to use the standard systems with which he is familiar, as well as newer techniques, including pedicular fixation.

Middle Burst Fracture Without Neurologic Injury. Injuries to the L-2–L-3 vertebral levels are relatively common. In this area, the conus medullaris has given way to the cauda equina. The canal dimensions have also increased, accounting for the number of patients who are neurologically normal despite dramatic levels of canal compromise.

The choices for decompression of middle burst fractures are the same as for upper burst fractures. Once again, indirect methods may be used. A higher degree of canal clearance can be obtained if reductions are performed early. Iatrogenic injury is less likely to occur at this level because neither the cord nor conus is present. Direct methods may also be applied to these fractures. At the middle level, anterior decompression offers a slight advantage in safety and a higher degree of decompression can be achieved. In a neurologically normal patient, these advantages must be balanced with the unknown factor of how much clearance is necessary below the level of the conus.

The selection of instrumentation in middle burst fractures is more crucial than in upper lumbar injuries. Instrumentation that permits fixation of only one level below the fracture will preserve necessary lumbar mobility (Fig. 8-45). The injury to the anterior and middle column will put considerable stress on posterior instrumentation. Posterior column involvement will produce three-column instability, significantly stressing any instrumentation system. Serious consideration should be given to anterior grafting procedures, either with or without instrumentation, to provide an additional biomechanical buttress in cases in which excellent anatomic restoration of fragments has not been achieved. Anterior grafting may be performed using a primary or secondary anterior approach to place the bone strut. Struts can take the form of iliac crest, fibula, or allograft bone. A form of anterior grafting for body reinforcement may also be accomplished by adding morselized

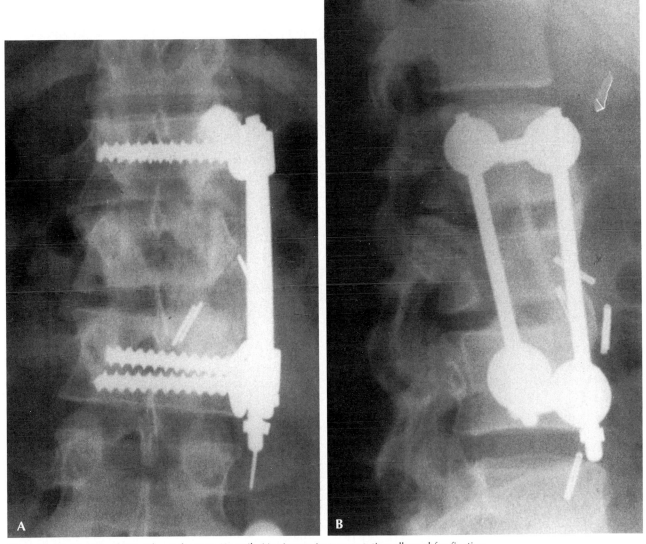

Figure 8-45. (*A, B*) In this L-2 burst fracture Kostuik–Harrington instrumentation allowed for fixation of the fracture from L-1–L-3, preserving motion for the lower lumbar spine.

bone via the transpedicular route prior to pedicular fixation.[61,175]

When a primary anterior decompression, instrumentation, and fusion has been selected, the concomitant posterior approach can often be avoided. The exception to this is the highly unstable burst fracture with complete disruption of one or more facets posteriorly (i.e., the Denis type D burst fracture). Translation on the anteroposterior radiograph or documentation of posterior element destruction on the CT scan are signs of the highly unstable injury, and should alert the surgeon that a concomitant posterior approach should be performed. This will avoid instrument failure, progressive deformity, or neurologic injury.

The surgeon's final choices are much more restricted than in upper lumbar lesions. Surgical decompression, however, is indicated less often because the incidence of significant neurologic impairment is lower. The primary consideration in choosing a system of instrumentation should be the surgeon's decision not to fuse lower than L-3 or L-4. Conservative management is a far better solution for the patient, preserving more future options, than a long lower lumbar fusion with loss of lumbar lordosis and preservation of only the L-5–S-1 disk space.[150]

Lower Burst Fracture.   Although burst compression fractures of L-4 and L-5 are uncommon injuries,[49,87,172] they deserve consideration apart from burst fractures of the upper and middle lumbar spine because of their unique position at the lumbosacral junction (Fig. 8-46). Personal experiences of each surgeon with the various techniques available will undoubtedly influence the decision-making process, as will the specific circumstances of each patient and fracture.

Several authors have shown that residual bony deformity after conservative care in a cast or brace causes less morbidity than a reduction with Harrington rods (Fig. 8-47) or Luque instrumentation.[49,145,172] There is a loss of lordosis common to all patients, whether treated conservatively or with instrumentation. The loss of lordosis in spines instrumented with Harrington distraction instrumentation is greater than in those of patients treated conservatively.[49] Recently, several au-

thors have reported better results using posterior instrumentation for this injury. Byrd reports solid fusion and preservation of lordosis after decompression, posterolateral fusion, and Steffee plating.[38] Edwards advocates use of rod–sleeve instrumentation with pedicular fixation in the middle segment for burst fractures of L-4–L-5. This system restricts fusion to two levels, with preservation of lordosis. Sacral screw fixation to S-1 is available with this system for use after burst fractures of L-5.[156]

Neurologic deficit is usually minor after burst fractures of L-4 or L-5, despite significant neural encroachment.[49] If progressive neural loss corresponds to radiologic evidence of canal or foraminal stenosis, the patient should be treated operatively with posterior decompression and fusion.[172] Decompression may be performed via a transabdominal approach; however, there are hazards in leaving metallic fixation near vascular structures. At these lower levels of the lumbar spine, laminectomy is sufficient for posterior decompression. There is room for access to the anterior fragments of bone, and the cauda can be retracted out of the way more easily than the conus.[22,177]

DISTRACTIVE EXTENSION

Distractive extension fractures are uncommon (Fig. 8-48). These injuries occur when major compressive forces act on the posterior elements at the same time that tension forces act on the anterior elements. The result is a low lumbar pars interarticularis fracture or laminar fractures.[36] After injury these lesions may completely reduce and be difficult to appreciate on radiographs. These injuries are very rare in the thoracolumbar spine[36,48] and are considered to have no propensity for the progression of deformity or neurologic injury.[77,241] Since these injuries are stable in flexion, they can be treated in an orthosis.[36] If operative therapy becomes necessary for other reasons, patients have been treated successfully with bilateral Harrington distraction rods.[48] Other types of posterior instrumentation used in a distraction or stabilization mode would probably be equally successful.

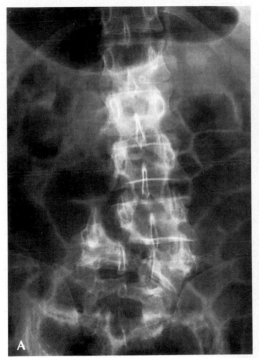

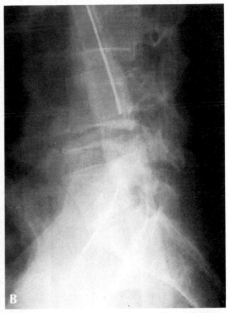

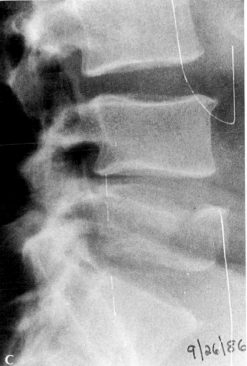

Figure 8-46. *(A, B)* Severe burst fracture of L-5 with three-column disruption. *(C)* A less severe L-5 burst injury. A 37-year-old man sustained this injury while mountain climbing. He slid approximately 40 feet down a steep rocky incline. He walked down the mountain after the injury. Three weeks later his back pain continued to worsen and he presented for radiographs. He refused a brace. He returned to full activity, including mountain climbing, within 3 months. He continued the sport for 2 more years until his death in a mountain climbing accident.

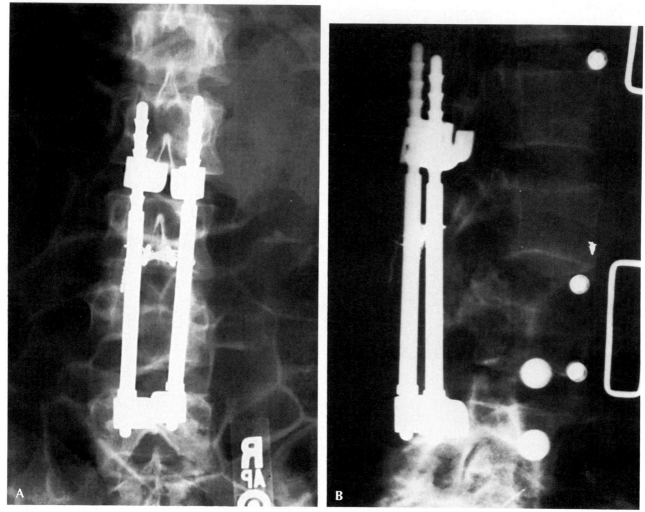

Figure 8-47. (*A, B*) Harrington instrumentation ill-advisedly used to treat an L-4 burst fracture. While body height was restored, there was significant loss of lordosis and incomplete canal decompression. The canal decompression was remedied with an anterior decompression and strut graft. The lordosis, however, was still lost.

LUMBOSACRAL DISLOCATION

Lumbosacral dislocation is another rare injury resulting from major trauma. The mechanisms are flexion, rotation, and compression. It is not a simple distractive flexion injury and does not fit simply into the Ferguson and Allen classification.

Patients who sustain this injury were either crushed in a stooped position[52] or had heavy weights land on them. The bony injury they sustain is either a pure dislocation or a dislocation with facet fracture.[246] It can be unilateral[20,185,253] or bilateral. The application of this force to the lumbosacral junction results in a traumatic anterior spondylolisthesis.[246]

The pathognomonic feature of this injury is the presence of multiple transverse process fractures above the lumbosacral fracture.* This may be the

* Reference numbers 52, 59, 75, 117, 185, 190, 216, 246, 253.

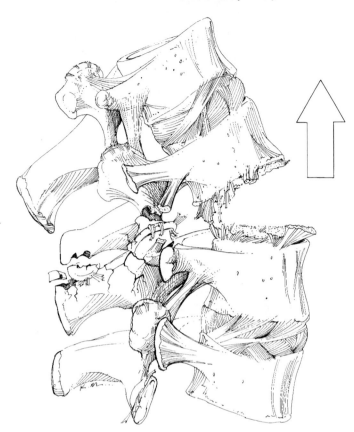

Figure 8-48. Distractive extension fracture.

key to the early diagnosis of lumbosacral fracture-dislocations.[75] The lateral radiograph most commonly demonstrates the anterior spondylolisthesis, which varies in degree.[52,75,216,246] The anteroposterior radiograph may demonstrate lateral subluxation of the lumbar spine on the sacrum[208] or deviation of the spinous process in the direction of the unilateral dislocation.[20] Computed tomography is most helpful, and demonstrates the absence of articulation between the lumbar and sacral facets.[246]

Many patients demonstrate neurologic compromise, most commonly with cauda equina syndrome. Reduction is associated with neurologic return. Most patients gain at least a partial return.[52,59,101,117,246] This injury may also be associated with abdominal injuries,[246] perineal lacera-

tions,[52] other long bone fractures, and facial trauma.[52,75,216,246]

This ligamentous injury requires surgical intervention to achieve successful treatment.[119] Conservative treatment has been only partially successful,[20,59,190,253] and the dislocation often cannot be reduced by closed methods. Reduction of the dislocation has been achieved by flexion of the fracture (using the operating table) and reduction of the facets, followed by extension, which locks the fracture in the reduced position.[52,75,117,185,216,246] The displacement required in the operative unlocking of the facets is not greater than what occurred at the moment of injury, and does not cause additional neurologic injury. Partial facetectomy may facilitate reduction and may be required to reduce the dislocation.[52,59,117,216,246] Laminectomy is required only if the dislocation is irreducible[59] or if there is material within the canal causing neural compromise.[117] Decompression and reduction should be followed by posterior or posterolateral fusion. Fixation was in the past obtained by wiring the bases of the spinous processes together[52,185,246] or by use of Harrington instrumentation.[117] The majority of current fixation techniques are stressed significantly when placed to fix the lumbosacral junction. The best choice is probably the specially designed Roy-Camille lumbosacral plate[214] or other pedicular systems.[156]

MINOR ISOLATED INJURIES

Minor injuries should be considered separately only if they occur in isolation from other fractures and fit none of the patterns described above. If they occur in conjunction with other fractures, they are considered as part of the more major injury.[55]

Injuries to the transverse processes, spinous processes, pars interarticularis, and articular processes may occur as isolated injuries. Frequently these occur secondary to direct trauma or as a result of a fall on the back or extreme muscle pull. Transverse process fractures also occur with Malgaine fractures of the pelvis, violent lateral flexion injuries, and lumbosacral dislocations. These lesions must be ruled out either by plain film or by CT scan.[55,206] Pars interarticularis fractures can occur acutely in young individuals involved in sports activities, although they are more commonly the result of chronic, repeated stresses.[55,155]

Isolated injuries are almost never associated with neurologic injury. Transverse process fractures may be associated with brachial plexus lesions in the high thoracic spine (T-1–T-2).[55] Spinous process fractures may be associated with contusions of the conus, which recuperate rapidly.[55] These injuries do not tend to be involved in progressive deformity. Nicoll[191] believed that bilateral pars interarticularis fractures below L-3 will progress, but most authors do not agree with him. These isolated injuries have little or no likelihood for progression of the spinal deformity or neurologic injury. They should be treated conservatively with bed rest until pain has resolved, then by immobilization until there is radiologic evidence of bony union, perhaps best demonstrated on the CT scan.[77]

SUMMARY

In this chapter we have attempted to give an overview of the different types of injuries that occur in the thoracolumbar spine. Vigilance in detection is crucial. Associated injuries must be discovered and cared for. Careful, systematic examination of radiographs will lead to the correct diagnosis. Treatment should be predicated on the mechanism of injury.

There is often no one best treatment plan for any specific injury. Without doubt the best choice for each patient should be strongly guided by the surgeon's familiarity with each of the instrumentation techniques. While we all wish to offer patients the rapid mobilization afforded by surgical techniques, conservative management can yield better or more salvageable results than a poorly performed sophisticated technique.

REFERENCES

1. Aaro S, Ohlen G: The effect of Harrington instrumentation on the sagittal configuration and mobility of the spine in scoliosis. Spine 8:570–575, 1983
2. Aebi M, Etter C, Kehl T, Thalgott J: The internal skeletal fixation system: A new treatment of thoracolumbar fractures and other spinal disorders. Clin Orthop 227:30–43, 1988
3. Aebi M, Etter C, Kehl T, Thalgott J: Stabilization of the lower thoracic and lumbar spine with the internal spinal skeletal fixation system: Indications, techniques and first results of treatment. Spine 12:544–551, 1987
4. Aebi M, Mohler J, Zack G, Morscher E: Analysis of 75 operated thoracolumbar fractures and fracture dislocations with and without neurologic deficit. Arch Orthop Trauma Surg 105:100–112, 1986
5. Akbarnia BA, Fogarty JP, Smith KR: New trends in surgical stabilization of thoraco-lumbar spinal fractures with emphasis for sublaminar wiring. Paraplegia 23:27–33, 1985

6. Akbarnia BA, Fogarty JP, Tayob AA: Contoured Harrington instrumentation in the treatment of unstable spinal fractures: The effect of supplementary sublaminar wires. Clin Orthop 189:186–194, 1984

7. Allen BL, Tencer AF, Ferguson RL: The biomechanics of decompressive laminectomy. Spine 12:803–808, 1987

8. Andén U, Lake A, Nordwall A: The role of the anterior longitudinal ligament in Harrington rod fixation of unstable thoracolumbar spinal fractures. Spine 5:23–25, 1980

9. Angtuaco EJ, Binet EF: Radiology of thoracic and lumbar fractures. Clin Orthop 189:43–57, 1984

10. Atlas SW, Regenbogen V, Rogers LF, Kim KS: The radiographic characterization of burst fractures of the spine. AJR. 147:575–582, 1986

11. Bedbrook GM: Fracture dislocations of the spine with and without paralysis: The case for conservatism and against operative techniques. In Leathe KE, Hoaglund FT, Riseborough EJ (eds): Controversies in Orthopedic Surgery. Philadelphia, WB Saunders, 1982

12. Bedbrook GM: Spinal injuries with tetraplegia and paraplegia. J Bone Joint Surg [Br] 61:267–284, 1979

13. Bedbrook GM: Treatment of thoracolumbar dislocation and fractures with paraplegia. Clin Orthop 112:27–43, 1975

14. Bedbrook GM, Clark WB: Thoracic spine injuries with spinal cord damage. J R Coll Surg Edinb 26:264–271, 1981

15. Beerman R, Batt HD, Green BA: Lumbar vertebral reformation after traumatic compression fracture. AJNR. 6:455–456, 1985

16. Bentley G, McSweeney T: Multiple spinal injuries. Br J Surg 55:565–570, 1968

17. Benzel EC, Larson SJ: Functional recovery after decompressive operation for thoracic and lumbar spine fractures. Neurosurgery 19:772–778, 1986

18. Blasier RD, LaMont RL: Chance fracture in a child: A case report with non-operative treatment. J Pediatr Orthop 5:92–93, 1985

19. Boechat MI: Spinal deformities and pseudofractures. AJR 148:97–98, 1987

20. Boger DC, Chandler RW, Pearce PG, Balciunas A: Unilateral facet dislocation at the lumbosacral junction. J Bone Joint Surg [Am] 65:1174–1178, 1983

21. Böhler J: Operative treatment of fractures of the dorsal and lumbar spine. J Trauma 10:1119–1122, 1970

22. Bohlman HH: Current concepts review: Treatment of fractures and dislocations of the thoracic and lumbar spine. J Bone Joint Surg [Am] 67:165–169, 1985

23. Bohlman HH: Traumatic fractures of the upper thoracic spine with paralysis. J Bone Joint Surg [Am] 56:1299, 1974

24. Bohlman HH, Eismont FJ: Surgical techniques of anterior decompression and fusion for spinal cord injuries. Clin Orthop 154:57–67, 1981

25. Bohlman HH, Freehafer A, Dejak J: The results of treatment of acute injuries of the upper thoracic spine with paralysis. J Bone Joint Surg [Am] 67:360–369, 1985

26. Boynton LW, Kalb R: Double lumen sign as demonstrated by computerized tomography in spine dislocation. Spine 8:910–912, 1983

27. Braakman R: The value of more aggressive management in traumatic paraplegia. Neurosurg Rev 9:141–147, 1986

28. Bradford DS, Akbarnia BA, Winter RB, Seljeskog EL: Surgical stabilization of fracture and fracture dislocations of the thoracic spine. Spine 2:185–196, 1977

29. Bradford DS, McBride G: Thoracic/lumbar spine fractures with incomplete neurologic deficit: A correlative study on the adequacy of decompression vs. neurologic return. Orthopaedic Transactions 8:159–160, 1984

30. Bradford DS, McBride GG: Surgical management of thoracolumbar spine fractures with incomplete neurologic deficits. Clin Orthop 218:201–216, 1987

31. Bradford DS, Thompson RC: Fractures and dislocations of the spine: Indications for surgical intervention. Minn Med 59:711–720, 1976

32. Brant-Zawadzki M, Jeffrey RB, Minagi H, Pitts LH: High resolution CT of thoracolumbar fractures. AJR 138:699–704, 1976

33. Brant-Zawadski M, Miller EM, Federle MP: CT in the evaluation of spine trauma. AJR 136:369–375, 1981

34. Brisco CHW: Thoracolumbar fractures. S Afr Med J 70:321–324, 1986

35. Bryant CE, Sullivan JA: Management of thoracic and lumbar spine fractures with Harrington distraction rods supplemented with segmental wiring. Spine 8:532–537, 1983

36. Bucholz RW, Gill K: Classification of injuries to the thoracolumbar spine. Orthop Clin North Am 17:67–73, 1986

37. Burke DC, Murray DD: The management of thoracic and thoraco-lumbar injuries of the spine with neurologic improvement. J Bone Joint Surg [Br] 58:72–78, 1976

38. Byrd JA: The treatment of L5 burst fractures with

neurologic deficit. Poster exhibit at the 55th annual meeting of the American Academy of Orthopedic Surgeons, Atlanta, Georgia, February 1988

39. Calenoff L, Chesare JW, Rogers LF et al: Multiple level spinal injuries: Importance of early recognition. AJR 130:665–669, 1978

40. Carragher AM, Cranley B: Seat belt stomach transection in association with "Chance" vertebral fracture. Br J Surg 74:397, 1987

41. Casey MP, Asher MA, Jacobs RA, Orrick JM: The effect of Harrington rod contouring on lumbar lordosis. Spine 12:750–753, 1987

42. Chance CQ: Note on a type of flexion fracture of the spine. Br J Radiol 21:452–453, 1948

43. Cochran T, Irstam L, Nachemson A: Long term anatomic and functional changes in patients with adolescent idiopathic scoliosis treated with Harrington rod fusion. Spine 8:576–584, 1983

44. Colley DP, Dunsker SB: Traumatic narrowing of the dorsolumbar spinal canal demonstrated by computed tomography. Radiology 129:95–98, 1978

45. Convery FR, Minteer MA, Smith RW, Emerson SM: Fracture-dislocation of the dorsal-lumbar spine: Acute operative stabilization by Harrington instrumentation. Spine 3:160–166, 1978

46. Cook WA: Transthoracic vertebral surgery. Ann Thorac Surg 12:54–68, 1971

47. Cope R, Salmon A, Gaines R: Association of a thoracic distraction fracture and an unusual avulsion fracture. Spine 12:943–945, 1987

48. Cotler JM, Vernace JV, Michalski JA: The use of Harrington rods in thoracolumbar fractures. Orthop Clin North Am 17:87–103, 1986

49. Court-Brown CM, Gertzbein SD: The management of burst fractures of the fifth lumbar vertebra. Spine 12:308–312, 1987

50. Daffner RH, Deeb ZL, Rothfus WE: The posterior vertebral body line: Importance in the detection of burst fractures. AJR 148:93–96, 1987

51. Daffner RH, Deeb ZL, Rothfus WE: Thoracic fractures and dislocations in motorcyclists. Skeletal Radiol 16:280–284, 1987

52. Das De S, McCreath SW: Lumbosacral fracture-dislocations. J Bone Joint Surg [Br] 63:58–60, 1981

53. Davies WE, Morris JH, Hill V: An analysis of conservative nonsurgical management of thoracolumbar fractures and fracture-dislocations with neural damage. J Bone Joint Surg [Am] 62:1324–1328, 1980

54. Denis F: Spinal instability as defined by the three

column spine concept in acute spinal trauma. Clin Orthop 189:65–76, 1984

55. Denis F: The three column spine and its significance in the classification of acute thoracolumbar spinal injuries. Spine 8:817–831, 1983

56. Denis F, Armstrong GWD, Searls BA, Matta L: Acute thoracolumbar burst fractures in the absence of neurologic deficit: A comparison between operative and non-operative treatment. Clin Orthop 189:142–149, 1984

57. De Oliviera JC: A new type of fracture-dislocation of the thoracolumbar spine. J Bone Joint Surg [Am] 60:481–488, 1978

58. Dewald RL: Burst fractures of the thoracic and lumbar spine. Clin Orthop 189:150–161, 1984

59. Dewey P, Browne PSH: Fracture dislocation of the lumbosacral spine with cauda equina lesion. J Bone Joint Surg [Br] 50:635–638, 1968

60. Dick W: The "fixateur interne" as a versatile implant for spine surgery. Spine 12:882–900, 1987

61. Dick W, Kluger P, Magerl F et al: A new device for internal fixation of thoracolumbar and lumbar spine fractures. Paraplegia 23:225–232, 1985

62. Dickson JH, Harrington PR, Erwin WD: Harrington instrumentation in the fractured, unstable thoracic and lumbar spine. Tex Med 69:91–98, 1973

63. Dickson JH, Harrington PR, Erwin WD: Results of reduction and stabilization of the severely fractured thoracic and lumbar spine. J Bone Joint Surg [Am] 60:799–805, 1978

64. Dodd CAF, Fergusson CM, Pearcy MJ, Houghton GR: Vertebral motion measured before and after Harrington rod removal for unstable thoracolumbar fractures of the spine. Spine 11:452–455, 1986

65. Dolan EJ, Taotor CH, Endrenyi L: The value of decompression for acute spinal cord compression injury. J Neurosurg 53:749–755, 1980

66. Dommisse GF: The blood supply of the spinal cord: A critical vascular zone in spinal surgery. J Bone Joint Surg [Br] 56:225–235, 1974

67. Drummond D, Guadagni J, Keene JS et al: Interspinous process segmental spinal instrumentation. J Pediatr Orthop 4:397–404, 1984

68. Dunn HK: Anterior spine stabilization and decompression for thoracolumbar injuries. Orthop Clin North Am 17:113–119, 1986

69. Dunn HK: Neurologic recovery following anterior spinal canal decompression in thoracic and lumbar injuries. Orthopaedic Transactions 8:160, 1984

70. Durward QJ, Schweigel JF, Harrison P: Management of fractures of the thoracolumbar and lumbar spine. Neurosurgery 8:555–561, 1981

71. Edwards CC, Levine AM: Early rod–sleeve stabilization of the injured thoracic and lumbar spine. Orthop Clin North Am 17:121–145, 1986

72. Edwards CC, York JJ, Levine AM, Weigel MC: Determinants of spinal hook dislodgement. Orthopaedic Transactions 10:8, 1986

73. Erickson DL, Leider LL, Brown WE: One-stage decompression: Stabilization for thoracolumbar fractures. Spine 2:53–56, 1977

74. Farcy JP, Weidenbaum M, Michelsen CB et al: A comparative biomechanical study of spinal fixation using Cotrel–Dubousset instrumentation. Spine 12:877–881, 1987

75. Fardon DF: Displaced fracture of the lumbosacral spine and delayed cauda equina deficit. Clin Orthop 120:155–158, 1976

76. Ferguson RL, Allen BL: An algorithm for the treatment of unstable thoracolumbar fractures. Orthop Clin North Am 17:105–112, 1986

77. Ferguson RL, Allen BL: A mechanistic classification of thoracolumbar spine fractures. Clin Orthop 189:77–88, 1984

78. Fidler MW: Posterior instrumentation of the spine: An experimental comparison of various possible techniques. Spine 11:367–372, 1986

79. Fidler MW: Remodeling of the spinal canal after burst fracture: A prospective study of two cases. J Bone Joint Surg [Br] 70:729–732, 1988

80. Fidler MW, Plasmas CMT: The effect of four types of support on the segmental mobility of the lumbosacral spine. J Bone Joint Surg [Am] 65:943–947, 1983

81. Fife D, Kraus J: Anatomic location of spinal cord injury: Relationship to the cause of injury. Spine 11:2–5, 1986

82. Fister JS, Savino AW, DeWald RL: The management of unstable burst fractures of the thoracolumbar spine. Orthopaedic Transactions 7:15–16, 1983

83. Flesch JR, Leider LL, Erickson DL et al: Harrington instrumentation and spine fusion for unstable fractures and fracture-dislocations of the thoracic and lumbar spine. J Bone Joint Surg [Am] 59:143–153, 1977

84. Floman Y, Fast A, Pollack D et al: The simultaneous application of an interspinous compressive wire and Harrington distraction rods in the treatment of fracture dislocation of the thoracic and lumbar spine. Clin Orthop 205:207–215, 1986

85. Fountain SS: A single-stage combined surgical approach for vertebral resections. J Bone Joint Surg [Am] 61:1011–1017, 1979

86. Frankel HL, Hancok DO, Hyslop G et al: The value of postural reduction in the initial management of closed injuries of the spine with paraplegia and tetraplegia. Paraplegia 7:179–192, 1969

87. Frederickson BE, Yuan HA, Miller H: Burst fractures of the fifth lumbar vertebra: A report of four cases. J Bone Joint Surg [Am] 64:1088–1094, 1982

88. Gaines RW, Breedlove RF, Munson G: Stabilization of thoracic and thoracolumbar fracture-dislocations with Harrington rods and sublaminar wires. Clin Orthop 189:195–203, 1984

89. Gaines RW, Humphreys WG: A plea for judgment in management of thoracolumbar fractures and fracture-dislocations: A reassessment of surgical indications. Clin Orthop 189:36–42, 1984

90. Gaines RW, Leatherman KD: Benefits of the Harrington compression in lumbar and thoracolumbar idiopathic scoliosis in adolescents and adults. Spine 6:483–488, 1981

91. Gaines RW, Munson G, Satterlee C et al: Harrington distraction rods supplemented with sublaminar wires for thoracolumbar fracture dislocations: Experimental and clinical investigation. Orthopaedic Transactions 7:15, 1983

92. Garfin SR, Mowery CA, Guerra J, Marshall LF: Confirmation of the posterolateral technique to decompress and fuse thoracolumbar spine burst fractures. Spine 10:218–223, 1985

93. Gelderman PW: The operative stabilization and grafting of thoracic and lumbar spinal fractures. Surg Neurol 23:101–120, 1985

94. Gertzbein SD, Court-Brown CM: Flexion-distraction injuries of the lumbar spine: Mechanisms of injury and classification. Clin Orthop 227:52–60, 1988

95. Gertzbein SD, Court-Brown CM, Marks P et al: The neurologic outcome following surgery for spinal fractures. Spine 13:641–644, 1988

96. Gertzbein SD, Macmicheal D, Tile M: Harrington instrumentation as a method of fixation in fractures of the spine: A critical analysis of deficiencies. J Bone Joint Surg [Br] 64:526–529, 1982

97. Gertzbein SD, Offierski C: Complete fracture dislocation of the thoracic spine without spinal cord injury. J Bone Joint Surg [Am] 61:449–451, 1979

98. Golimbu C, Firooznia H, Rafii M, Delman A: Computed tomography of thoracic and lumbar

spine fractures that have been treated with Harrington instrumentation. Radiology 151:731–733, 1984

99. Grant JMF, Sears WR: Spinal injury and computed tomography: A review of fracture pathology and a new approach to canal decompression. Aust NZ J Surg 56:299–307, 1986

100. Gregerson GG, Lucas DB: An in vivo study of the axial rotation of the human thoracolumbar spine. J Bone Joint Surg [Am] 49:247–262, 1967

101. Griffin JB, Sutherland GH: Traumatic posterior fracture-dislocation of the lumbosacral joint. J Trauma 20:426–428, 1980

102. Gumley G, Taylor TKF, Ryan MD: Distraction fractures of the lumbar spine. J Bone Joint Surg [Br] 64:520–525, 1982

103. Gurr KR, McAfee PC: Cotrel–Dubousset instrumentation in adults: A preliminary report. Spine 13:510–520, 1988

104. Guttman L: Spinal deformities in traumatic paraplegics and tetraplegics following surgical procedures. Paraplegia 7:38–58, 1969

105. Guttman L: Surgical aspects of the treatment of traumatic paraplegia. J Bone Joint Surg [Br] 31:399–403, 1949

106. Hadley MN, Zabramski JM, Browner CM et al: Pediatric spinal trauma: Review of 122 cases of spinal cord and vertebral column injuries. J Neurosurg 68:18–24, 1988

107. Handel SF, Lee YY: Computed tomography of spinal fractures. Radiol Clin North Am 19:69–89, 1981

108. Handelberg F, Bellemans MA, Opdecam P, Casteleyn PP: The use of computerized tomographs in the diagnosis of thoracolumbar injury. J Bone Joint Surg [Br] 63:336–341, 1981

109. Hannon KM: Harrington instrumentation in fractures and dislocations of the thoracic and lumbar spine. South Med J 69:1269–1273, 1976

110. Hardcastle P, Bedbrook G, Cutis K: Long term results of conservative and operative management in complete paraplegics with spinal cord injuries between T10 and L2 with respect to function. Clin Orthop 224:88–96, 1987

111. Harris JH: Radiographic evaluation of spinal trauma. Orthop Clin North Am 17:75–86, 1986

112. Harryman DT: Complete fracture dislocation of the thoracic spine associated with spontaneous neurologic decompression: A case report. Clin Orthop 207:64–69, 1986

113. Hazel WA, Jones RA, Morrey BF, Stauffer RN: Vertebral fractures without neurological deficit:

A long term follow-up study. J Bone Joint Surg [Am] 70:1319–1321, 1988

114. Hearon BF, Thomas HA, Raddin JH Jr: Mechanism of vertebral fracture in the F/FB-111 ejection experience. Aviat Space Eviron Med 53:440–448, 1982

115. Herrlin K, Ekelund L, Sundëen G: Radiologic and clinical evaluation of Harrington instrumentation in the injured dorsolumbar spine. Acta Radiol [Diagn] 24:289–295, 1983

116. Herron LD: Lateral flexion-distraction fracture: A variant of the seat-belt fracture. Spine 12:398–400, 1987

117. Herron LD, Williams RC: Fracture dislocation of the lumbosacral spine. Clin Orthop 186:205–211, 1984

118. Holdsworth F: Review article: Fractures, dislocations and fracture-dislocations of the spine. J Bone Joint Surg [Am] 52:1534–1551, 1970

119. Holdsworth FW, Hardy A: Early treatment of paraplegia from fractures of the thoraco-lumbar spine. J Bone Joint Surg [Br] 35:540–550, 1953

120. Huekle DF, Kaufer H: Vertebral column injuries and seat belts. J Trauma 15:304–318, 1975

121. Jackson RH, Quisling RG, Day AL: Fractures and complete dislocation of the thoracic or lumbosacral spine: Report of three cases. Neurosurgery 5:250–253, 1979

122. Jacobs RR: Bilateral fracture of the pedicles through the fourth and fifth lumbar vertebrae with anterior displacement of the vertebral bodies. J Bone Joint Surg [Am] 59:409–410, 1977

123. Jacobs RR, Asher MA, Snider RK: Thoracolumbar spinal injuries: A comparative study of recumbency and operative treatment in 100 patients. Spine 5:463–477, 1980

124. Jacobs RR, Casey MP: Surgical management of thoracolumbar spinal injuries: General principles and controversial considerations. Clin Orthop 189:22–35, 1984

125. Jacobs RR, Dahners LE, Gertzbein SD et al: A locking hook-spinal rod: Current status of development. Paraplegia 21:197–200, 1983

126. Jacobs RR, Schlaepfer F, Mathys R et al: A locking hook spinal rod system for stabilization of fracture-dislocations and correction of deformities of the dorsolumbar spine: A biomechanical evaluation. Clin Orthop 189:168–177, 1984

127. Jelsma RK, Kirsch PT, Rice JF, Jelsma LF: The radiographic description of thoracolumbar fractures. Surg Neurol 18:230–236, 1982

128. Jodoin A, Dupuis P, Fraser M, Beaumont P: Un-

stable fractures of the thoracolumbar spine: A 10-year experience at the Sacr-Coeur Hospital. J Trauma 25:197–202, 1985

129. Johnson JR, Leatherman KD, Holt RT: Anterior decompression of the spinal cord for neurological deficit. Spine 8:396–405, 1983

130. Kachoie A, Bloch R, Banna M: Post-traumatic dorsal pseudomeningocele. J Can Assoc Rad 36:262–263, 1985

131. Kahanovitz N, Arnoczky SP, Levine DB, Otis JP: The effects of internal fixation on the articular cartilage of unfused canine facet joint cartilage. Spine 9:268–272, 1984

132. Kahanovitz N, Bullough P, Jacobs RR: The effect of internal fixation without arthrodesis on human facet joint cartilage. Clin Orthop 189:204–208, 1984

133. Kaneda K, Abumi K, Fujiya M: Burst fractures with neurologic deficits of the thoracolumbar–lumbar spine: Results of anterior decompression and stabilization with anterior instrumentation. Spine 9:788–795, 1984

134. Karlström G, Olerud S, Sjöoström L: Transpedicular segmental fixation: Description of a new procedure. Orthopedics 11:689–700, 1988

135. Kaufer H, Hayes JT: Lumbar fracture dislocation: A study of 21 cases. J Bone Joint Surg [Am] 48:712–730, 1966

136. Keene JS: Radiographic evaluation of thoracolumbar fractures. Clin Orthop 189:58–64, 1984

137. Keene JS: Thoracolumbar fractures in winter sports. Clin Orthop 216:39–49, 1987

138. Keene JS, Goletz TH, Benson RC: Undetected genito-urinary dysfunction in vertebral fractures. J Bone Joint Surg [Am] 62:997–999, 1980

139. Keene JS, Goletz TH, Lilleas F et al: Diagnosis of vertebral fractures: A comparison of conventional radiography, conventional tomography, and computed axial tomography. J Bone Joint Surg [Am] 64:586–595, 1982

140. Keene JS, Wackwitz DL, Drummond DS, Breed AL: Compression-distraction instrumentation of unstable thoracolumbar fractures: Anatomic results obtained with each type of injury and method of instrumentation. Spine 11:895–902, 1986

141. Kelly RP, Whitesides TE: Treatment of lumbodorsal fracture-dislocations. Ann Surg 167:705–717, 1968

142. Kewalrami LS, Taylor RG: Multiple noncontiguous injuries to the spine. Acta Orthop Scand 47:52–58, 1976

143. Kilcoyne RF, Mack LA, King HA et al: Thoracolumbar spine injuries associated with vertical plunges: Reappraisal with computed tomography. Radiology 146:137–140, 1983

144. King AG: Burst compression fractures of the thoracolumbar spine: Pathologic anatomy and surgical management. Orthopedics 10:1711–1719, 1987

145. King AG: Spinal column trauma. In Anderson LD (ed): Instructional Course Lectures, Vol 35. St. Louis, CV Mosby, 1986

146. Kinnard P, Ghibely A, Gordon D et al: Roy-Camille plates in unstable spinal conditions: A preliminary report. Spine 11:131, 1986

147. Kostuik JP: Anterior fixation for fractures of the thoracic and lumbar spine with or without neurologic involvement. Clin Orthop 189:103–115, 1984

148. Kostuik JP: Anterior spinal cord decompression for lesions of the thoracic and lumbar spine, techniques, new methods of internal fixation results. Spine 8:512–531, 1983

149. Kostuik JP, Errico TJ, Gleason TF: Techniques of internal fixation for degenerative conditions of the lumbar spine. Clin Orthop 203:219–231, 1986

150. Kostuik JP, Hall BB: Spinal fusions to the sacrum in adults with scoliosis. Spine 8:489–500, 1983

151. Krompinger WJ, Frederickson BE, Mino DE, Yuan HA: Conservative treatment of fractures of the thoracic and lumbar spine. Orthop Clin North Am 17:161–170, 1986

152. Lantz SA, Schultz AB: Lumbar spine orthosis wearing: I. Restriction of gross body motions. Spine 11:834–837, 1986

153. Lantz SA, Schultz AB: Lumbar spine orthosis wearing: II. Effect on trunk muscle myoelectric activity. Spine 11:838–842, 1986

154. Larson SJ, Holst RA, Hemmy DC, Sances A: Lateral extracavitary approach to traumatic lesions of the thoracic and lumbar spine. J Neurosurg 45:628–637, 1976

155. Letts M, Smallman T, Afansiev R, Gouw G: Fracture of the pars interarticularis in adolescent athletes: A clinical–biomechanical analysis. J Pediatr Orthop 6:40–46, 1986

156. Levine A: Modular instrumentation of lumbar spine fractures. Presented at Specialty Day, Orthopedic Trauma Association, at the 55th annual meeting of the American Academy of Orthopedic Surgeons. Atlanta, Georgia, February 1988

157. Levine A, Bosse M, Edwards CC: Bilateral facet

dislocations in the thoracolumbar spine. Orthopaedic Transactions 10:12–13, 1986

158. Levine A, Bosse M, Edwards CC: Bilateral facet dislocations in the thoracolumbar spine. Spine 13:630–640, 1988

159. Levine A, Edwards CC: Complications in the treatment of acute spinal injury. Orthop Clin North Am 17:183–203, 1986

160. Levine A, Edwards CC: Lumbar spine trauma. In Camins M, O'Leary P (eds): The Lumbar Spine. New York, Raven Press, 1987

161. Lewis J, McKibbin B: The treatment of unstable fracture-dislocations of the thoracolumbar spine accompanied by paraplegia. J Bone Joint Surg [Br] 56:603–612, 1974

162. Lifeso RM, Arabie KM, Kadhi SKM: Fractures of the thoracolumbar spine. Paraplegia 23:207–224, 1985

163. Lindahl S, Willén J, Irstam L: Computed tomography of bone fragments in the spinal canal: An experimental study. Spine 8:181–186, 1983

164. Lindahl S, Willén J, Irstam L: Unstable thoracolumbar fractures: A comparative radiologic study of conservative treatment and Harrington instrumentation. Acta Radiol [Diagn] 26:67–77, 1985

165. Lindahl S, Willen J, Nordwall A, Irstam L: The crush cleavage fracture: A "new" thoracolumbar unstable burst fracture. Spine 8:559–569, 1983

166. Louw JA: Unstable fractures of the thoracic and lumbar spine treated with Harrington distraction instrumentation and sublaminar wires. S Afr Med J 71:759–762, 1987

167. Luque ER: Segmental spinal instrumentation in the treatment of fractures of the spine. Orthopaedic Transactions 6:22, 1982

168. Luque ER, Cassis N, Ramirez-Wiella G: Segmental spinal instrumentation in the treatment of fractures of the thoracolumbar spine. Spine 7:312–317, 1982

169. Maiman DJ, Larson SJ, Benzel EC: Neurologic improvement associated with late decompression of the thoracolumbar spinal cord. Neurosurgery 14:302–307, 1984

170. Maiman DJ, Sances A, Larson SJ et al: Comparison of the failure biomechanics of spinal fixation devices. Neurosurgery 17:574–580, 1985

171. Malcolm BW, Bradford DS, Winter RB, Chou SN: Post-traumatic kyphosis: A review of forty-eight surgically treated patients. J Bone Joint Surg [Am] 63:891–899, 1981

172. Manaster BJ, Osborne AG: CT patterns of facet fracture dislocations in the thoracolumbar region. AJR 148:335–340, 1987

173. McAfee PC, Bohlman HH: Complications following Harrington instrumentation for fractures of the thoracolumbar spine. J Bone Joint Surg [Am] 67:672–686, 1985

174. McAfee PC, Bohlman HH, Yuan HA: Anterior decompression of traumatic thoracolumbar fractures with incomplete neurological deficit using a retroperitoneal approach. J Bone Joint Surg [Am] 67:89–104, 1985

175. McAfee PC, Werner FW, Glisson RR: A biomechanical analysis of spinal instrumentation systems in thoracolumbar fractures: Comparison of traditional Harrington distraction instrumentation with segmental spinal instrumentation. Spine 10:204–217, 1985

176. McAfee PC, Yuan HA, Frederickson BE, Lubicky JP: The value of computed tomography in thoracolumbar fractures: An analysis of one hundred consecutive classes and a new classification. J Bone Joint Surg [Am] 65:461–473, 1983

177. McAfee PC, Yuan HA, Lasda NA: The unstable burst fracture. Spine 7:365–373, 1982

178. McBride GG, Bradford DS: Vertebral body replacement with femoral neck allograft and vascularized rib strut graft: A technique for treating post-traumatic kyphosis with neurologic deficit. Spine 8:406–415, 1983

179. McGahan JP, Benson D, Chehrazi B et al: Intraoperative sonographic monitoring of reduction of thoracolumbar burst fractures. AJR 145:1229–1232, 1985

180. Meyer PR: Complications of treatment of fractures and dislocations of the dorsolumbar spine. In Epps CH (ed): Complications in Orthopedic Surgery. Philadephia, JB Lippincott, 1986

181. Meyer PR: Posterior stabilization of thoracic, lumbar and sacral injuries. In Anderson LD (ed): Instructional Course Lectures. St. Louis, CV Mosby, 1986

182. Miller CA, Dewey RC, Hunt WE: Impaction fracture of the lumbar vertebra with dural tear. J Neurosurg 53:765–771, 1980

183. Miller F, Reger SI, Wang GJ, Boychuck L: Biomechanical analysis of segmental spinal fixation in a fracture model. Orthopaedic Transactions 6:23, 1982

184. Morgan TH, Wharton GW, Austin GN: The results of laminectomy in patients with incomplete spinal cord injuries. Paraplegia 9:14–23, 1973

185. Morris BDA: Unilateral dislocation of a lumbosacral facet: A case report. J Bone Joint Surg [Am] 63:164–165, 1981

186. Morris JM: Biomechanics of corsets and braces for

the low back. In Brown FW (ed): Symposium on the Lumbar Spine. St. Louis, CV Mosby, 1981

187. Munson G, Satterlee C, Hammond S et al: Experimental evaluation of Harrington rod fixation supplemented with sublaminar wires in stabilizing thoracolumbar fracture-dislocations. Clin Orthop 189:97–102, 1984

188. Murphy MJ, Southwick WO, Ogden JA: Treatment of the unstable thoraco-lumbar spine with combination Harrington distraction and compression rods. Orthopaedic Transactions 6:9, 1982

189. Nash CL, Schatzinger LH, Brown RH, Brodkey J: The unstable thoracic compression fracture: Its problems and the use of spinal cord monitoring in the evaluation of treatment. Spine 2:261–265, 1977

190. Newell RLM: Lumbosacral fracture-dislocation: A case managed conservatively, with a return to heavy work. Injury 9:131–134, 1977

191. Nicoll EA: Fractures of the dorso-lumbar spine. J Bone Joint Surg [Br] 31:376–394, 1949

192. Norton PL, Brown T: The immobilizing efficiency of back braces: Their effect on the posture and motion of the lumbosacral spine. J Bone Joint Surg [Am] 39:111–139, 1957

193. Nykamp PW, Levy JM, Christensen F et al: Computed tomography for a bursting fracture of the lumbar spine. J Bone Joint Surg [Am] 60:1108–1109, 1978

194. O'Callaghan JP, Ullrich CG, Yuan HA, Kieffer SA: CT of facet distraction in flexion injuries of the thoracolumbar spine: The "naked" facet. AJR 134:563–566, 1980

195. O'Laoire SA, Thomas DGT: Surgery in incomplete spinal cord injury. Surg Neurol 17:12–15, 1982

196. Olerud S, Karlström G, Sjöström L: Transpedicular fixation of thoracolumbar vertebral fractures. Clin Orthop 227:44–51, 1988

197. Osebold WR, Weinstein SL, Sprague BL: Thoracolumbar spine fractures: Results of treatment. Spine 6:13–34, 1981

198. Pang D, Wilberger JE: Spinal cord injury without radiographic abnormalities in children. J Neurosurg 57:114–129, 1982

199. Paul RL, Michael RH, Dunn JE, Williams JP: Anterior transthoracic surgical decompression of acute spinal cord injuries. J Neurosurg 43:299–307, 1975

200. Pay NT, George AE, Benjamin VB et al: Positive and negative contrast myelography in spinal trauma. Radiology 123:103–111, 1977

201. Pierce DS: Long term management of thoracolumbar fractures and fracture dislocations. In American Academy of Orthopedic Surgeons (ed): Instructional Course Lectures. St. Louis, CV Mosby, 1972

202. Post MJD, Gren BA, Quencer RM et al: The value of computed tomography in spinal trauma. Spine 7:417–431, 1982

203. Purcell GA, Markolf KL, Dawson EG: Twelfth thoracic-first lumbar vertebral mechanical stability of fractures after Harrington-rod instrumentation. J Bone Joint Surg [Am] 63:71–78, 1981

204. Quencer RM, Montalvo BM, Eismont FJ, Green BA: Intraoperative spinal sonography in thoracic and lumbar fractures: Evaluation of Harrington rod instrumentation. AJR 145:343–349, 1985

205. Reid DC, Henderson R, Saboe L, Miller JDR: Etiology and clinical course of missed spine fractures. J Trauma 27:980–985, 1987

206. Reis ND, Keret D: Fracture of the transverse process of the fifth lumbar vertebra. Injury 16:421–423, 1985

207. Rennie W, Mitchell N: Flexion distraction fractures of the thoracolumbar spine. J Bone Joint Surg [Am] 55:386–390, 1973

208. Resnick CS, Scheer CE, Adelaar RS: Lumbosacral dislocation. J Can Assoc Radiol 36:259–261, 1985

209. Riska EB: Antero-lateral decompression as a treatment of paraplegia following vertebral fracture in the thoraco-lumbar spine. Int Orthop 1:22–32, 1977

210. Riska EB, Myllynen P, Böstman O: Anterolateral decompression for neural involvement in thoracolumbar fractures. J Bone Joint Surg [Br] 69:704–708, 1987

211. Roberts JB, Curtiss PH: Stability of the thoracic and lumbar spine in traumatic paraplegia following fracture or fracture-dislocation. J Bone Joint Surg [Am] 52:1115–1130, 1970

212. Roy-Camille R, Saillant G, Beraux D, Salgado V: Osteosynthesis of thoraco-lumbar spine fractures with metal plates screwed through the vertebral pedicles. Reconstr Surg Traumatol 15:2–16, 1976

213. Roy-Camille R, Saillant G, Mazel CH: Internal fixation of the lumbar spine with pedicle screw plating. Clin Orthop 206:7–17, 1986

214. Roy-Camille R, Saillant G, Mazel CH: Plating of thoracic, thoracolumbar, and lumbar injuries with pedicle screw plates. Orthop Clin North Am 17:147–159, 1986

215. Ruge JR, Sinson GP, McLone DG, Cerullo LJ: Pediatric spinal injury: The very young. J Neurosurg 68:25–30, 1988

216. Samberg LC: Fracture-dislocation of the lumbo-sacral spine. J Bone Joint Surg [Am] 57:1007–1008, 1975

217. Sasson A, Mozes G: Complete fracture-dislocation of the thoracic spine without neurologic deficit. Spine 12:67–70, 1987

218. Scher AT: Double fractures of the spine: An indication for routine radiographic examination of the entire spine after injury. S Afr Med J 53:411–413, 1978

219. Shuman WP, Rogers JV, Sickler ME et al: Thoracolumbar burst fractures: CT dimensions of the spinal canal relative to post-surgical improvement. AJR 145:337–341, 1985

220. Smith GR, Northrop CH, Loop JW: Jumper's fractures: Patterns of thoracolumbar spine injuries associated with vertical plunges. Radiology 122:657–663, 1977

221. Smith WS, Kaufer H: Patterns and mechanisms of lumbar injuries associated with lap seat belts. J Bone Joint Surg [Am] 51:239–254, 1969

222. Soreff J, Axdorph G, Bylund P et al: Treatment of patients with unstable fractures of the thoracic and lumbar spines: A follow-up study of surgical and conservative treatment. Acta Orthop Scand 53:369–381, 1982

223. Spielholz NI, Benjamin NV, Ransohoff J: Somatosensory evoked potentials and clinical outcome in spinal cord injury, pp 217–222. In Popp AJ (ed): Neural Trauma. New York, Raven Press, 1979

224. Stauffer ES: Current concepts review: Internal fixation of fractures of the thoracolumbar spine. J Bone Joint Surg [Am] 66:1136–1138, 1984

225. Steiner ME, Herndon WA, Sullivan AJ: Stabilization of thoracolumbar spine fractures: Indications for referral, timing of surgery, and type of instrumentation. Orthop Trans 10:13, 1986

226. Sullivan JA: Sublaminar wiring of Harrington distraction rods for unstable thoracolumbar spine fractures. Clin Orthop 189:178–185, 1984

227. Sullivan JA, Bryant CE: Management of thoracic and lumbar spine fractures with Harrington rods supplemented with segmental wires. Orthopaedic Transactions 7:15, 1983

228. Svensson O, Aaro S, Öhlén G: Harrington instrumentation for thoracic and lumbar vertebral fractures. Acta Orthop Scand 55:38–47, 1984

229. Tearse DS, Keene JS, Drummond DS: Management of noncontiguous vertebral fractures. Paraplegia 25:100–105, 1987

230. Tencer AF, Allen BL, Ferguson RL: A biomechanical study of thoracolumbar spinal fractures with bone in the canal: Part I. The effect of laminectomy. Spine 10:580–585, 1985

231. Tencer AF, Allen BL, Ferguson RL: A biomechanical study of thoracolumbar spinal fractures with bone in the canal: Part III. Mechanical properties of the dura and its tethering ligaments. Spine 10:741–747, 1985

232. Uriarte E, Elguezabal B, Tovio R: Fracture-dislocation of the thoracic spine without neurologic lesion. Clin Orthop 217:261–265, 1987

233. van Hanswyck EP, Yuan HA, Eckhardt WA: Orthotic management of thoracolumbar spine fractures with a "total contact" TLSO. Orthotics and Prosthetics 33:10–19, 1979

234. Vincent KA, Benson DR, McGahan JP: Intraoperative sonography for thoracolumbar burst fractures. Poster exhibit at the 55th annual meeting of the American Academy of Orthopedic Surgeons, Atlanta, Georgia, February 1988

235. Walters CL, Schmidek HH, Krag MH, Brier L: The management of thoracolumbar fractures. In Dunsker SB, Schmidek HH, Frymoyer J, Kahn A (eds): The Unstable Spine: Thoracic, Lumbar and Sacral Regions. New York, Grune and Stratton, 1986

236. Wang GJ, Whitehill R, Stamp WG, Rosenberger R: The treatment of fracture dislocations of the thoracolumbar spine with halofemoral traction and Harrington rod instrumentation. Clin Orthop 142:168–175, 1979

237. Waters RL, Morris JM: Effect of spinal supports on the electrical activity of muscles of the trunk. J Bone Joint Surg [Am] 52:51–60, 1970

238. Weber SC, Sutherland GH: An unusual rotational fracture-dislocation of the thoracic spine without neurologic sequelae internally fixed with a combined anterior and posterior approach. J Trauma 26:474–479, 1986

239. Weinstein JN, Collalto P, Lehmann TR: Thoracolumbar "burst" fractures treated conservatively: A long-term follow-up. Spine 13:33–38, 1988

240. Weisz GM: Post-traumatic spinal stenosis. Arch Orthop Trauma Surg 106:57–60, 1986

241. Weitzman G: Treatment of stable thoracolumbar spine compression fractures by early ambulation. Clin Orthop 76:116–122, 1971

242. Wenger DR, Carollo JJ: The mechanics of thoracolumbar fractures stabilized by segmental fixation. Clin Orthop 189:89–96, 1984

243. White AA, Panjabi MM: Clinical Biomechanics of the Spine. Philadelphia, JB Lippincott, 1978

244. White RR, Newberg A, Seligson D: Computerized

tomographic assessment of the traumatized dorsolumbar spine before and after Harrington instrumentation. Clin Orthop 146:150–156, 1980

245. Whitesides TE, Shah SGA: On the management of unstable fractures of the thoracolumbar spine: Rationale for the use of anterior decompression and fusion and posterior stabilization. Spine 1:99–107, 1976

246. Wilchinisky ME: Traumatic lumbosacral dislocation: A case report and review of the literature. Orthopedics 10:1271–1274, 1987

247. Willén J, Lindahl S, Nordwall A: Unstable thoracolumbar fractures: A comparative clinical study of conservative treatment and Harrington instrumentation. Spine 10:111–122, 1985

248. Wilmot CB, Hall KM: Evaluation of acute surgical intervention in traumatic paraplegia. Paraplegia 24:71–76, 1986

249. Yngve DA, Harris WP, Herndon WA, Sullivan JA: Spinal cord injury without fracture. Orthopaedic Transactions 10:12, 1986

250. Yocum TD, Leatherman KD, Brower TD: The early rod fixation in treatment of fracture-dislocations of the spine. J Bone Joint Surg [Am] 52:1257, 1970

251. Yosipovitch Z, Robin GC, Makin M: Open reduction of unstable thoracolumbar spinal injuries and fixation with Harrington rods. J Bone Joint Surg [Am] 59:1003–1015, 1977

252. Young B, Brooks WH, Tibbs PA: Anterior decompression and fusion for thoracolumbar fractures with neurological deficits. Acta Neurochir 57:287–298, 1981

253. Zoltan JD, Gilula LD, Murphy WA: Unilateral facet dislocation between the fifth lumbar and first sacral vertebrae: A case report. J Bone Joint Surg [Am] 61:767–768, 1979

254. Zwimpfer TT, Gertzbein SG: Ultralight aircraft crashes: Their increasing incidence and associated fractures of the thoracolumbar spine. J Trauma 27:431–436, 1987

9

INSTABILITY AND MECHANICS OF IMPLANTS AND BRACES FOR THORACIC AND LUMBAR FRACTURES

Mark Lorenz
Avinash Patwardhan
Michael Zindrick

It is generally accepted that surgical management of unstable spinal fractures offers advantages over postural reductions. The goals of operative fixation of unstable fractures should be to restore normal anatomic alignment of the spine, to protect neurologic structures, and to obtain early mobilization of the patient. In order to achieve these goals, the surgeon must understand the instability patterns of various spinal fractures and become familiar with the strengths and weaknesses of the many devices currently available for internal fixation.

EFFECT OF INJURY ON BIOMECHANICAL STABILITY

The various anatomic components of a spinal segment contribute in different amounts to load bearing and provide inherent stability to the spinal segments. The traditional concept of instability was proposed by Holdsworth.[10] He defined spinal instability as "rupture of the posterior ligaments." The spinal segment was grouped into two load-bearing columns: anterior and posterior. The posterior column consisted of the posterior ligamentous complex. The anterior column was defined as "elements anterior to and including the posterior longitudinal ligament."

Subsequent investigators have tried to more precisely define for the clinician the elusive concept of instability. Jacobs and associates[11] simulated three types of injuries in fresh human cadaver spines. Posterior ligamentous injury was simulated by disrupting the supraspinous, interspinous, ligamentum flavum, and facet capsule ligaments at T-11–T-12 and by performing a single-plane osteotomy through the upper portion of the T-12 vertebral body. The anterior longitudinal ligament was preserved. Anterior injury was simulated by inducing a comminuted fracture of the entire T-12 vertebral body but preserving the anterior longitudinal ligament. The combined injury was simulated by both the posterior ligamentous injury and anterior comminuted vertebral body fracture. Both anterior and posterior injuries caused a decrease in stiffness of the segment in flexion by 70% to 80% of normal. The combined injury resulted in a significant flexion deformity (43 ± 7 degrees) at no load.

The effect of progressive disruption of the posterior ligamentous complex, facet joints, and part of the annulus fibrosus on the range of motion at the L-1–L-2 interspace was studied by Nagel and associates.[22] The range of motion in flexion increased with statistical significance following severing of facet joints. In the fully disrupted joint that simulated a seat belt type injury, the range of motion in flexion and lateral bending increased to twice the value of the intact segment; in axial rotation the increase was nearly 10-fold.

Denis[1] reclassified acute thoracolumbar fractures, proposing a three-column spine theory. In his model the anterior column was formed by the anterior longitudinal ligament, anterior annulus fibrosus, and anterior part of the vertebral body. The middle column was formed by the posterior longitudinal ligament, posterior annulus fibrosus, and posterior wall of the vertebral body. The posterior column was formed by the posterior arch, supraspinous ligament, interspinous ligament, capsule, and ligamentum flavum. In this model the compression fracture involves failure of the anterior column with the middle column being totally intact. In severe compression fractures, failure under tension of the posterior ligamentous complex is possible. The hallmark of the compression fracture, however, is the intact middle column, which prevents subluxation of the motion segment. The burst fracture involves failure of both the anterior and middle column under an axial load. The seat belt type injury represents failure of the posterior and middle columns. Finally, the fracture-dislocation injury represents failure of all three columns. The three-column concept, therefore, allows us to accurately recognize injury patterns, their mechanism, and the ensuing instabilities.

Axial load carrying capacity of the thoracolumbar spine as a function of injury to the three columns of the spine was studied by Haher and associates[8] using 10 human thoracolumbar spines.

Five specimens were loaded axially and in 20 degrees flexion with all three columns intact, and following sequential destruction of the anterior and middle columns. The remaining five specimens were loaded axially and in extension in an intact mode, and following sequential disruption of the posterior and middle columns. Disruption of the anterior column reduced the load carrying capacity (LCC) of the spine by 20%. The reduction of the LCC of the spine was 80% with disruption of both the anterior and middle columns of the spine. Disruption of the posterior column reduced the LCC by 35%, while the reduction in LCC was 60% with disruption of both the posterior and middle columns.

Ferguson and associates[3] found that a two-column injury involving the anterior and posterior columns, as in a severe compression fracture, can cause 70% to 80% reduction in segmental stiffness in both flexion and torsion, while a three-column injury such as a fracture-dislocation can render the spinal segment completely unstable in all modes of loading. Disruption of two columns in the three-column model, therefore, can lead to significant instability.

The results of these tests illustrate that the stability of the spine, measured by the load displacement behavior of the injured spinal segments and the overall LCC of the spine, is affected by an injury. Further, the extent of residual stability is a function of the type of injury, that is, the anatomic components or columns disrupted by the injury. Disruption of two adjacent columns in the three-column model, therefore, leads to significant instability.

BIOMECHANICAL STUDIES OF SPINAL INSTRUMENTATION SYSTEMS

The goal of a spinal instrumentation system is to maintain anatomic alignment of injured spinal segments by sharing the loads acting on the spine until a solid biologic fusion has taken place. The ability of an instrumentation system to stabilize the injured segments can be evaluated by quantifying two important characteristics of the system: failure load and stiffness. The failure load defines the magnitude of the load at which the construct will fail. Biomechanical failure can occur either within the fixation device itself or by failure at the bone–metal interface.

The second biomechanical characteristic of the construct is its stiffness, which is a measure of the resistance of the construct to deformation when the construct is subjected to a load. The clinical relevance of stiffness is that the greater the stiffness of the construct, the smaller the displacement that occurs in individual spinal segments spanned by the construct under physiologic load. Since maintaining anatomic alignment of the spinal segments under normal physiologic loads during the process of fusion is important, theoretically, the stiffer the construct the better the chances of an early solid fusion in normal anatomic alignment.

Both the failure load and the stiffness of the construct will depend on the type of load acting on the spine. In order to have all of the relevant information, these characteristics must be quantified in axial compression, flexion, extension, lateral bending, and torsion. Finally, the ability of an instrumentation system to stabilize the spinal segments has an indirect bearing on the mechanical integrity of the instrumentation system itself. Once a strong fusion develops, the load-sharing requirement on the fixation device is not as stringent as that immediately after surgery.

Several biomechanical studies have compared different types of instrumentation systems used to stabilize fractures of the thoracic and lumbar spine.[3,5-7,9,11,12,17,24] The strength of the bone–metal interface has been measured for the Harrington system,[12] segmental instrumentation with wires,[27] and interpeduncular fixation of plates and rods.[13,28]

STRENGTH OF BONE–METAL INTERFACE

Quantification of the strength of bone–metal interface is critical to determining the strength of the construct. Often the strength of the bone where the fixation devices attach to the spine is the limiting factor in governing the failure strength of the construct. Biomechanical studies of Harrington distraction rods have shown that in axial load the construct fails due to hook cut-out at the upper hook site. Jacobs and associates[12] compared the upper hook pull-out strength of the Harrington hook to that of a locking hook. The Harrington hook failed at 800 N force applied perpendicular to the rod, while the locking hook required 1275 N force for failure, representing an improvement of 60%. Wenger and associates[27] determined the strength of different fixation sites for segmental instrumentation with wires. The peak pull-out loads ranged from 1035 N in the midthoracic region to 1970 N in the lumbar vertebrae. Fixation to the spinous processes resulted in lower pull-out strengths (ranging from 285 to 420 N).

The strength of a construct using pedicular screw fixation depends on strength of screw fixation in the pedicles. Zindrick and associates[28] as well Krag and associates[13] measured screw pull-out strength for interpedicular fixation of plates and/or rods to the spine. The mean pull-out strengths ranged from 750 to 1980 N. Their data showed that the greater the major diameter of the screw, the higher the pull-out strength. In general, the pull-out strength was not a function of the minor diameter, pitch, or tooth profile. An increase in the depth of penetration of the screw increased the strength of fixation against a load applied perpendicular to the long axis of the screw. The mean pull-out force ranged from 365 to 1185 N for the five commercially available screw designs tested. Increased depth of screw insertion was found to increase screw–bone purchase in cyclic loading tests. Methyl methacrylate augmentation significantly improved the pull-out strength of the pedicular screw.[28]

STRENGTH AND RIGIDITY OF THE CONSTRUCT

Jacobs and associates[11] evaluated Harrington rods and Roy-Camille plates in stabilizing anterior, posterior, and combined injuries at the T-11–T-12 level. Both the Roy-Camille plates and the Harrington compression system with hooks in the lamina provided satisfactory reduction and stabilization of posterior injury in flexion, although the Harrington system allowed more deformation. Stabilization of the anterior injury with a longer Harrington distraction rod resulted in a failure load in flexion (moment) that was one third greater than with the short rod, with less deformity. In combined injury the long Harrington distraction rod method resisted twice the load with less angulation at the fracture site than did the short rod construct.

Jacobs and associates[12] also compared the long Harrington distraction rod method with the Synthes system and a three-above, three-below construct for stabilization of fracture-dislocation injury at the T-11–T-12 level. The failure load in flexion for the locking hook rod system was nearly three times that of the Harrington rod without locking hooks, with less deformity and more energy absorption at failure.

The stability of eight different constructs was compared by Panjabi and associates[24] for a seat belt type injury at T-12–L-1. The injury was simulated by disrupting the middle and posterior columns and leaving the anterior half of the disk and anterior longitudinal ligament intact. In the flexion–extension mode, the Harrington distraction plus compression rod system yielded the most rigid construct as compared to the Dunn device, Harrington compression alone, Harrington distraction alone, Harrington distraction with Edwards sleeves, the Luque system, the Luque rectangle, and the Luque short device. The Luque system with two rods resulted in the most stable construct in lateral bending, while in axial rotation none of the eight devices was more stable than the intact spine.

For stabilization of translational fracture-dislocation injuries with three-column disruption, the Harrington distraction rods were found to have the least ability to resist torsion.[17] Segmental fixation of the rods resulted in some improvement over the distraction rods alone, whereas the Luque segmental spinal instrumentation (SSI) resulted in the stiffest construct to resist torsion.

Stabilization of an L-1 slice fracture with seven instrumentation systems was studied by Gaines and associates.[5] Harrington rods with sublaminar wires resulted in the most stable construct in flexion loading, followed by the variable slotted plate (VSP Steffee). On the other hand, the Harrington construct was found to be notably unstable for torsional loading. The Kaneda device with and without the transverse fixator and the Luque system gave satisfactory stability to the construct in torsion, with a pedicle fixation system (VSP Steffee system) resulting in the most stable construct in torsion.

Posterior stabilization of L-1 burst fractures was compared by Gepstein and associates[7] using three different systems: Harrington distraction rods, three vertebrae above and two below; Harrington–Luque, three above and two below; and Cotrel-Dubousset (CD), two above and one below the fracture level. These constructs were tested under combined loading in axial compression and flexion. Both of the Harrington systems failed with upper hook cut-out, while in the CD construct failure occurred outside the instrumented area without any change of the burst fracture alignment. The failure load for the CD construct was approximately 3.5 times that of the Harrington rod construct and 2.5 times the Harrington–Luque construct. Furthermore, the CD construct allowed only half as much deformation, and therefore was twice as rigid as the other two constructs.

Similar results for burst fracture stabilization were found by Hoeltzel and associates.[9] Tested under combined loading in axial compression and flexion, the CD system instrumented two vertebrae above and two below the fracture site was found to give the stiffest construct as compared to Harrington rods alone, Harrington rods with segmental wiring, and the Luque system instrumented over the same level. However, in torsional loading the CD (two above, two below) construct was only half as stiff as the Luque. A shorter CD construct (one above, one below) gave the most stable construct in torsion.

McAfee and associates[17] compared stabilization of unstable burst fractures with the Harrington distraction rod with and without segmental fixation and the Luque SSI system. In axial loading, the Harrington rods with segmental wire fixation resulted in the most stable construct, with the Luque SSI being the least stable.

PEDICULAR SYSTEMS

Stabilization of L-1 burst fracture with five different fixation systems using pedicular fixation at T-12 and L-2 was studied by Galpin and associates.[6] All five systems significantly improved the stability of the uninstrumented spine in axial loading. There was no significant difference in axial stiffness of the five constructs; however, the Zielke system, with only two posterior bars without the anterior bar, was only slightly stiffer than the uninstrumented spine. In torsion all five systems performed equally well and significantly improved the stability of the construct as compared to the uninstrumented spine.

Ferguson and associates[3] compared the stability achieved by Roy-Camille plates to the stability achieved by more traditional systems in two simulated injuries. Greater stiffness was achieved overall when using Roy-Camille plates compared to conventional rod systems. This result is in concert with the findings of Gaines[5] and Galpin.[6]

SUMMARY OF BIOMECHANICAL DATA

For an easier overview, we have tabulated the results of various investigations of clinically available posterior instrumentation systems. Table 9-1 represents the fracture-dislocation model (anterior, middle, and posterior column injury), while Table

Table 9-1. A M P Model (Fracture Dislocation Simulation)*

FLEXION/COMPRESSION LOAD	TORSION LOAD
Gaines	
H W	VSP
VSP/H E	$= \dfrac{L}{H\ W} =$
$= = \dfrac{H}{L} = -$	H E
	H
Ferguson	
$= \dfrac{R\ C\ P}{J} =$	$= \dfrac{R\ C\ P}{H\ W} =$
H W	L
L	J
McAffee	
No data	$= \dfrac{L}{H\ W}$
	H

H—Harrington Rod
H F—Harrington Rod Edward's Sleeve
H W—Harrington Rod Sublaminar Wires
L—Luque Rod
J—Jacob's Rod
VSP—Steffee Plate
RCP—Roy Camille Plate
= = =—Indicates significant performance drop

* This table is a summary of biomechanical test results by various authors. Systems are listed in decreasing order of restoring stiffness to the injured segment.

Table 9-2. A M Model (Burst Fracture Simulation)*

AXIAL/FLEXION/COMPRESSION LOAD	TORSION LOAD
Galpin	
L P, VSP, AO	L P, VSP, AO
Gepstein	
$= = \dfrac{CD\ (2+1)}{H\ W} - - -$	No data
H	
Hoeltzel	
$= = \dfrac{CD\ (2+2)}{H\ W} - - -$	$= = \dfrac{CD\ (1+1)}{L} - -$
L	CD (2 + 2)
H	

H—Harrington Rod
H W—Harrington Sublaminar Wires
L—Luque Rod
CD—Cotrell Dubousset
VSP—Steffee Plate
L P—Luque Plate
AO—AO Internal Fixator
= = =—Indicates significant performance drop

* This table is a summary of biomechanical test results by various authors. Systems are listed in decreasing order of restoring stiffness to the injured segment.

9-2 shows results for the burst fracture model (anterior and middle column injury). Tables 9-3 and 9-4 show results for the distractive flexion (posterior and middle column injury) and compression fracture (anterior and posterior column injury) models, respectively. Since the methods used by various authors differ substantially, direct comparison among all studies is difficult. However, we have ranked the different systems within each study based on the authors' data on the overall rigidity of these systems in flexion–compression and torsional loading modes.

The results of biomechanical testing of instrumentation systems indicate that fixation devices using interpedicular screw fixation through the spine result in the most stable construct in all modes of loading and, therefore, can potentially stabilize injury to all three load-bearing columns. It seems reasonable to expect that patients with these systems have sufficient stability to obtain a solid fusion without the need for an external support. The improved rigidity of these constructs is

Table 9-3. P M Model (Flexion Distraction Simulation)*

FLEXION/COMPRESSION	ROTATION
Punjabi	
H C	All poor
H + H C	
H E	
— L —	
H	

H—Harrington rod
H C—Harrington Compression
H E—Harrington Edward's Sleeves
L—Luque Rods
= = =—Indicates significant performance drop

* This table is a summary of biomechanical test results by various authors. Systems are listed in decreasing order of restoring stiffness to the injured segment.

Table 9-4. A P Model (Compression Fracture Simulation)*

FLEXION/COMPRESSION LOAD	TORSION LOAD
Ferguson	
R C P	R C P
— ——— —	— ——— —
H W	H W
L	L
J	J

R C P—Roy Camille Plate
H W—Harrington Rod Sublaminar Wires
L—Luque Rod
J—Jacobs Rod
= = =—Indicates significant performance drop

* This table is a summary of biomechanical test results by various authors. Systems are listed in decreasing order of restoring stiffness to the injured segment.

derived from the fixation of screws in the pedicles. The screws provide a greater control on the three-dimensional motion of the vertebral body due to the fact that the bone–metal interface has the ability to transmit not only forces, but moments. In contrast, the interface between the lamina and the standard Harrington hook or segmental wire cannot transmit moments and, as a result, does not provide as much control over the three-dimensional motion of the vertebrae. Since these constructs can adequately stabilize the injured segments with a shorter fusion than the traditional systems, they offer a distinct advantage, particularly in the lumbar region, by preserving normal mobile segments. However, it should be kept in mind that both the strength and rigidity of these constructs will be adversely affected by the lack of good bony purchase of pedicular screws, such as in osteoporotic bone.

The Harrington distraction rod can carry the axial load in the physiologic range. However, it is vulnerable to forward flexion and rotation. Postoperative orthoses that restrict these motions will minimize the chances of hook dislodgement or fracture. The Harrington distraction rod, when used in the lumbar spine, can cause a loss of lumbar lordosis, a phenomenon referred to as "flat back syndrome." Attempts to control this problem include contouring the rod through the lordotic curvature of the lumbar spine and using a square

hook, and using sleeves that provide a transverse force on the lamina and counteract the tendency of the spine to become hypolordotic due to the distraction force.

Segmental fixation of Harrington rods using wires improves the failure strength and rigidity of the construct in flexion and rotation, because segmental fixation distributes the load over multiple fixation points. The Luque system benefits from this principle, but it is notably weak in axial loading. The CD system combines the axial load-carrying ability of the Harrington rod with the improved torsional rigidity of segmental fixation.

Finally, it is essential to appreciate that an instrumentation system does not work in isolation, but relies on the biologic system to share the loads. Thus a posterior fixation device is much more likely to "survive" if there is an adequate anterior load path that acts to reduce the bending loads and motions of the device.

BIOMECHANICAL STUDIES OF SPINAL ORTHOSES

Spinal orthoses have traditionally played a role in the management of thoracic and lumbar fractures with or without surgical stabilization. A variety of orthoses of different functional designs have been used over the past several decades. The traditional approaches to orthotic stabilization have been leather body braces and plaster body casts. Recent approaches include the use of a hyperextension brace, total-contact thoracolumbosacral orthoses (TLSOs) such as those with an anterior or posterior opening or a bivalve design, and a recently reported anterior shell design. Biomechanical studies of spinal orthoses have documented the ability of various orthoses to limit segmental motion and overall motion of the trunk. Others have investigated the effect of these orthoses on the myoelectric activity of trunk muscles and on intradiscal and intra-abdominal pressures and loads acting on the spine.

Segmental immobilization with spinal orthoses was studied by Norton and Brown.[23] They found there to be little effect on segmental motion with any of the orthoses. Orthoses were found to be relatively more effective in limiting motion at the upper levels than at lower levels. Some of the orthoses occasionally increased motion at the lumbosacral joint when compared to normal motion. Lumsden and Morris[16] confirmed this observation for axial rotation at the lumbosacral joint. They noted that a chairback brace was more effective than a corset, and that the orthoses in general were more effective at upper levels than at the lumbosacral joint.

The effectiveness of three braces on stabilization of a seat belt type injury at L-1–L-2 was studied by Nagel and associates[22] using human cadavers. Range of motion at the joint space was measured in flexion–extension, lateral bending, and axial rotation before and after the intervention. The three-point hyperextension brace was fair in limiting flexion–extension motion but had little effect on motion in lateral bending or axial rotation. The Taylor-Knight brace was effective in lateral bending and fair in flexion–extension, but had little effect in limiting axial rotation. The body cast performed satisfactorily in limiting motion in all three modes.

The effectiveness of the canvas corset, Raney jacket, baycast jacket, and baycast spica on limiting segmental motion in flexion was studied in normal adults by Fidler and Plasmans.[4] The canvas corset was found to reduce segmental motion by 33% of normal. The Raney jacket and baycast jacket reduced segmental motion by about two thirds at midlumbar levels. The baycast spica was the only brace that was effective in limiting motion at the lower lumbar levels.

In a recent study, Patwardhan and associates[25] used a computer model of the spine to evaluate the effect of injury and orthotic stabilization on the load-carrying ability of the spine. An injury of variable severity was simulated at the T-11–L-1 segments. The progression of angular and translational deformities at the injured segments was calculated with and without a hyperextension orthosis when the model spine was subjected to flexion moments in addition to gravitational loads. Under gravitational loads and small flexion moments, the hyperextension orthosis was found to be effective in limiting displacements at the injury site to within the levels of a normal spine for injuries that caused about 60% reduction in segmental stiffness. However, for higher flexion moments (10 Nm), the segmental motions at the injury site in the braced spine exceeded the normal levels for much less severe injuries (those that caused about 25% reduction in segmental stiffness).

Based on these results the authors proposed three zones of spinal stability. Zone 1 represents injuries that cause up to 25% reduction in segmental stiffness. This most likely includes injuries with single-column disruptions, such as most compression fractures. The hyperextension orthosis appears to adequately limit the progression of deformity in these injuries with little or no restriction of activities. Zone 2 represents injuries that cause a 25% to 60% reduction in segmental stiffness, such as severe compression fractures and some burst fractures. These injuries may be adequately stabilized in the hyperextension orthosis when the activity level is restricted to maintain near-normal resistance to progression of deformity. Finally, Zone 3 represents injuries that cause greater than 60% reduction in segmental stiffness at the injury site, such as severe burst fractures and fracture-dislocation injuries. The hyperextension orthosis is unable to limit the progression of deformities to within normal levels under gravitational load that simulates standing.

The effectiveness of spinal orthoses in limiting overall trunk motion in flexion–extension, lateral bending, and axial rotation was studied by Dorsky and associates.[2] All subjects were tested with four braces: the Raney jacket, molded polypropylene TLSO, Camp lace-up corset, and elastic corset. The Raney jacket and molded TLSO were found to provide the most overall restriction of trunk motion. The Camp corset provided an intermediate degree of restriction and the elastic corset was only minimally restrictive. All braces were more effective in controlling lateral bending of the lumbar spine than they were in flexion–extension motion.

Lantz and Schultz[14] studied the effects of wearing a lumbosacral corset, a chairback brace, and a molded plastic TLSO on restriction of gross body motions. Trunk movements in flexion, extension, lateral bending, and torsion were examined in five healthy men when standing and sitting. The molded TLSO resulted in the most mean-motion restriction across all eight movements for all subjects, while the corset resulted in the least restriction of gross upper body motions.

A number of investigators have studied the effect of spinal orthosis wearing on the myoelectric activities of the trunk muscles. Morris and Lucas[18] found that myoelectric activity in the abdominal muscles decreased when braces were worn, although there was no change in intra-abdominal and intrathoracic pressures. Waters and Morris[26] measured the effects of brace wearing on the myoelectric activity of trunk muscles during level walking at different speeds. The chairback brace and the lumbosacral corset had no significant effect on the myoelectric activity of the erector spinae muscles and the internal and external oblique muscles when the subjects stood upright or walked at a comfortable speed. During walking at a fast pace while wearing the chairback brace, the activity in the oblique abdominal muscles was not significantly altered, but the activity in the back muscles was increased in most subjects.

Lantz and Schultz[15] studied the effects of the lumbosacral corset, chairback brace, and molded plastic TLSO on the myoelectric activity of back muscles and oblique abdominal muscles as the subjects performed 19 isometric tasks involving a moderate degree of exertion. None of the orthoses was consistently effective in reducing measured myoelectric activity. In many cases the signal levels increased when the orthoses were worn. Overall, the chairback brace was the most effective in reducing myoelectric activity in the sym-

metrical anterior weight-holding tasks, while the molded plastic TLSO was the most effective in the lateral bending and twist-resisting tasks. Further, the study concluded that lumbar orthosis wearing is mechanically effective only sometimes, and even then its effect on reducing the loads on the lumbar trunk structures is not significant.

A few studies have examined the effect of orthosis wearing on intradiscal and intra-abdominal pressures in an attempt to evaluate the effectiveness of spinal orthoses in reducing the loads on the spine. Nachemson and Morris[20] measured the effect of an inflatable corset on intradiscal pressures in the lumbar spine while the subjects stood upright. When the corset was worn but not inflated, intradiscal pressures were nearly the same as when no corset was worn. However, the disk pressures decreased by 25% when the corset was inflated. In a later study, Nachemson and associates[21] monitored intradiscal pressures along with intra-abdominal pressures and myoelectric activity of trunk muscles while subjects wearing a spinal brace performed eight different activities. The braces included the Camp canvas corset, Raney flexion jacket, and Boston brace. Tests were performed with subjects experiencing 0, 15, and 30 degrees of lumbar extension. The spinal braces did not have any consistent effect on reducing the myoelectric activity in the erector spinae. The effect of orthoses on the small intra-abdominal pressures measured was also inconsistent. Orthosis wearing decreased the intradiscal pressures in some activities studied while increasing it in others.

Krag and associates[13] measured the intra-abdominal pressure and myoelectric activity in the erector spinae muscles in normal subjects who performed isometric extension pulls in upright and flexed postures with no brace and while wearing a Camp lumbosacral corset and a Raney flexion jacket. They observed that the resting intra-abdominal pressure was voluntarily increased well above the normal level.

Nachemson and Elfstrom[19] studied the effect of external immobilization (using a Milwaukee brace and body cast) following a Valsalva maneuver on the loads acting on spinal instrumentation in patients with idiopathic scoliosis. Loads in the Harrington rod were monitored using strain gages with the patients in supine, sitting, and relaxed standing positions as well as during level walking. Both the Milwaukee brace and body cast reduced the axial force in the Harrington rod during standing and walking.

SUMMARY

Biomechanical studies of simulated injuries help us in achieving a better understanding of the three-dimensional nature of instability, which may not be obvious from radiographic evaluation alone. The data on strength and rigidity of instrumentation systems provide a way of objectively comparing the efficacy of different constructs in stabilizing different thoracolumbar injuries, and understanding why some constructs fail.

Studies on bracing have shown that braces function primarily as range of motion restrictors, thereby decreasing loads on the injured segments under physiologic conditions. This is particularly important for flexion and rotation, which are modes in which the surgical constructs are shown to be most vulnerable.

However, one must exercise caution in making clinical decisions based solely on biomechanical data. Although these studies help us eliminate the grossly inadequate surgical constructs and braces from the wide range of choices available to date, they do not point to a single system as an answer to all of our problems. Clearly, clinical experience has shown satisfactory results with many different constructs which, according to the biomechanical studies, are not necessarily the stiffest constructs in all modes of testing. Clinical success, therefore, does not appear to lie in finding the stiffest possible system, but rather in achieving a balance between a construct that is stiff enough to restore the biologic load path in conjunction with appropriate motion restriction, and the use of postoperative bracing until fusion healing occurs.

REFERENCES

1. Denis F: The three column spine and its significance in the classification of acute thoracolumbar spinal injuries. Spine 8:817, 1983
2. Dorsky S, Buchalter D, Kahanovitz N, Nordin M: A three dimensional investigation of lumbar brace immobilization utilizing a noninvasive technique. Presented at the 33rd annual meeting of the Orthopaedic Research Society, San Francisco, California, 1987
3. Ferguson RL, Tencer AF, Woodard P et al: Biomechanical comparison of spinal fracture models and the stabilizing effects of posterior instrumentations. Spine 13:453–460, 1988
4. Fidler MW, Plasmans CMT: The effect of four types of support on the segmental mobility of the lumbosacral spine. J Bone Joint Surg Am 65:943–947, 1983
5. Gaines RW, Carson WL, Satterlee CC, Groh GI: Improving quality of spinal internal fixation: Evolution toward ideal immobilization. A biomechanical study. Presented at the 21st annual meeting of the Scoliosis Research Society, Hamilton, Bermuda, September 1986
6. Galpin RD, Corin JD, Ashman RB, Johnston CE: Biomechanical testing of pedicle screw instrumentation in a burst fracture model. Presented at the 22nd annual meeting of the Scoliosis Research Society, Vancouver, British Columbia, Canada, September 1987
7. Gepstein R, Latta L, Shufflebarger IIL: Cotrel–Dubousset instrumentation for lumbar burst fractures: A biomechanical study. Presented at the 21st annual meeting of the Scoliosis Research Society, Hamilton, Bermuda, September 1986
8. Haher TR, Lospinuso M, Tozzi J et al: The contribution of the three columns of the spine to spinal stability: A biomechanical model. Presented at the 22nd annual meeting of the Scoliosis Research Society, Vancouver, British Columbia, Canada, September 1987
9. Hoeltzel DA, Athanasiou KA, Farcy JP et al: A standardized comparison of mechanical stability and stiffness for the Cotrel–Dubousset, Harrington distraction, and Moe and Luque spinal fixation systems. Advances in Bioengineering 52–53, 1986
10. Holdsworth F: Fractures, dislocations, and fracture dislocations of the spine. JBJS 52A:1534–1551, 1970
11. Jacobs RR, Nordwall A, Nachemson A: Reduction, stability, and strength provided by internal fixation systems for thoracolumbar spinal injuries. Clin Orthop 171:300–308, 1982
12. Jacobs RR, Schlaepfer F, Mathys R et al: A locking hook spinal rod system for stabilization of fracture-dislocations and correction of deformities of the dorsolumbar spine: A biomechanic evaluation. Clin Orthop 189:168–177, 1984
13. Krag MH, Beynnon BD, Pope MH et al: An internal fixator for posterior application to short segments

of the thoracic, lumbar, or lumbosacral spine. Clin Orthop 203:75–98, 1986

14. Lantz SA, Schultz AB: Lumbar spine orthosis wearing: I. Restriction of gross body motions. Spine 11:834–837, 1986

15. Lantz SA, Schultz AB: Lumbar spine orthosis wearing: II. Effect on trunk muscle myoelectric activity. Spine 11:838–842, 1986

16. Lumsden RM, Morris JM: An in vivo study of axial rotation and immobilization at the lumbosacral joint. J Bone Joint Surg [Am] 50:1591, 1968

17. McAfee PC, Werner FW, Glisson RR: A biomechanical analysis of spinal instrumentation systems in thoracolumbar fractures: Comparison of traditional Harrington distraction instrumentation with segmental spinal instrumentation. Spine 10:204–217, 1985

18. Morris JM, Lucas DB: Physiological considerations in bracing of spine. Orthop Prosth Appl 37–44, 1963

19. Nachemson A, Elfstrom G: Intravital wireless telemetry of axial forces in Harrington distraction rods in patients with idiopathic scoliosis. J Bone Joint Surg [Am] 53:445–465, 1971

20. Nachemson A, Morris JM: In vivo measurements of intradiscal pressure. J Bone Joint Surg 46A:1077–1092, 1964

21. Nachemson A, Schultz AB, Andersson GBJ: Mechanical effectiveness studies of lumbar spine orthoses. Scand J Rehabil Med [Suppl] 9:139–149, 1983

22. Nagel DA, Koogle TA, Pinziali RL, Perkash I: Stability of the upper lumbar spine following progressive disruptions and the application of individual internal and external fixation devices. J Bone Joint Surg 63A:62–70, 1981

23. Norton PL, Brown T: The immobilizing efficiency of the back braces: Their effect on the posture and motion of the lumbosacral spine. J Bone Joint Surg [Am] 39:111–139, 1957

24. Panjabi MM, Abumi K, Duranceau JS, Crisco JJ: Studies in the biomechanical stabilization of internal thoraco-lumbar fixation devices. Presented at the 22nd annual meeting of the Scoliosis Research Society, Vancouver, British Columbia, Canada, September 1987

25. Patwardhan AG, Li S, Gavin T et al: Orthotic stabilization of thoracolumbar injuries. Presented at the 4th annual meeting of the North American Spine Society, Quebec City, Canada. June 29–July 2, 1989

26. Waters RL, Morris JM: Effects of spinal supports on the electrical activity of muscles of the trunk. J Bone Joint Surg 52A:51–60, 1970

27. Wenger D, Miller S, Wilkerson J: Evaluation of fixation sites for segmental instrumentation of the human vertebra. Presented at the 16th annual meeting of the Scoliosis Research Society, Montreal, Quebec, Canada, September 1981

28. Zindrick MR, Wiltse LL, Widell EH et al: A biomechanical study of intrapeduncular screw fixation in the lumbosacral spine. Clin Orthop 203:99–112, 1986

10

ANTERIOR TECHNIQUES OF STABILIZATION IN THORACIC AND LUMBAR TRAUMA

John P. Kostuik

History records that the first surgical procedure for a spinal cord injury was performed by Paul of Aegina (AD 625–690). Since that time, the treatment of injuries of the spine with or without neurologic deficit, and in particular those involving the thoracic and lumbar spine, has moved from bed rest to postural reduction to laminectomy with or without posterior fusion. The fusion, when done, has sometimes been in conjunction with varying forms of posterior internal fixation, such as wires, plates, and springs.

Because of the high failure rate of posterior fixation devices such as wires and plates, the conservative postural reduction approach of Guttman, Frankel, and Bedbrook[2,12,15,16] for fractures of the spinal column was adopted in many spinal centers throughout the world. However, reduction was not universally obtained by this method.[25,28,32]

The reports of Harrington[19] in 1962 and Dickson and associates[9] in 1978 led to considerable efforts in an attempt to achieve stabilization of fracture-dislocations of the thoracic and lumbar spine. An important development was Harrington distraction rods, which provided three-point fixation. Their use resulted in a more anatomic reduction of the vertebral column, particularly the anterior column, obviating the need for laminectomy. Laminectomy not infrequently increased the neurologic deficit and resulted in an increasing kyphosis.[25,27,39]

In most centers in North America, Harrington instrumentation has become the preferred mode of treatment for stabilization of injuries of the thoracic and lumbar spine. This form of fixation has enhanced the speed with which rehabilitation of patients with spinal injury may commence.

Although accepted by many as a panacea, Harrington instrumentation has not proven to be so, with particular reference to burst injuries of the thoracic and lumbar spine. Initial reports on the use of Harrington distraction rods with three-point fixation failed to differentiate between different fracture patterns.[5,9,41] It was felt that application of a distractive force would result in bony fragments being cleared from the neural canal and realigned. This was based on the assumption that the fragments would remain attached to the posterior or anterior longitudinal ligament. Numerous reports have now indicated that this is not the case, particularly with reference to burst injuries of the spine.[4,6,8,21,21a,23,24,26,29,31,40] As a result of such reports and similar cases in the author's experience, together with cases of late onset of neurologic deficit after old burst injuries, which subsequently required anterior cord decompression and fusion to obtain beneficial results, it has become the author's policy to perform anterior surgery together with anterior fixation for some burst injuries of the spine.

With modern anterior fixation devices, there is no need in most cases for posterior fusion and instrumentation in the treatment of either the acute injury or late post-traumatic kyphosis, with or without neurologic involvement, unless there is an associated severe comminution and instability of the posterior elements.

DEVELOPMENT OF ANTERIOR TECHNIQUES

Royle in 1928[33] was the first to describe anterior spinal cord decompression. The technique, however, remained unpopular until Hodgson and Stock[20] in 1956 reported on anterior decompression for tuberculous lesions of the spine that had resulted in paraplegia.

Since then there has been an increasing number of reports of anterior decompression for related problems, such as tuberculosis, pyogenic osteomyelitis, rigid kyphotic deformities, and, more recently, both primary and metastatic tumors and burst fractures.[34,35] Most reports have described anterior débridement and resection, and fusion without the use of internal fixation.

Wenger* in 1953 was first to describe the use of an anterior distractive device. Unfortunately, this failed. The use of anterior devices still remains unpopular largely because of their lack of ready availability and fear of complications.

Dwyer[10] in 1969 was the first in the modern era to report on the use of an anterior corrective device in the treatment of a spinal deformity, namely scoliosis in the thoracolumbar spine. Hall[17] in 1977 reported on the use of modified Dwyer instrumentation and anterior stabilization of the spine. Dunn† reported on the use of an anterior distractive stabilizing device for the treatment of burst injuries of the spine. Unfortunately, in the hands of others this resulted in a significant series of traumatic aneurysms of the aorta or the common iliac system, which resulted in the discontinuance of this rigid device (Fig. 10-1). Zielke[42] in 1977 reported on the use of his device to replace

* Dunn H: Personal communication, 1983.
† Milgram J, Hospital for Joint Diseases, New York: Personal communication, 1982.

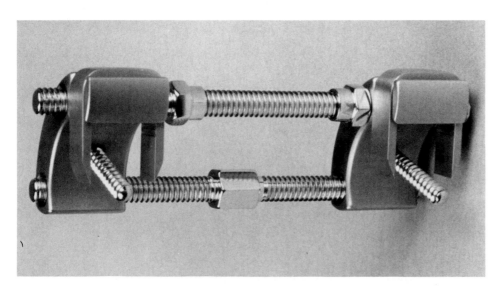

Figure 10-1. Dunn's device.

Dwyer instrumentation for the treatment of scoliosis. He together with Slot[36] reported on the use of an anterior distractor for the treatment of kyphotic deformities and kyphosis as a result of acute burst injuries of the thoracic and lumbar spine (Fig. 10-2). Others have reported on the use of AO plates anteriorly, but have reported a high incidence of screw backout. Kaneda[21] reported in 1982 on the use of his instrumentation for the correction of kyphotic deformities and the achievement of anterior stabilization in acute burst fractures (Fig. 10-3). Subsequent reports have indicated a high degree of success.

This author reported in 1983 and subsequently[22,23] on modified Harrington instrumentation used anteriorly with screws for the stabilization of deformity of the spine and the correction of kyphotic deformities. The anterior Harrington system[21a] has been used in 350 cases over 9 years for a variety of reasons, including the correction of acute kyphosis in burst injuries, late post-traumatic kyphosis, Scheuermann's kyphosis, acute angular kyphosis, and anterior fixation for posterior pseudarthrosis.[22] There has been a high rate of success, with only 26 screw fractures in the first 350 cases: 15 in acute fractures, three in late post-traumatic kyphosis, three used anteriorly for correction of Scheuermann's kyphosis, one used anteriorly for congenital kyphosis, three used posteriorly for pedicle fixation in degenerative disease, and one in a case of previous posterior decompression for tumor over three levels. Four rods have broken anteriorly, two of these in acute bursting injuries. A total of 1400 screws and 700 rods have been used to date.

In the treatment of acute burst injuries or late post-traumatic kyphosis, anterior Harrington devices serve to readily correct the kyphosis, provide stability, and allow for early rehabilitation and ambulation. The ease of application allows for its variable use in many areas of the spine. The uppermost level of vertebral body insertion has been T-2, and the lowest level, L-5. Although the screws are available in three lengths, they can be readily shortened by cutting the tips. The use of washers or staples serves to prevent toggling of the screw within the cancellous vertebral body. In cases of severe osteopenia, methyl methacrylate bone cement can be used to enhance screw fixation.

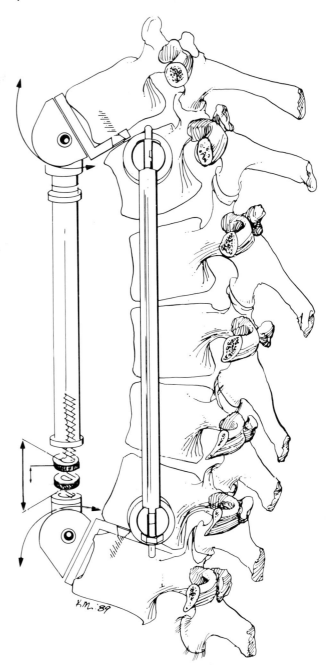

Figure 10-2. Slot and Zielke's anterior distractive device.

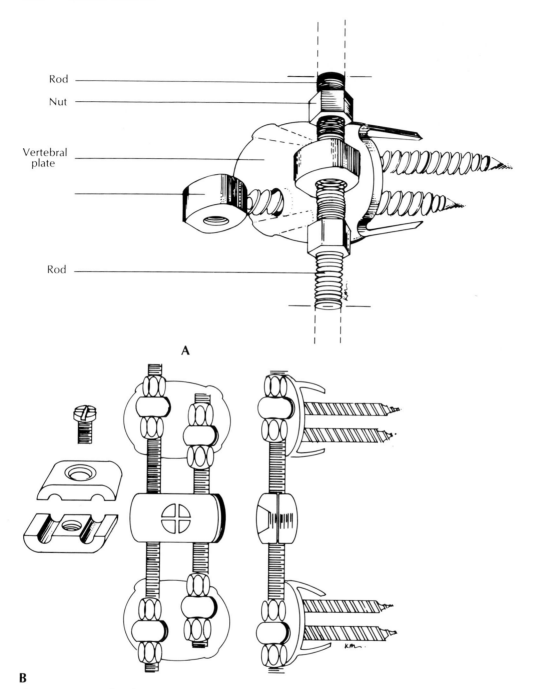

Rod

Nut

Vertebral plate

Rod

A

B

Figure 10-3. Kaneda's device. (*A*) Close-up of end-plate screw device. (*B*) Kaneda's device on profile and anteriorly.

Armstrong* has recently reported on the development of an anterior plate, but this is as yet experimental (Fig. 10-4).[2a] Rezaian[30] has reported on an interbody distractive device for treatment of acute burst injuries (Figs. 10-5, 10-6). In the author's experience this device is bulky and leaves little room for an anterior interbody graft.

Anterior distractive devices or fixation devices generally fall into the following categories:

1. Plates
2. External devices, in which the rods lie outside of the vertebral bodies. Distractive devices include the Kostuik–Harrington,[23] Dunn,[9a] Slot,[36] and Zielke[42] devices and plates, the AO plate, the Armstrong* plate, and Yuan's I beam plate (Fig. 10-7).†
3. Interbody devices such as the Rezaian device or temporary devices such as the Pinto distractor (Fig. 10-8)

Plates provide fixation only, whereas most distractive devices are corrective as well. Reports on anterior interbody fusion in the lumbar spine indicate varying rates of union, ranging from 100% to 18%.[1,3,4,11,13,14,18,33,35,37] In most series the average has been 10% to 20% nonunion. As a result there has been a somewhat general reluctance to perform anterior surgery in the lumbar spine. In the author's experience the incidence of nonunion has been 5% with the use of Kostuik–Harrington[22] devices for kyphotic deformities that are either acute, as in burst injuries, or late, as in long fusions for Scheuermann's kyphosis corrected anteriorly with anterior distraction. The incidence of nonunion using double Zielke instrumentation anteriorly, where posterior surgery was felt not to be reasonable or feasible, was 12% in salvage surgery for degenerative lumbar disk disease in the author's hands.

Malcolm and associates[25] reported on the use of interbody grafts. In the case of post-traumatic kyphosis, they found a 50% incidence of nonunion and loss of correction with the use of interbody

(Text continued on p. 288)

* Armstrong G: Personal communication, 1987.
† Yuan H: Personal communication, 1987.

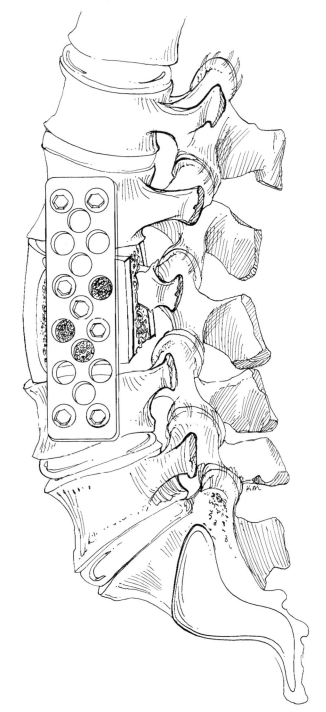

Figure 10-4. Armstrong's plate.

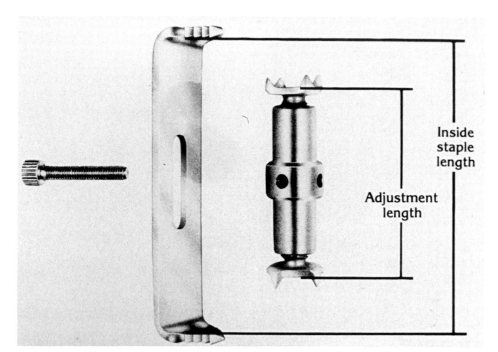

Figure 10-5. Rezaian's device.

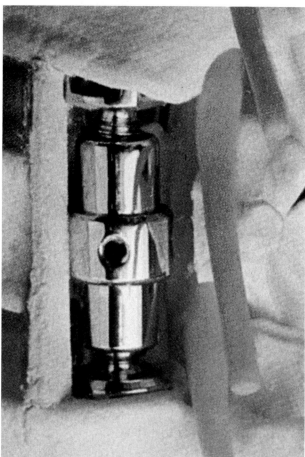

Figure 10-6. Rezaian's device in place. Device is bulky and leaves little room for bone grafted noted anteriorly.

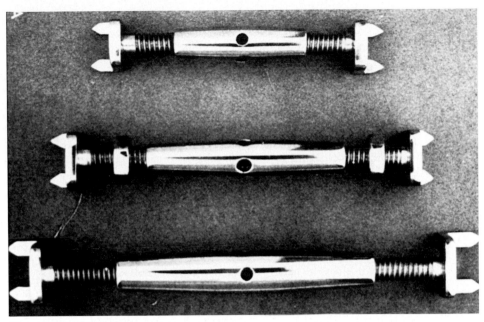

Figure 10-7. Pinto temporary distractor.

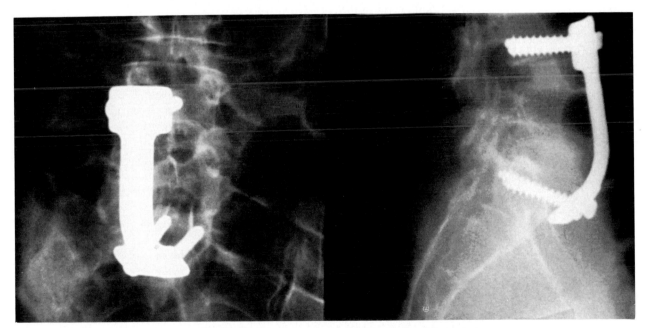

Figure 10-8. Yuan's I beam plate. Used here in a salvage case of posterior pseudarthrosis in a previous posterior fusion for degenerative disk disease, the plate has been contoured for the sacral promontory.

grafts without fixation or second-stage posterior surgery. They recommended the use of supplementary posterior fixation and fusion, as they felt that anterior fusion alone was insufficient. Morscher* stated that interbody grafts were unable to withstand physiologic loads without fixation. White[38] reported that iliac crest interbody grafts cannot withstand the loads in the erect position, although they may in the recumbent position. Fibular cortical strut grafts may withstand these loads; however, revascularization does not take place until approximately 6 months after surgery.

The author feels that with the advent of anterior fixation devices, particularly anterior distraction devices, supplementary fixation and fusion is no longer necessary, since the device serves to correct the kyphosis and is under a compressive load. The anterior lumbar spine supports three to four times the body weight. Bicortical or tricortical iliac crest grafts cannot support these loads in the erect position. Hence, anterior fixation devices are needed.

While testing in a cyclical and dynamic fashion in the laboratory using calf spines, the author has noted that a single anterior fixation rod device used alone does not provide good control over rotation and lateral bending. As a result, when rod systems are to be used, supplementary fixation with a second rod as a neutralization rod is recommended, preferably with coupling of the two rods. Laboratory testing indicates that rod systems, although not as rigid in rotation as segmental wiring or posterior Harrington instrumentation, do provide sufficient stability to allow for early rehabilitation and ambulation, generally with the use of an external orthosis rather than a body cast.

The use of anterior fixation devices precludes the need for posterior fusion or instrumentation in the majority of cases, provided that the posterior elements are intact (i.e., not comminuted in the burst fracture or not resected in the other cases). The use of these devices shortens hospitalization and lessens the need for a second procedure, with its possible morbidity. However, if the posterior elements are absent or comminuted or if more than one vertebral body has been resected, a sec-

* Morscher E: Personal communication, 1975.

ond-stage posterior stabilization and fusion, in addition to the anterior fixation, is necessary.

SURGICAL APPROACHES

For anterior spinal cord decompression the author prefers the use of the left side. The advantages to this approach are that the aorta tends to protect the left common venous iliac system and that damage to arterial vascular structures can easily be repaired. Damage to venous structures, on the other hand, is more difficult to repair and such injury frequently results in greater blood loss.

The only indication for an anterior approach in trauma is for burst injuries or late post-traumatic kyphosis.

With injuries to L-5 and occasionally to L-4, posterior decompression can be done by removing the posterior elements, preferably en bloc, and pushing the bony fragments anteriorly and removing any disk fragments, or by using employed distraction and lordosis by means of an internal fixator. Generally, in fractures proximal to L-5 the author prefers an anterior approach. A left flank approach is satisfactory for lesions of L-3–L-4 and L-5. In this approach the iliolumbar and segmental vessels must be ligated and the psoas resected at the lateral aspect of the vertebral bodies. For approaches to L-2 and L-3 frequently the approach is through the 12th rib, which is often subdiaphragmatic. If it is not, at the most a small part of the diaphragm must be released. For approaches to T-12 and occasionally L-1 and T-11, a thoracoabdominal approach must be used.

For more proximal approaches in the thoracic spine, generally an incision is made two ribs above the desired vertebral level (i.e., a fracture of T-9 is approached through the bed of the 7th rib). If the ribs are horizontal one can make the approach one rib proximal to the affected vertebral body.

Ligation of the segmental vessels two levels proximal and distal to the affected site at any level allows for satisfactory mobilization of the major vascular structures, and prevents their abutment against any foreign materials that might be used. Care must be taken to avoid the abutment of any screw heads or prominent metal components against the aorta or common iliac artery.

INDICATIONS FOR ANTERIOR FIXATION

Current indications for anterior fixation of spinal fractures with or without decompression of the spinal cord are:

1. Acute burst fractures with neurologic injury involving the anterior and middle column, with retropulsion of bony fragments into the canal (Figs. 10-9, 10-10).
2. Late burst injuries (i.e., those occurring 10 days or more post-injury) with or without neurologic injury. These are analogous to a Colles' fracture, which in cancellous bone is difficult to reduce by standard means 10 days or more following injury. This has also been the author's experience with posterior attempts at reduction of late burst injuries using Harrington distraction, or, more recently, posterior pedicle fixation devices such as the AO internal fixator, described in Chapter 11.
3. Burst injuries without neurologic injury that on computed tomography show significant retropulsion of material into the spinal canal. At the present time retropulsion causing occlusion of greater than 50% of the canal is considered to be significant. However, the amount of retropulsion required before anterior fixation is indicated is dependent on the bony level of the injury. The region of the cauda equina will tolerate much greater bony intrusion into the canal than the more proximal cord level. As much as 85% canal occlusion has been noted in the area of the cauda equina without neurologic sequelae, whereas as little as 20% has resulted in severe paraparesis in the area of the cord.[21a] There is no available data on the long-term sequelae of significant bony intrusion of the canal, although this author,[23] Bohlman[3] and Malcolm[25] have reported on the late development of spinal stenosis following such injuries.
4. Lumbar fractures at L-2 or lower. Harrington instrumentation or its modifications used posteriorly necessitates the immobilization of at least five levels. Although current methods employing these techniques advo-cate fusion of two to three levels only, the subsequent immobilization of the remaining levels, despite rod removal at 9 to 12 months, may result in premature facet degeneration. Moreover, prolonged distal immobilization to L-4 or L-5 may result in precocious degenerative changes below the levels of fusion, as noted in the long-standing effect of such immobilization in scoliosis patients.[7]

Anterior fusion of a maximum of two levels precludes such complications, but could possibly be supplanted by pedicle fixation techniques. The advent, however, of distractive devices that include the building in of lordosis, such as the AO internal fixator, may decrease the need for anterior surgery for acute burst injuries.

ANTERIOR KOSTUIK–HARRINGTON INSTRUMENTATION

Prior to the development of the anterior Kostuik–Harrington instrumentation (Fig. 10-11), 17 patients underwent anterior dural decompression and grafting using iliac crest bicortical grafts with or without internal fixation. These consisted of six patients with no anterior fixation, two of whom underwent secondary posterior fixation; four patients with anterior fixation using AO heavy compression plates; and seven patients with anterior fixation using Dwyer–Hall rods. These cases were done prior to 1979.

This author has previously reported[21a,23,24] on the use of anterior Kostuik screws together with a round-ended Harrington rod to distract the kyphotic deformity and a secondary Dwyer–Hall rod for neutralization. The latter rod has been replaced by the heavy Harrington compression rod since 1983.

The preferred technique of fixation in recent years has been using the modified anterior Kostuik–Harrington distractive device (see Fig. 10-11). Surgery is performed using an anterolateral approach. The left side is preferred. Segmental vessels are ligated in the midline. The ligation of segmental vessels two levels proximal and one

(Text continued on p. 295)

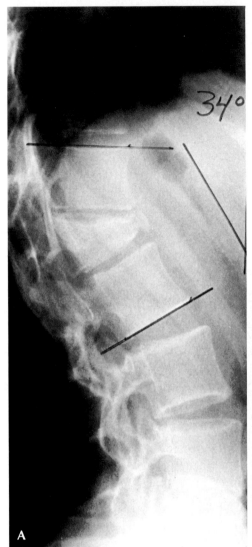

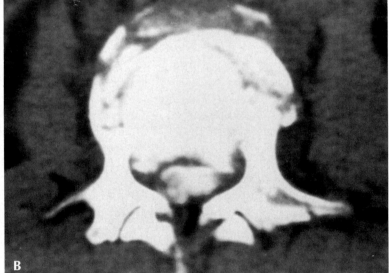

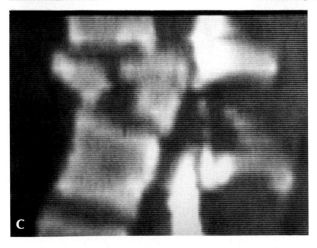

Figure 10-9. Operation of an acute bursting fracture. (*A*) Preoperative lateral radiograph shows loss of anterior column height or greater than 50% and kyphosis of 34 degrees. (*B*) Preoperative CT scan shows marked canal occlusion, Frankel grade B. (*C*) Lateral CT reconstruction. Note instability.

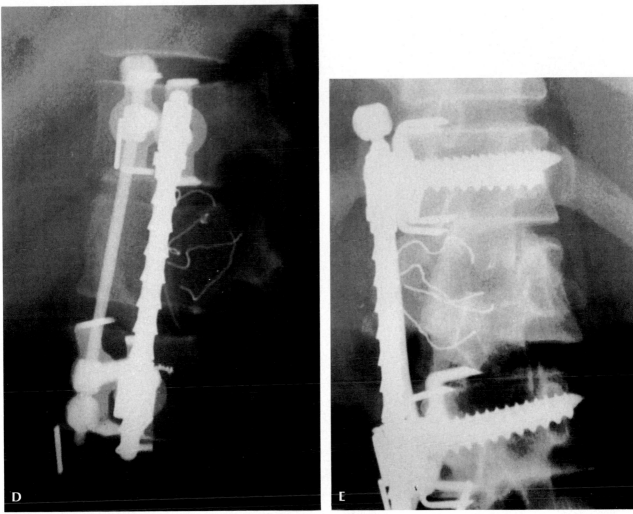

Figure 10-9. (*continued*). (*D*) Postoperative lateral radiograph shows complete restoration of height of vertebral body. (*E*) Postoperative anteroposterior radiograph. Patient was restored to Frankel grade D. This case was completed in 6 hours.

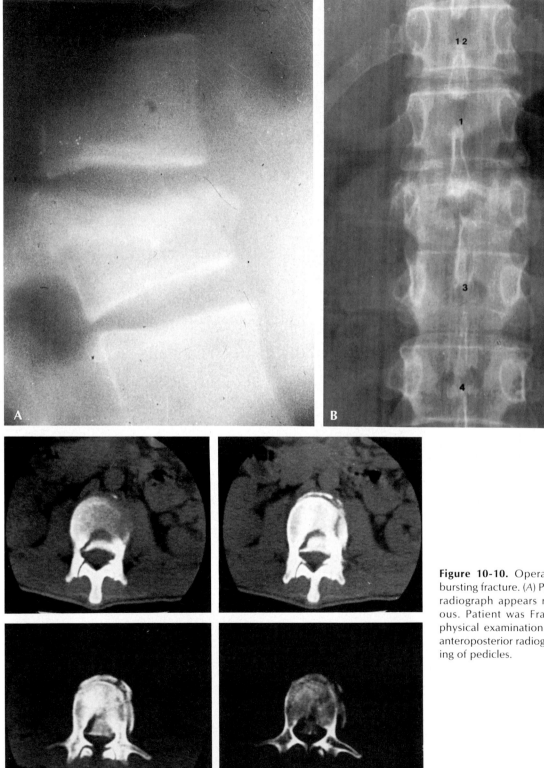

Figure 10-10. Operation of an acute bursting fracture. (A) Preoperative lateral radiograph appears relatively innocuous. Patient was Frankel grade C on physical examination. (B) Preoperative anteroposterior radiograph shows splaying of pedicles.

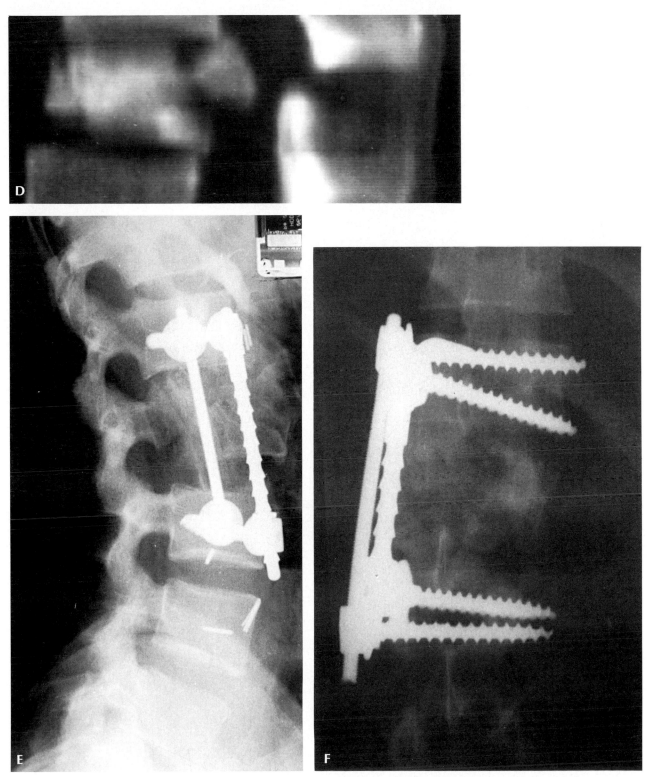

Figure 10-10. (*continued*). (*C, D*) Computed tomographic reconstruction. Note the sharp angulatory fragment unattached to soft tissue at the time of surgery. Axial cuts showed marked occlusion. (*E*) Postoperative lateral radiograph. Patient has recovered to Frankel grade D. (*F*) Postoperative antero-posterior radiograph.

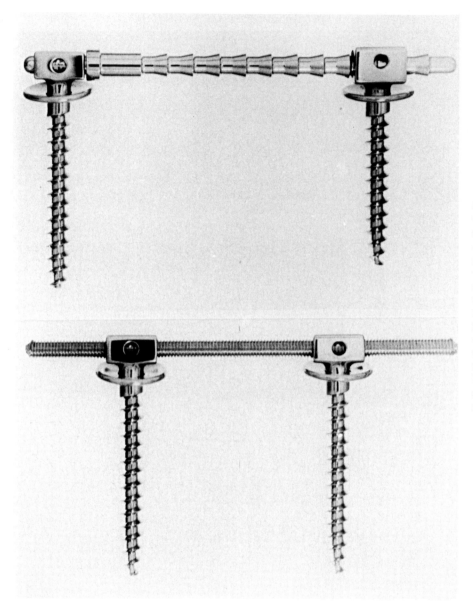

Figure 10-11. Kostuik–Harrington instrumentation used with standard Harrington round-ended rods and equipment staples. Rods and staples are preferred to washers because they aid in coupling. Larger-holed (distraction) screw is used for the rachet end of the distraction rod. Smaller-holed (collar) screws are used for the collar end of the distraction rod and heavy Harrington compression rods. Screw heads on the compression rods are usually crimped. Nuts may be used.

to two levels distal allows the large vessels to fall away from the fixation devices and prevents vascular sequelae. No coagulation near intervertebral foramina is done in order to avoid possible vascular compromise to neural structures. If decompression is required, this is carried out first, with the anterior quarter of the body being preserved with soft-tissue attachments in order to provide a viable graft (Fig. 10-12*A*). The dura is completely decompressed anteriorly and to the right and left, and is allowed to float forward. If the dura is thick, as it may be in cases of chronic compression, it may be opened as well.

In cases in which dural compression is not required, the disk spaces and end-plates are removed on either side of the fracture back to the posterior longitudinal ligament. Following this, Kostuik spinal screws of appropriate length are inserted into the vertebral bodies. A distraction-ended screw is used for the rachet end and a collar-ended screw for the butt end of the Harrington rod. Staples are preferred to enhance screw fixation. A round Harrington rod is inserted and a distractive force sufficient to restore normal vertebral body height is employed. The rachet end of the rod is secured with "C" clamps (Fig. 10-12*B*). The iliac crest is then exposed and iliac crest with cortices on two sides is removed in the form of a block slightly longer than the space to be grafted. This is inserted under compression (Fig. 10-12*C*). If osteopenia is present a tricortical iliac crest graft is used. Following this, appropriate Kostuik collar-ended screws are inserted into the vertebral body above and below the site of the fracture or decompression, and a heavy Harrington compression rod is inserted and the screw heads crimped in order to enhance stability (Fig. 10-12*D*). This rod acts as a neutralization rod and enhances rotational control. Iliac crest graft is preferred and may be supplemented with rib if this is removed at the time of the surgical approach.

Postoperative immobilization is usually with a plastic molded orthosis, or in less accommodating patients, a body cast. Ambulation is dependent on the degree of neurologic damage. Early transfers and walking are permitted.

CASE STUDY

Between 1979 and 1987, 80 patients were treated by the author using an anterior approach for bursting injuries of the thoracic and lumbar spine. These can be subdivided into two groups: those requiring dural decompression for neurologic compromise together with anterior correction of deformity and stabilization (57 patients), and those in whom no neurologic deficit occurred but because of significant partial canal occlusion anterior decompression together with anterior stabilization was done (23 patients).

Procedures were performed as soon as possible in order to enhance root sparing and recovery; early decompression does not aid in cord recovery but may aid in cauda equina (or root) injury. All 57 patients with neurologic injury were treated with decompression within 72 hours of injury. Of these, 22 were treated at between 48 and 72 hours and 3 were treated between 6 and 48 hours of injury (four patients were treated within 6 hours of injury).

The age range was 17 to 63 years, with an average of 32 years. The levels of injury were from T-4 to L-5. Only one patient underwent planned two-stage surgery. The second stage was to stabilize the spine posteriorly after anterior stabilization and decompression, as it was recognized that there was severe posterior comminution.

Preoperatively, routine radiographs were done. Myelography was used prior to 1976, but computed tomography has been used since then. In the past 7 years sagittal reconstruction has been added.

UNION

Nonunion occurred in only two cases of Kostuik–Harrington instrumentation, both of which, in retrospect, would have benefited from early second-stage posterior fixation, as a review of computed tomographic scans revealed extensive comminution of the posterior bony elements. Today in similar cases, posterior fixation is carried out within 10 days of primary anterior surgery.

(*Text continued on p. 298*)

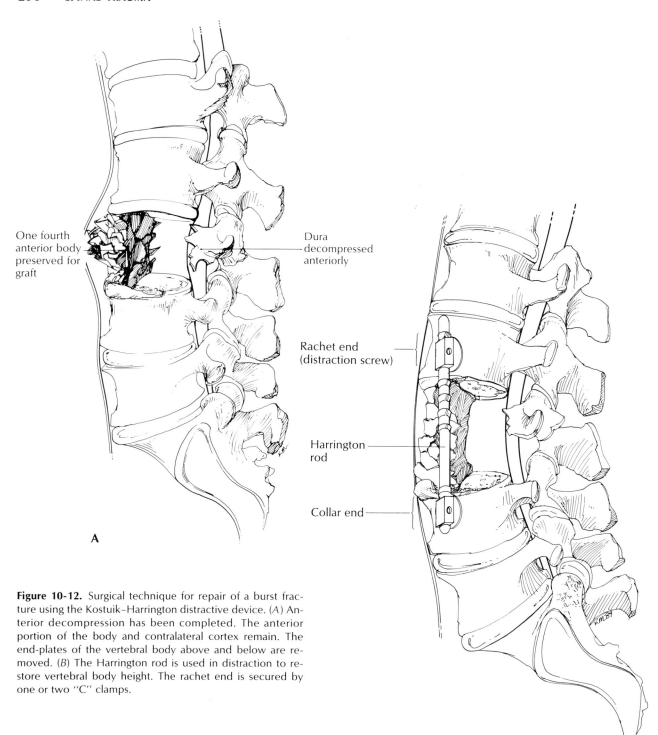

One fourth
anterior body
preserved for
graft

Dura
decompressed
anteriorly

Rachet end
(distraction screw)

Harrington
rod

Collar end

A

B

Figure 10-12. Surgical technique for repair of a burst fracture using the Kostuik–Harrington distractive device. (*A*) Anterior decompression has been completed. The anterior
portion of the body and contralateral cortex remain. The
end-plates of the vertebral body above and below are removed. (*B*) The Harrington rod is used in distraction to restore vertebral body height. The rachet end is secured by
one or two "C" clamps.

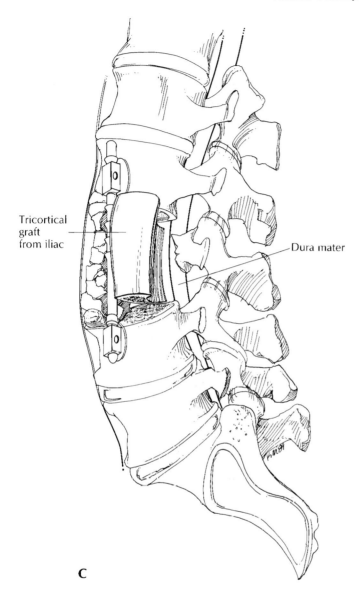

Tricortical
graft
from iliac

Dura mater

C

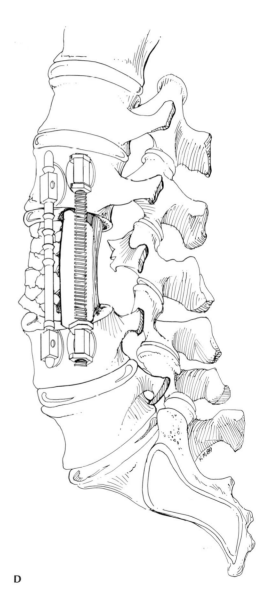

D

Figure 10-12. (*continued*). (*C*) Bone graft is added. Usually one iliac crest bicortical graft slightly larger than the defect is used. (The graft is tricortical in the presence of osteopenia.) In addition, rib struts or small fragments of iliac crest graft are added. (*D*) A second heavy Harrington compression rod is added posterior to the distraction rod to enhance stability. The screw heads on this rod are usually crimped.

Two early cases of nonunion occurred prior to 1979, when AO broad plates were used for anterior immobilization.

NEUROLOGIC RECOVERY

Of the 35 patients who were treated within 48 hours, four were complete paraplegics, with lesions at T-11, T-12, L-1, and L-2, respectively. No root recovery occurred despite early decompression (within 24 hours). The remaining 31 patients, who were partial paraplegics, recovered an average of 1.6 Frankel grades. Of these, four patients, with levels of injury at T-12, L-1, L-2, and L-3, were treated within 6 hours. All improved from Frankel grade B to Frankel grade D, with return of bowel and bladder function. No correlation as to the degree of canal intrusion was possible, except that in each case compromise was greater than 50%.

In the 22 partial paraplegic patients treated between 48 and 72 hours after injury, the average recovery was 1.0 grades. These figures suggest that the earlier the decompression, perhaps the greater the neurologic recovery. However, the numbers are far to few to be of statistical significance. Considering the variables of age, sex, level of injury, degree of injury, and time of decompression, approximately 1000 cases would be necessary to be conclusive.

Thirty-six of the 57 patients with neurologic injury presented with loss of bowel and bladder function. Four of these were complete paraplegics and remained so. Of the remaining 32 cases, the 10 who had lesions in the area of the conus medullaris (L-1) required continued intermittent catheterization. The rest regained satisfactory bladder control, with either fully normal control or regular timed use of urinary facilities.

PAIN RELIEF

Four patients complained postoperatively of severe incisional flank pain and dysthesia (post-thoracotomy syndrome). Two were relieved by extradural rhizotomies, one was relieved by phenol intercostal blocks, and one refused further treatment.

Six patients complained of significant late low back pain in the lumbosacral area. In four this was disabling and prevented their return to their employment. All six, because of their pain, underwent diskography. Two were found to have reproducible symptoms at L-4–L-5, and four at L-5–S-1. All disks showed early radiographic changes of degeneration. All patients were 22 years of age or younger—an age when these changes are not normally found. No patient had a prior history of low back pain. Two patients have undergone L-5–S-1 fusions, one with complete relief of pain. The other patient continues to complain of pain.

The etiology of the pain and disk degeneration is felt to be directly due to the spinal injury. Burst injuries are essentially axial loading injuries with a secondary component of anterior flexion moment. Distal soft-tissue (disk) injuries are felt to be possible, similar to multiple-level bony injuries that may occur with such a mechanism of injury.

COMPLICATIONS

Osteomyelitis occurred in one patient, necessitating removal of the anterior fixation devices once union occurred. A partial sequestrectomy of the grafted area was necessary. The fixation devices were not loose at the time of removal. Wound healing occurred by secondary intention.

Superficial wound or donor site infection occurred in six cases and was treated by local wound care.

Pulmonary embolism occurred in one case. This occurred prior to the current routine administration of an anticoagulant.

Atelectasis occurred in seven cases, two of which required ventilation for 48 hours.

Routine urinary antisepsis was used in all cases, but despite this most paraplegics at some stage of their acute hospitalization developed a urinary tract infection, requiring appropriate antibiotic treatment.

No major pressure sores developed during the acute care period, which lasted from 10 to 30 days (an average of 24 days) until admission to a convalescent or paraplegic rehabilitation center.

There were no early or late neurologic or vascular injuries.

Of the 13 cases in which screw breakage occurred, two developed a nonunion, as described earlier. Two cases were associated with rod breakage. No broken screws have been removed.

One early case of a severe T-12 bursting injury, Frankel grade A, with significant posterior element comminution failed when the patient started transfers in the early postoperative rehabilitation period. Additional second-stage posterior pedicle fixation in cases of severe posterior comminution is now recommended.

SUMMARY

This chapter described the uses for anterior fixation in the treatment of fractures of the thoracic and lumbar spine. The role of decompression in neurologic injury remains controversial. The results of neurologic improvement using anterior Kostuik–Harrington instrumentation were extremely gratifying, with an average improvement of 1.6 Frankel grades in all incomplete cases.

REFERENCES

1. Batchelor JS: Anterior interbody spinal fusion. Guy's Hosp Rep 112:61, 1963
2. Bedbrook GM: Spinal injuries with tetraplegia and paraplegia. J Bone Joint Surg [Br] 61:267, 1979
2a. Black RC, Eng P, Gardner MD et al: A contoured anterior spinal fraction plate. Clin Orthop 227:135–142, 1988
3. Bohlman HH, Eismont FJ: Surgical techniques of anterior decompression and fusion for spinal cord injuries. Clin Orthop 154:57–67, 1981
4. Bohlman HH, Freeajfel A, Dejak J: Spinal cord injuries: Late anterior decompression of spinal cord injuries. J Bone Joint Surg [Am] 57:1025, 1975
5. Bradford DS, Akbarnia BA, Winter RD, Seljescog EL: Surgical stabilization of fracture and fracture dislocation of the thoracic spine. Spine 2:185, 1977
6. Breig A: The therapeutic possibilities of surgical bioengineering in incomplete spinal cord lesions. Paraplegia 9:173, 1972
7. Cochran T, Irstam L, Nachemson A: Long term anatomic and functional changes in patients with adolescent idiopathic scoliosis treated by Harrington rod fusion. Spine 8:576–584, 1983
8. Dewald RL, Fister JS, Savino AW: The management of unstable burst fractures of the thoracolumbar spine. Presented at the annual meeting of the Scoliosis Research Society, Denver, Colorado, September 1982
9. Dickson JH, Harrington PR, Erwin WD: Results of reduction and stabilization of the severely fractured thoracic and lumbar spine. J Bone Joint Surg [Am] 60:799, 1978
9a. Dunn HK: Anterior spine stabilization and decompression for thoracolumbar injuries. Orthop Clin North Am 17:113–119, 1986
10. Dwyer AF: Experience of anterior correction of scoliosis. Clin Orthop 93:191, 1973
11. Flynn JC, Hoque MA: Anterior fusion of the lumbar spine. J Bone Joint Surg [Am] 61:1143, 1979
12. Frankel HL, Hancock DO, Hyslop G et al: The value of postural reduction in the initial management of closed injuries of the spine with paraplegia and tetraplegia: Part 1. Paraplegia 7:179, 1969
13. Freebody B, Bendal R, Taylor RD: Anterior transperitoneal lumbar fusion. J Bone Joint Surg [Br] 53:617, 1971
14. Goldner JL, McCollum DE, Urbaniak JR: Anterior disc excision and interbody spine fusion for chronic low back pain. In American Academy of Orthopaedic Surgeons (ed): Symposium of the Spine III. St. Louis, CV Mosby, 1969
15. Guttmann L: Initial treatment of traumatic paraplegia. Proceedings of the Royal Society of Medicine 47:1103, 1954
16. Guttmann L: Spinal deformities in traumatic paraplegics and tetraplegics following surgical procedures. Paraplegia 7:38, 1969
17. Hall JE, Micheli LJ: The use of modified Dwyer instrumentation in anterior stabilization of the spine. Presented at the annual meeting of the Scoliosis Research Society, Hong Kong, October 1977
18. Harmon PH: Anterior extra peritoneal disc excision and vertebral body fusion. Clin Orthop 18:169, 1960
19. Harrington PR: Treatment of scoliosis. J Bone Joint Surg [Am] 44:591, 1962
20. Hodgson AR, Stock FE: Anterior spinal fusion: A preliminary communication on radical treatment of Pott's disease and Pott's paraplegia. Br J Surg 44:266–275, 1956
21. Kaneda K, Abume K, Fujiya M: Burst fractures with

neurologic defects of the thoracolumbar-lumbar spine: Results of anterior decompression and stabilization with anterior instrumentation. Spine 9:788–795, 1984

21a. Kostuik JP: Anterior fixation for burst fractures of the thoracic and lumbar spine with or without neurological involvement. Spine 13:286–293, 1988

22. Kostuik JP: Anterior Kostuik–Harrington distraction systems for the treatment of kyphotic deformities. The Iowa Orthopedic Journal 8:68–77, 1988

23. Kostuik JP: Anterior spinal cord decompression for lesions of the thoracic and lumbar spine: Techniques, new methods of internal fixation, results. Spine 8:512–531, 1983

24. Kostuik JP: Anterior fixation for fractures of the thoracic and lumbar spine with or without neurologic involvement. Clin Orthop 189:103–115, 1984

25. Malcolm BW, Bradford DS, Winter RB, Chou SN: Post-traumatic kyphosis. J Bone Joint Surg [Am] 63:891, 1981

26. Moon MS, Kim I, Woo YK et al: Anterior interbody fusion in fractures and fracture dislocations of the spine. Int Orthop 5:143, 1981

27. Morgan TH, Wharton GW, Austin GN: The results of laminectomy in patients with incomplete spinal cord injuries. Paraplegia 9:14, 1971

28. Nicholl EA: Fractures of the dorso-lumbar spine. J Bone Joint Surg [Br] 31:376, 1949

29. Paul RL, Michael RH, Dunn JE, Williams JP: Anterior transthoracic surgical decompression of acute spinal cord injuries. J Neurosurg 43:299, 1975

30. Rezaian SM, Dombrowski ET, Ghista DN: Spinal fixator for the management of spinal injury: The mechanical rationale. Eng Med 12:95, 1983

31. Riska EB: Antero-lateral decompression as a treatment of paraplegia following a vertebral fracture in the thoraco-lumbar spine. Int Orthop 1:22, 1977

32. Roberts JB, Curtis PH Jr: Stability of the thoracic and lumbar spine in traumatic paraplegia following fracture or fracture dislocation. J Bone Joint Surg [Am] 52:1115, 1970

33. Royle ND: The operative removal of an accessory vertebra. Australian Medical Journal 1:467, 1928

34. Sacks S: Anterior interbody fusion of the lumbar spine. J Bone Joint Surg [Br] 47:211, 1965

35. Sacks S: Anterior interbody fusion of the lumbar spine: Indications and results in two hundred cases. Clin Orthop 44:163, 1966

36. Slot GH: A new distraction system for the correction of kyphosis using the anterior approach. Presented at the Scoliosis Research Society, Montreal, Quebec, Canada, September 1981

37. Stauffer RN, Coventry MB: Anterior interbody lumbar spine fusion: Analysis of Mayo Clinic series. J Bone Joint Surg [Am] 54:756, 1972

38. White AA III, Panjabi M, Thomas CL: The clinical biomechanics of kyphotic deformities. Clin Orthop 128:8–17, 1977

39. Whitesides TE Jr.: Traumatic kyphosis of the thoracolumbar spine. Clin Orthop, 128:78, 1977

40. Whitesides TE Jr., Shah SGA: The management of unstable fractures of the thoracolumbar spine. Spine 1:99, 1976

41. Yosipovitch Z, Robin GC, Makin M: Open reduction of unstable thoracolumbar spinal injuries and fixation with Harrington rods. J Bone Joint Surg [Am] 59:1003, 1977

42. Zielke K: Ventral derotation spondylodese: Behandlungsergebnisse bein idiopathischen lumbarskoliosen. Orthopade 120:320–329, 1982

11

POSTERIOR PEDICULAR SCREW TECHNIQUES

Stephen I. Esses

Drew A. Bednar

ANATOMY OF THE PEDICLE

The pedicle is a tubelike bony structure that connects the anterior and posterior columns of the spine. The angle between the long axis of the pedicle and the sagittal plane varies considerably at the different thoracic and lumbar levels.[3] For example, at T-12 the pedicle is almost parallel to the sagittal plane, whereas at L-5 the angle measures approximately 30 degrees. There is a general trend for the angle between the pedicle and sagittal plane to increase as one proceeds cranially or caudally from the T-12 level. The pedicle in cross section is not a circle; the horizontal diameter is smaller than the vertical diameter. The horizontal or minor diameter increases in the lower lumbar vertebrae. The mean minor diameter at L-1 is approximately 7 mm and at L-5 is about 10 mm.[13]

Medial to the medial wall of the pedicle lies the dural sac. Inferior to the pedicle is the nerve root in the intervertebral foramen. Because the lumbar roots are usually situated in the upper one third of the foramen, it is more dangerous to penetrate the pedicle inferiorly as compared to superiorly.

LOCALIZATION OF THE PEDICLE

A variety of techniques have been used to localize the pedicle intraoperatively for screw insertion. Many surgeons continue to use an image intensifier when drilling and placing screws down the pedicle. This method has the advantage of allowing the surgeon to be certain of correct screw placement in both the anteroposterior and lateral planes while performing the procedure. There are, however, disadvantages. These include the awkwardness of obtaining biplanar image intensifier views during surgery, increased risk of infection, radiation exposure to patient and surgeon, and a tendency to rely on imaging rather than anatomy during this step of surgery.

We have relied on anatomic landmarks for localizing the starting points during pedicular drilling and screwing. Static radiographs are taken to confirm accurate placement of the fixation device. We routinely use three techniques for localization of the pedicular starting points. These are referred to as the intersection technique, pars technique, and accessory process technique.

INTERSECTION TECHNIQUE

The transverse processes and pedicles lie in the same axial plane. This is easily appreciated when looking at an anteroposterior radiograph of the lumbar spine or an axial computed tomographic scan at the level of the pedicle. The pedicle is located in a sagittal plane just lateral to the lumbar facet joints. For this reason a line dropped from the lateral aspect of the facet joint will intersect a line that bisects the transverse process at a spot overlying the pedicle (Fig. 11-1). Because there is

variability in the relevant anatomy from patient to patient, it is essential that the surgeon examine the radiographs preoperatively to assess the relationship of the pedicle both to the transverse process and to the facet joint. In this way an accurate intersection can be assessed intraoperatively. We routinely move the facet joints in question in order to more thoroughly assess their orientation intraoperatively.

PARS TECHNIQUE

The pars interarticularis is that area of bone where the pedicle coalesces to the lamina. Since the lamina and the pars interarticularis can be easily identified at the time of surgery, they provide landmarks by which a pedicular starting point can be made. Intraoperatively a cob is swept up the lamina of the vertebra in question and out to the pars interarticularis. Drilling from this point permits easy entry into the pedicle.

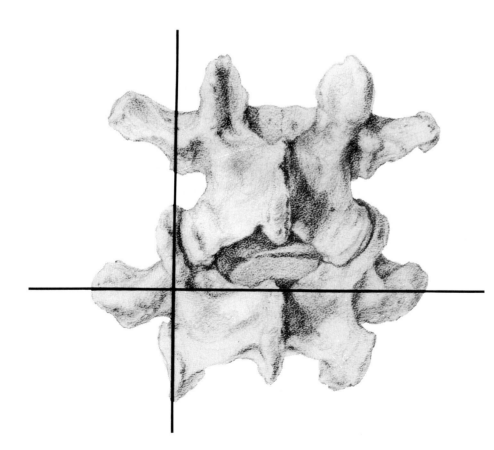

Figure 11-1. The intersection technique. A line bisecting the transverse process and a line marking the lateral aspect of the facet joint intersect at a spot overlying the pedicle.

ACCESSORY PROCESS TECHNIQUE

In many patients there is a small prominence of bone at the base of the transverse process. This accessory process can be used as a starting site for pedicular drilling (Fig. 11-2). It must be appreciated, however, that the accessory process is a more lateral starting point than that identified using the intersection technique, which is in turn a more lateral starting point than the pars interarticularis. For this reason, a different angle must be used when drilling from these three sites (Fig. 11-3). The computed tomographic scan is an invaluable aid in assessing the angle of the pedicle to the sagittal plane. This information is invaluable in deciding what angle to drill at.

PEDICULAR DRILLING

The most important aspect of pedicular fixation is adequate preoperative planning. As previously mentioned, an anteroposterior radiograph allows the surgeon to accurately identify the relationship of the pedicle to both the transverse process and the facet joint. A computed tomographic scan, if available, allows assessment of the angle of the pedicle to the sagittal plane. Both of these imaging studies should be displayed in the operating room for easy reference. We routinely draw the pedicle, transverse process, and facet joint in grease pencil on the radiographs preoperatively. At the time of

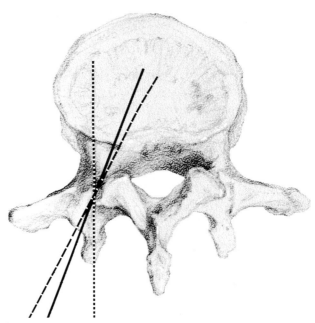

Figure 11-3. The drill angle will vary depending on the starting point selected. The pars technique uses a medial starting point and the drill approximates the sagittal plane (short-dotted line). The accessory process technique is the most lateral, and the drill must, therefore, aim medially (long-dotted line). The intersection technique starts between the other two (solid line).

surgery, all three anatomic methods of localization are used for each pedicle. In this way, a clear image of the pedicle and its orientation can be imagined by the surgeon.

A hand drill is placed at the starting point and is used to perforate the posterior cortex. The use of a hand drill provides tactile feedback to the surgeon. By drilling a small portion and then pushing with the drill, the surgeon can ensure that he remains in bone.

When the hand drill is removed, a depth gauge is placed in the hole. The depth gauge is used to palpate the hole and ensure that it is in the pedicle. Palpation medially ensures that there is no breach of the cortex into the spinal canal. Palpation inferiorly ensures that the neural foramen has not been embarrassed. Palpation laterally ensures that the drill has not gone out the side of the pedicle or vertebral body. With palpation the surgeon should be confident that the drilled hole is within the bony confines of the pedicular tube.

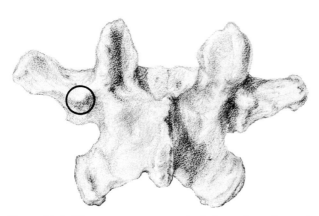

Figure 11-2. The accessory process technique. A small prominence of bone at the base of the transverse process marks a drilling point for the pedicle.

The appropriate screw is now inserted down the drilled hole. Depending upon which instrumentation system is being used, the screw length may be predetermined. In instances in which screw length is variable, an assessment of the distance from the posterior arch of the vertebral body to its anterior cortex must be estimated. Studies have shown that in the lumbar spine this distance is rarely less than 40 mm.[3] There has been some question in the past as to the necessity of breaching the anterior cortex to gain additional screw purchase. We believe that the anterior cortex should not be drilled or screwed. This avoids any possible injury to the great vessels anteriorly. As the screw is being placed down the pedicle and into the vertebral body, the surgeon will feel increased purchase as the screw tip enters the anterior third of the vertebral body. Cancellous bone is most dense in this area of the vertebral body and provides more than adequate fixation.

Radiographs are now taken in the anteroposterior and lateral planes. These radiographs are used for confirmation of accurate screw placement. As previously mentioned, the surgeon should be well aware that he is in the pedicle by palpation with the depth gauge prior to screw insertion. Radiographs provide confirmation and documentation for the patients' records.

SCREW–ROD SYSTEMS

FIXATEUR INTERNE

The prototype of the pedicle screw and rod systems is the external spinal skeletal fixator, which was designed by Fritz Magerl.[12] This instrumentation system was used initially in the treatment of thoracolumbar fractures, and allowed reduction of fractures while immobilizing only one level above and below the affected vertebra. The advantages of this implant were readily apparent and thus, together with Walter Dick, the instrumentation was modified so that it became completely implantable.[5] The fixateur interne (internal fixator) uses 5.0 mm Schantz screws placed down the pedicles and connected with 7.0 mm flattened stain-

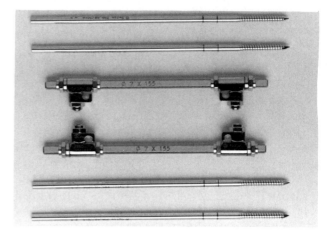

Figure 11-4. The AO spinal internal fixator.

less steel rods (Fig. 11-4). The coupling mechanism between the Schantz screws and the rods is mobile in the sagittal plane and thus allows for restoration of kyphosis and lordosis. The system itself can be maintained in distraction, compression, or neutralization.

The stability of this instrumentation has been tested by Dick and associates.[5] They found that the range of elasticity of the device itself was approximately 40 Nm anterior bending moment. It is interesting to note that between 40 and 70 nm a slight permanent deformation occurs without loosening at the coupling device. This has been noted in one of our clinical cases.

The great advantage of the fixateur interne is that the Schantz screws provide very long lever arms, facilitating reduction maneuvers. By opposing the posterior ends of these screws, lordosis can be created. Distraction of the Schantz screws restores vertebral body height without causing concomitant kyphosis.

The fixateur interne has been used most successfully for the treatment of thoracolumbar fractures.[2,4] There have been very few technical complications with this system. There has been an attempt to increase the indications for this system. It would appear that the fixateur interne also provides very stable fixation in cases of multilevel segmental instability and following multilevel decompression.[1] There has also been some work using the fixateur interne for the correction of spondylolisthesis.[6] The results are not as impressive as those for fractures. In one series it was possible to improve the slippage grade in only 50% of cases.

OTHER SCREW–ROD SYSTEMS

A number of new screw–rod systems are emerging from the biomechanics laboratories of several major centers. Notable are the so-called Long Beach system being developed by Wiltze, on which there is as yet no design or biomechanical data available[7]; the pedicular screw–rod coupling component of Eduardo Luque's new system[11]; the Kostuik–Harrington system as adapted for pedicular fixation, for which preliminary clinical data, but no biomechanics are available;[*] and the Vermont spinal fixator, or VSF, described by Krag and associates,[8] for which again no clinical data is presented. All of these systems remain in the preliminary stages of development at the time of writing, and they will therefore not be described in detail; the reader should be aware of ongoing alternate system development and be prepared to follow the literature scrupulously as these systems are pioneered.

SCREW–PLATE SYSTEMS

ROY-CAMILLE PLATES

This French-designed spinal plating system, designed to be used in conjunction with pedicular and facet screws, is the predecessor of most modern pedicular screw–plate fixation systems. This system has been in clinical use since 1963, and a generous body of clinical material with an impressive follow-up has evolved to support its merits.[14]

The Roy-Camille system consists of precontoured spinal plates that are designed for use throughout the length of the thoracic and lumbosacral spine. These plates are perforated by screw holes at intervals of 13 mm, felt anatomically to correspond to alternate pedicle and facet purchase points. The screw holes are collared to min-

imize the mechanical stress necessarily engendered by creating a screw hole in a plate and to increase the uniformity of stiffness of the plates.

The pedicular screw design to complement this plating system is a 4- or 4.5-mm diameter screw ranging in length from 32 to 46 mm. Optional 18-mm screws designed for facet purchase in alternate screw holes are available.[13]

The Roy-Camille plate is a rather flexible device with a plastic deformation limit of only 11.3 Nm.[9,10] This is significantly less than the probable maximum in vivo bending moment in the lumbar spine.

System rigidity is also compromised by the lack of a fixed couple between the screws and plate. This system is intended for application using the 4-point fixation principle, which necessarily immobilizes normal motion segments above and below any index level.[13,14] This system is intended to be used in conjunction with posterior and/or posterolateral grafting of index motion segments, with a normal motion segment above and below that is immobilized but not fused and theoretically regains mobility at the time of implant removal.[13]

This system is also intended for use with a postoperative thoracolumbar corset or Minerva jacket. Relevant clinical material is scantily reviewed in the North American literature.[14] This system's originator reports a 75% rate of acceptable fracture reduction with less than 5 degrees of residual kyphotic deformity in a series of 84 fractures, virtually uniform success in posterior lumbosacral fusion, and similarly impressive results in spondylolisthesis and the surgical management of tumors. There is a 25% incidence of proximal or distalmost screw failure occurring between 5 and 24 months postoperatively, suggesting that the implant should be removed at approximately 6 months.

This is a flexible system designed for 4-point fixation and postoperative orthotic immobilization. There is no definitive long-term clinical follow-up material available in the North American literature.

This system does not appear to be in very widespread use despite its longevity. The requirement for multilevel instrumentation and postoperative use of heavy casts or braces may be factors.

* Kostuik JP: Personal communication.

STEFFEE PEDICULAR SCREW–PLATE SYSTEM

The Steffee system is one of specialized plates and modified cancellous pedicular screws. It has evolved over the past decade in response to the perceived limitations of standard fracture plates as a posterior spinal fixation modality.

Despite a specialized double nut fixation of the screw to the plate in an attempt to increase rigidity, the rigidity of the Steffee system remains such that it must be used with a 4-point fixation system.[17] This necessitates immobilization of normal motion segments above and below any index level. There is also the theoretical problem of a plate limiting the bony surface area available for fusion.

The screw is a modified cancellous bone screw, ranging in diameter from 5.5 to 7.0 mm and in length from 55 to 110 mm. It is mated through a pair of specialized nuts to a nested slotted plate system (Fig. 11-5). The plates are 16 mm wide and range in length from 44 to 196 mm. Early designs were constructed of standard surgical steel, but ongoing implant development with the study of titanium-based components is in progress.

This system has been used primarily in North America and seems to be gaining popularity in the orthopedic community. It remains a relatively new system, and clinical material in the literature and follow-up are limited.

Early results are, however, encouraging. The developers cite an average operating time of 3 to 4 hours with a hospital stay of 11.8 days for fusions of long lumbosacral segments after decompression in cases of spinal stenosis. Preliminary results of the developers' series indicate a rate of 90% excellent to good functional clinical results. Complications cited in the initial 120 cases include eight cases of implant failure and five pseudarthroses.[17] There were seven deep wound infections and two cases of nerve root impingement attributed to bone graft. The clinical results of the application of this implant system to spinal surgery remain, at this point, extremely preliminary. There is no well-documented series of even short-term results in the literature at this time.

A series of 14 cases of reduction and fusion for high grade spondylolisthesis has recently been published.[16] The Steffee plate has proven effective in obtaining reduction of slippage, but an interbody fusion is necessary for maintenance of this reduction. Four-point implant fixation and two-point sacral fixation are required. The follow-up in this series is indeterminant.[16] In a series of 36 posterior lumbar interbody fusions performed with

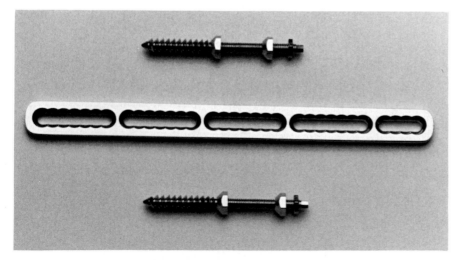

Figure 11-5. The Steffee screw–plate system.

the Steffee plate having a minimum follow-up of 6 months, there was a 92% success rate, with three patients continuing to have back pain after fusion, two dural tears incurred, and one screw breakage.[15] The maximum follow-up in this series is again only 1 year and results remain preliminary.

OTHER SCREW–PLATE SYSTEMS

Notched plates have been developed by the AO/ASIF group (Fig. 11-6). They come in a variety of lengths, with a profile measuring 6 × 11 mm. These plates have been designed to accept 4.5-mm cortical screws and 6.5-mm cancellous bone screws. There is a very short distance between the screw holes, so that there is rarely a very big discrepancy between the starting point for a pedicle screw and a hole in the plate through which the screw must be inserted.

Luque has recently developed a screw–plate system.[11] The distinguishing characteristic of his design is that the screws are cannulated. Blunt-ended wires are drilled down the pedicle. The blunt tip ensures that the wire does not penetrate the cortex of the pedicle. After radiographs are taken to ensure proper location of the wires, screws can be placed down the pedicle over the guide wire. Long screwdrivers are used to manipulate the position of the vertebral column once the screws have good purchase. These "joysticks" allow restoration of lordosis in cases of burst fractures.

SUMMARY

Systems incorporating pedicular fixation are still in a state of evolution. In order to avoid any catastrophic complications due to misplacement of the pedicle screw, the ideal system must allow the screw insertion site to be unrestricted. This is not achieved with plate systems, as obviously every pedicle screw must go through a plate hole. The Steffee and Luque systems both have modified plate designs in an effort to overcome this problem.

Screw–rod systems have the advantage of allowing the screw insertion site to be unrestricted. This, however, results in each system needing to have a coupling apparatus to attach the screw end to the rod. Many of these are bulky and thus increase the risk of wound healing problems. The coupling system of the AO fixateur interne is palpable in the upper lumbar spine if the patient is thin.

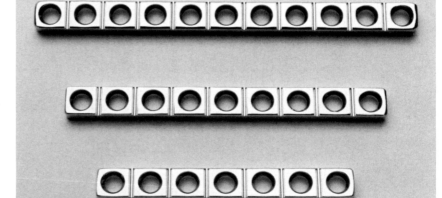

Figure 11-6. AO notched spinal plates.

Biomechanical data demonstrates the superiority of pedicular screw fixation over any hook design. It remains a challenge to perfect an instrumentation system that uses this biomechanical strength in a simple and safe manner.

REFERENCES

1. Aebi M, Etter C, Kehl T, Thalgott J: The internal spinal skeletal fixation system: A new treatment of thoracolumbar fractures and other spinal disorders. Clin Orthop 227:30–43, 1988
2. Aebi M, Etter C, Kehl T, Thalgott J: Stabilization of the lower thoracic and lumbar spine with the internal spinal skeletal fixator system: Indications, techniques and first results of treatment. Spine 12:544–551, 1987
3. Berry JL, Moran JM, Berg WS, Steffee AD: A morphometric study of human lumbar and skeletal thoracic vertebrae. Spine 12:362–367, 1987
4. Dick W: The "fixateur interne" as a versatile implant for spine surgery. Spine 12:882–900, 1987
5. Dick W, Kluger P, Magerl F et al: A new device for internal fixation of thoracolumbar and lumbar spine fractures: The fixateur interne. Paraplegia 23:225–232, 1985
6. Esses SI: The spinal internal fixator. Presented at the annual meeting of the North American Spine Society, Colorado Springs, July 1988
7. Field BT, Wiltse LL, Zindrick MR et al: The Long Beach spinal fixation system. Presented at the 2nd annual meeting of the North American Spine Association. Niguel, California, July 1985
8. Krag MH, Beynnon BD, Pope MH et al: Internal fixator for posterior application to short segments of the thoracic, lumbar or lumbosacral spine. Clin Orthop 203:75–98, 1986
9. Lavaste F: Biomechanique du rachis dorso-lumbaire, pp 19–23. In Deuxieme Journees d'Orthopedie de la Pitie. Paris, Masson, 1980
10. Lavaste F: Etude des implant rachibiens: Memoire de biomechanique. Engineering thesis. Ecole Nationale des Arts et Metiers à Paris, 1979
11. Luque ER: Interpeduncular segmental fixation. Clin Orthop 203:54–57, 1986
12. Magerl FP: Stabilization of the lower thoracic and lumbar spine with external skeletal fixation. Clin Orthop 189:125, 1984
13. Roy-Camille R, Saillant G, Mazel CH: Internal fixation of the lumbar spine with pedicle screw plating. Clin Orthop 203:7–17, 1986
14. Roy-Camille R, Saillant G, Mazel CH et al: Posterior spinal fixation with transpedicular screws and plates. Display handout for American Academy of Orthopaedic Surgeons. Paris, Groupe Hospitalier la Pitie Salpetiere, 1987
15. Steffee AD, Sitkowski DJ: Posterior lumbar interbody fusion and plates. Clin Orthop 227:99–102, 1988
16. Steffee AD, Sitkowski DJ: Reduction and stabilization of grade IV spondylolisthesis. Clin Orthop 227:82–89, 1988
17. Steffee AD, Biscup RS, Stitlowski DJ et al: Segmental spine plates with pedicle screw fixation: A new internal fixation device for disorders of the lumbar and thoracolumbar spine. Clin Orthop 203:45–54, 1986

12

STANDARD POSTERIOR TECHNIQUES IN THE TREATMENT OF THORACIC AND LUMBAR SPINE FRACTURES

Thomas J. Errico
James O'Neill

The surgical management of thoracic and lumbar spine fractures is an exciting and evolving area of spinal surgery. The decision-making process involves judgments regarding present and potential neurologic deficits as well as short- and long-term stability of the spinal column. This requires precise understanding and evaluation of neurologic function, neuropathologic compression, and pathomechanics of injury patterns as evidenced by existing levels of bony disruption.

The function of the spine is to provide bony support to house and protect the neural elements. When applied pathologic forces disrupt the structural integrity of the spine, the prevailing deforming forces produce the specific fracture pattern. Fracture patterns vary not only with respect to the amount and duration of the applied force but also with respect to the level of the spine to which the force is applied. Simplistically, reversing the deforming forces should reduce spinal fracture deformity. The accomplished spinal surgeon, with his implant armamentarium, seeks to restore appropriate anteroposterior and lateral translational and rotational correction while maintaining reasonable sagittal plane contours. Solid fusions for long-term stability are performed over the minimum necessary motion segments, preserving as much normal spinal motion as possible. When successfully completed and combined with appropriate decompression, the spinal injured patient is left with the maximum potential for neurologic recovery and the least likelihood for acute or chronic instability.

EVOLUTION OF POSTERIOR TECHNIQUES

The modern era of instrumentation of spinal fractures began with the use of the dual Harrington distraction rod in traumatic injuries.[15] Without doubt, the use of Harrington instrumentation allowed for effective restoration of vertebral body height.[3,17,25,38,40,45] However, shortcomings of the system became readily apparent. While distraction in the lumbar spine adequately restored collapsed vertebral body height, it also eliminated normal lumbar lordosis. The result was iatrogenic lumbar kyphosis ("flat back syndrome").[33] Various modifications to Harrington distraction rods were performed in order minimize the loss of lordosis. The addition to a Harrington construct of a heavy-gauge stainless steel tension band between adjacent spinous processes has been used to help preserve lordosis in the lumbar region.[21] Similarly, in the lumbar region a single midline compression rod has been used between a dual Harrington rod construct to help preserve lordosis.[30,45] The use of lordotically contoured square-ended rods in square hooks, however, was judged to be not sufficient in preserving lordosis.[7]

A further shortcoming of the Harrington system was lack of segmental fixation to the spine and loss of correction. Because the spine is viscoelastic, a distraction system anchored at each end of several spinal segments loses fixation with time. As the spine relaxes there may be translational motion between segments and loss of sagittal plane contours. The adaptation of Luque rod instrumentation and sublaminar wiring represents an attempt to solve these problems (Fig. 12-1).[36] Segmental instrumentation as popularized by Eduardo Luque permits direct application of transverse forces, which helps reduce deformity and maintain alignment in each plane.[49] While there is no inherent distraction mechanism in the instrumentation, use of a Harrington outrigger to supply distraction at the time of reduction is suggested. In burst injuries, however, the inability of the system to maintain distraction has led to unacceptably high complication rates.[1]

The use of sublaminar wires with Harrington distraction rods represented a compromise construct (Fig. 12-2).[49] This proved to have biome-

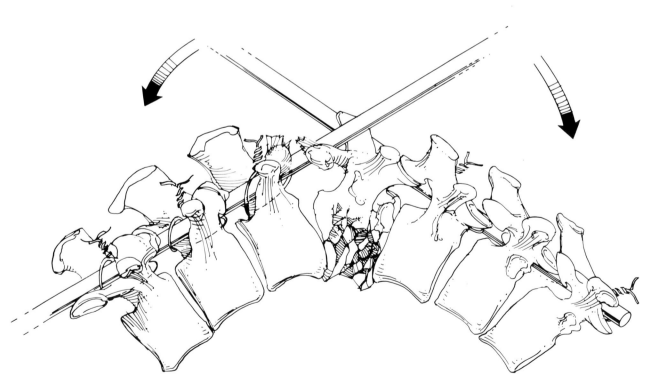

Figure 12-1. Reduction Maneuver using L rods and sublaminar wires.

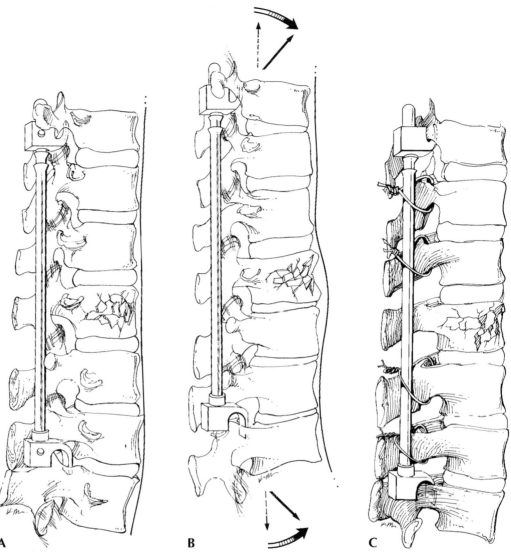

Figure 12-2. (*A*) Correction of the fracture deformity with distraction rods. (*B*) Settling of the fracture fragments after viscous and elastic relation of the anterior longitudinal ligament. (*C*) Prevention of settling of fracture fragments by the addition of segmental wire fixation to the Harrington rods. (From Wenger DR, Carollo JJ: The mechanics of thoracolumbar fractures stabilized by segmental fixation. Clin Orthop 189:89–96, 1984.)

chanical advantages in stability over the simple dual rod technique with regard to resisting axial loading, lateral bending, and forward flexion loading. The rotational stability was particularly improved.[41] The passage of sublaminar wires, however, must be approached with special skill and caution in spinal injury in which there are swollen neural structures or areas of canal compromise. This potential complication may be sidestepped with the use of segmental interspinous process wiring.[16]

A further refinement of three-point fixation with standard Harrington rods has been the addition of high-density polyethylene sleeves to the rod (Fig. 12-3).[17] The rod sleeves are potential space fillers that slide over the rod at strategic locations. The rod sleeve corrects post-traumatic kyphosis by producing an extension moment at the apex of the deformity. Theoretically, a dynamic anterior force is maintained as the spinal rod is bent within its elastic range, compensating for anterior ligament stress–relaxation. Additionally, proponents state, the anterior force from the sleeve is directed through the underlying pedicle to push the posteriorly displaced vertebral body forward. Obviously, the sleeves must not be placed over areas of fractured posterior arches due to possible impalement of laminar fragments into the canal. In this type of situation the sleeves must bridge the fractured segment on intact lamina above and below.

In a clever total departure from the Harrington rod, the locking hook spinal rod was devised by Jacobs (Fig. 12-4).[27,28] This system has several attractive concepts. The rod is locked to the hooks by a system of nuts that prevents spinning of the rod in the hooks. The contour of the rod can thus be kept in the proper plane. Also, the upper hook has a sliding cover that locks the lamina in the hook, providing security against upper hook cutout. Distraction is provided in gentle gradations by the threaded portion of the rod. The potential for overdistraction where the anterior longitudinal ligament is disrupted is therefore avoided. Without the notches of the Harrington distraction rod, the Jacobs rod is stronger, and rod fractures well-known to occur at the rod–rachet junction are avoided.

Cotrel–Dubousset instrumentation is not a totally new instrumentation system. Rather, it represents a confluence of concepts evolved from experience with preceding instrumentations. The instrumentation consists of a knurled rod featuring a diamond cross-cut pattern. The system allows for a wide variety of closed and open hooks that be can attached to the rod in any direction or rotation. Parallel rods are cross-connected by transverse loading devices to form a rectangular construct. The versatility of hook placement and hook fixation to the rod allows for selective and three-dimensional correction of spinal malalignment and maintenance of the correction. The capabilities of the system allow it to be used in a wide variety of fracture patterns. Because the system is relatively new, a large experience with fractures has not yet been reported.

As can be seen, the surgeon has a wide range of choices in preoperative selection of an implant system for any given fracture. By recognizing the mechanisms of each injury pattern the surgeon can select an appropriate implant and reduction maneuver. It is important to recognize that there is no one best implant system or reduction method for every fracture type. More than one system can be used in any given fracture pattern. As long as the operating surgeon reverses the prevailing deforming forces without creating iatrogenic injury, restores proper spinal alignment, and stabilizes the spine until fusion can take place, clinical success can be accomplished.

The mechanistic classification of thoracolumbar spine fractures proposed by Ferguson and Allen,[20] as well as the three-column theory of Denis,[12] will serve as a framework for the discussion of specific fracture patterns in which posterior rod techniques may be used.

COMPRESSIVE FLEXION INJURIES

Spinal fractures induced by eccentric loading of the flexed spine result in compressive stress through the anterior spinal column and tension strain through the middle and posterior columns. Stage 1 (CFS1) injuries spare the middle and posterior column.[20] If there is less than 50% loss of anterior body height and lack of posterior disruption, these fractures are usually treated conservatively.[31,34,38,46,50]

Stage 2 (CFS2) involves the posterior column in addition to the anterior column (Fig. 12-5). The *(Text continued on p. 315)*

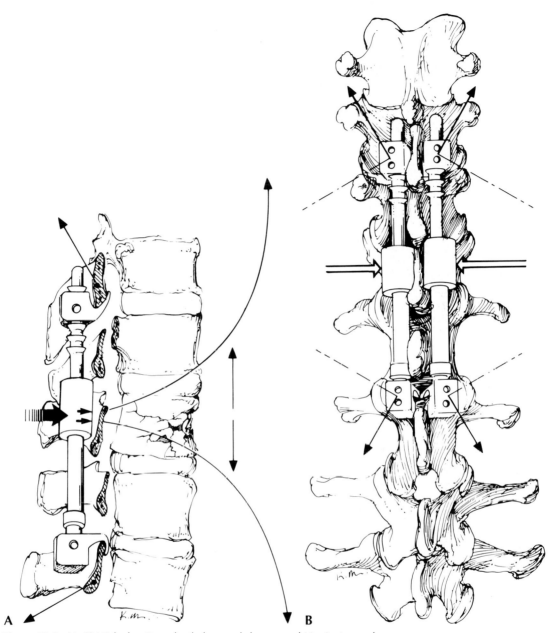

Figure 12-3. (*A, B*) High-density polyethylene rod sleeves and Harrington rods.

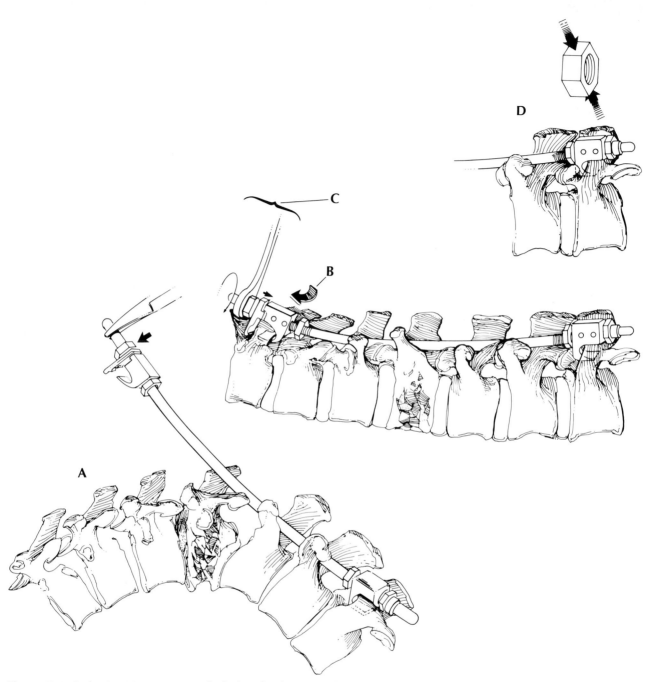

Figure 12-4. Reduction Maneuver using the locking hook spinal rod. (*A*) The lower hook is inserted first and reduction is performed by downward force on the top of the rod. (*B*) The upper hook is inserted under the lamina and advanced along the rod. (*C*) After radiographic confirmation of reduction the sliding cover is advanced along the top of the lamina, locking it to the hook. (*D*) The nut collars are crimped onto the flat sides of the rod.

key element of this fracture is the integrity of the middle column. Instability results when there is greater than 50% loss of anterior vertebral height or disruption of posterior elements, as evidenced on plain radiographs or computed tomography. Surgical stabilization is performed to prevent early or late deformity.[32] Harrington distraction rods have been used to successfully stabilize this injury.[16,21,28,30,38] Three-point fixation is relied on to help restore anterior body height and to stabilize the posterior disruption. However, as long as the middle column remains intact a simple compression system will reduce the anterior kyphotic deformity. The intact middle column is used as a hinge to reverse the tensile disruption of the posterior elements (Fig. 12-6).

Compressive flexion stage 3 (CFS3) injuries include middle column disruption, for a highly unstable three-column injury pattern. Characteristically, the middle column fails in tension, resulting in distraction of the posterior vertebral wall (Fig. 12-7).[19,20] The posterosuperior margin of the vertebral body may be rotated into the canal to various degrees, causing confusion with a burst fracture. Harrington distraction instrumentation has most commonly been used in these fractures.[20,22,47,51] A reduction maneuver with three-point fixation is necessary to reduce the kyphotic deformity without pushing the disrupted middle column into the canal (Fig. 12-8). When properly performed, ligamentaxis should partially reduce

(*Text continued on p. 319*)

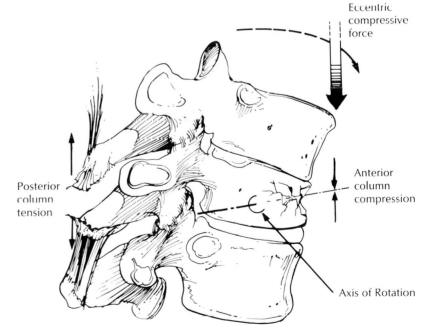

Figure 12-5. An example of a CFS2 injury in the thoracic spine, in which greater than 50% compression of the anterior column has occurred. There is failure of the posterior ligamentous structures under tension, resulting in spinous process widening. The key to this fracture is integrity of the middle column.

Eccentric compressive force

Posterior column tension

Anterior column compression

Axis of Rotation

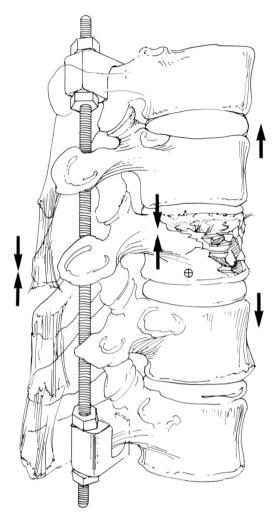

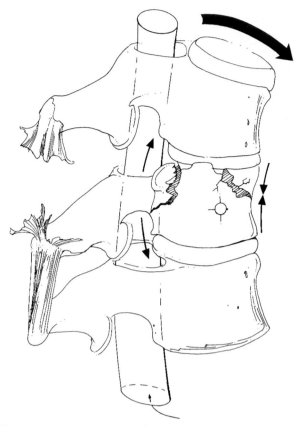

Figure 12-6. Compression instrumentation reduction of a CFS2 injury. Compression of the posterior elements provides a pivoting force anteriorly, with the middle column serving as a fulcrum. There must be no bony or disk disruption in the middle column because compression could produce disk or bony retropulsion into the canal. Preoperative evaluation with adequate bone and soft-tissue imaging of the middle column is imperative. During intraoperative reduction consideration should be given to spinal cord monitoring and/or a wake-up test.

Figure 12-7. In a CFS3 injury there is tension failure of the middle column in addition to anterior and posterior disruption. The posterosuperior margin of the vertebral body may be rotated into the canal to various degrees. Any extension with compression posteriorly may cause the middle fragment to be forced deeper into the neural canal. An extension moment with distraction is necessary to reduce this fracture and prevent further neurologic injury.

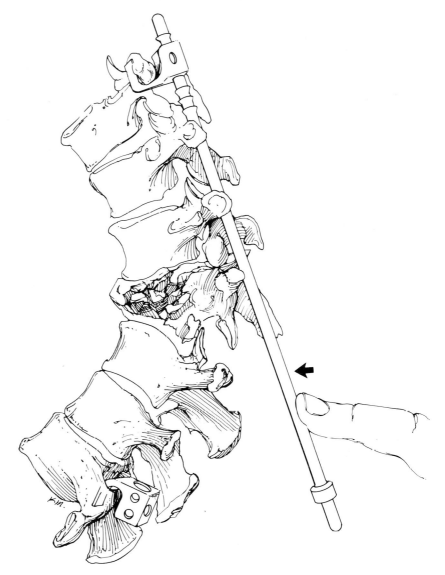

Figure 12-8. Three-point fixation using Harrington distraction rods. Each individual rod provides three points of fixation to the spine. Two are at the hook sites and the third is on an intact lamina at the apex of the deformity. Proper contouring of the rods will allow for sufficient anteriorly directed force at the apex of the kyphos to perform reduction. It will also allow insertion of the collar end of the rod into the hook with laminar failure. To create adequate lever arms for reducing and stabilizing these fractures it is best to secure the hook sites at least three segments above and two segments below the fracture site.

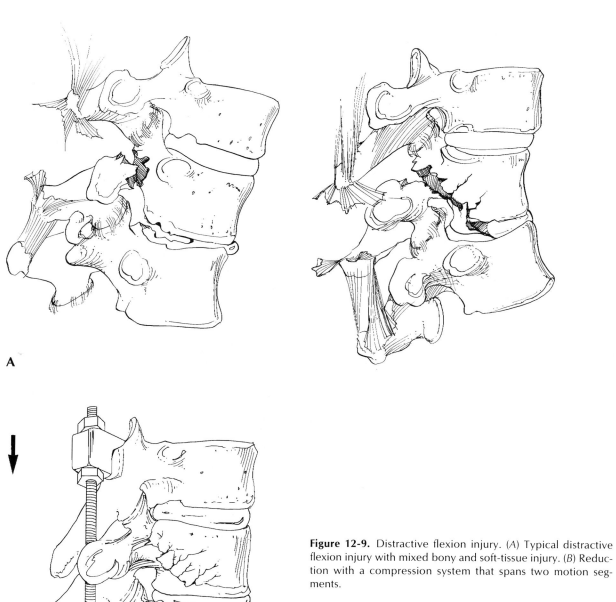

A

B

Figure 12-9. Distractive flexion injury. (*A*) Typical distractive flexion injury with mixed bony and soft-tissue injury. (*B*) Reduction with a compression system that spans two motion segments.

retropulsed fragments in the canal.[34] Other posterior rod techniques can be used with equal effectiveness.

DISTRACTIVE FLEXION INJURIES

A spinal fracture or dislocation occurring as a result of a distractive flexion force demonstrates tension failure of all three columns of the spine (Fig. 12-9A). Characteristically, the levels involved are located in the upper lumbar spine, usually ranging between T-12 and L-3.[12,23,24,29,35,44] The axis of rotation is anterior to the vertebral body, with rotation occurring in the sagittal plane.[4,9,26] The injury may go purely through bone, as in the original Chance fracture,[8,24] or through ligaments and disks alone. More commonly it is a combination of the two. Injuries completely or nearly completely through bone may be treated conservatively; they do not require surgical intervention.[24] The majority of distractive flexion injuries, however, are better treated with operative intervention.

A compression apparatus is obviously the treatment of choice. In its simplest conceptual form, an interspinous wire applies compression and creates a tension band across the injured segment. Harrington compression instrumentation will reduce the deformity in a more secure fashion and provide secure fixation (Fig. 12-9B).[5] Any stable compression system, such as Cotrel–Dubousset instrumentation applied in compression or Harrington reverse rachet rods, should be equally useful.

LATERAL FLEXION INJURIES

When lateral bending of the spine results in compression of the vertebral body and posterior elements unilaterally, a lateral flexion fracture may result.[20] There is unilateral shortening of vertebral body height with compressive failure of the posterior elements on the ipsilateral side (Fig. 12-10). Contralaterally, one sees tension failure of the bony and ligamentous structures on the convex side. A facet dislocation on the convexity may often be noted. With posterior element disruption the potential for long-term instability exists.

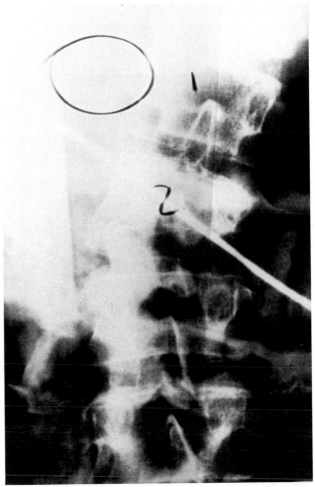

Figure 12-10. An L-2 lateral flexion injury in an 18-year-old man following a motor vehicle accident. There is a loss of vertebral body height in the concavity of the deformity. On the convex side a tension-induced fracture line through the pars interarticularis, lamina, and spinous process is noted. The patient was neurologically intact.

Biomechanically, the most logical construct is the combined use of a Harrington distraction rod on the concave side with a Harrington compression system on the convexity (Fig. 12-11).[10] Conceptually, the spinal injury model is loosely akin to a traumatically induced scoliotic deformity. Therefore, the myriad of constructs devised for correction and stabilization of the scoliotic deformity could all be useful in this injury pattern (Fig. 12-12).

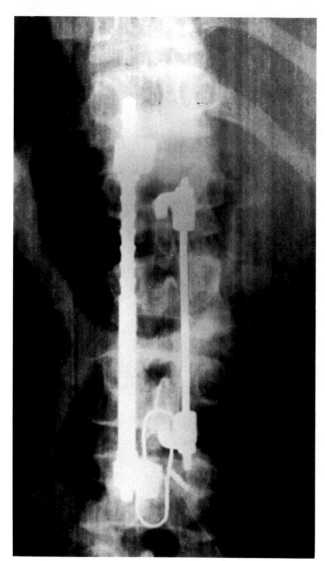

Figure 12-11. Same patient as in Figure 12-10. Postoperative restoration of alignment with a Harrington distraction rod placed in the concavity of the curve from T-12 to L-4 and a small Harrington threaded rod loaded in compression on the convexity of the curve from L-1 to L-3. The instrumentation provides reversal of the deforming forces. Note also the use of an interspinous wire between L-3 and L-4 in an effort to preserve lumbar lordosis. A posterolateral fusion was performed from L-1 to L-4. The lateral flexion deformity as measured from L-1–L-3 improved from 30 degrees to 9 degrees.

TRANSLATIONAL OR SHEAR TYPE FRACTURE-DISLOCATIONS

Injuries in which the spinal column is displaced directly anteriorly (Fig 12-13), posteriorly (Fig. 12-14), or laterally are termed translational fracture-dislocations.[4,11,12,20] These severely unstable injuries are often significantly displaced, with rupture of the anterior longitudinal ligament and all other ligaments and articulations of the spine. All of these injuries are highly unstable lesions that will require operative stabilization to prevent chronic instability.[2,4,11,12,32,48]

Posterior distraction instrumentation is less secure in this setting in the presence of a disrupted anterior longitudinal ligament and in the face of concomitant rotational instability. Also, because normal constraints to distraction are ruptured, use of the Harrington outrigger alone may overdistract the spinal cord and further damage neural elements. One possible option is the simultaneous application of compressive and distractive forces. In this procedure, the Harrington outrigger is mounted, and progressive distraction is applied slowly, without full correction. A double 18-gauge wire may then be applied to bridge the fracture-dislocation. A hyperextension force is thus applied. With the compression wire securely tightened, further distraction of the outrigger can be performed. With appropriate reduction verified by radiographs, distraction rods replace the outrigger.[21] A midline compression rod may be used in place of the compression wire (Fig. 12-15). With this option, overdistraction is prevented and greater stability of rotation is afforded.[30,42] Despite precautions there is still a significant rate of hook dislodgement and pseudarthrosis.[10,37,43] Therefore, segmental fixation should be used. Harrington rods with segmental fixation, Luque instrumentation, or Cotrel–Dubousset instrumentation will all improve rotational stability.

(*Text continued on p. 323*)

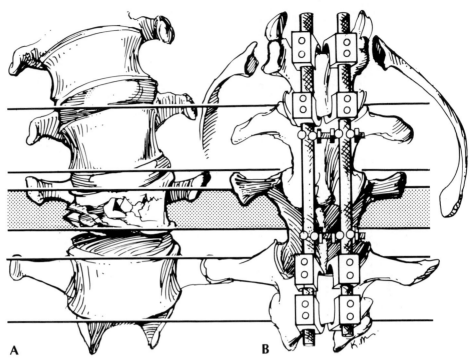

Figure 12-12. (*A, B*) Reduction of a lateral flexion injury with Cotrel–Dubousset instrumentation. A diagrammatic lateral flexion injury of L-2 is shown. Cotrel–Dubousset instrumentation can be configured to reduce and maintain the deformity. Instrumentation from T-12 to L-3 affords approximately equal lever arms above and below the unstable area. An extra motion segment is preserved over the use of Harrington instrumentation in the same injury, depicted in Figure 12-11. The hook configuration consists of bilateral claws at T-12 and L-3. In addition, up-going laminar hooks may be placed under L-1 should there be adequate room in the canal. However, these hooks would lie roughly posterior to the site of the L-2 vertebral body middle column comminution and should be omitted if the canal is compromised anteriorly. Following appropriate sagittal plane contouring, the concave rod is inserted first and distraction is applied. The convex rod is then inserted and compression is applied. Two devices for transverse loaders finish the rectangular construct.

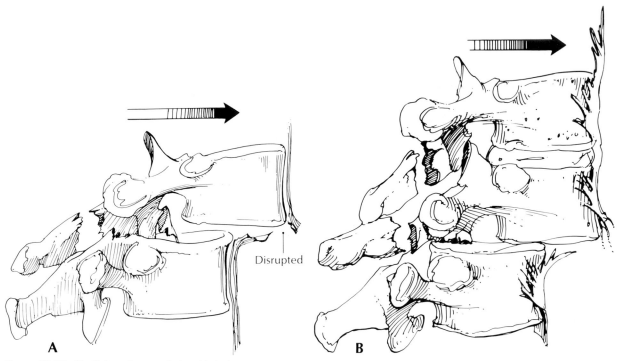

Disrupted

Figure 12-13. (*A, B*) Anterior translational injuries.

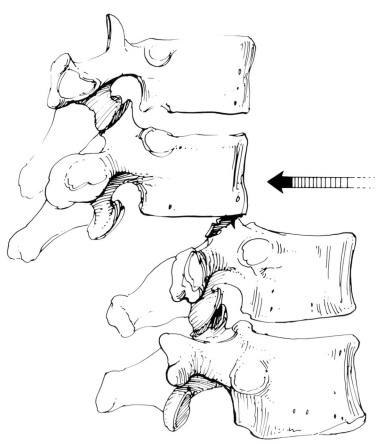

Figure 12-14. Posterior translational injuries.

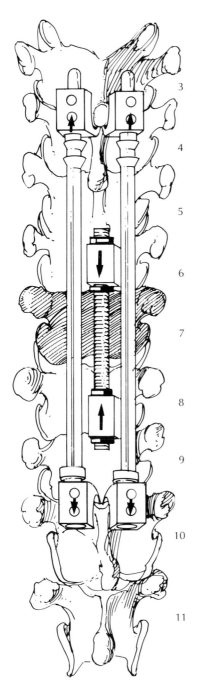

3

4

5

6

7

8

9

10

11

Figure 12-15. Midline compression rod between dual distraction rods in a translational fracture-dislocation.

TORSIONAL FLEXION OR ROTATION–FLEXION DISLOCATIONS

Torsional flexion injuries of the spine occur when there is torsion and compression in the anterior column and torsion and tension in the middle and posterior columns (Fig. 12-16).[6,11,12,20] The flexion moment often spares the anterior longitudinal ligament, which may be stripped off the anterior border of the vertebral body but not ruptured. The facets are usually fractured and dislocated, and the superior vertebral body may be sliced off. The injury is most commonly seen in the thoracic spine with a complete neurologic injury pattern (Fig. 12-17).

The most commonly used system to treat these injuries has been Harrington instrumentation.[4,5,10,15,20,22,45] Reduction is usually achieved by applying the outrigger in the concavity of the fracture in the coronal plane, and gently disengaging the fracture fragments. Because the anterior longitudinal ligament is characteristically intact in these fractures, there is less chance of overdistraction. Reduction is performed by placing the distraction rod though the ratchet hook and levering down on the apex of the deformity to seat the collar-end of the rod, achieving three-point fixation (Fig. 12-18).

Similarly, Cotrel-Dubousset instrumentation may be used to reduce and stabilize torsional flexion injuries (Fig. 12-19). A Cotrel–Dubousset rod is contoured to the desired thoracic kyphosis, less than the angulation of the deformity. With the rod securely anchored to the proximal spine segment via two sets of closed pedicle and transverse process hooks, a closed pedicle hook is mounted on the end of the rod. The fracture is reduced by levering the rod into the open hooks of the segment of spine distal to the fracture, while simultaneously seating the closed pedicle hook on the end of the rod. Hook blockers are inserted into all open hooks, and bolts are applied. In this way the sagittal plane deformity is reduced and secured by

(*Text continued on p. 327*)

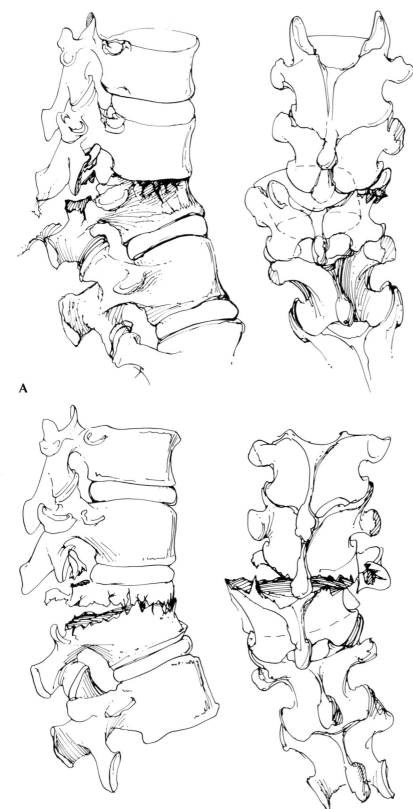

A

B

Figure 12-16. (*A, B*) Torsional flexion injury.

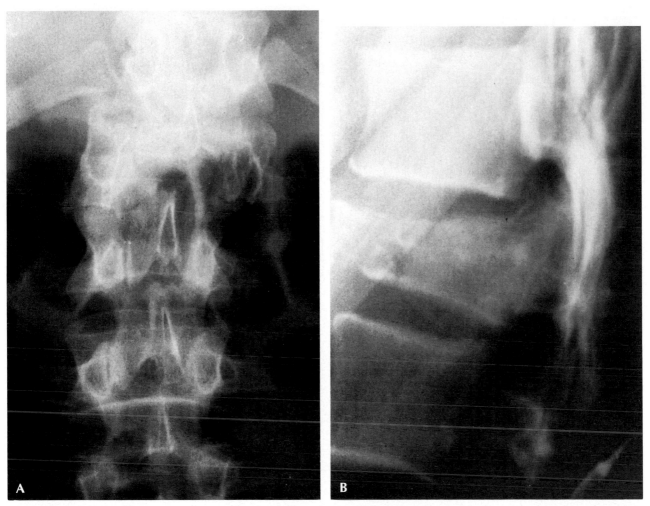

Figure 12-17. (*A, B*) This 18-year-old man suffered a thoracic fracture-dislocation with complete paraplegia secondary to a motor vehicle accident. There were concomitant rib and sternal fractures as well. A midthoracic gibbus deformity was noted.

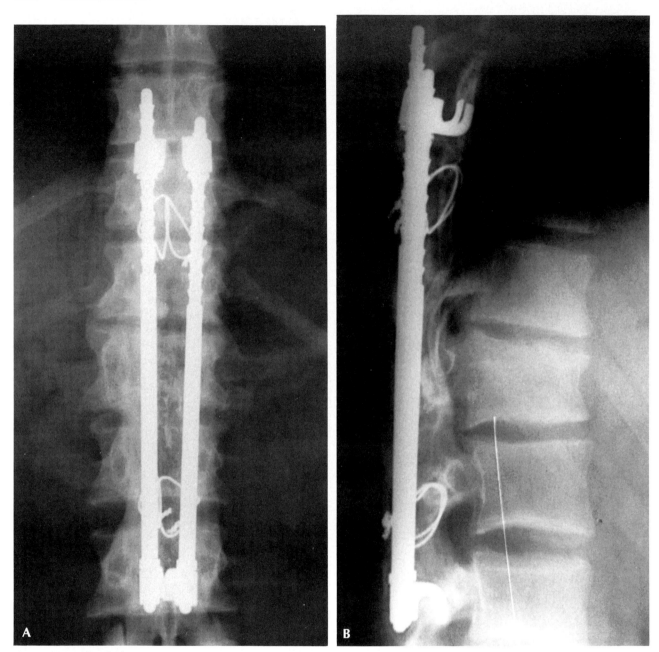

Figure 12-18. (*A, B*) Same patient as in Figure 12-17. Reduction was achieved by engaging the distraction rod through the ratchet hook and levering down on the apex of the deformity to seat the collar end of the rod. (Three-point fixation is also shown in Figure 12-8.)

four "claw" configurations, two each above and below the fracture site. Further improvement in alignment may, if necessary, be achieved by in situ rod benders. With the other rod placed in a similar fashion and connected by means of a pair of transverse loaders, a strong rectangular construct is created.

VERTICAL COMPRESSION INJURIES

When a vertebral body undergoes failure by vertical compressive loading, a spectrum of injury may occur, ranging from a failure of one or both end-plates to compression of the anterior and middle column, occasionally with posterior column involvement.[12] As the entire vertebral body is shortened, the posterior vertebral wall may burst into the neural canal, as documented on computed tomography.[13,26,38,39] The pedicles are widened and often posterior bony elements are fractured, with vertical laminar fractures or facet disruptions.[14]

Traditionally, Harrington distraction instrumentation has been used to stabilize these fractures. Distraction may partially or fully restore vertebral body height. The distraction rods, to a limited extent, indirectly reduce retropulsed fragments and prevent recollapse. As previously mentioned, Harrington rods have shortcomings, and in no other fracture pattern are these more glaring. Harrington rods used in the lumbar spine for burst injuries have poor fixation to the spine, create "flat back" deformity, create multi-segment loss of mobility, and can incompletely reduce canal impingement. In an attempt to improve upon these recognized shortcomings, rod sleeves, locking rods, the rod long–fuse short method, squareended rods and hooks, and the addition of contoured rods and sublaminar wires have been suggested. Pedicular fixation techniques are being explored as a possible means of avoiding these problems (see Chapter 11).

The use of Cotrel–Dubousset instrumentation in a rod and hook configuration may prove to be a useful tool in the treatment of vertical compression injuries.[18] The specific configuration used will depend on the location of the burst injury (Fig. 12-20). In the thoracic spine the rod will be contoured for the normal kyphosis. In the lumbar spine a lordosis will have to be restored and contoured into the rod. In the transitional area of the thoracolumbar region a gentle "S" curve will have to be achieved (Figs. 12-21, 12-22). Hook placements are dictated by the desire to achieve roughly equal lever arms proximal and distal to the fracture and to maximize available motion segments in the lumbar spine (Fig. 12-23). Secure fixation of the instrumentation system requires either single or double "claw" configurations above or below the injury level. In order to avoid further canal compromise, care must be taken not to place laminar hooks at levels where the dural tube is impinged by bony fragments anteriorly.

SUMMARY

This chapter has attempted to elucidate some of the problems, pitfalls, and possible technical solutions in the application of nonpedicular posterior instrumentation for thoracolumbar spine fractures. The successful clinical treatment of a specific spinal fracture does not start with technical knowledge of complex instrumentations, but with recognition of the fracture pattern and understanding of the prevailing forces that caused the injury. By recognizing the extent of spinal column defects, reversing the deforming forces, and achieving and maintaining proper spinal alignment with a rationally selected spinal implant, the chances of clinical success are maximized.

(*Text continued on p. 333*)

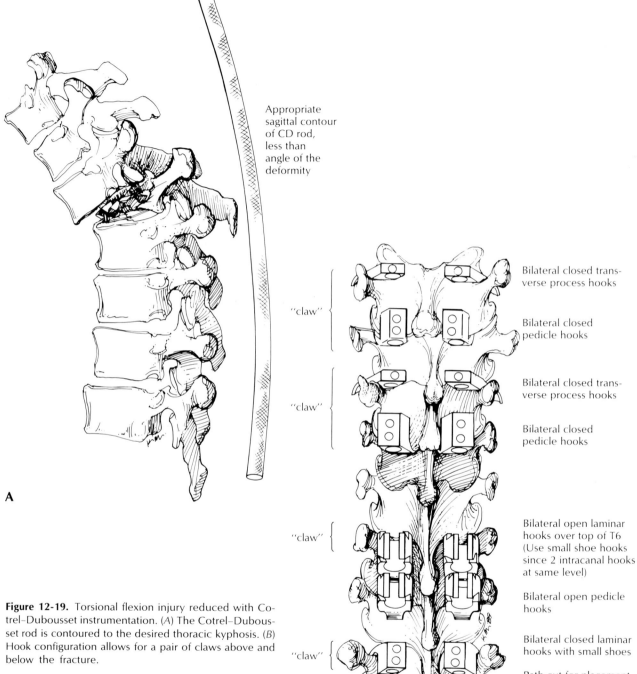

Appropriate sagittal contour of CD rod, less than angle of the deformity

"claw"

Bilateral closed transverse process hooks

Bilateral closed pedicle hooks

"claw"

Bilateral closed transverse process hooks

Bilateral closed pedicle hooks

"claw"

Bilateral open laminar hooks over top of T6 (Use small shoe hooks since 2 intracanal hooks at same level)

Bilateral open pedicle hooks

Bilateral closed laminar hooks with small shoes

"claw"

Path cut for placement of closed pedicle hook upon placement of rod

A

B

Figure 12-19. Torsional flexion injury reduced with Cotrel–Dubousset instrumentation. (*A*) The Cotrel–Dubousset rod is contoured to the desired thoracic kyphosis. (*B*) Hook configuration allows for a pair of claws above and below the fracture.

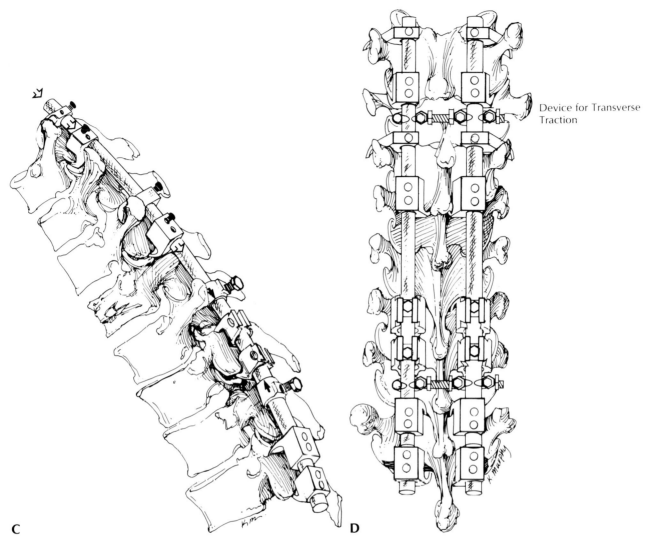

Device for Transverse
Traction

C   D

Figure 12-19. (*continued*). (*C*) Reduction maneuver. (*D*) Final rectangular construct. As the rod is levered into open hooks, the distal-most closed pedicle hook is seated. Bushings are slid over the rod, into the open hooks, converting the hooks to closed. All hooks are reseated and secured with bolts. The spine is reduced. Contralateral rod is placed. Two DTTs are placed and bolts are tightened to shear. If necessary, further improvement in sagittal plane alignment is achieved with in-situ rod bending.

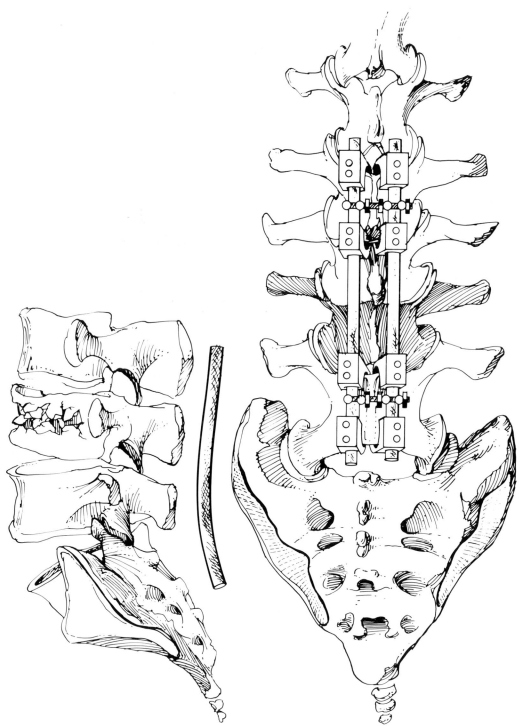

Figure 12-20. Stabilization of an L-4 burst fracture with Cotrel–Dubousset instrumentation. In an attempt to preserve lumbar spine motion a configuration is designed to instrument two levels above and one level below the fracture site. With anterior canal impingement at the top of the involved fractured vertebra, upgoing hooks on the superior adjacent lamina is not advised. The lamina are securely grasped by a pair of "claws" above and below the fracture site. The exact construct pattern would work as well for an L-3 burst fracture with an L-1–L-4 construct.

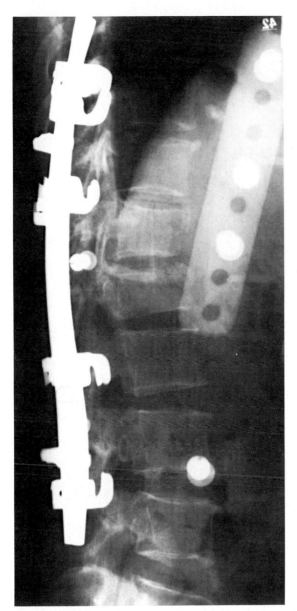

Figure 12-21. L-1 burst fracture in a 47-year-old woman with incomplete neurologic function. Shown is gentle "S"-shaped contouring of the rod in the thoracolumbar junction with Cotrel–Dubousset instrumentation.

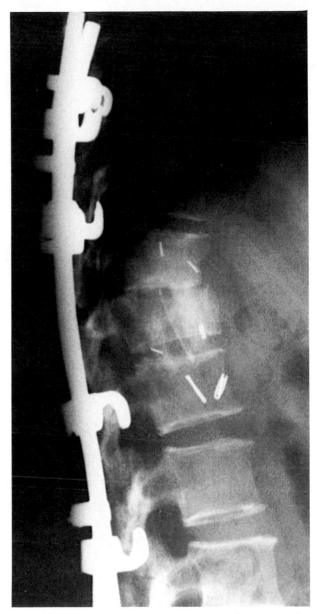

Figure 12-22. Same patient as in Figure 12-21. A postoperative myelogram revealed a persistent anterior dural compression. An anterior decompression and strut grafting was performed 1 week later.

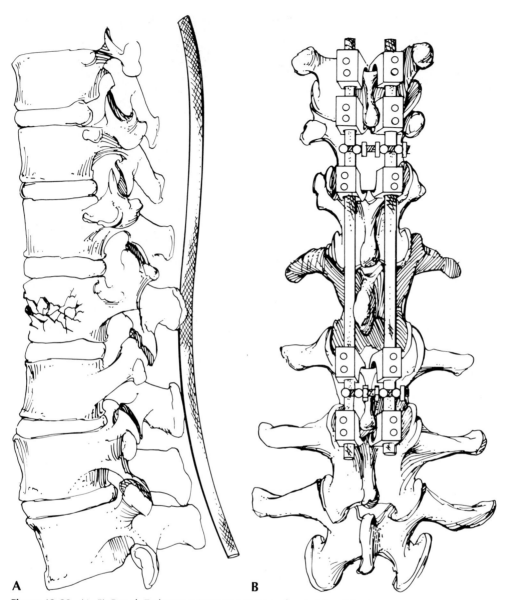

A   **B**

Figure 12-23. (*A, B*) Cotrel–Dubousset instrumentation of an L-1 burst fracture.

REFERENCES

1. Aebi M, Mohler J, Zack G, Morscher E: Analysis of 75 operated thoracolumbar fractures and fracture dislocations with and without neurologic deficit. Arch Orthop Trauma Surg 105:100–112, 1986

2. Antuaco EJ, Binet EF: Radiology of thoracic and lumbar fractures. Clin Orthop 189:43–57, 1984

3. Beerman R, Batt HD, Green BA: Lumbar vertebral reformation after traumatic compression fracture. AJNR 6:455–456, 1985

4. Bohlman HH: Current concepts review: Treatment of fractures and dislocations of the thoracic and lumbar spine. J Bone Joint Surg [Am] 67:165–169, 1985

5. Bradford DS, Akbarnia BB, Winter RB, Seljeskog EL: Surgical stabilization of fracture and fracture dislocations of the thoracic spine. Spine 2:185–196, 1977

6. Bucholz RW, Gill K: Classification of injuries to the thoracolumbar spine. Orthop Clin North Am 17:67–73, 1986

7. Casey MP, Asher MA, Jacobs RA, Orrick JM: The effect of Harrington rod contouring on lumbar lordosis. Spine 12:750–753, 1987

8. Chance CQ: Note on a type of flexion fracture of the spine. Br J Radiol 21:452–453, 1948

9. Cope R, Salmon A, Gaines R: Association of a thoracic distraction fracture and an unusual avulsion fracture. Spine 12:943–945, 1987

10. Cotler JM, Vernace JV, Michalski JA: The use of Harrington rods in thoracolumbar fractures. Orthop Clin North Am. 17:87–103, 1986

11. Denis F: Spinal instability as defined by the three column spine concept in acute spinal trauma. Clin Orthop 189:65–76, 1984

12. Denis F: The three column spine and its significance in the classification of acute thoracolumbar spinal injuries. Spine 8:817–831, 1983

13. Denis F, Armstrong GWD, Searls BA, Matta L: Acute thoracolumbar burst fractures in the absence of neurologic deficit: A comparison between operative and non-operative treatment. Clin Orthop 189:142–149, 1984

14. Dewald RL: Burst fractures of the thoracic and lumbar spine. Clin Orthop 189:150–161, 1984

15. Dickson JH, Harrington PR, Erwin WD: Harrington instrumentation in the fractured, unstable thoracic and lumbar spine. Tex Med 69:91–98, 1973

16. Drummond D, Guadagni J, Keene JS et al: Interspinous process segmental spinal instrumentation. J Pediatr Orthop 4:397–404, 1984

17. Edwards CC, Levine AM: Early rod–sleeve stabilization of the injured thoracic and lumbar spine. Orthop Clin North Am 17:121–145, 1986

18. Farcy JP, Weidenbaum M, Michelson CB et al: A comparative biomechanical study of spinal fixation using Cotrel–Dubousset instrumentation. Spine 12:877–881, 1987

19. Ferguson RL, Allen BL: An algorithm for the treatment of unstable thoracolumbar fractures. Orthop Clin North Am 17:105–112, 1986

20. Ferguson RL, Allen BL: A mechanistic classification of thoraco-lumbar spine fractures. Clin Orthop 189:77–88, 1984

21. Flesch JR, Leider LL, Erickson DL et al: Harrington instrumentation and spine fusion for unstable fractures and fracture-dislocations of the thoracic and lumbar spine. J Bone Joint Surg [Am] 59:143–153, 1977

22. Floman Y, Fast A, Pollack D et al: The simultaneous application of an interspinous compressive wire and Harrington distraction rods in the treatment of fracture-dislocation of the thoracic and lumbar spine. Clin Orthop 205:207–215, 1986

23. Gertzbein SD, Courtney-Brown CM: Flexion-distraction injuries of the lumbar spine: Mechanisms of injury and classification. Clin Orthop 227:52–60, 1988

24. Gumley G, Taylor TKF, Ryan MD: Distraction fractures of lumbar spine. J Bone Joint Surg [Br] 64:520–525, 1982

25. Hannon KM: Harrington instrumentation in fractures and dislocations of the thoracic and lumbar spine. South Med J 69:1269–1273, 1976

26. Herrlin K, Ekelund L, Sunden G: Radiologic and clinical evaluation of Harrington instrumentation in the injured dorsolumbar spine. Acta Radiol [Diagn] 24:289–295, 1983

27. Jacobs RR, Dahners LE, Gertzbein SD et al: A locking hook-spinal rod: Current status of development. Paraplegia 21:197–200, 1983

28. Jacobs RR, Schlaepfer F, Mathys R et al: A locking hook spinal rod system for stabilization of fracture dislocations and correction of deformities of the dorsolumbar spine: A biomechanical evaluation. Clin Orthop 189:168–177, 1984

29. Kaufer H, Hayes JT: Lumbar fracture dislocation: A study of 21 cases. J Bone Joint Surg [Am] 48:712–730, 1966

30. Keene JS, Wackwitz DL, Drummond DS, Breed AL: Compression-distraction instrumentation of unstable thoracolumbar fractures: Anatomic results obtained with each type of injury and method of instrumentation. Spine 11:895–902, 1986

31. Kelly RP, Whitesides TE: Treatment of lumbodorsal fracture-dislocations. Ann Surg 167:705–717, 1968

32. King AG: Spinal column trauma. In Anderson LD (ed): Instructional Course Lectures, Vol 35. St Louis, CV Mosby, 1986

33. Kostuik JP, Errico TJ, Gleason TF: Techniques of internal fixation for degenerative conditions of the lumbar spine. Clin Orthop 203:219–231, 1986

34. Levine A, Edwards CC: Lumbar spine trauma. In Camins M, O'Leary P (eds): The Lumbar Spine. New York, Raven Press, 1987

35. Lewis J, Mckibbin B: The treatment of unstable fracture-dislocations of the thoracolumbar spine accompanied by paraplegia. J Bone Joint Surg [Br] 56:603–612, 1974

36. Luque ER, Cassis N, Ramirez-Qiella G: Segmental spinal instrumentation in the treatment of fractures of the thoracolumbar spine. Spine 7:312–317, 1982

37. McAfee PC, Bohlman HH: Complications following Harrington instrumentation for fractures of the thoracolumbar spine. J Bone Joint Surg [Am] 67:672–686, 1985

38. McAfee PC, Yuan HA, Frederickson BE, Lubicky JP: The value of computed tomography in thoracolumbar fractures: An analysis of one hundred consecutive cases and a new classification. J Bone Joint Surg [Am] 65:461–473, 1983

39. McAfee PC, Yuan HA, Lasda NA: The unstable burst fracture. Spine 7:365–373, 1982

40. Meyer PR: Posterior stabilization of thoracic, lumbar and sacral injuries. In Anderson LD (ed): Instructional Course Lectures. St Louis, CV Mosby, 1986

41. Munson G, Satterlee C, Hammond S et al: Experimental evaluation of Harrington rod fixation supplemented with sublaminar wires in stabilizing thoracolumbar fracture-dislocations. Clin Orthop 189:97–102, 1984

42. Murphy MJ, Southwick WO, Ogden JA: Treatment of the unstable thoraco-lumbar spine with combination Harrington distraction and compression rods. Orthopaedic Transactions 6:9, 1982

43. Osebold WR, Weinstein SL, Sprague BL: Thoracolumbar spine fractures: Results of treatment. Spine 6:13–34, 1981

44. Smith WS, Kaufer H: Patterns and mechanisms of lumbar injuries associated with lap seat belts. J Bone Joint Surg [Am] 51:239–254, 1969

45. Svensson O, Aaro S, Ohlen G: Harrington instrumentation for thoracic and lumbar vertebral fractures. Acta Orthop Scand 55:38–47, 1984

46. Van Hanswyck EP, Yuan HA, Eckardt WA: Orthotic management of thoracolumbar spine fractures with a "total contact" TLSO. Orthotics and Prosthetics 33:10–19, 1979

47. Wang GJ, Whitehill R, Stamp WG, Rosenberger R: The treatment of fracture dislocations of the thoracolumbar spine with halofemoral traction and Harrington rod instrumentation. Clin Orthop 142:168–175, 1979

48. Weber SC, Sutherland GH: An unusual rotational fracture-dislocation of the thoracic spine without neurologic sequelae internally fixed with a combined anterior and posterior approach. J Trauma 26:474–479, 1986

49. Wenger DR, Carollo JJ: The mechanics of thoracolumbar fractures stabilized by segmental fixation. Clin Orthop 189:89–96, 1984

50. Whitesides TE, Shah SGA: On the management of unstable fractures of the thoracolumbar spine: Rationale for the use of anterior decompression and fusion and posterior stabilization. Spine 1:99–107, 1976

51. Yosipovitch A, Robin GC, Makin M: Open reduction of unstable thoracolumbar spinal injuries and fixation with Harrington rods. J Bone Joint Surg [Am] 59:1003–1015, 1977

SACRAL SPINE

13

SACRAL SPINE FRACTURES

Allen Carl

BACKGROUND

The sacral bone, or "os sacrum," as coined by the Romans, was so called because of the "sacred" protective function it affords the genitals. Ancient Egyptians and Greeks revered the sacrum. It is thought to have been an important bone in sacrificial rites and resurrection ceremonies. Ancients incorrectly believed that the sacrum was the first bone to ossify and the last to disintegrate, thus explaining its involvement in religious rites.[44]

ANATOMY

The sacrum, triangular in shape, is composed of five fused vertebrae. It articulates superiorly with L-5, inferiorly with the coccyx, and laterally with the ilia. The sacroiliac joints span S-1 and S-2 in females and S-1 to S-3 in males. Dorsally, spinous processes are united to form the medial sacral crest (Fig. 13-1). The position of the sacral ala makes the sacrum wider dorsally than ventrally. This wedging phenomenon provides stability. Posterior sacroiliac and iliolumbar ligaments also enhance stability.

The anterior and posterior sacral foramina communicate with the sacral canal and allow the transit of the spinal nerves. The anterior sacral foramina are twice the diameter of the exiting nerve root. The foramina are the weakest structural part of the sacrum.[1] The dorsal root ganglia divide in the sacral canal rather than outside the foramina, as is found in the more proximal spine. The lower lumbar and upper sacral roots innervate the distal lower extremities, and the lower sacral roots control genital, bladder, and anorectal function (Table 13-1). The lumbosacral plexus is composed of the fourth lumbar to the third sacral nerve roots. There is functional overlap of the lower sacral roots, making localization difficult. Loss of bladder and urethral sphincter function occurs with injury to the second sacral root and below. Bilat-

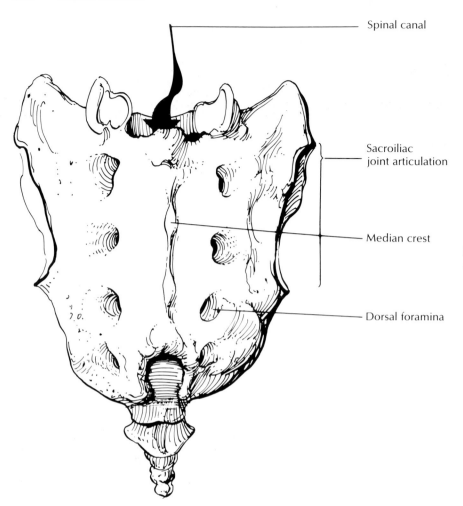

Spinal canal

Sacroiliac
joint articulation

Median crest

Figure 13-1. Dorsal view of the sacrum.

Dorsal foramina

Table 13-1. Neurologic Evaluation

LEVEL	MOTOR FUNCTION	SENSORY DISTRIBUTION	REFLEXES
L-5	Foot dorsiflexion and inversion	Dorsal first web space	
	Hip abduction and internal rotation	Lateral calf	
S-1	Hip extension, plantar flexion	Sole, lateral foot	Achilles tendon
S-2	External urethral and external anal sphincter control	Posterior leg, genitalia	
S-3	Perineal muscle control	Superior medial thigh, perineum	Bulbocavernous
S-4 and S-5		Perineum	

eral nerve root injury causes bowel and bladder dysfunction. Unilateral sacral root damage may lead to loss of sensation but no functional debility.

EPIDEMIOLOGY

The first report of a sacral fracture was by Malgaigne in 1847. He recorded one such injury in 2,358 patients.[4] Bonnin[1] was the first to classify sacral fractures.

Sacral fractures comprise 1% of all of spinal fractures. They are commonly associated with pelvic fractures, but are often overlooked when treating severe life-threatening injuries.[15,30,39-41,47] Most commonly, the fractures are sustained in motor vehicle accidents and falls. Radiographic documentation requires a sharp eye and quality radiographs, which may often be suboptimal in the emergency situation. Up to 61% of sacral fractures are missed initially.[24,33] Transverse sacral fractures are uncommon, comprising 4% to 5% of all sacral fractures.[1,2,16,29,30,40,47] Purser[36] was the first to report a transverse sacral fracture. A high level of suspicion is needed to diagnose a sacral fracture in a trauma victim. This explains the wide diversity of sacral fracture statistics, which may vary from 4%[46] to 74%.[18] The most commonly recorded value of sacral fractures in multiple-trauma victims is 40% to 50%.[1,16,29]

DIAGNOSIS

Most patients complain of severe low back and buttock pain. There may be an ecchymosis over the buttock, and sacral pain on rectal examination. Occasionally, there may be radiculopathic symptoms. An altered level of consciousness may be one reason for delayed diagnosis. Injury to lower lumbar or upper sacral roots may manifest itself in motor weakness in foot and ankle function. Low sacral root injuries reveal weakened sphincter strength and tone. Early urinary catheter placement in severe trauma may mask bladder dysfunction for several days. Perineal numbness may not be deduced in the emergency room. Rectal examination may be overlooked during the early evaluation of major trauma.

It is imperative to obtain an adequate history and perform a thorough physical examination. Clinical examinations should focus on pain and deformity. Neurologic evaluation requires examination for perineal deficits and anal and vesical sphincter dysfunction. Once urinary difficulties are noted, postvoid residuals must be monitored. Motor function of both lower extremities needs to be documented. In lucid patients, sensory dermatomic defects help in the diagnosis. Asymmetry or absence of reflex in the bulbocavernosus muscle and ankle are helpful in diagnosis of the uncooperative patient. Damage to nerve roots from stretching or from direct pressure caused by bone, hemorrhage, or callous or fibrous tissue may explain the nerve injury. Neurologic injury in sacral fractures was described initially in 1936 by Lam,[26] and was further identified by Patterson and Morton[34] and Peltier.[35] Cerebrospinal fluid leaks, rectal injuries, presacral venous and arterial lacerations, and delayed neurologic injury due to premature mobilization in the presence of instability have all been reported.[16,19,38,47]

CLASSIFICATION

Many classifications for sacral spine fractures have been published. Most classification systems deal with the type and degree of bony disruption. In general, fracture patterns proceed along stress flow lines, and disruption is often through the foramina. The first and second anterior and posterior sacral foramina weaken the bone connecting the lateral sacral mass, making it the most frequently broken link between the ilium and the vertebral column. The sacrum is strong in compression, but fails in tension, rotation, and shear.[1] These fracture patterns are most often longitudinal or oblique.

The most commonly used classification subdivides the injuries into direct and indirect trauma (Table 13-2). Gunshot wounds (penetrating trauma) are the most common direct sacral traumatic injuries. Most are structurally stable. Direct severe blunt trauma results in a comminuted sacral fracture. This injury is rare, and is often accompanied by first and second sacral nerve root injury, which usually resolves. Low transverse fractures

Table 13-2. Sacral Fracture Classifications

DIRECT TRAUMA	INDIRECT TRAUMA
Penetrating	High Transverse
Comminuted	Type I
Low transverse	Type II
	Type III
	Vertical
	Lateral mass
	Juxta-articular
	Cleaving
	Avulsion

Adapted from Schmidek HH, Smith DA, Kristiansen TK: Sacral Fractures. Neurosurgery 15:735–746, 1984

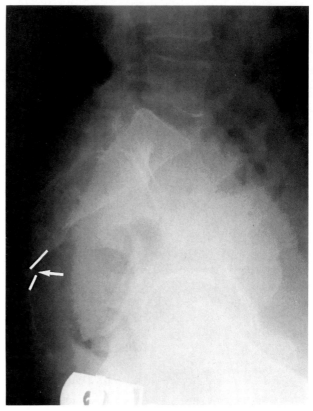

Figure 13-2. Transverse fracture of the fourth sacral vertebra (lateral radiograph).

are due to a direct blow to the coccyx (Fig. 13-2). This causes forward displacement of the sacrococcygeal fragment. Levering of the distal sacrum and coccyx causes fracture below S-3 at the site of sacroiliac fixation. The injury level is below the thecal sac, and neurologic damage is uncommon unless the bony fragments displace upward into neurologic structures. Rectal perforation and cerebrospinal fluid leaks have been reported.[19,47] Low transverse fractures are stable, as they are below the area of weight bearing (Fig. 13-3).

Most sacral fractures occur by indirect injury. Ninety percent occur with an associated pelvic fracture;[1,16,41,46] 25% to 50% have an accompanying neurologic deficit.[1] These deficits are due to direct sacral root compression, stretching, lumbosacral plexus injury, or cauda equina lesion. The sacrum can play an important role in pelvic injuries.

Pelvic fractures with dual sites of ring disruption lead to instability.[23,31] Instability is seen most commonly with vertical shear lesions, but also occurs with lateral and anteroposterior compression pelvic injuries. Most Malgaigne fractures associated with sacral lesions are unstable.[17] These sacral fractures are usually longitudinal or oblique. The pelvic disruption that causes the instability is treated with reduction and external or internal fixation.[23] The accompanying sacral fracture, especially when associated with neurologic deficit, must be included in the treatment plan.

Vertical fractures are the most common injuries resulting from indirect forces. Categorization of these vertical injuries into oblique and longitudinal lines allows for anatomic subclassification.[1] Vertical fractures include:

Lateral mass fractures that extend through the sacral foramina on one side (Fig. 13-4)

Juxta-articular fractures involving the lateral sacral mass adjacent to the sacroiliac joint (Fig. 13-5)

Longitudinal cleaving fractures that extend from the proximal sacral foramina to the coccyx and may or may not involve multiple neuroforamina[48]

Avulsion fractures occurring at sacrotuberal or sacrospinal ligament insertions (Fig. 13-6)[3]

Fractures that do not fit into these categories may be a mixture of any of the aforementioned patterns.

(*Text continued on p. 343*)

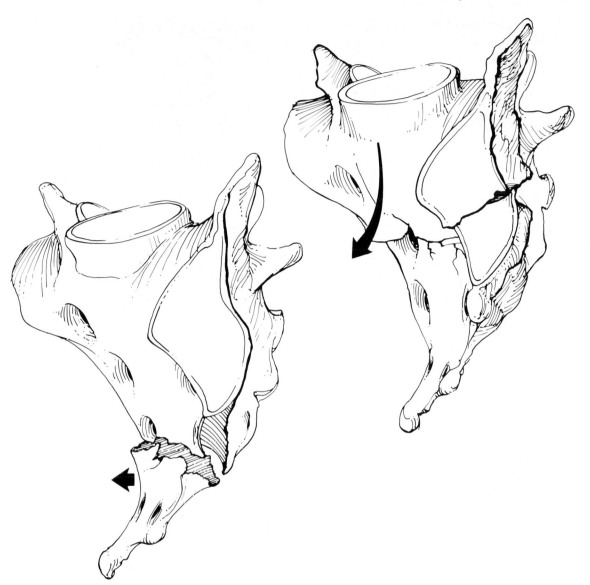

Figure 13-3. Transverse sacral fractures.

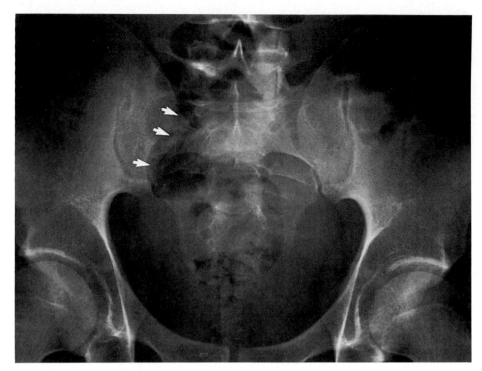

Figure 13-4. Lateral sacral mass fracture (Ferguson's frontal radiograph). In Ferguson's view the radiographic beam is angled down at 50 degrees from the horizontal, clearly showing the sacral arcuate lines.

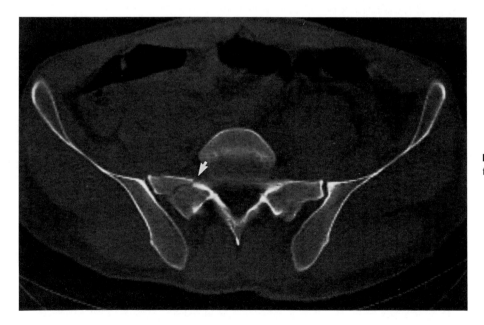

Figure 13-5. Juxta-articular sacral fracture (CT).

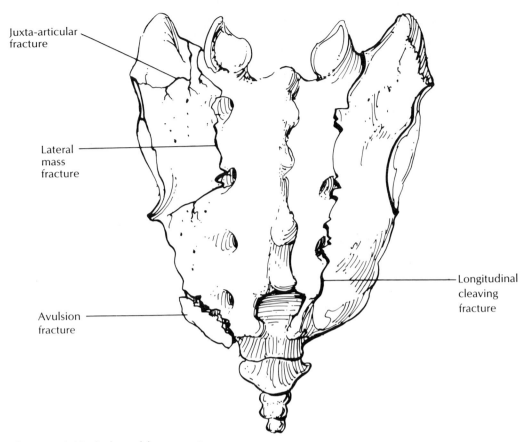

Juxta-articular fracture

Lateral mass fracture

Avulsion fracture

Longitudinal cleaving fracture

Figure 13-6. Vertical sacral fracture patterns.

The second type of indirect injury is the uncommon high transverse sacral fractures (see Fig. 13-3). Only 42 have been reported in the literature.[2,4,5-7,11,13,15,16,36,38-40,45,47,50] The fracture occurs with a forward force on a flexed lumbosacral spine with the knees fixed in extension and the hips flexed.[2] Upper transverse sacral fractures usually occur as isolated injuries, but seven patients had associated pelvic fractures.[4,5,11,16,45] They are unstable and frequently displaced. The most common site of these transverse fractures occurs between S-2 and S-3. Forty-one patients had associated neurologic deficit.

Upper transverse sacral fractures have been subdivided by Roy-Camille into three types (Fig. 13-7). Type I is a flexion force fracture with an anterior bend to the upper sacral segment (Fig. 13-8). Type II is a flexion force fracture with posterior displacement of the upper fragment that becomes horizontally displaced and settles on the lower segment fracture surfaces, resulting in lumbar kyphosis. Type III is an extension force fracture with an anterior displacement of the upper fragment that remains vertical and slips anteriorly in front of the lower segment, causing lumbar lordosis (Fig. 13-9).

Francis Denis devised a new classification system that divides the sacrum into three zones, from peripheral at the alae to central at the medial crest.[10] Of 236 patients, there was a 32% inci-

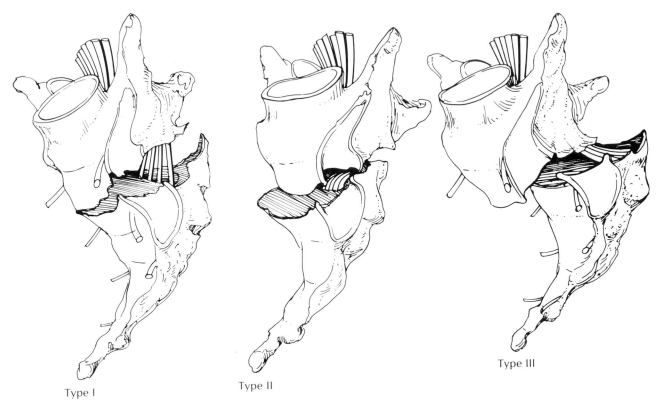

Type I　　　Type II　　　Type III

Figure 13-7. Upper transverse sacral fracture patterns.

dence of neurologic deficit. Incidence of nerve damage was 5.9% in zone 1, 28% in zone 2, and 87% in zone 3. Damage was more frequent when the fracture was close to the spinal canal. This classification system does not take injury mechanism or degree of bony disruption into account (Fig. 13-10).

A very rare injury is bilateral sacral fracture-dislocation. Only two cases have been reported.[25,28] One was treated operatively, and the other nonoperatively. Both patients had good results. I treated a third patient nonoperatively with prolonged bedrest, and also had a good result[6] (Fig. 13-11). Three sacral fractures in children have been reported.[11,22,38]

LABORATORY TESTS

A sacral fracture may be masked on plain anteroposterior radiographs of the pelvis due to overlying intestinal gas and lumbosacral lordosis. Denis has gone so far as to state that this radiographic view is useless.[10] Subtle findings, such as low lumbar transverse process fractures, asymmetrical sacral foramina, or irregular trabeculae at the lateral sacral masses, may be tip-offs to investigate for a sacral fracture. The fracture force may propagate through the foramina and proceed proximally, resulting in lower lumbar transverse process fractures. Hallgrimsson[20] and Byrnes[4] noted difficulties in radiologic diagnosis, and suggested that the

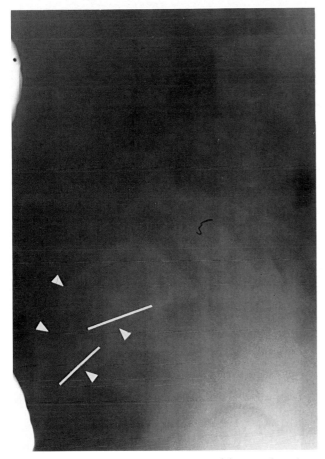

Figure 13-8. Type I upper transverse sacral fracture (lateral radiograph).

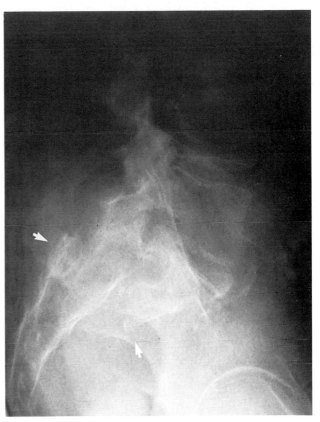

Figure 13-9. Type III upper transverse sacral fracture (lateral radiograph).

beam be angled down at 50 degrees from the horizontal, which is known as "Feurgeuson's view" (Fig.13-12). This allows the best view of the sacral arcuate lines, which outline the neuroforamina. The diagnosis is made by evaluating for asymmetry of the anterosuperior sacral foraminal lines (Fig. 13-13). Pelvic inlet, outlet, and oblique views are helpful.[2] A lateral radiograph is best for diagnosing a displaced transverse sacral fracture (see Fig. 13-2).[10,11]

Tomography, sacral myelography, and computed tomography enhance fracture pattern identification. Myelography to the thecal sac termina-tion at S-2 helps to evaluate for canal and nerve root impingement. Offending fracture fragments or angulation can be identified. Traumatic irreversible meningoceles due to nerve root avulsions can also be identified. Computed tomography shows the extent of spinal canal compromise (Fig. 13-14). Bone scanning has been used to detect sacral fractures in elderly osteopenic patients with mild trauma.[8,27,37]

Urodynamics in the form of cystometrography can be used to evaluate conus and lower sacral root lesions.[32] With complete lesions, there is a detrusor muscle paralysis. Incomplete cauda

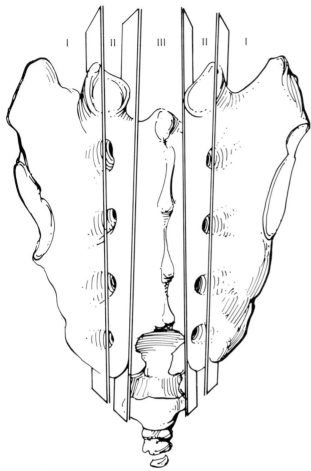

Figure 13-10. Neurologic deficit by sacral fracture location (zones I, II, and III).

equina damage can also be detected by urologic testing. Serial examinations are useful in evaluating neurologic return. Electromyography and evoked potentials are useful tools that also give insight into identification of neurologic injury.[48] Sacral root paralysis with normal electromyography performed 3 to 6 weeks after injury most often indicates neuropraxia. Patchy neurologic changes that spare paraspinal muscle activity indicate lumbosacral plexus damage outside the spinal canal, while the presence of paraspinal abnormalities are due to pathology within the spinal canal.

Pudendal nerve evoked potentials are new clinical tests that can be added to the diagnostic armamentarium.[9] They allow direct measurement of certain peripheral and central neurogenic pathways involved in bowel, bladder, and sexual function. As these tests become more sophisticated, they may surpass others used for neurologic evaluation.

TREATMENT

The three major treatment goals for sacral spine fractures are pain relief, neurologic improvement, and stable bone healing. Nonoperative and operative management have been used to achieve these goals. In cases with instability but no neurologic deficit, conservative management is the treatment of choice. This includes bed rest for 8 to 12 weeks and occasional traction and fracture reduction in cases with significant displacement. Attempts at closed and postural reduction are less than satisfactory. Use of the hip spica was reported in several cases.[41] Patients without instability require 4 to 8 weeks of bed rest, and digital rectal reduction for those fractures found to be displaced.[47] Sacral fractures associated with unstable pelvic injuries may be improved by operative (external or internal) fixation or nonoperative stabilization of the pelvis. Delayed neurologic injury from increasing fracture deformity, callus, consolidating hematoma, and fibrous scarring can occur.[12,14,16,42,47] In cases of transverse fractures, surgical and nonsurgical treatment gave similar results. In most cases, motor function improved satisfactorily, but bowel or bladder return was often poor regardless of treatment.[4,11,38,39,45]

Presently, surgical management is indicated for cases with neurologic impairment and persisting pressure from fracture fragments, deformity, callus, or hematoma. Sacral unroofing allows for hematoma evacuation, restoration of bony alignment, and nerve root exploration and decompression. In most cases, the injury at impact determines the eventual outcome. Surgery did not help bowel and bladder dysfunction unless it was a partial lesion. Surgical cases were those with the

(*Text continued on p. 349*)

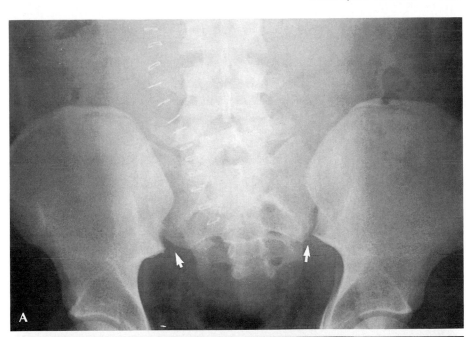

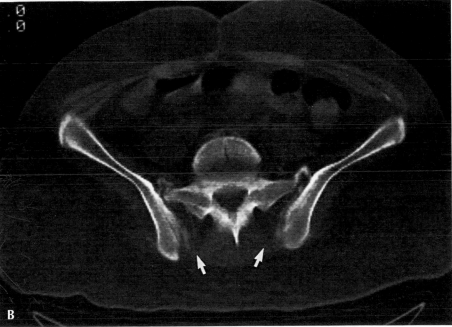

Figure 13-11. (*A*) Bilateral sacral fracture-dislocation (Ferguson's frontal radiograph). (*B*) Bilateral sacroiliac joint disruption (CT).

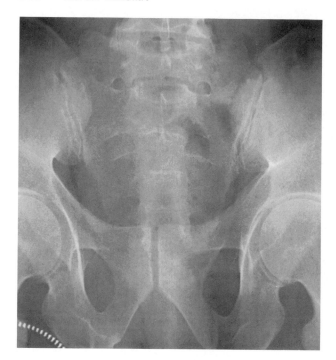

Figure 13-12. Ferguson's radiographic view of the sacrum.

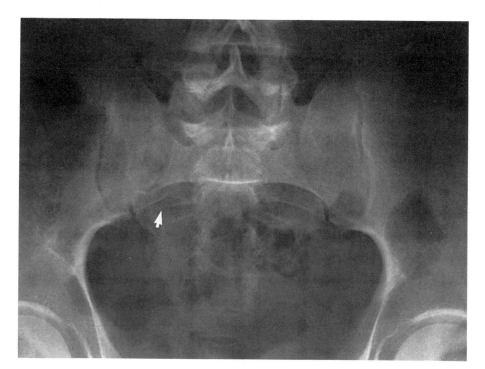

Figure 13-13. Asymetrical sacral arcuate lines.

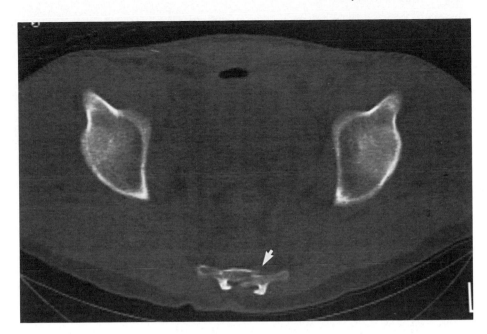

Figure 13-14. Computerized axial tomography shows the extent of spinal canal compromise.

most severe damage, and these results led to only partial recovery. Bony fusion and instrumentation was performed in four patients, two with Harrington rods, and two with pedicle screws.[13,39] The results were good, but the surgical procedure is demanding. In those cases with dural injury, watertight repair of the lesion is required.[11]

Anterior sacral surgery in the form of fusion has revealed promising results,[43] but bleeding from retroperitoneal hematoma is a concern in those cases subjected to early surgery.[41] Observation for delayed neurologic deficit is important, and late surgery may be required. Rehabilitation problems may involve gait, sexual function, and bowel and bladder function.

REFERENCES

1. Bonnin JG: Sacral fracture and injuries to the cauda equina. J Bone Joint Surg 27:113–127, 1945
2. Bucknill TM, Blackburn JS: Fracture-dislocation of the sacrum. J Bone Joint Surg [Br] 58:467–470, 1976
3. Burman MP: Tear of the sacrospinous and sacrotuberous ligaments. J Bone Joint Surg [Am] 34:331–339, 1952
4. Byrnes DP, Russo GL, Ducler TB, Cowley RA: Sacrum fractures and neurological damage. J Neurosurg 47:459–462, 1977
5. Carl A, Delman A, Engler G: Displaced transverse sacral fractures. Clin Orthop 194:195–198, 1985
6. Carl A, Thomas S: Bilateral sacroiliac joint fracture dislocation: A case report. J Trauma, in press
7. Chiaruttini M: Transverse sacral fracture with transient neurologic complication. Ann Emerg Med 16:111–113, 1987
8. Cooper KL, Beabout JW, Swee RG: Insufficiency fractures of the sacrum. Radiology 156:15–20, 1985
9. Cracco RQ, Bodis-Wollner I: Evoked Potentials, pp 68–75. New York, Alan R Liss, 1986
10. Denis F, Davis S, Comfort T: Sacral fractures: An important problem though frequently undiagnosed and untreated. Presented at the 21st annual meeting of the Scoliosis Research Society. Hamilton, Bermuda, September 1986
11. Dowling T, Epstein JA, Epstein NE: S1-S2 sacral fracture involving neural elements of the cauda equina. Spine 9:851–853, 1985

12. Epstein NE, Epstein JA, Carras R: Unilateral S-1 root compression syndrome caused by fracture of the sacrum. Neurosurgery 19:1025–1027, 1986

13. Fardon DF: Displaced transverse fracture of the sacrum with nerve root injury: Report of a case with successful operative management. J Trauma 19:119–122, 1979

14. Fardon DF: Sacral fractures. Correspondence. J Neurosurg 48:316, 1978

15. Ferris B, Hutton P: Anteriorly displaced transverse fracture of the sacrum at the level of the sacro-iliac joint. J Bone Joint Surg [Am] 65:407–409, 1983

16. Fountain SS, Hamilton RD, Jameson RM: Transverse fracture of the sacrum. J Bone Joint Surg [Am] 59:486–489, 1977

17. Fredrickson BE, Yuan HA, Miller HE: Treatment of painful long-standing displaced fracture-dislocations of the sacrum. Clin Orthop 186:93–95, 1982

18. Furey WW: Fractures of the pelvis, with special reference to associated fractures of the sacrum. AJR 47:96, 1942

19. Hadley MD, Carter LP: Sacral fracture with pseudomeningocele and cerebrospinal fluid fistula: Case report and review of the literature. Neurosurgery 16:843–846, 1985

20. Hallgrimsson S: Three cases of fracture of the sacrum. Acta Orthop Scand 9:100–114, 1938

21. Heckman JD, Keats PK: Fracture of the sacrum in a child. J Bone Joint Surg [Am] 60:404–405, 1978

22. Jackson H, Kam J, Harris JH, Harle TS: The sacral arcuate lines in upper sacral fractures. Radiology 145:35–39, 1982

23. Kellman JF, McMurtry RY, Daley D, Tile M: The unstable pelvic fracture. Orthop Clin North Am 18:25–41, 1987

24. Laasonen EM: Missed sacral fractures. Ann Clin Res 9:84–87, 1977

25. Lafollette BF, Levine MI, McNiesh LM: Bilateral fracture-dislocation of the sacrum. J Bone Joint Surg [Am] 68:1099–1101, 1986

26. Lam CR: Nerve injury in fracture of the pelvis. Ann Surg 104:945–951, 1936

27. Lourie H: Spontaneous osteoporotic fracture of the sacrum. JAMA 248:715–717, 1982

28. Marcus RE, Hansen ST: Bilateral fracture-dislocation of the sacrum. J Bone Joint Surg [Am] 66:1297–1299, 1984

29. Mendelman JP: Fractures of the sacrum. AJR 42:100–103, 1939

30. Miller C, Rechtine GR: Sacral fractures. Orthopaedic Review 14:681–687, 1985

31. Moed BR, Morawa LG: Displaced midline longitudinal fracture of the sacrum. J Trauma 24:435–437, 1984

32. Mundy AR, Stephenson TP, Wein AJ: Urodynamics: Principles, Practice and Application, pp 259–272. Edinburgh, Churchill Livingstone, 1984

33. Northrop CH, Eto RT, Loop JW: Vertical fracture of the sacral ala: Significance of non-continuity of the anterior superior sacral foraminal line. AJR 124:102–106, 1975

34. Patterson FP, Morton KS: Neurologic complications of fractures and dislocation of the pelvis. Surg Gynecol Obstet 112:702–706, 1961

35. Peltier LF: Complications associated with fractures of the pelvis. J Bone Joint Surg [Am] 47:1060–1069, 1965

36. Purser DW: Displaced fracture of the sacrum. J Bone Joint Surg [Br] 51:346–347, 1969

37. Ries T: Detection of osteoporotic sacral fracture with radionuclides. Radiology 146:783–785, 1983

38. Rowell CE: Fracture of sacrum with hemisaddle anesthesia and cerebrospinal fluid leak. Med J Aust 1:16–19, 1965

39. Roy-Camille R, Saillant G, Gagna G, Mazel C: Transverse fracture of the upper sacrum: Suicidal jumper's fracture. Spine 10:838–845, 1985

40. Sabiston CP, Wing PC: Sacral fractures: Classification and neurologic implications. J Trauma 26:1113–1115, 1986

41. Schmidek HH, Smith DA, Kristiansen TK: Sacral fractures. Neurosurgery 15:735–746, 1984

42. Schnaid E, Eisenstein SM, Drummond-Webb J: Delayed post-traumatic cauda equina compression syndrome. J Trauma 25:1099–1101, 1985

43. Simpson LA, Leighton RK, Waddell JP: Anterior approach and stabilization of the disrupted sacroiliac joint. Presented at the 53rd annual meeting of the AAOS, New Orleans, Louisiana, February 1986

44. Sugar O: How the sacrum got its name. JAMA 257:2061–2063, 1987

45. Tomaszek DE: Sacral fractures and neurologic deficit: Diagnosis and management. Contemporary Orthopaedics 11:51–55, 1985

46. Wakeley CPG: Fractures of the pelvis: An analysis of 100 cases. Br J Surg 17:22–29, 1929

47. Weaver EN, England GD, Richardson DE: Sacral fracture: Case presentation and review. Neurosurgery 9:725–728, 1981

48. Weis EB: Subtle neurological injuries in pelvic fractures. J Trauma 24:983–985, 1984

49. Weisel SW, Zeide MS, Terry RL: Longitudinal fractures of the sacrum: Case report. J Trauma 19:70–71, 1979

50. Woodward AH, Kelly PJ: An unusual fracture of the sacrum. Minn Med 57:465–66, 1974

14

SACROILIAC JOINT INJURIES

Justin G. Lamont

Disruption of the pelvic ring complex is usually the product of high energy injuries. Associated injuries are common. Aggressive treatment can be lifesaving and can improve the late functional outcome. This chapter will explore subjects relevant to a surgeon treating a patient with sacroiliac joint (SIJ) fractures and dislocations. Sacroiliac joint injuries have been receiving more attention in recent years as more surgeons try to improve the results of treatment with early stabilization. More work needs to be done to help clarify what treatment protocol should be used.

The focus of this chapter is SIJ injuries; related sacral fractures are addressed in Chapter 13. Other pelvic injuries, such as wing fractures, acetabular fractures, and pubic diastasis injuries are beyond the scope of this chapter and will not be covered. This chapter is not intended to be a self study course in the treatment SIJ injuries. It will hopefully stimulate interest in the treatment of such injuries by a review of the techniques involved in assessing, treating, and caring for patients with SIJ injuries.

The reader is cautioned that while isolated SIJ injuries do occur, they are frequently seen in combination with other pelvic injuries. One should not attempt the treatment of SIJ injuries without being skilled in the treatment of pelvic and acetabular fractures. This is especially important for the surgeon who is considering treating an SIJ injury and then referring the patient for treatment of other pelvic or acetabular fractures. Without proper knowledge and techniques, optimum treatment options for other fractures could be unknowingly eliminated or made more difficult by the SIJ injury approach taken.

OVERVIEW

HISTORY

In the treatment of SIJ injuries the past coexists with the present. Patients with massive injuries frequently die or are considered too "sick" to be able to tolerate major surgical procedures to stabilize pelvic fractures. Much of the morbidity and mortality has been associated with the trauma and not with the treatment or lack of it. In part this has been due to the lack of successful surgical alternatives. The earliest attempts at internal fixation, in general, suffered from the lack of modern advances in anesthesia, aseptic technique, antibiotics, and metallurgy. Instrumentation has been improving as people try new ideas and reinvent old ones. Various types of traction and slings have been a time-honored method of dealing with SIJ injuries.

External fixation has enjoyed a popularity due to less operative exposure, time, and risk. It continues to be a mainstay of treatment for initial resuscitative measures. However, it is much less popular for definitive fixation, especially at major trauma centers where a large number of these injuries are seen. This is largely due to poor outcomes in unstable pelvic injuries and in part due to the confidence gained from the volume of cases. Unstable posterior pelvic ring injuries cannot be controlled by external fixation. Internal fixation is indicated in these cases, although the most appropriate methods are as yet not well documented by long-term studies.

Internal fixation on a delayed basis has been gaining popularity. It is associated with a high operative complication rate but affords more stable fixation. Surgical approaches are more involved and may be compromised by other required procedures (e.g., colostomies) or severely traumatized soft tissues. Soft-tissue considerations and the need for improved visualization have fostered interest in anterior approaches to the SIJ for internal fixation. Until recently, posterior approaches to the SIJ predominated. An assortment of devices, including screws, special plates, and threaded bars, have been used. In addition, combinations of internal and external fixation have been used with success.

CHANGES

Experience has shown that certain injury patterns are well suited for a specific type of internal fixa-

tion. The collective experience of the larger trauma centers using internal fixation has helped to formulate protocols of treatment. While by no means universally agreed upon, these protocols for internal fixation have been major change in recent years from the traction methods used by a majority of surgeons treating SIJ injuries. In the past, there was a very limited number pioneers in the field using internal fixation on the often difficult cases. Treating surgeons have benefited from the "cross-fertilization" from the increasing number of colleagues working in the field.

More attention to the late outcomes of SIJ injuries in the follow-up of different treatments has been a helpful change. A better restoration of anatomy can result in considerable improvement of late function, and has been found to have a significantly beneficial effect on the short-term improvement of the patient. There are not enough long-term studies yet to define acceptable parameters of treatment. More work is needed in this area.

TRENDS

A general trend of treatment that has evolved among surgeons who treat SIJ injuries on a regular basis is the use of external fixation as an acute resuscitative procedure and then definitive internal fixation on a delayed basis. The acute stabilization of spinal and long bone fractures has improved the lot of the multiple-trauma patient in recent years. Potentially fatal complications are reduced by early, aggressive stabilization of such fractures. This treatment trend has influenced the thinking of surgeons treating patients with pelvic fractures as well. Prolonged bed rest in traction has a detrimental effect on multiple-trauma patients. The timing of the stabilization of fractures is important for the resuscitation of patients. However, extensive surgery on pelvic fractures in the acute setting can lead to washout coagulopathies and other complications, and actually increase morbidity and mortality. It is dangerous to approach every case in a "cookbook" fashion. Close cooperation among the members of the trauma team caring for a multiple-trauma patient is critical. Knowing when to proceed and when not to is largely a matter of experience. There is no ethical substitute today for proper training at a major trauma center in order to gain this experience.

FUTURE DEVELOPMENTS

As more collective experience is gained and disseminated, answers to some current questions should be forthcoming: What is the optimal time to perform pelvic fixation, and what are the parameters for choosing that time? Which SIJ injuries should be reconstructed and which should be acutely fused? What are the best techniques to facilitate the placement of hardware? Diagnostic imaging techniques are constantly improving, and will continue to help in the understanding of SIJ injuries and facilitation of treatment plans. Further development may include the use of imaging techniques in the placement of hardware. The lack of widespread use of the most expensive, state-of-the-art, technologies will continue to be a stimulus to working with standardly available tools in developing treatment protocols.

CLASSIFICATION

Classifications of injuries should serve several purposes. One is to define the injury in order to facilitate communication. A description of a fracture should be understandable and useful to those who cannot review the patient or all pertinent background data personally. As a classification becomes more detailed it ceases to facilitate communication and can actually become a hindrance. It is expected that a certain lexicon has to be mastered in any field. However, overly detailed classifications are often more trouble than they are worth. The second purpose of a classification is to help indicate what would be an appropriate treatment method for a given injury. Third, there should be some prognostic value in the classification to help one assess the outcome.

There is no current standard classification of SIJ injuries used by previous authors in the field. In fact, most authors to date have devised their own classification schemes for use in their writings. Sacroiliac joint injuries are usually addressed as a subset of pelvic ring injuries. The following are among the classifications that have been devised.[1,6,7]

PENNAL

Pennal and Sutherland studied pelvic ring injuries and proposed three main types of force vectors that cause injury: anteroposterior compression, lateral compression, and vertical shear. Their analysis has been accepted for many years and is commonly used to describe the types of injuries. Anteroposterior forces may cause the pubic symphysis to split apart or be pushed inward. This results in either a diastasis or a "straddle" fracture of all four pubic rami. If the pubis separates far enough, the iliac wings can fracture or the SIJ can open (Fig. 14-1). If only the anterior SIJ ligaments yield, an "open book" type of injury results.

A lateral compression force causes some type of compression fracture of the sacral ala, with fracture or separation of the posterior SIJ. In addition, some type of anterior pelvic lesion is present (Fig. 14-2). This anterior lesion can be a pubic symphysis diastasis, a ramus fracture of the ipsilateral or contralateral side of the SIJ, or both.

In a vertical shear type of injury, the sacrotuberal and sacrospinal ligaments must be disrupted for displacement of more than a few centimeters to occur. This injury type involves a high energy level and carries a worse prognosis, usually due to associated injuries. Further, the likelihood of neural injury by traction on nerve roots is higher. The vertical shear force disrupts either the symphysis or rami anteriorly as well. There can be significant posterior displacement of the hemipelvis without superior displacement. Bilateral vertical shear injuries involve more energy and carry a worse prognosis. Variants of these general types occur, but the general principles apply.

LETOURNEL

Letournel classifies pelvic ring injuries by anatomic site (Fig. 14-3). There are therefore six sites of injury: the symphysis, rami, acetabulum, ilium, SIJ, and sacrum. Numerous variations in each category, as well as many combinations, are possible.

(*Text continued on p. 356*)

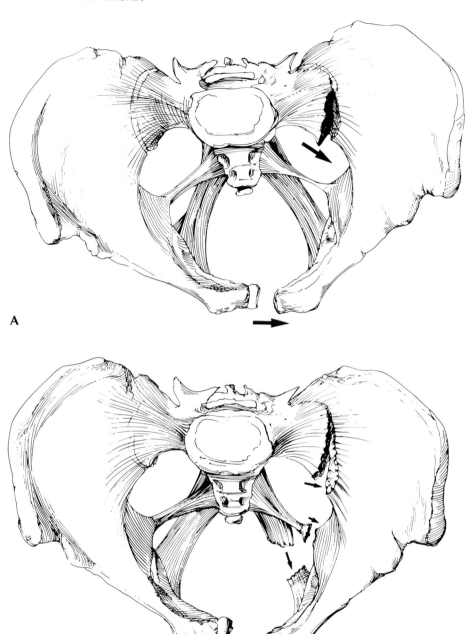

Figure 14-1. (*A*) Anteroposterior compression injuries. Sacrospinous and sacrotuberous ligaments are intact. (*B*) Only posterior ligaments are intact.

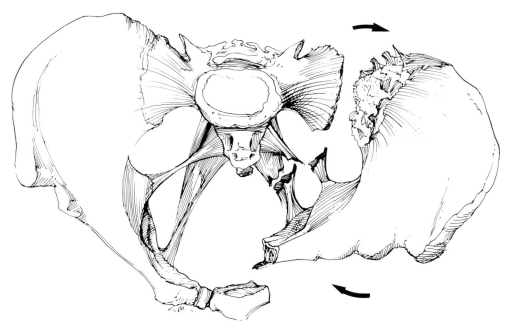

Figure 14-2. Lateral compression injury. Complete disruption, unstable.

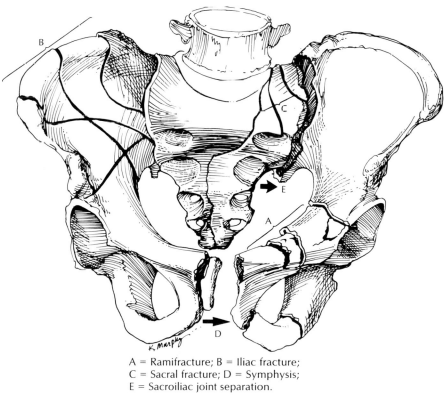

A = Ramifracture; B = Iliac fracture;
C = Sacral fracture; D = Symphysis;
E = Sacroiliac joint separation.

Figure 14-3. Letournel's classification.

Letournel's is a unified scheme in which site and magnitude as well as direction of displacement are used to assess stability. The exact threshold of stability is not defined. It does direct one's attention to the area potentially needing fixation.

BUCHOLZ

Bucholz proposed a classification scheme that attempts to combine the site of injury with the degree of displacement.[1] His scheme defines the areas needing fixation and offers prognostic value according to the magnitude of the forces involved to create the injury. Bucholz noted three types of injuries. First is the mild symphysis disruption with a nondisplaced vertical shear or mild open book type injury. Second is the more severe type of open book injury, in which the sacrotuberal and sacrospinal ligaments are torn. Finally, there is symphysis disruption with complete posterior separation.

This classification leaves out bilateral SIJ injuries, iliac wing fractures, and acetabular fractures. All of these omitted injuries have an important bearing on the degree of total injury and the treatment needed. This has been pointed out by Mears and Rubash, who have added a fourth category to include these injuries.

There is no classification that fulfills all the goals mentioned above completely. Any significant disruption of the SIJ, which includes the posterior ligaments, is a major injury and is unstable. Early reduction is necessary for successful restoration of anatomy. Late cases have a higher complication rate and a lower success rate compared to cases treated within 2 weeks of injury. Open injuries should serve as a alarm to the treating surgeon to look for life-threatening associated injuries prior to focusing on the SIJ injuries. There is an additional challenge of acute and delayed sepsis prevention.

EVALUATION

Evaluation of a patient with an SIJ injury must proceed according to Advanced Trauma Life Support (ATLS) principles.[2] Because of the possibility of concomitant life-threatening injuries, it is im-

perative to thoroughly examine the patient before focusing on a specific skeletal injury. After this is done, basic studies should be ordered, and then more detailed studies as needed. A therapeutic decision should be the basis for ordering more sophisticated and expensive studies.

CLINICAL EXAMINATION

The examination of a patient in the acute setting should focus on the discovery of occult life-threatening injuries and the triage of obvious injuries. Advanced Trauma Life Support principles should be followed. A patent functioning airway must take initial priority. The basic steps for the rest of the initial examination are well covered in ATLS courses and texts. The reader is encouraged to make use of these resources. In a patient is transferred after the acute setting the clinician is still responsible to make sure that no injuries were missed by the referring institution.

Once the general evaluation of the patient is complete and a triage of injuries has been done, attention can be focused on the pelvis. The focus of evaluation for SIJ injuries is pelvic instability and the associated complications. It is important to try to establish the neurologic status of the patient prior to any therapeutic intervention. This is helpful in gauging the severity of an injury, such as a vertical shear fracture-dislocation of the SIJ with potential neurologic compromise. The greater the displacement of the iliac wing or the greater the involvement of the sacral fracture, the more likely it is that there will be a neurologic injury.

If a patient is to be operated on for other injuries or to receive a related procedure, such as a laparotomy, that is an ideal time to asses the clinical stability of an SIJ injury. The patient will be relaxed and will experience no pain during the examination. One must be careful not to examine an unstable pelvis too vigorously in order to avoid causing further injury. Gross instability of the iliac wing should alert one to the need for some type of provisional fixation in the acute setting. Anteroposterior and mediolateral compression should be applied to the pelvis by hand, and the amount of motion or presence of crepitus should be noted. This can then be compared with radiographic studies to more accurately define the injury.

The presence of open pelvic fractures should alert the treating physician to the magnitude of the injury. Open pelvic fractures are high energy injuries. Along with associated injuries, they have a significant rate of morbidity and mortality. Hemorrhage is the major cause of death in pelvic fractures. In only a small minority of cases is the bleeding arterial. The massive venous plexus of the pelvis and large cancellous surfaces are the most common sources of bleeding. The best way to control this type of bleeding is stabilization of the fracture fragments. Diverting colostomies should be performed if open fracture wounds are near the perineum. Damage to the soft tissues in regions where surgical exposures may be required should be noted. There is a high association of wound breakdown and postoperative infection with posterior approaches through traumatized tissue. Severe skin contusions, in addition to obvious abrasions and lacerations, should be a relative contraindication to incisions. Underlying muscle necrosis is an unforeseen problem when open reductions are attempted.

PLAIN FILMS

Much information can be obtained from plain films about unstable SIJ injuries. Anteroposterior and 40-degree inlet and outlet views should be taken. The vertical displacement of an iliac wing is an obvious way to spot an unstable injury. Fractures of the lateral processes of L-5 and L-4 are suggestive of instability. Avulsion of the bone is caused by the iliolumbar ligaments. A widening of the SIJ can be seen on a film of the pelvis. Bilateral injuries may make the widening less obvious, but marked asymmetry should be apparent. Other pelvic fractures should alert one to the possibility of SIJ injuries. Any pubic symphysis diastasis greater than 2 to 3 cm should be an indication to further evaluate the posterior pelvis. A pure open book type of injury with disruption of only the anterior sacroiliac ligaments will not have any vertical displacement of the ilium, even though there will be some anteroposterior instability on compression. Marked widening of the pubic symphysis indicates more extensive SIJ injury with possible posterior sacroiliac ligament involvement and instability.

COMPUTED TOMOGRAPHY

Due to overlying gas shadows and the geometry of the bony architecture, plain films are limited in their ability to portray an SIJ injury. Up to 60% of sacral fractures are missed on plain films. While multiple views can better define the injury, a computed tomographic (CT) scan is considered the best way to define the SIJ by most people treating these injuries. Unlike in acetabular or some other pelvic fractures, three-dimensional imaging is not as necessary or even useful for examining the SIJ specifically. The angulation of the iliac wings is clearly evident. Small fractures of the articular surfaces of the SIJ are apparent. The involvement of the sacrum is well defined. This is especially important if one is considering using the sacrum for an implant in fixing the SIJ. Computed tomography will be helpful in diagnosis of areas near the SIJ as well. Plain films will show other fractures, such as spinal fractures, needing CT studies. Also, a CT scan of the abdomen may be indicated for soft-tissue evaluation in the case of blunt abdominal trauma.

The two most important criteria on the CT scan with respect to the SIJ are joint incongruity and degree of displacement. As with most joint surfaces, several millimeters of displacement does not warrant surgical intervention. In addition, if the displacement is an anterior opening of the SIJ, more displacement can be tolerated. Vertical displacement is more critical to reduce because of the shape of the joint surfaces. Vertical displacement quickly leads to joint incongruity.

BONE SCANS

Bone scans are of little use in the acute evaluation of SIJ injuries. Historically, the pelvis has been compared to a Lifesaver candy: it cannot be broken in only one place. Bone scans have shown occult injuries in the SIJ in association with anterior fractures, giving credence to the "ring" theory. However, if a bone scan is required to find an SIJ injury, the injury will probably not require any treatment. Treatment would usually consist of restricted weight bearing until the pain decreases. Pathologic fractures of the SIJ would warrant the routine use of the bone scan.

MAGNETIC RESONANCE IMAGING

Magnetic resonance imaging has little, if any, role in the evaluation of SIJ injuries. In general, it is much more useful for evaluating soft tissues than bone. The advantages of magnetic resonance imaging are that no ionizing radiation is used and better quality sagittal reconstructions are possible. However, it is not routinely used for SIJ injury evaluations.

TREATMENT

The treatment for SIJ injuries is varied. There is conflicting data on the best way to manage these injuries. A distinction should be made between early resuscitative measures and definitive treatment with long-term follow-up. Absence of pain and pelvic symmetry are the long-term goals. The least dangerous method should be employed toward that end. However, severely injured patients have different requirements than patients with isolated injuries.

BED REST

For patients who have not suffered multiple trauma and whose injury is stable, simple bed rest is usually adequate. Fracture consolidation is usually rapid, and ambulation is usually possible by several weeks. However, the fracture must be stable or there may be unacceptable displacement even with bed rest. Weight bearing should be progressive, with initial protection based on the severity of the injury. Prolonged bed rest should be avoided. With an isolated injury that is marginal, it is important to remember that a fusion can be done at a later time for pain. However, correction of malunions and nonunions is difficult and is often more dangerous than an initial stabilization. For these problems the best treatment is prevention.

Bed rest will require some type of prophylaxis against thromboembolism. The risk of internal bleeding has to be evaluated in light of associated injuries. The "best" type of protection is still debated in the literature. Sodium warfarin (Coumadin) has been used with success, but requires careful monitoring. Complications can be lethal on both extremes of dosage. It is important for the physician to use a method with which he is familiar. Older patients are at an increased risk while at bed rest; early mobilization, even if it is bed to chair, should be stressed.

SLINGS

Pelvic slings have been used to try to reduce open book type injuries of the pelvis. They are not indicated for vertical shear type injuries. The type of reduction obtained with this technique is questionable. A narrowing of the pubic diastasis is of little functional importance. The incongruity of the SIJ is of more importance for the prevention of late sacroiliac pain. Unless a CT scan shows an acceptable reduction of the SIJ, this type of treatment is difficult to justify. Furthermore, a sling seldom increases the patient's level of comfort. Turning the patient is still difficult, and therefore nursing care is not facilitated.

TRACTION

Traction is used to pull down a vertically displaced ilium. It does not correct posterior displacement. As with slings, the reduction of the SIJ is important to assess. Marked leg length discrepancies and sitting imbalance can result if vertical displacement is not corrected. A patient can be treated in traction until cleared for operative reduction and stabilization. Traction does help minimize motion at the injury site and thus helps prevent blood loss. Skeletal traction in a supine position is not well tolerated by a patient with lung injuries. Therefore, traction should not be used as a first-line treatment in a multiple-trauma patient. Soft-tissue problems or osteoporosis may be indications for traction. Because of the weights required, femoral pins are usually used. It is important to keep the pins extracapsular to avoid the complication of a septic joint. Pins placed in the ilium or trochanter should not be used to aid in reduction if surgical approaches may be planned in that area.

The time in traction will vary, depending on the degree of injury and the degree of bony callus formation, as seen in serial radiographs. The time is also dependent on clinical stability. Wheelchairs can be used to keep patients from bearing weight while still permitting mobilization. Six weeks of traction will often be required to obtain sufficient stability.

INSTRUMENTATION

The use of instrumentation for SIJ injuries should be based on the degree of instability and the presence of associated soft-tissue injuries. The patient is usually not operated on until 5 to 7 days after the injury if major posterior instrumentation is going to be used. External fixators are used acutely. Pin tract infections can preclude the use of an anterior approach to the SIJ. If an anterior approach is planned, an anterior frame should be avoided if possible. A plate can be used to keep a pubic diastasis together. Plate fixation can be done by itself or in conjunction with a laparotomy. Use of Pfannenstiel's incision is preferred for a plate fixation alone.

EXTERNAL

External fixation is the mainstay of initial treatment of unstable SIJ injuries at this time. A surgeon should be well versed in this technique if treating these injuries. Many configurations of frames have been devised to treat unstable SIJ injuries. Rigid constructs were used to try deal with posterior instability. These frames required more extensive exposure and multiple pin clusters. Although they are more stable than simple frames, later posterior fixation obviates their need. A main disadvantage of the very rigid external fixation frame is the inability to get an accurate reduction of an unstable SIJ.

Therefore, many surgeons use a simple frame of one or two 5-mm half pins connected by a simple crossbar type of frame. Six-millimeter half pins are sometimes used for more rigidity, but 5-mm pins will usually suffice. There is a thick column of bone in the ilium approximately three finger breadths back from the anterosuperior iliac spine. There is also an overhang of the lateral lip of the iliac crest. These two points must be kept in mind when inserting the pins. The crests are usually predrilled with a 5/32-inch drill bit. They can be placed percutaneously using a Steinmann pin carefully inserted along the inner table of the crest as a guide. Small incisions can also be used. Large hematomas will drain through incisions during the insertion process. This may appear to constitute a large blood loss. While this is blood already lost from the intravascular space, it does decompress the retroperitoneal hematoma. This results in loss of tamponade, and the retroperitoneal space will refill. Reducing the pelvic fracture will decrease the volume available for the hematoma to fill. Also, the shearing of the clotting pelvic veins is decreased by the relative stability afforded by the frame.

It is important to realize that the wings are displaced when planning the skin incisions for the pins. An attempt should be made to reduce the iliac wings by manual means before starting pin insertion. Excessive "closing of the book" anteriorly will result in a widening posteriorly, and should be avoided. The time required for application should be no more than 20 to 30 minutes by an experienced operative team. This can be done in conjunction with a laparotomy. The frame can be angled downward to permit any abdominal procedure, and then tilted upward at the end. It is important to remember the patient's sitting posture when placing the pins and assembling the frame. An angle of about 60 degrees between the iliac crest and the pins is usually appropriate.

Postoperatively, the pins should have daily care with some type of cleaning protocol. Continued use of pin dressings is not needed after several days. Any infected, draining pin should be replaced or removed. Erythema, drainage, and pain, even without fever or large elevations of the white blood count, are sufficient cause for pin removal. Weight bearing is not permitted for 4 to 6 weeks at a minimum with an external fixator and a potentially unstable fracture. Further procedures to provide posterior fixation do not appreciably change the time course for the earliest allowable weight bearing. Bilateral injuries will require a wheelchair. With bilateral SIJ injuries, anterior external fixators provide little stability indeed.

Wing fractures may make the use of half pin placement impossible. In this situation, internal fixation of the anterior ring injury may be required.

INTERNAL

Internal fixation can be carried out in a variety of ways. The two basic types of implants are screws and plates. Large cancellous screws are usually used with some type of washer to prevent the screw head from cutting into the bone. Sometimes a two-hole plate is used as a large washer for two screws. This type of fixation is usually used for transiliac fixation of SIJ injuries from the posterior approach. Independently placed screws can be used for fixing wing fractures and fracture-dislocations through the SIJ. These are placed between the inner and outer tables of the iliac crest. The most commonly done type of internal fixation is posteriorly applied screws with washers, or plates and screws.

Posterior

The posterior approach to the SIJ is usually carried out through a longitudinal incision centered 2 cm lateral to the posterosuperior iliac spine. If the incision is made lateral to the spine, this facilitates exposure of the iliac wing for hardware placement. The gluteus maximus is elevated subperiosteally from the ilium. It is almost futile to try to assess the reduction of the SIJ just from looking at the posterior aspect of the joint. The ilium is angled and overhangs the joint, which is also covered by the thick posterior sacroiliac ligaments. If one carefully dissects over the top of the sacrum onto the ala, the top of the joint can be palpated. The inferior portion of the SIJ is palpable through the greater sciatic notch. This should be done in a blunt fashion with care taken not to injure the L-5 nerve root. If the surgeon's finger is long enough, the anterior SIJ can be palpated on its superior portion. Retraction of the gluteal structures is often difficult when attempting to place screws from the lateral ilium into the sacrum. Either the ala of the sacrum or the body of S-1 may be used,

depending on the injury. Percutaneous screw insertion endangers the gluteal neurovascular structures, and care must be taken (Figs. 14-4, 14-5, 14-6).

Bilateral posterior crest exposure can be done through two parallel longitudinal incisions or through one long transverse one. The transverse incision is used for the double cobra plate popularized by Mears[6] or any other bilateral plating instrumentation. A plate can also be tunneled beneath the skin bridge between two longitudinal incisions (Fig. 14-7). Some type of bilateral fixation is mandatory with bilateral SIJ injury. There must be sufficient purchase of the hardware into both iliac wings and the sacrum. With extensive comminution of the sacrum, the bodies of S-1 or even S-2 must be used.

When placing screws into the sacrum, iatrogenic damage to nerve roots and blood vessels can be minimized by palpating landmarks and using the image intensifier, as described by Matta.[4] It is imperative to practice on pelvic models to gain a feel for the orientation of the screws and to try to simulate what the actual surgical exposure permits one to see. Four cortices can be felt when drilling from the lateral ilium to the anterior sacrum. First is the lateral wall at the starting point. This is usually two finger breadths anterior to the posteroinferior iliac spine and about 1.5 cm above the top of the sciatic notch. A second screw is placed about 2 cm superior to this, parallel to a line connecting the back edge of the two posterior spines. These screws should not be parallel in the transverse plane, but rather angled about 10 degrees. The next two cortices are those of the joint surfaces of the SIJ. The last cortex is the anterior sacrum. Penetration of this cortex to any significant degree by either a drill bit or screw should be avoided. Unexplained sudden massive drops in blood pressure should alert the surgeon to a possible iliac vessel injury. These landmarks are guides, and the individual patient's anatomy must dictate actual screw placement. Although one can read an account of this procedure and see illustrations, seeing an actual case is invaluable.[4]

The image intensifier can be very helpful, but the patient must be on a radiolucent table to use it. The image intensifier must be able to yield a sharp

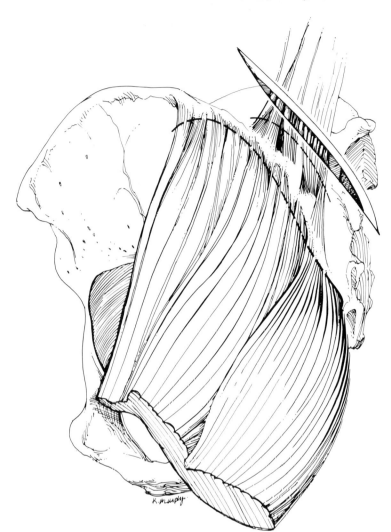

Figure 14-4. Posterior internal fixation, approach. Skin incision; dotted line = fascial incision.

picture, which is difficult in obese and large persons. The surgeon directs the technician to obtain the necessary views. Penetration of the caudal canal is often hard to appreciate, and a postoperative CT scan is useful if this is suspected. Cannulated screws are useful in avoiding injury by misdirected screws.

The paraspinal muscles must be elevated off the sacrum for the placement of bilateral plating in the SIJ. Care must be taken to avoid injuring the dorsal nerve roots. The L-5 nerve root lies on the groove in the superior ala of the sacrum. The iliac vessels lie anterior to the sacrum. These structures are at risk when drilling or inserting screws. The inferior margin of the SIJ can be exposed to facilitate the palpation of a reduction and the location of landmarks such as the sacral foramina. The foramina are used as guides to avoid nerve root injury when placing screws. A finger is kept over the

(*Text continued on p. 364*)

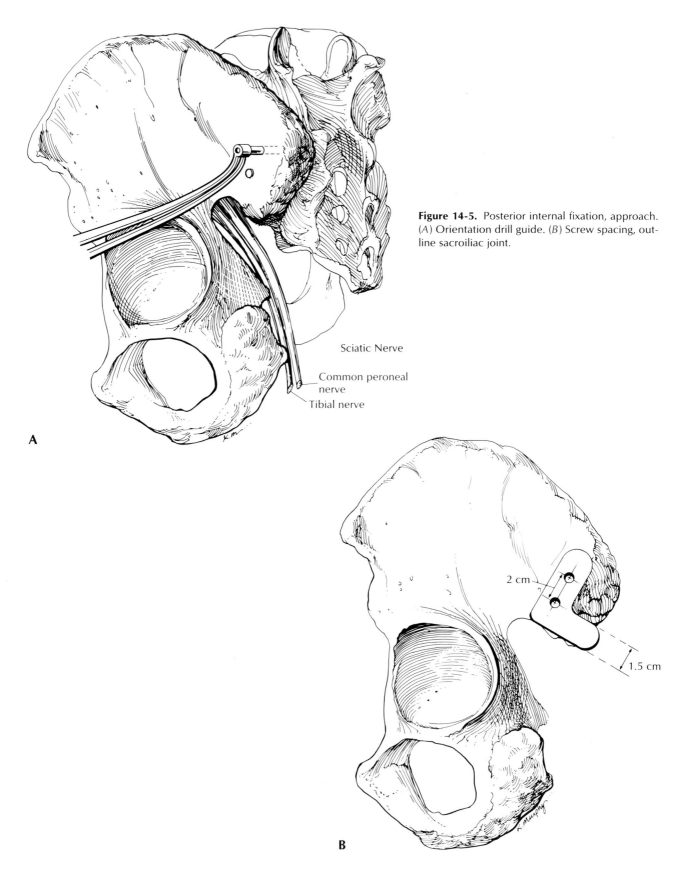

Figure 14-5. Posterior internal fixation, approach. (A) Orientation drill guide. (B) Screw spacing, outline sacroiliac joint.

Sciatic Nerve

Common peroneal nerve

Tibial nerve

A

2 cm

1.5 cm

B

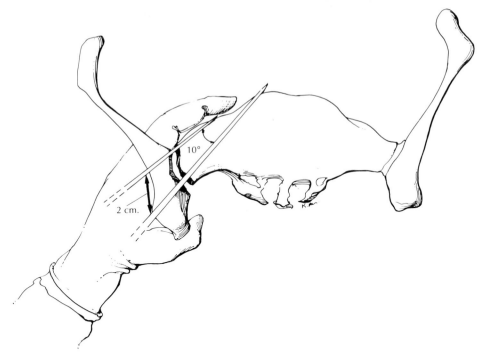

Figure 14-6. Posterior internal fixation, placement. Angle of drill bit for sacroiliac fixation.

Figure 14-7. Posterior plate, bilateral sacroiliac joints.

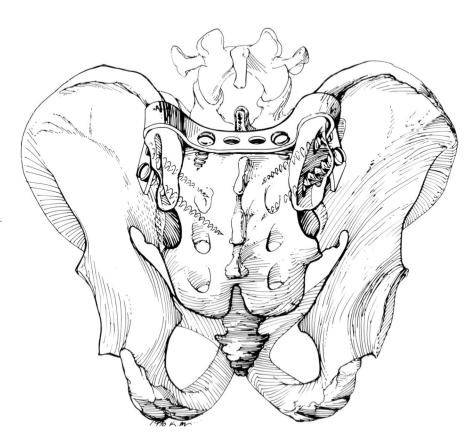

foramen while drilling. When exposing the inferior SIJ, care must be taken not to injure the superior gluteal artery in the greater sciatic notch.

Threaded bars and nuts or long screws can be used to help stabilize the iliac wings (Figs. 14-8, 14-9). Compression can be applied across the sacrum to aid in stabilization. Care must be taken to avoid nerve root compression in the presence of sacral comminution. One or two bars can be inserted through the two posterior crests. A two-hole plate can be used as a washer on each side to make the construct more rigid. The posterior spines of the upper sacrum can be used as another fixation point. The approach can be either two longitudinal incisions or one transverse one. The threaded bars will work better if used as an adjunct to screws placed across the SIJ as described above (Fig. 14-10).

Anterior

Interest in anterior instrumentation arose in part because of postoperative wound complications and iatrogenic neurovascular injuries with the posterior approach. However, the anterior surgical approach is more formidable. The articular surface of the SIJ can be inspected under direct vision. This is difficult if not often impossible from the back. If one sees extensive damage to the articular surfaces of the SIJ, a primary fusion can be considered. While several special plates for the anterior plating of the SIJ are being developed, their suitability cannot be determined until they become more widely used.

The anterior approach to the SIJ is done by using the upper portion of the ilioinguinal approach as described by Letournel and, more re-

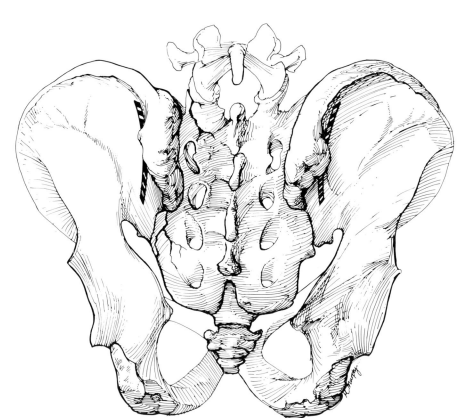

Figure 14-8. Posterior internal fixation, skin incisions.

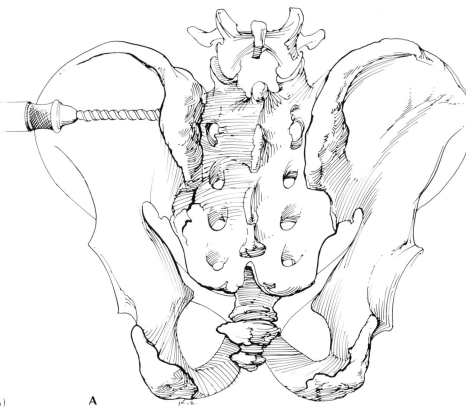

Figure 14-9. Threaded bars. (A) Before drilling. (B) Rod bolted to each posterior iliac spine.

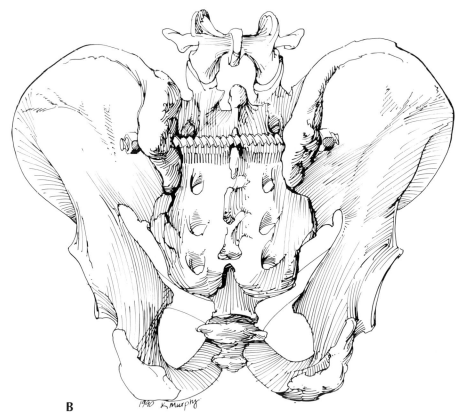

A

B

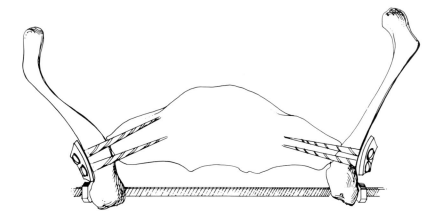

Figure 14-10. Bilateral combined fixation of the sacroiliac joint.

cently, by Matta.[5] The lower portion of this approach is used for open reduction and internal fixation of acetabular fractures and will not be discussed. The patient is placed supine with a bolster under the buttock. This permits the incision to be carried out over the superiormost portion of the iliac brim and back toward the sacrum. The muscles are detached from the iliac crest from the superior spine anteriorly to the posterior third of the crest. The inner surface of the ilium is stripped subperiosteally. Bone bleeders may require bone wax for control. The internal iliac fossa is exposed over to the SIJ. A retractor is then placed medially on the quadrilateral surface of the pelvis. The iliopsoas and femoral nerve are thus displaced medially, permitting plates and screws to be placed across the SIJ.

A plate can be placed on the pubic symphysis through a Pfannenstiel approach or a midline approach (Fig. 14-11). The spermatic cords are identified by vessel loops in the male. The round ligament is found in the female. The attachment of the rectus abdominus is often avulsed off one or both sides of the symphysis, facilitating hardware placement. Several different plating configurations have been used by various authors with success. Two plates can be used at right angles to each other. However, a simple plate on the symphysis is sufficient if posterior instrumentation is planned. Care must be taken not to injure the bladder or

the urethra during reduction of a diastasis. This is easily checked by a ribbon retractor and lap pad protecting the bladder and a foley catheter identifying the urethra. Reduction is done using a reduction forceps to close the symphysis. Accurate reduction is important; just coapting the pubis in a haphazard fashion will compromise an accurate reduction posteriorly. Care must be taken not to injure the obturator neurovascular bundle with the tips of the reduction forceps during placement of the instrument. Repair and closure of the rectus abdominus is helped by flexing the operating table to take tension off the muscle.

Regardless of the type of fixation used for the SIJ, reduction of the joint can be difficult. Using a small, temporary external fixator "handle" on the iliac brim will help a great deal. Smooth Steinmann pins can be used as provisional fixation while the definitive plate and screws are being applied. The space available to work in the internal iliac fossa is quite limited, and planning of the placement retractors, instruments, and implants to avoid obstruction is well rewarded.

Once the SIJ is reduced and temporarily held, definitive fixation can be applied. This usually consists of two plates contoured to the surface of the ilium and sacrum. It is important to cross the SIJ with a plate in two places to prevent toggling. This type of fixation is not possible from the anterior approach if there is extensive sacral alar comminution. Failing to identify this with preoperative studies may be an invitation to disaster. This situation may be salvaged by closing and using a posterior approach, or by inserting percutaneous screws posteriorly. This is difficult but possible.

Combined Anterior and Posterior

Combined anterior and posterior internal fixation of the SIJ is quite well supported from a biomechanical viewpoint. This would usually entail some type of pubic symphysis plating with either an anterior plating of the SIJ or screws, plates, or threaded bars in the back. This type of surgery should not be attempted in a patient in the acute period, when the patient is marginally stable. Because there can be significant blood loss, a cell saver is useful any time this type of approach is taken.

COMBINED INTERNAL AND EXTERNAL

Combined internal and external fixation of the SIJ is often staged. The external fixation is applied anteriorly as a resuscitative procedure. Five to seven days later, the posterior internal fixation is applied. If open reduction and internal fixation of the SIJ is planned in conjunction with any type of pubic symphysis fixation, the SIJ should be done first. This will help avoid a malreduction of the more important SIJ caused by a symphysis fixation that was not properly reduced first. If the posterior fixation is tenuous, internal fixation of the symphysis may be preferable. An external fixator applied anteriorly may become infected or loose, and thus cannot be relied on to last until healing is sufficient for removal.

POSTOPERATIVE COURSE

Postoperative treatment is often critical for the achievement of optimal results. If premature weight bearing is started, the fixation may loosen or fail. In addition, the injuries often associated with fixation must be aggressively mobilized to facilitate maximal recovery.

PAIN CONTROL

Pain is one of the major obstacles to mobilization and hence must be controlled as quickly and as thoroughly as possibly. Large doses of narcotics on an around-the-clock schedule may control pain, but such treatment is not desirable. The patient must try to develop a diurnal pattern of sleep and activity. More activity during the day and more pain medication at night is one way to help bring about a functional daily pattern. The dosages and frequency of administration of narcotics has to be modified according to the patient's age, weight, drug history, liver function, degree of injury and surgery, and personality.

One way to control the amount of pain medication the patient gets and still let the patient have control of when it is administered is to use a patient-controlled analgesia system. This is a pump with a calibrated amount of narcotic that is injected intravenously by a patient-controlled switch. The amount of medication that can be administered in a given time period is controlled. The patient gets a quick response to the medication because it is an intravenous narcotic. Also, because the medication can be given rapidly after the onset of more severe pain (within the preset limits), less total medication is needed. A protocol of intramuscular injections, oral narcotics, and then other analgesics must be established and adhered to. Epidural opiates are another option.

BED REST

Bed rest is in general undesirable for the treatment of musculoskeletal injuries. Function breeds function, as well as prevents new problems. It is usually resorted to when the fixation of fractures is not stable enough to permit mobilization of the patient. Significant stresses are applied to the hip and pelvis in a patient in bed, largely due to muscular contractions. Skeletal traction pins can help counteract these muscular forces. When traction is used, joint mobilization should not be forgotten. Passive assist cords can help the patient move the hip and knee in traction. Decisions about when to discontinue bed rest are based on clinical examination and serial radiographic studies. Callus forma-

(*Text continued on p. 370*)

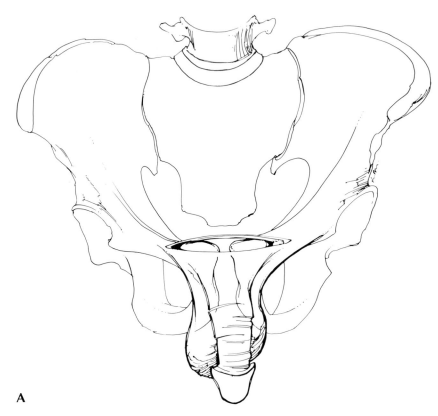

Figure 14-11. Anterior plate. (A) Skin incision. (B) Deep dissection.

A

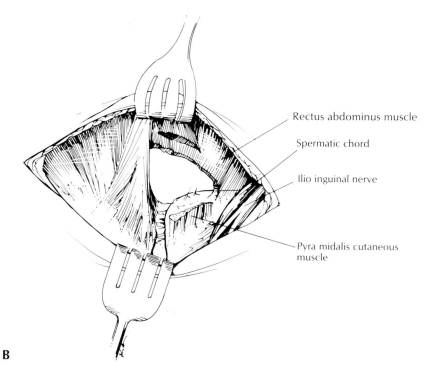

Rectus abdominus muscle

Spermatic chord

Ilio inguinal nerve

Pyra midalis cutaneous muscle

B

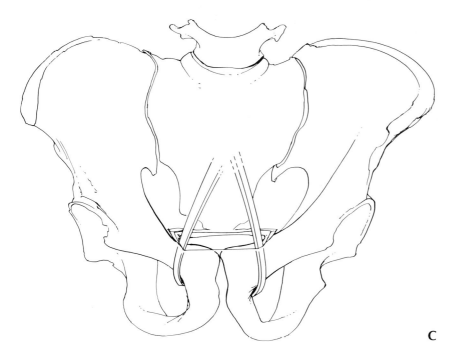

C

Figure 14-11. (*continued*). (*C*) Reduction. (*D*) Plating.

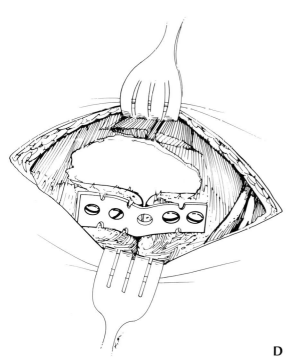

D

tion is one clinicial criterion. Heterotopic bone may sometimes confuse the radiographic picture by obscuring a nonunion but not providing stability. Sitting out of bed in a chair requires transfers that may not be possible early on. Also, the patient must be compliant if transfers are done. Full weight bearing is often a consequence of first attempts at transfers. It is better for the treating surgeon to witness the first transfers and evaluate if they should be continued. This is obviously most important in tenuous situations.

PASSIVE MOTION

The work of Salter[8] has forever drawn attention to the importance of keeping joints mobile. Further studies on articular cartilage have confirmed this. The SIJ injury and its surgical treatment limit a patient's activities. It is important to mobilize nearby joints to promote faster recovery and limit complications. Continuous passive motion machines have greatly helped in the postoperative care of trauma and arthroplasty patients. However, the protective effect of muscular contraction on venous return should not be overlooked. Patients should be instructed on exercises to be done while in bed, with or without the use of continuous passive motion machines.

PHYSICAL THERAPY

Physical therapy should not proceed in a vacuum in regard to the surgeon. Rote orders do not routinely lead to routine results. Mistakes in weight-bearing orders can be catastrophic. It is impossible for the therapist to decide on the proper status according to postoperative films; input from the surgeon is essential. Variables such as bony quality, hardware purchase, and occult fracture lines must be taken into account. Initial physical therapy efforts are usually directed at mobilization of the patient. Later, more attention is paid to improving range of motion and, finally, strength. Feedback from the therapist is helpful on deciding whether to trust patients to comply with their the weight-bearing status. This is quite relevant in light of the average trauma patient's age and educational and employment background. The fre-

quently associated musculoskeletal injuries make physical therapy a vital part of the treatment of SIJ injuries.

WEIGHT BEARING

The forces transmitted across the SIJ preclude full weight bearing on an unstable injury. However, when stability is questionable, decisions regarding weight bearing can be difficult. If radiographs show no signs of gross displacement or the fixation is felt to be sound, some type of partial weight bearing can usually be started. The clinical response is useful but not reliable enough, especially in the early stages. If there is a question, and the patient can cooperate, no weight bearing should be allowed for 6 weeks in most cases. At 6 weeks, in stable situations weight bearing can be progressed as tolerated. If the SIJ was grossly unstable at the time of injury, only partial weight bearing (usually, less than half of body weight) should be allowed for 2 to 4 more weeks. Radiographs should be taken shortly after any major change in weight bearing status or if there is sudden onset of increased pain. Any change in hardware or fracture position warrants a reduction in weight bearing status. Healing is often difficult to assess on plain films. Computed tomographic scans are compromised by scatter in the region of the hardware, making fine detail hard to read. Therefore, prudent use of the clinical response with a cautious approach is safest. Bilateral injuries that are unstable preclude ambulation.

WHEELCHAIR

When ambulation is contraindicated because of the instability of the fracture site, wheelchairs are needed to get patients moving around in preparation for discharge. Careful transfers with assistance are usually well tolerated. However, once out of the surgeon's direct supervision, pain will often be the limiting factor for the patient. If the SIJ injury was an isolated one, patients will mobilize more rapidly. Upper extremity injuries make wheelchair use difficult if not impossible. If companions are available this is not a problem. However, because the need for a wheelchair is short-term, the cost of an electric wheelchair is not justified. If patients are not reliable or are not able to use a wheelchair, an intermediate care facility should be arranged.

COMPLICATIONS

Complications are defined here as deleterious effects on the patient as a result of either the injury or treatment. Complications should not be equated with malpractice. Malpractice is a legal issue that involves adherence to the standard of care in a community. Deciding how to define malpractice is beyond the scope of this chapter and practically all medical publications. It is decided in a court. Nevertheless, one should bear in mind when making contributions to the medical record or corresponding with other physicians that the use of new technology and new procedures may not be legally considered optimal care.

Many complications are preventable by proper awareness. The anatomy of the SIJ makes hardware placement difficult and sometimes dangerous. The more familiar one is with the anatomy through practice, the less likely one is to get into trouble. Pelvic models are invaluable for this training. Knowing the type of associated injuries helps in their identification. Knowing the proper treatment and starting it promptly can often minimize the damage. The chronologic division of complications is a logical way to approach the subject.

PREOPERATIVE

Preoperative complications are either direct results of the trauma that cannot be prevented or missed injuries. Trauma studies show a trimodal distribution of mortality.[9] The initial peak is not preventable in most circumstances, as it occurs almost immediately after injury due to massive central nervous system injury or great vessel rupture. The next peak occurs when the treating physician is able to address preoperative preventable complications. The most likely surgically preventable cause of death is abdominal bleeding.

Neurologic and urologic emergencies require prompt attention. Therefore, designated trauma centers that are prepared to handle the spectrum of injuries are the only appropriate treatment places for patients with major pelvic injuries. Pelvic fractures occur in blunt multiple trauma at least 20% of the time. As previously mentioned, open pelvic fractures are associated with a very high morbidity and mortality rate.

Initial resuscitative efforts are directed at airway and bleeding problems. Spinal injuries must always be kept in mind when moving patients. Fluid resuscitation is an important step after the primary survey, as is outlined in Advanced Trauma Life Support texts. Rectal exams for tears or high-riding prostates are important. Bleeding from the vagina or urethra indicate occult open pelvic fractures. Urethrograms should be done in males prior to passing a foley catheter if any blood can be milked from the urethral meatus. Cystograms and an intravenous pyelogram are then indicated. The laparotomy will often be lifesaving in a hypotensive patient. A peritoneal lavage may be used to compliment the physical exam, or a computed tomographic scan may be used. Nasogastric tubes should not be inserted in patients with facial fractures, to prevent intracranial placement.

The pneumatic antishock garment or military antishock trousers are being used to help stabilize patients with pelvic fractures. The time they are inflated and the injuries they are covering up must be kept in mind. Compartment syndromes secondary to this treatment may result in amputation with indiscriminate use. Spica casts are helpful for a lengthy transport of a patient to a tertiary care facility. Angiography can be diagnostic and therapeutic. Small arterial bleeding is amenable to selective embolization. However, long delays in beginning this treatment are counterproductive. Large bore vessel injury can only be treated by open means. Venous bleeding from the pelvis is made worse by open exploration and decompression of the closed space the patient is bleeding into. Stabilization of the fractures by external fixation is very helpful in this setting. On rare occasions, radical amputations may be the only lifesaving procedure in the face of uncontrolled bleeding.

PERIOPERATIVE

A major cause of death in pelvic fractures is bleeding. In the patient with washout coagulopathy, attempts at major posterior reconstructive surgery in the acute setting are unwise at the very least. Even in a delayed setting, washout coagulopathy is a real threat. The patient may have been resuscitative in the acute period with massive quantities of blood. A delay of several days will not bring the patient's coagulation status back to normal. Coagulation profiles and studies of bleeding times may be done to help decide on what blood products will help the most for planned surgery. The rare case of a pre-existing bleeding diasthesis may also change the treatment plans.

Pulmonary complications can ensue shortly after the patient arrives. In addition to pulmonary bleeding and a pneumothorax, shock lung or aspiration pneumonia can quickly change the condition of the patient. Fat emboli can cause rapid pulmonary compromise and necessitate abandoning definitive bony stabilization.

IATROGENIC

Iatrogenic complications are among the most disturbing complications to all concerned. Their prevention is best accomplished by proper training and diligence. Good fortune is never unwelcome, but often fails to save the unwitting surgeon. Direct injury to nerves and blood vessels is the result of dissection or hardware placement. Clotted vessels may open up again in the course of dissection. Unstable fractures distort anatomy, making intact cadavers deceptive road maps. The preoperative understanding of the extent of the injury will help in the dissection. "Exploring" the fracture without some idea of its configuration and surrounding structures is inviting trouble. It is obvious that the "learning curve" is best done in a supervised setting. Another complication is failing to accomplish what one sets out to do with reduction and fixation. While this is influenced by the degree of injury, the surgeon must realistically assess his own abilities. Planning an intervention before a problem occurs is a necessary part of any surgery.

Nowhere is this more necessary than in the pelvis, where large bore vessels, nerves, and viscera are millimeters from pins, drill bits, and screws.

POSTOPERATIVE

Many postoperative complications can be prevented by controlled early mobilization. Sepsis is dependent on initial wounds, prophylaxis, sterile technique, and patient nutrition. Thromboembolic disease, decubiti, and contractures are activity-related. Prolonged use of urinary catheters and poor pulmonary therapy increase the risk of infection. Later, persistent pain identifies treatment failures.

SHORT-TERM

Wound breakdown and infection is more common in posterior approaches than in most other orthopedic approaches. It has been reported as high as 50%.[3] Patient positioning and nutrition must be properly managed to help prevent this complication. Water and air mattresses, sheepskin, and a dietary consult are helpful. Getting the patient to sit up is important for a number of reasons, including facilitation of wound care, enhancement of pulmonary function, and relief of orthostatic changes from prolonged bed rest. Superficial infections need to be drained if a collection is present, and antibiotics should be used based on cultures and sensitivities. Drains should not be left in for more than a few days. Deep infections require débridement of necrotic tissue. If hardware is affording stability, it is best left in until healing of the bone proceeds. Posterior skin breakdowns may require flaps for coverage. Skin grafts over poor tissue beds will compound the problem. Getting the patient to lie prone is helpful for breakdown problems.

The usual litany of postoperative complications, such as phlebitis, deep venous thrombosis, urinary tract infections, pulmonary atelectasis and infection, decubiti, pulmonary emboli, drug reactions, substance abuse, and psychological problems, need to be dealt with according to the institution's usual protocol. These protocol are by no means universal, and consultants are highly recommended for optimal results when available.

Pain management and discharge planning are items that are best attacked early and often. Sticking to a protocol makes it easier on the staff when dealing with difficult patients.

Early loss of fixation is usually best dealt with by immediate revision. If the reason for failure was noncompliance of the prescribed weight bearing status, having the patient document his refusal of treatment may be a better alternative for all concerned. Revision surgery has less chance of success and a repeated failure may leave the patient worse off. If the hardware appears to be failing despite the best of efforts, one may try limiting the patient's activities. A consultation with a colleague more experienced in these techniques is always advisable before revision surgery is undertaken.

LONG-TERM

After the patient gets over the short-term onslaught of complication, the late complications rear their ugly heads. Infection continues to be the bane of many orthopedic procedures on a delayed as well as acute basis. With late infections, hardware may be removed to rid the infection site of any nonviable materials. Débridement and antibiotics based on cultures are, of course, routine. Even in the late period, soft-tissue coverage may be a problem with a surgical solution.

Pain is probably the king pin of late complications. If the SIJ is a source of pain, it may require fusion. Fusion is very effective if the pain is from the SIJ. Injection of a local anesthetic is useful. Other sources of late pain are nonunions, nerve root impingement, infection, mechanical low back pain, and workmen's compensation insurance. The latter is not intended to be derogatory; rather, it is a well-documented phenomenon that must be dealt with. Computed tomographic scans are indicated to evaluate the pain. Pain clinic consultations may be obtained. However, there is a finite failure rate in every series, and this is higher in litigation and compensation cases. Labels can be detrimental, and are best earned, not applied on a whim.

Malunions of pelvic fractures can cause sitting imbalance, leg length discrepancy, back pain, dyspareunia, major gait abnormalities, loss of self-esteem, and the list goes on. Most of these problems are caused by skeletal deformities, which are identifiable with radiographic imaging techniques early on in the course of treatment. Sometimes they are not treated due to other overriding circumstances. In these cases, it is important to have some salvage plan or find someone who does. The patient should be kept informed of the decision-making process as much as possible. Unrealistic goals with high risks should not be undertaken to try to salvage a situation even if the patient wants to "give it a try."

SUMMARY

Sacroiliac joint injuries are challenging problems. The anatomy is not easily accessible. The geometry is difficult. Long-term follow-up is needed to evaluate results. The immediate resuscitative benefits must weighed against long-term functional results. Fixation techniques have improved and methods will continue to become more standardized. Trauma organizations have a responsibility to further collaborative efforts in defining optimal treatment. There is no substitute for experience, but poor experiences need not be repeated. Better communication and dissemination of developments in the field in training programs will help all concerned. The current database is growing, but much more work needs to be done.

REFERENCES

1. Bucholz RW: The pathological anatomy of Malgaine fracture-dislocations of the pelvis. J Bone Joint Surg [Am] 63:400–404, 1981
2. Committee on Trauma of the American College of Surgeons: Advanced Trauma Life Support Handbook. Chicago, 1988
3. Kellam JF, McMurtry RY, Paley D et al: The unstable pelvic fracture: Operative treatment. Orthop Clin North Am 18:25, 1987
4. Matta JM: Orthopaedic knowledge update 2: Home study syllabus. AAOS 345–346, 1987

5. Matta JM, Letournel E, Browner BD: Surgical management of acetabular fractures: Instructional course lectures. AAOS 35:382, 1986
6. Mears D, Rubash H: Pelvic and Acetabular Fractures. New Jersey, Slack Publications, 1986
7. Pennal GF, Tile M, Wadell JP et al: Pelvic disruption: Assessment and classification. Clin Orthop 151:12, 1980
8. Salter RB, Simmonds DF et al: The effects of continued passive motion on the healing of articular cartilage defects. J Bone Joint Surg [Am] 57:570, 1975
9. Trunkey DD: Trauma Management: Early Management of Visceral, Nervous System, and Musculoskeletal Injuries. Chicago, Year Book Medical Publishers, 1988

SPINAL CORD
INJURY

15

NEURO-PHYSIOLOGY OF SPINAL CORD INJURY

Wise Young

Motor and sensory deficits in spinal cord injury have traditionally been attributed to axonal loss at the lesion site. Spinal axons are believed to be unable to regenerate.[75] Together, these two beliefs have led to the widely held view that the only hope for spinal cord injury lies either in preventing axonal loss or regenerating lost axons.[91] Clinical management of spinal cord injury echoes this pessimistic view. The primary rationale for early surgery and pharmacologic therapy of acute spinal cord injury has been prevention of further injury[99] and not restoration of function. Clinicians are reluctant to operate on spinal-injured patients, especially those with so-called "complete" lesions, because such patients are perceived to be incapable of recovery. Everyone is waiting with bated breath for researchers to find out why spinal axons do not regenerate and how to make them regenerate.

Animal studies[10,37-43,87,97] and even human studies,[86] however, suggest that remarkably few spinal axons can support motor and sensory recovery in spinal cord injury. Pathologic examinations of injured spinal cords indicate that some axonal preservation is common, even in severe injuries leading to complete loss of sensory and motor function below the lesion level.[57] Recent clinical studies have shown that most so-called "complete" spinal-injured patients have residual, albeit subclinical, evidence of descending and ascending activity.[30] Neurophysiologic studies have shown that most axons surviving spinal cord injury are likely to be dysfunctional[9] owing to demyelination.[11]

The observation that even severely injured spinal cords have residual axons and that these axons may be dysfunctional owing to demyelination suggests the possibility of several nonregenerative therapeutic approaches to spinal cord injury. First, treatments that improve axonal conduction may improve function. Second, increasing the excitability of proximal and distal neural structures may reduce the number of axons required for sensory and motor function. Third, regenerating axons suffer from the same constraints that limit the function of surviving axons, such as demyelination. Treatments that improve conduction in surviving injured axons may well improve conduction in regenerated axons as well. Combined, these considerations provide hope that effective therapies for spinal cord injury may be possible within our lifetime.

A detailed understanding of the neurophysiology of injured spinal cords is essential for developing treatments. Treatments aimed at improving conduction presume the presence of dysfunctional axons in the patients. Successful application of therapy will require careful selection of patients for treatment. Treatments that manipulate the excitability of the spinal cord must be appropriately directed. Since the regenerative therapy of the future will be unlikely to regenerate the entire spinal cord and probably will add relatively few axons to an already existing population of axons, the therapy must be selectively aimed at restoring specific pathways. Finally, the efficacy of treatments must be documented. Neurophysiologic testing will be essential for identifying subclinical effects.

The neurophysiology of the spinal cord is probably better understood than that of any other part of the central nervous system. The concepts of reflex, neuron, synapse, interneuron, motor neuron, and presynaptic and postsynaptic inhibition were first proposed and elucidated in the spinal cord. The neurophysiology of the spinal cord will not be reviewed here since the subject has been extensively covered elsewhere.

This chapter is divided into four sections. The first reviews the theoretical bases of surface recorded potentials and common pitfalls associated with interpreting evoked potentials. The second describes four major classes of neurophysiologic responses used for assessing spinal conduction: somatosensory evoked potentials, spinal cord evoked potentials, motor evoked potentials, and sensorimotor reflexes. The third section deals with morphologic and physiologic mechanisms underlying evoked potential changes, with emphasis on demyelination as a cause of axonal dysfunction. The fourth section focuses on clinical use of evoked potentials, comparing neurophysiologic tests and neurologic examinations and then describing evoked potential changes after spinal cord injury and during intraoperative spinal cord monitoring.

THEORETICAL BASES OF EVOKED POTENTIALS

Neurons generate electrical signals. These signals provide a unique window into the brain, allowing us to observe and measure neuronal activity underlying motor and sensory responses. Traditional neurophysiologic methods have emphasized electrodes inserted directly into the tissue generating the electrical activity. The signals, however, can be detected from the body surface. For example, electroencephalographic signals recorded from the scalp represent spontaneous cortical activity. To test specific pathways, it is necessary to stimulate the appropriate activity. Stimulated neuronal signals are called evoked potentials.

ORIGINS OF EVOKED POTENTIALS

Evoked potentials are field potentials.[90] Field potentials are generated by extracellular ionic currents in tissues when membrane ionic channels open.[62] Owing to their gradients across neuronal membranes, sodium (Na) and calcium (Ca) ions enter cells, while potassium (K) ions leave cells. Where Na and Ca channels are open, ions enter neurons and produce an extracellular negativity commonly called a "sink." Conversely, where K channels are open, K ions leave the cells, producing an extracellular positivity called a "source." Some membrane channels allow chloride (Cl) ions to move into the cells, producing extracellular positivity. Ionic movements that depolarize cells tend to produce sinks, and those that hyperpolarize cellular membranes yield sources.

The law of electroneutrality stipulates that current entering or leaving a cell must complete the circuit. The current must leak in or out somewhere else in the cell, resulting in "passive" sources or sinks. An active sink must be balanced by a passive source, and an active source must likewise be associated with an equivalent passive sink. Since the circuit must be completed within the cell, this tends to make part of an active neuron negative and the other parts positive, or vice versa. For this reason, the sources of field potentials are often referred to as current "dipoles," which are approximately the dimensions of the active neurons. The polarity of the resulting potential depends on the location of the electrodes relative to the current dipoles.

Synaptic currents that depolarize neurons (i.e., excitatory postsynaptic potentials [EPSPs]), are active sinks, whereas hyperpolarizing inhibitory postsynaptic potentials (IPSPs) tend to be active sources.[35,36] Although there is no easy way to distinguish between active and passive current sinks or sources in signals recorded from the body surface, some conventions are helpful. For example, if the synaptic activity is excitatory and situated on dendrites, and the dendrites are oriented toward the body surface, the resulting potentials on the brain surface should be negative and largest close to the neurons. On the other hand, owing to convolutions of the cortical surface, neurons may well be oriented parallel to the organ surface. In such a case, negativities and positivities may appear over wide areas of the cortex far from the dipoles.

Action potentials present a special case because they propagate long distances within the tissue. A conducted action potential is a propagating wave of Na channel openings followed by K channel openings. Consider an action potential conducting in a linearly oriented bundle of axons. A monopolar recording of the action potential will sense initially a passive current source as the action potential approaches the recording site, an active sink as the action potential reaches the recording site, and then passive sources and active sinks (owing to K channel opening) as the action potential passes beyond the recording site. Figure 15-1 illustrates current sources and sinks associated with an action potential propagating in an axon past the recording electrode, generating a positive–negative–positive waveform, shown in Figure 15-2. The leading positivity is smaller than the trailing positivity because K channels open shortly after the Na channels, producing an active current source. When two electrodes are used to record the action potential differentially, a complex waveform results from the subtraction of the two waveforms because of the time delay (Fig. 15-3).

Current sinks propagating within neurons produce biphasic negative–positive waveforms. For example, consider the case of an afferent volley activating dorsal horn neurons in the spinal cord. Recorded from the spinal cord dorsum, the first event is activation of presynaptic structures, generating either a positive–negative–positive or a negative–positive waveform. A large negative potential then follows, resulting from excitatory synaptic potentials in neuronal dendrites in the dorsal horn. As the excitation spreads to the cell bodies, the dendrites become current sources and produce a large positivity. Figure 15-4 illustrates the waveforms of segmental responses activated either by peripheral nerve stimulation or stimulation of the dorsal columns.

Figure 15-1. The distribution of sources and sinks produced by a conducting action potential in an axon. Active current sinks occur where cations (positively charged ions) enter cells, creating an extracellular negativity. Active sources are where cations leave cells, creating an extracellular positivity. Passive sources and sinks result from current leaving and entering cells to complete the circuit, creating extracellular positivities and negativities, respectively.

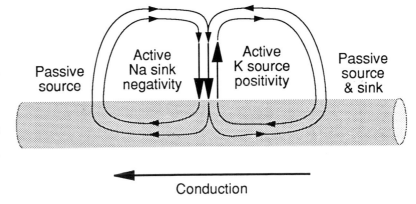

Passive source

Active Na sink negativity

Active K source positivity

Passive source & sink

Conduction

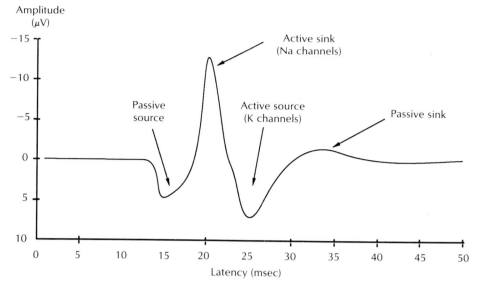

Figure 15-2. Waveform of a theoretical conducting action potential recorded with a single electrode with respect to a distant ground electrode. Note the positive-negative-positive configuration of the waveform, representing the passage of the action potential.

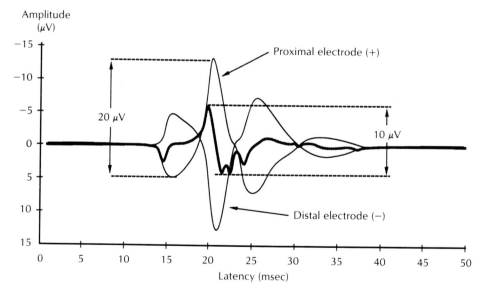

Figure 15-3. Differential recording of an action potential. The same waveform shown in Figure 15-2 was inverted and delayed by 0.5 msec for the distal electrode (or negative channel of the amplifier). The sum of the two waveforms is illustrated by the bold trace. The original waveform has a peak-to-peak amplitude of 20 μV, whereas the peak-to-peak amplitudes of the differentially recorded action potential is only 10 μV.

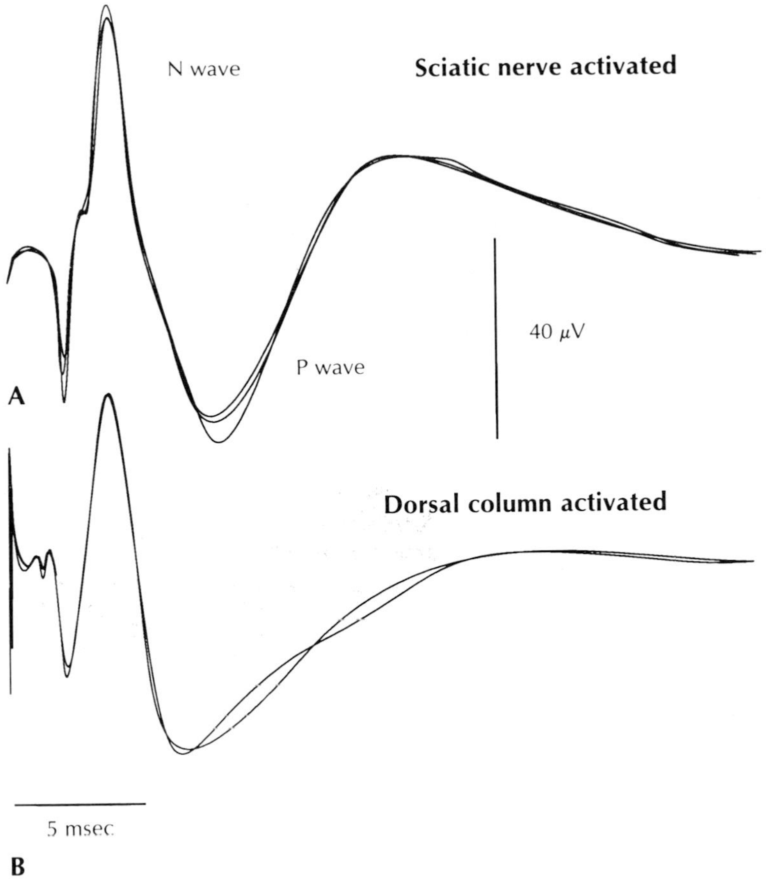

Figure 15-4. Waveform of synaptic potentials resulting from dendritic activation that invades the cell bodies. The dendrites are assumed to be facing the recording electrode and to be the first to be activated by an afferent volley. In this and all sequential figures we follow the convention of showing negative polarity up. The dendritic sink produces an initial negativity (N-wave) followed by a large positivity (P-wave). The top trace (A) illustrates the waveform of spinal cord segmental activation resulting from an afferent volley, while the bottom trace (B) illustrates the response resulting from stimulation of the dorsal column. Both were recorded from the spinal cord of a 3 week old Wistar rat.

SPATIAL AND TEMPORAL SUMMATION

Individual neurons generate too little current to produce detectable field potentials outside of the tissue. Many neurons have to be activated synchronously in order to generate field potentials large enough to be detected from the body surface. Evoked potential amplitudes increase when neuronal events are tightly synchronized and decrease if neuronal events vary in latency. For example, variability of conduction time in injured spinal axons may result in asynchronous afferent signals, thereby causing smaller evoked potentials, even though all of the axons may still be conducting. Conversely, injury may slow down conduction in some axons, making conduction velocity more uniform, paradoxically increasing the amplitude of evoked potentials.

Synaptic activity generally produces larger field potentials than action potentials in white matter for the following reasons. First, synaptic currents are typically of longer duration than action currents (10 to 15 msec vs. 1 to 2 msec). The likelihood of temporal summation, that is, the ionic currents occurring at the same time, is significantly greater with synaptic activity than action potentials. Second, action currents do not form well-defined dipoles in axons. For example, a patch of opened Na channels will produce a local sink surrounded on two sides by passive sources. Electrodes may not detect action potentials unless they pass or end in the vicinity of the recording site. As a general rule, synaptic currents dominate evoked potentials recorded from the body surface.

Field potential amplitudes are also influenced by the spatial distribution of current sinks and sources.[63] Two simple principles govern the amplitude of field potentials emanating from a neuronal population. First, juxtaposed current sources and sinks cancel. For example, a tissue containing neurons with random orientations will not generate large fields. Second, the neural structure must be "open." An example of an open structure is a flat sheet of tissue with all the neurons oriented in one direction perpendicular to the sheet. An open structure generates large fields, whereas a "closed" structure will not emanate field potentials beyond the borders of the structure.[58] For example, a spherical nucleus with the neurons oriented perpendicular to the surface of the sphere is a closed structure. Figure 15-5 illustrates open and closed neuronal ensembles.

Currents associated with neuronal activity consequently may not manifest in field potentials detectable from the body surface. Most cortical structures are partially closed structures owing to convolutions of the hemispheric surface. Within the cortical sulci, for example, the cortical layers are parallel to the brain surface and constitute a more or less closed structure, except to electrodes situated at or within the sulcus. Subcortical nuclei are typically closed structures generating small or no evoked potentials outside of the nucleus. For this reason, most subcortical activity does not show up in evoked potential studies. When small potentials are seen, they frequently represent the action potential volleys or presynaptic currents rather than the postsynaptic currents of nuclear neurons. Thus, absence of evoked potentials does not necessarily mean that no activity is present in the structure.

PITFALLS IN INTERPRETING AVERAGED WAVEFORMS

Most tests of spinal cord function use electrical pulses to stimulate neuronal activity. Electrical stimulation is an unnatural means of activating the nervous system. Normally, central nervous system activity is mediated by temporally modulated bursts of activity that sequentially turn on overlapping excitatory and inhibitory circuits. Electrical stimuli tend to produce supramaximal, synchronous, and repeated unitary activations of both

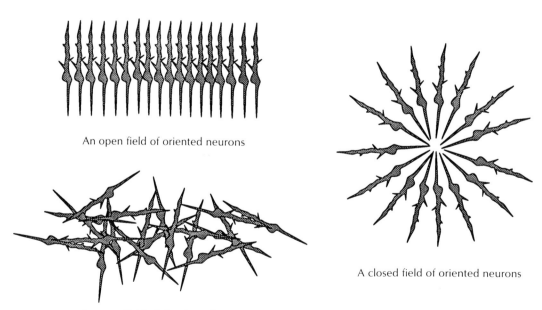

An open field of oriented neurons

An open field of disoriented neurons

A closed field of oriented neurons

Figure 15-5. Open and closed neuronal fields. The upper left array of open field oriented neurons will generate the largest external field potentials. The lower left array of open field disoriented neurons will generate small potentials. The right array represents a closed field, which should generate little or no external field potentials.

excitatory and inhibitory connections. A neuronal circuit that responds to electrical stimulation may not be able to support function. Conversely, a circuit that does not respond to electrical stimulation may be able to support some function. Thus, the presence of electrically activated responses does not necessarily imply function and vice versa.

Even under favorable recording conditions, evoked potentials recorded from the body surface are typically small, on the order of 2 to 5 μV, compared with background noise levels of 50 to 500 μV. To resolve such small signals from background noise, two techniques of noise reduction are popular: signal averaging and differential recording. Signal averaging is based on the assumption that noise is random with respect to the stimulus. Repeated averaging of the signal should reduce all signals that are not time-locked to the stimulus. The technique of differential recording simply subtracts the electrical potentials recorded with one electrode from another. Although differential recording is not usually regarded as a noise reduction technique, it is actually more effective than signal averaging. Differential recordings are based on the assumption that electrical potentials that simultaneously affect both electrodes will

cancel. Differential recording can eliminate as much as 99% of background noise.

Signal averaging has strict theoretical and practical limitations. Assuming random noise of sufficiently high frequency, averaging at best enhances signal-to-noise ratio by $\sqrt{n}$, where n is the number of responses averaged. Figure 15-6 shows the reduction in noise-to-signal ratio as a function of n. Averaging larger numbers of response does not linearly decrease noise. For example, averaging 100 responses will reduce noise by a factor of 10, but averaging 900 responses will reduce noise by only a factor 30. Since 1000 responses is essentially the practical limit for evoked potentials in clinical situations, signal averaging is effective only in situations in which the noise-to-signal ratio is less than 30:1, assuming optimal noise cancellation conditions and consistent signals.

Averaging can eliminate signal as well as noise. In addition, averaging will distort the waveform of the signal. Figure 15-7 illustrates what can happen to an averaged waveform when the latencies of individual responses are varied during averaging. The individual waveforms have a constant peak-to-peak amplitude of 20 μV, while latency is progressively delayed by 0.5 msec over a 5 msec

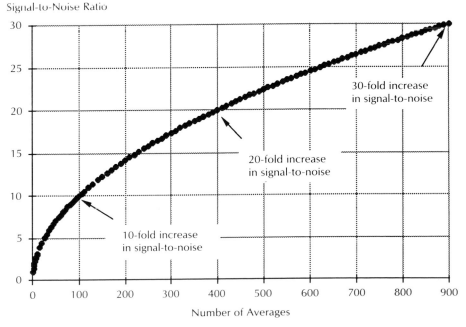

Figure 15-6. Decreasing benefits of signal averaging with increasing number of responses averaged. Signal averaging increases the signal-to-noise ratio by a factor of $\sqrt{n}$ where n is the number of responses averaged. Averaging 100 responses will reduce noise 10-fold. One has to average 400 and 900 responses to get a 20-fold and 30-fold reduction in noise.

Signal-to-Noise Ratio

10-fold increase in signal-to-noise

20-fold increase in signal-to-noise

30-fold increase in signal-to-noise

Number of Averages

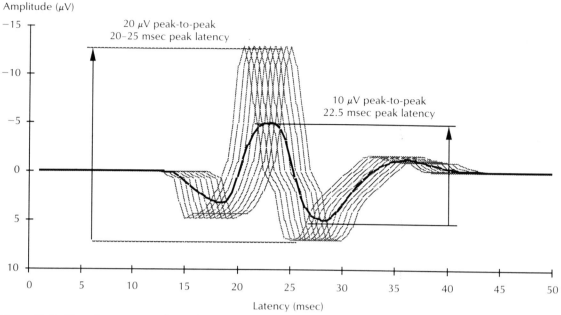

Figure 15-7. Distortion in averaged waveforms resulting from latency variations. The gray waveforms represent the responses contributing to the final average (*bold line*). The latencies of the response were successively increased from 20 to 25 msec in 0.5 msec increments. Note that the peak-to-peak amplitude of the original waveforms is 20 μV while the final averaged waveform is only 10 μV.

range. The peak-to-peak amplitude of the averaged waveform is reduced by 50%, to 10 μV. Variations in both amplitude and latency can produce even more dramatic distortions of the averaged waveform. Figure 15-8 shows an example of latency and amplitude effects on the averaged waveform. The same waveform used in Figure 15-7 was used for the individual responses. The responses were successively delayed in latency by 0.5 msec over a 5 msec range and reduced 10% in amplitude. The individual waveforms have peak-to-peak amplitudes of 20 to 7.7 μV (an average of 13.8 μV), nearly twice the 6.9 μV peak-to-peak amplitude of the averaged waveform. The latency of the largest negative peak on individual responses ranges from 20 to 25 msec (an average of 22.5 msec), compared with a peak latency of 21.5 msec of the averaged waveform. Clearly, the averaged waveforms may not be representative of the original waveforms that represent the average.

NEAR AND FAR FIELD POTENTIALS

One of the primary techniques of noise reduction in electrophysiologic tests is differential recording. When electrical potentials are recorded differentially, two electrodes are referenced to a ground electrode. By convention, one of the inputs is called "positive" and the other is called "negative." The signal at the negative input is inverted and subtracted from the signal at the positive input. All potentials that occur simultaneously at both electrodes, therefore, cancel, and the output represents the difference in the two electrodes. This is a highly effective means of eliminating noise and, in fact, is the chief noise-reduction technique used in electroencephalograms and electrocardiograms.

If the electrodes are situated close to each other, the output of the differential recording tends to be very small in amplitude. Since poten-

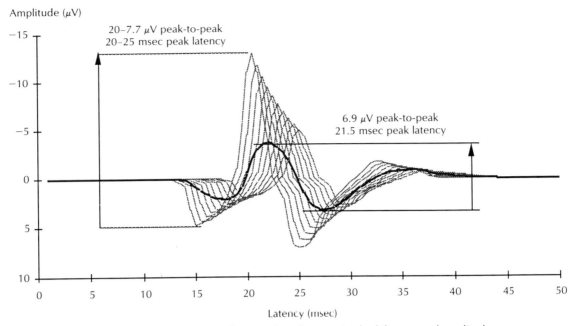

Figure 15-8. Distortion in the averaged waveform resulting from varying both latency and amplitude of the response. The gray waveforms represent the responses contributing to the final average (*bold line*). The latencies of the responses were successively increased from 20 to 25 msec in 0.5 msec increments. The amplitudes of the responses were decreased 10% with each successive response. Note that the peak-to-peak amplitude of the averaged waveform is 6.9 μV, less than the smallest individual response. Also note that the peak latency (21.5 msec) of the averaged waveform is different from the averaged peak latencies of the original responses (22.5 msec).

tials that are generated from distant dipoles will tend to affect both electrodes and hence will cancel, only local current dipoles that affect one electrode more than the other will be reflected in differential recordings. The signals resulting from closely spaced differential recordings are called "near" field potentials. If the electrodes are situated far apart, the differential recording will detect electrical potentials resulting from current dipoles that are further away. The signals from widely separated electrodes are called "far" field potentials. With electrodes that are sufficiently separated (e.g., recordings between the skull vertex and a knee), entire sequences of neuronal events from the afferent volley to the cortical activation can be recorded simultaneously.[21,25,27]

Differential recording can contribute artifacts. Consider the situation of a propagating action potential recorded with two electrodes placed side by side. Assume that the action potential is propa-

gating from right to left. The amplifier records the potential from the right (proximal) electrode at normal polarity, while it inverts the potential from the left electrode (distal). The output of the amplifier is the sum of the normal and inverted potentials. Figure 15-3 shows the results of summing two waveforms recorded differentially with two electrodes from an action potential that passes the proximal electrode 0.5 msec before the distal electrode. As the action potential approaches the electrode pair, a positive–negative–positive waveform is recorded by the proximal electrode. A similar but inverted and delayed waveform is recorded from the distal electrode. The sum of the normal and inverted channels yields a different and smaller waveform with multiple artifactual peaks. The peak-to-peak amplitude of the differentially recorded waveform is only 10 μV even though the monopolarly recorded waveforms each have peak-to-peak amplitudes of 20 μV.

Ideally, the negative input of the differential recording should placed on a "nonactive" recording site so that it senses background noise but not neuronal field potentials. Unfortunately, there are very few such sites on the body. Popular reference recording sites used in clinical work include the limb contralateral to the one being stimulated, the earlobes, abdomen, and even esophageal leads.[26] However, all these positions can and do contain active electrical field signals. Care must be taken to rule out the possibility that signals present at the negative recording site are not cancelling out a desired signal recorded from the positive input. By comparing potentials recorded from multiple sites to see which components of evoked potential are common to each site, investigators can determine the origins of far field potentials.[24]

EVOKED POTENTIALS USED FOR SPINAL CORD MONITORING

Evoked potentials are often classified and named according to the part of the nervous system that is stimulated and from where the responses are recorded. For spinal cord monitoring, four major types of evoked potentials are commonly used: somatosensory evoked potentials (SEP), spinal cord evoked potentials (SCEP), motor evoked potentials (MEP), and sensorimotor reflexes (SMR). SEPs represent the responses in the central nervous system that are elicited by peripheral nerve or receptor stimulation. These are often prefixed by the locations from which the responses are recorded (e.g., "cortical SEP"). SCEPs are activated by electrical stimulation of the spinal cord. MEPs are activated by cortical stimulation of the motor cortex. SMRs are motor responses resulting from sensory input: for example, segmental reflexes, long loop reflexes, vestibulospinal reflexes, and others.

SOMATOSENSORY EVOKED POTENTIALS

Cortical SEPs were among the first evoked potentials recorded in humans.[23] Recorded with electrodes glued to the scalp and activated by peripheral nerve stimulation, cortical SEPs are robust and can be consistently obtained from patients with intact sensory systems even under adverse recording conditions, which are often encountered in the hospital setting. In patients with thin skulls, the potentials can sometimes be detected without averaging. The amplitudes of the responses are on the order of electroencephalographic activity recorded from the scalp. Early studies of cortical SEPs simply used overlaid oscilloscope tracings of amplified potentials.

A standard cortical SEP test usually involves stimulations of the median nerve and posterior tibial nerves. Other popular stimulation sites include the radial nerve, brachial nerve, the peroneal nerve in the popliteal fossa, and even nerve endings in skin. Figure 15-9 illustrates the cortical SEPs activated by median nerve and posterior tibial nerve stimulations in the author. Note the W-shaped waveform of the posterior tibial SEP, with onset latency at about 37 msec. The median nerve evoked response is smaller (3 μV) and has an earlier onset latency (18 msec). The amplitudes and latencies vary depending on the height of the patient, the thickness of the skull and scalp, and the degree of axonal myelination. The last is important especially in children who have not yet completed myelination; their SEPs tend to have very long latencies despite their smaller body size.

Cortical SEPs have been extensively used to monitor spinal cord injury in animal studies. Figure 15-10 illustrate cortical SEPs obtained from a pentobarbital (40 mg/kg i.p.) anesthetized cat. The response was elicited by sciatic nerve stimulation (2.3 Hz, 0.1 msec duration, twice the twitch threshold) and recorded (average of 256 responses) differentially with two epidural electrodes, one placed on the vertex and the other overlying the somatosensory cortex 2 mm lateral to the midline and contralateral to the nerve stimulation site. The response is robust, with peak-to-peak amplitudes of >1 mV, consisting of a highly synchronized initial positivity at 17 msec onset followed by a negativity peaking at 25 to 30 msec, and sometimes a slow late positivity. Interrupting the dorsal column (bilateral dorsal column ablation) eliminated the response.

Animal studies indicate that the dorsal column ipsilateral to the stimulated side is necessary and sufficient to conduct a cortical SEP.[17] A unilateral isolated lesion of the ipsilateral dorsal column will

PT SEP

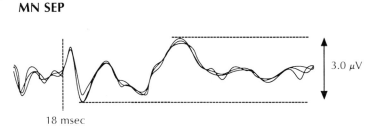

37 msec

6.3 μV

Figure 15-9. Cortical SEPs activated by median nerve (MN) and posterior tibialis (PT) stimulations in the author. The potentials represent averages of 100 responses activated at 2.3 Hz (in order to reduce 60 Hz electrical noise) and recorded differentially between the frontal midline and the vertex (for the PT SEP) and the frontal midline and C3′ (for the MN SEP).

MN SEP

18 msec

3.0 μV

Figure 15-10. Cortical SEPs activated by sciatic nerve stimulation in a cat before and after bilateral dorsal column (DC) interruptions. Note the shoulder on the falling phase of the negativity wave. This is common in both cats and humans. (Adapted from Cohen AR, Young W, Ransohoff J: Intraspinal localization of the somatosensory evoked potential. Neurosurgery 9:157–161, 1981).

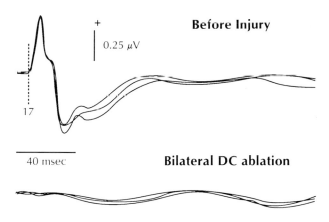

+

0.25 μV

Before Injury

17

40 msec

Bilateral DC ablation

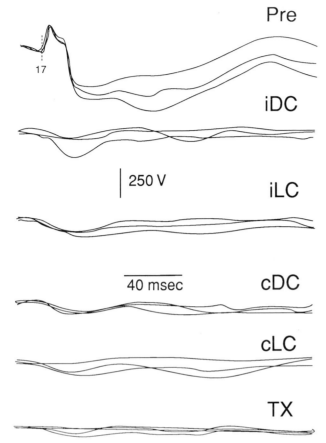

Pre

17

iDC

| 250 V

iLC

—— 40 msec

cDC

cLC

TX

Figure 15-11. Effect of a unilateral lesion of the ipsilateral dorsal column on cortical SEPs in the cat. Removing the dorsal column on one side immediately and completely abolished the cortical SEP. Further lesions do not restore the response. Pre = normal response, iDC = ipsilateral dorsal column, iLC = ipsilateral lateral column, cDC = contralateral dorsal column, cLC = contralateral lateral column, TX = transections. (Adapted from Cohen AR, Young W, Ransohoff J: Intraspinal localization of the somatosensory evoked potential. Neurosurgery 9:157–161, 1981).

abolish the cortical SEP, as shown in Figure 15-11. Sequential lesions of the contralateral dorsal column, lateral columns, and ventral columns do not eliminate the response, as shown in Figure 15-12. In fact, a robust cortical SEP can be seen even in a spinal cord in which all the white matter columns had been lesioned except for the dorsal column ipsilateral to the stimulation site. Note the remarkable preservation of both the waveform and amplitude of the cortical response despite four sets of lesions, which eliminated all the spinal tracts except for the ipsilateral dorsal column.

Many ascending spinal pathways carry sensory information to the brain. The major ones, summarized in Figure 15-13, can be categorized into two types: dorsal columns and interneuronal tracts. The dorsal columns are essentially extensions of peripheral nerve into the spinal cord. The cell bodies of dorsal column axons reside in the dorsal sensory ganglia. Dorsal sensory ganglia axons bifurcate when they enter the spinal cord. One branch synapses with neurons in the spinal gray. The other branch ascends the dorsal column to synapse on neurons of the dorsal column nuclei situated in the lower brainstem. Occasionally, dorsal column axons will give off descending branches. The dorsal column nuclear cells send axons to the ventral posterolateral nucleus in the contralateral thalamus, which in turn send axons to the somatosensory cortex. The dorsal column nuclei are complex structures.[85] Axons from the dorsal column activate not only the lemniscal relay cells but also the interneurons that inhibit the relay cells pre- and postsynaptically. In addition, the interneurons receive inputs from descending pyramidal tracts, which provide both feedforward and feedback inhibition.

The interneuronal tracts include the spinomedullary, spinocervical, spinothalamic, and spinoreticular paths. Stimulation of the peripheral nerves should activate all these ascending pathways to some degree. These pathways may, however, be gated such that they are unable to follow stimulation at the rates used for averaging responses. In any case, even if the interneuronal pathways do not contribute to cortical SEPs in normal animals, the possibility that the interneu-

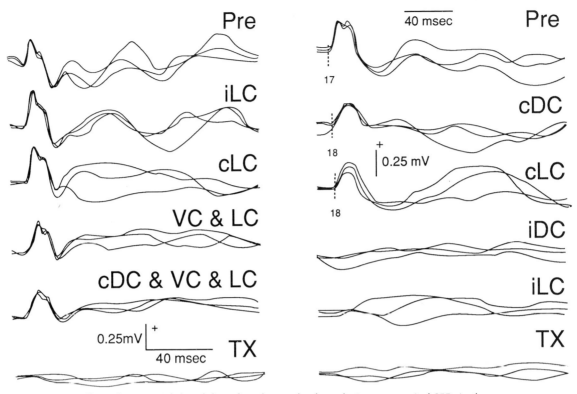

Figure 15-12. Effect of sequential dorsal, lateral, and ventral column lesions on cortical SEPs in the cat. Data from two experiments are shown. On the left, the normal response (Pre) is shown on the top. The SEPs were obtained after ipsilateral lateral column (iLC); contralateral lateral column (cLC); ventral and lateral column (VC & LC); and contralateral dorsal column, ventral column, and lateral column (cDC & VC & LC) ablations at different levels of the thoracic spinal cord. Note the survival of the response through these extensive multiple lesions. On the right, the cDC, cLC, and iDC were ablated; the cortical SEP disappeared with the iDC even though the iLC and VCs remain intact. Transections (TX) abolished the responses. (Adapted from Cohen AR, Young W, Ransohoff J: Intraspinal localization of the somatosensory evoked potential. Neurosurgery 9:157–161, 1981).

ronal pathways can carry SEPs in chronically injured spinal cords has not yet been ruled out. Some of these pathways may substitute for dorsal column pathways.

Somatosensory evoked responses can be recorded from many locations, both as near and far field potentials, after peripheral nerve or spinal root stimulation.[19,20,22] Figure 15-14 summarizes the stimulation and recording parameters of various popular electrode configurations used for recording somatosensory responses ascending the spinal cord. Figure 15-15 shows an example of

SEPs in a rat, recorded from the cortex, cervical cord, lumbar cord, and cauda equina. The potentials in the cervical and lumbar enlargements are largest, tend to be less affected by anesthesia, respond to high frequency stimulation of >100 Hz without fatigue, and can be recorded with electrodes inserted into the spinal epidural space, as well as from the spinous processes.[64] The epidurally recorded response has a characteristic waveform of three negative peaks at the low cervical level, with 14- to 22-msec latencies and 0.5- to 6.0-μV amplitudes.[55] Spinal SEPs have been exten-

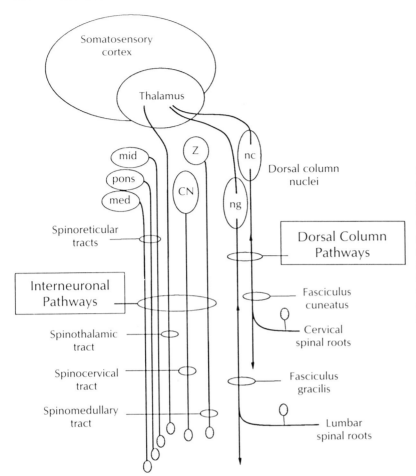

Figure 15-13. Ascending pathways of the spinal cord can be summarized as being of two types: interneuronal and dorsal column pathways. The interneuronal pathways include the spinoreticular (to the midbrain [mid], pons, and medulla [med]), spinothalamic (to the thalamus), spinocervical (to the cervical nucleus [CN]), and spinomedullary (to the interstitial nucleus of Cajal, or Z nucleus). The dorsal column pathways include the fasciculus gracilis (to the nucleus gracilis [ng]) and the fasciculus cuneatus (to the nucleus cuneatus [nc]).

sively used for monitoring scoliosis surgery[54] and other procedures.[65,66] Many variations of spinal SEPs have been described and used clinically, including descending lumbrosacral cord potentials evoked by median nerve stimulation,[78] representing propriospinal descending pathways.

SPINAL CORD EVOKED POTENTIALS

Spinal cord evoked potentials are responses that are recorded from the spinal cord and evoked by stimulation of the spinal cord. Spinal cord evoked potentials have long been studied in animals and are a part of the classic neurophysiology of the spinal cord. Although a number of exploratory efforts have been made since the 1950s to stimulate and record from the spinal cord directly, the technique was first applied clinically to relatively large patient populations in the 1970s.[80-82] Basically, the spinal cord is stimulated epidurally in the cervical or lumbrosacral region and the responses are recorded either above or below the stimulation site. The responses can be easily compared with those arising from peripheral nerve activated responses or stimulation of supraspinal structures.

It is important to distinguish between spinal SEPs activated by peripheral nerve stimulation and SCEPs activated by direct spinal cord stimulation. The latter should not be considered SEPs because spinal cord stimulation will activate both ascending and descending pathways. In addition, stimulation of a spinal tract will produce action potentials going both forward (orthodromic) and backward (antidromic) in the axons. Spinal cord

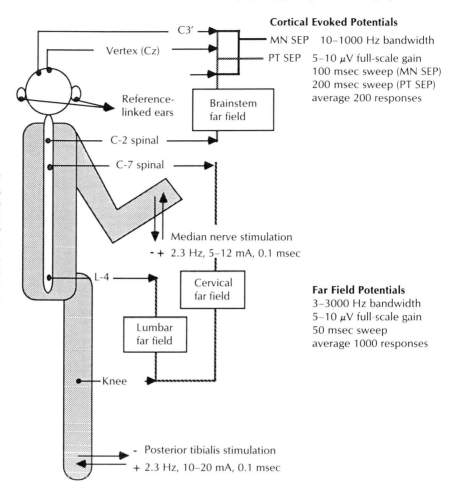

Figure 15-14. Diagram of the different types of recording and stimulation sites for SEPs. Cortical evoked potentials are recorded from the vertex (Cz), C3′, and frontal scalp locations. Brainstem far field potentials can be recorded with electrodes placed on the vertex referenced against the ears. Cervical and lumbar far field potentials can be recorded with electrodes placed at C-2, C-7, L-4, and the knee.

stimulation, for example, will activate action potentials conducting orthodromically and antidromically in the dorsal columns. The antidromic volley will invade the presynaptic terminations in the lumbrosacral spinal cord and produce local segmental reflex activity and motor activation. In addition, the antidromic volley will go directly out of sensory axons in the peripheral nerve.

Spinal cord stimulation activates responses that closely resemble segmental potentials evoked by peripheral nerve stimulation. The SCEP response is typically triphasic, with an initial small positive–negative–positive action potential complex, a negative wave, and a prolonged positive wave (see Fig. 15-4). Segmental somatosensory evoked responses tend to have relatively small initial action

potentials unless the recording electrode is situated right at the dorsal root entry zone. When the initial presynaptic component occurs, it usually is present at the rising phase of the negative wave. The SCEP response in the lumbar and cervical enlargement probably arises from antidromic activation of dorsal column axons, which then activate segmental responses in the same way peripheral nerve stimulation does.

Spinal cord evoked potentials possess several advantages over SEPs. First, the responses are very robust and require minimal averaging. Second, certain components of the SCEP can and will follow stimulus rates of 500 Hz or greater, enabling the tests to be carried out very rapidly. Finally, the stimulus and recording electrodes can

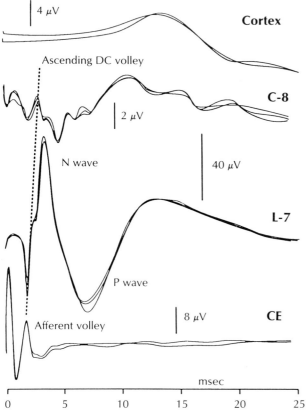

Figure 15-15. Ascending activity in the spinal cord of a juvenile (3-week-old) Wistar rat after sciatic nerve stimulation, recorded epidurally from the caudal equina (CE), lumbrosacral cord (L-7), cervical cord (C-8), and cortex. (DC = dorsal column, N-wave = negativity wave, P-wave = positivity wave).

be placed at various locations on the spinal cord, allowing the test to localize conduction defects. These advantages are balanced by the difficulties of placing epidural recording and stimulating electrodes for monitoring. Also, SCEP amplitudes depend critically on the location of the stimulating and recording electrodes. Electrode positions cannot always be reproduced exactly in every patient, especially when the electrodes are introduced via lumbar puncture and threaded into the epidural space. These difficulties have limited the use of SCEPs in the United States to the operating room setting, where the electrodes can be put directly onto exposed spinal cords.

MOTOR EVOKED POTENTIALS

Paralysis is the most obvious manifestation of spinal cord injury. Consequently, much effort has been devoted to developing techniques to monitor spinal motor pathways in humans[14,60,61,84] and animals.[5,47,83] The final common pathway of motor signals is, of course, the motor neuron. Most neurophysiologic tests of the motor system consequently rely on recordings of muscle potentials as the output of the motor stimulation. Electrical signals generated by muscles can be easily recorded without averaging from the skin surface or with needle electrodes placed in the muscles. Stimulating motor responses, however, presents a problem. Until 1980 most studies of MEPs have been carried out by direct electrical activation of surgically exposed cortical structures.[73] Spinal motor pathways can be activated in the brainstem or spinal cord. However, stimulation at these sites will almost invariably activate ascending, extrapyramidal, and other tracts owing to current spread to adjacent structures. Thus, the end result is a hodge-podge of activated systems, some of which may feed back indirectly to the pathway being monitored.

Merton and Morton showed in 1980[72] that the motor cortex can be stimulated directly with electrodes placed on the scalp. Very high voltages (500 V) are required for current to penetrate through the scalp and skull to the underlying cortex. Previous investigators[51] tried to activate the motor cortex with scalp stimulation but found such stimuli to be excessively painful. To reduce the risk of scalp burns and pain, stimuli durations must be very short. Merton and Morton used a very short duration (50 to 100 μsec exponential decay time constants), high amplitude electrical currents (500 μA), and electrodes with large surface areas.[71] Although these practices reduce the noxious effects somewhat, the stimulation can nevertheless be quite uncomfortable. Careful attention to electrode positioning and design are essential for reproducible results.[18,28,76]

Two developments in the field spurred MEPs into the clinical arena. First, Barker and associates[2–4] developed a means of producing intense focal magnetic fields that penetrate to the cortex with significantly less stimulation of the intervening cutaneous structures. Although the instruments require respectful handling owing to the enormous transient currents used to generate the magnetic fields (peak coil currents of 4000 A), they have been applied safely on hundreds of patients in the past three years. Specificity and localization of the stimulation still leave much to be desired, but magnetic transients do activate the motor cortex. Second, the threshold for motor cortex activation can be dramatically reduced by volitional activation of responding muscle groups.[6] The production of a motor twitch is gated by spinal segmental excitability.

Both electrical and magnetic stimulation of the motor cortex have attracted a great deal of interest. These stimulation techniques have allowed investigators to study conduction in the pyramidal tract electrophysiologically without surgical exposure of the cortex. The disadvantages of MEPs are, however, not sufficiently emphasized. First, MEPs are susceptible to changes in segmental excitability. The amplitudes of the MEPs are variable and consequently not particularly meaningful. The response can be recorded directly from the spinal cord, but this requires an epidural electrode, and the spinal signal tends to be small, multi-peaked, and variable in amplitude. Second, because of the smaller size and sagittal position of the hindlimb motor cortex (compared to the hand or face), consistent activation of MEP responses in the legs remains a problem even in healthy neurologically intact individuals. Finally, currently available magnetic stimulators do not focus the field sufficiently to activate the cortex in smaller animals such as cats and rats. However, the technique is still relatively young and improvements in stimulation and recording techniques are being made all the time. Many intriguing possibilities are just now starting to be explored. For example, MEPs can be used to condition segmental reflexes in the spinal cord. Vice versa, sensory input can be used to condition, stabilize, and test the extent of inhibitory or excitatory influences from descending axons.

SENSORIMOTOR REFLEXES

Sensory inputs can be used to activate motor responses. The monosynaptic stretch reflex is the best-known and best-understood example of this approach to testing the integrity and function of neural pathways. The neurophysiologic equivalent to the monosynaptic stretch reflex is the H-reflex, which is the segmental motor response from stimulating the Ia afferent sensory fibers to the lumbrosacral spinal cord. In the cervical region, there is the F-reflex, which apparently results from antidromic activation of motoneurons (since section of the dorsal roots does not eliminate this response). Finally, the withdrawal and cross-extensor reflexes can be elicited by noxious stimulation. In the latter, the ipsilateral limb withdraws and the contralateral limb extends. These reflexes are carried by localized segmental pathways. Their presence and absence allow conclusions about the integrity of the peripheral afferents, the segmental neuronal circuits, and the motor output of the system.

Reflexes with longer pathways can be used to assess the functional integrity of motor and sensory pathways simultaneously. Three that have been used extensively in both clinical and laboratory research include the vestibulospinal reflex, vibratory reflex, and long loop transcortical stretch reflex. These reflexes involve sensory and motor pathways, with at least two and probably more synaptic interactions. Tests examining these reflexes usually are based on muscle recordings after delivery of a sensory input. The long pathways of these reflexes are both advantageous and problematic. The responses are generally quite sensitive to small lesions situated almost anywhere in the spinal cord and brain. The responses usually have long latencies and variable amplitude. The tests do not allow accurate localization of lesion sites. Nevertheless, these tests are an important part of the armamentarium of clinical neurophysiologists interested in assessing spinal cord injury.

The vestibulospinal reflex is the shortest and most straightforward of the three listed. Electrical stimulation of the eighth nerve activates ventral spinal cord pathways,[1,16,44,100] producing short latency responses in postural trunk and limb muscles. Electrical stimuli can be delivered with electrodes placed in the ear. Unfortunately, such stimuli are uncomfortable and the responses are sensitive to anesthesia. Gruner and associates[50] recently found that brief acceleration produced by dropping an animal will reliably elicit stereotyped motor responses. Ketamine-sedated cats, rats, monkeys, and humans exhibit these free fall responses (FFRs). A typical set of FFRs is shown in Figure 15-16, recorded with bipolar electrodes inserted into the vastus lateralis, biceps femoris, semitendinosus, gastrocnemius, and tibialis anterior muscles in a ketamine-sedated cat dropped suddenly into free fall. The 200-msec records shown represent eight superimposed responses from each muscle. The responses were not averaged and typically exceeded 1 mV in amplitude. Two patterns of activity can be seen. In the vastus lateralis and tibialis anterior muscles, the response consists of a rapid unitary "spike" at 20 to 25 msec latency, followed by diffuse bursting activity. In

the biceps femoris, semitendinosus, and gastrocnemius muscles, the short latency response is followed by a period of electrical silence lasting 20 to 30 msec, a period of activity, and then a rhythmic bursting activity that can last 200 to 300 msec. The period of silence is of particular interest because segmental reflexes, such as the H-reflex, are suppressed during this period. This suggests an inhibitory phase of the response.

The vibratory reflex is essentially a tonic postural response. Vibration applied to a muscle or tendon will elicit a slow and long-lasting tonic muscle activation, which requires the integrity of both ascending and descending spinal pathways. Dimitrijevic and associates[32–34] used this reflex to assess sensory inputs to the bulboreticular system and the descending output of the reticulospinal and vestibulospinal systems. The vibratory reflex involves diffuse sensory and motor pathways and can persist even in severely spinal-injured patients. The vibratory reflex can be combined with neurologic examinations of patients and used to evaluate volitional capabilities by asking the patients to suppress or facilitate the response. Dimitrijevic used this approach to show that many so-called "complete" spinal cord injury patients are still capable of exerting descending motor influences on segmental activity below the level of injury.

Long latency motor response occurs after stretch stimulation of muscle receptors. Alternatively described as transcortical stretch reflex or long loop response,[45,67,68] this phenomenon has been the basis of much research into cortical control of motor activity. The presence of this response indicates the integrity of fast-conducting spinal pathways ascending to and descending from the motor cortex. It is absent in patients with paralysis or severe paresis. Like the MEP, the long loop response is very sensitive to volitional enhancement and thus is depressed by anesthesia. Lesions of either motor or sensory pathways will affect this response. These characteristics have made long loop reflexes less suitable for monitoring of spinal cord injury or for use in the operating room than the SEP or MEP. Nevertheless, the long loop reflex tests may detect small lesions of the spinal cord that would not be detected by standard

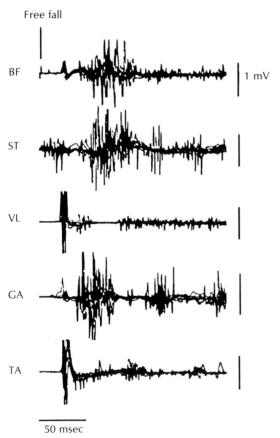

Figure 15-16. Free fall responses in a cat, recorded from the right biceps femoris (BF), semitendinosus (ST), vastus lateralis (VL), gastrocnemius (GA), and tibialis anterior (TA) muscles.

SEP or MEP tests. Long loop reflexes may also useful when combined with assessments of volitional capabilities of patients. For example, the degree to which a patient can voluntarily inhibit or enhance long loop responses may provide useful information concerning subtle changes in motor function.

AXONAL DYSFUNCTION IN INJURED SPINAL CORDS

Neurophysiologic studies of spinal cord injury have generally been aimed at documenting what has been lost. Actually, neurophysiologic tests are better for showing the behavior of axons that survive the injury rather than what was lost. This difference in perspective may seem trivial, but the distinction is an important one and can explain several seemingly paradoxical phenomena in spinal cord injury. The function of surviving axons depends on many factors. The behavior of the individual axons becomes more important in severe spinal cord injuries in which few axons remain, and the function of each axon plays a correspondingly greater-than-normal role in maintaining communication. In such cases, the tissue environment and myelination may become critical determinants of neurologic recovery. Understanding the causes of axonal dysfunction in injured spinal cords is critical to developing rational therapy for spinal cord injury.

AXONAL NUMBER AND FUNCTION IN INJURED SPINAL CORDS

Morphometric analyses of myelinated axons in spinal-injured animals suggest that remarkably few axons can support substantial functional recovery. More than three decades ago, Windle and associates[87] reported that cats recover useful locomotion even after lesions involving greater than 90% of the spinal tracts. Eidelberg and associates[37-43] have shown that selective preservation of ventral spinal tracts will allow locomotory recovery in cats and ferrets. In fact, a human case has been reported[86] in which a greater than 90% section of the spinal cord was observed at surgery and the patient recovered some motor and sensory function. The severity of the spinal cord injury was confirmed on autopsy. More recently, Blight[10] expressed these observations quantitatively by counting the number of axons crossing the lesion site in animals that are paralyzed or recovering from injury. Normal cats have approximately 500,000 myelinated spinal axons countable on light microscopy. After injury with a 20-g weight dropped 20 cm onto a spinal cord exposed by laminectomy, cats have 10,000 to 100,000 axons. Some cats with less than 50,000 axons were able to walk reasonably well. In general, 20,000 axons appears to be a lower limit for functional recovery. These findings suggest that survival of as little as 5% of the axons can support useful motor function in cats.

Very small differences in axon counts segregate animals that recover or do not recover from spinal cord injury. In a recent study of SEP, FFR, and locomotory recovery in 20 spinal-injured cats, we counted the number of myelinated axons crossing the lesion center on light microscopic examination. Figure 15-17 shows the proportions of animals that recovered FFRs, SEPs, both FFRs and SEPs, and unsupported locomotion for different categories of axon counts. In cats with more than 10,000 surviving axons, approximately 25% were able to walk and 50% had either SEPs and FFRs. In cats with more than 50,000 surviving axons, 60% were able to walk, 100% had SEP recovery, and 80% had FFR recovery. As might be expected, recovery of walking requires more axons than either SEP or FFR recovery. The mean axon count differences between recovering and nonrecovering animals were very small, on the order of 40,000 to 50,000, or less than 10% of the normal population of axons in cats.

These findings suggest an explanation for the hitherto puzzling tendency of many severely spinal-injured patients to recover substantial motor function if they have some minimal motor preservation during the acute stages. The difference between so-called "complete" and "incomplete" spinal cord injuries may depend on the survival of a small fraction of the axons in the spinal cord, perhaps as few as several thousand axons. A normal human spinal cord has perhaps 20 million

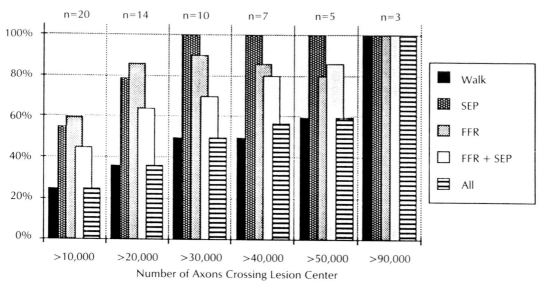

Figure 15-17. Proportion of cats that recover at 3 months after 13 g–20 cm supported T-8 contusion spinal cord injury. Axon counts represent myelinated axons crossing the lesion center. The number of animals in each axon-count category ranges from >10,000 to >90,000 axons (compared to >500,000 in normal cats). The percentage of animals in each category of axon count that recover walking, cortical SEPs, vestibular–spinal free fall responses (FFR), and both SEP and FFR are given in histogram form.

axons.[15] If we can extrapolate findings from cats to humans, as few as 1 million axons may be able to support function. Kakulas[56] examined more than 400 spinal cords of patients and found that complete transections of the spinal cord and losses of all axons crossing the lesion site are very rare.

Dimitrijevic and associates[28] have reported that as many as 70% of patients with neurologic diagnoses of complete spinal cord injury have neurophysiologic evidence of axonal conduction across the lesion site, a condition they called "discomplete"[29] to distinguish it from complete and incomplete spinal cord injury. Examining the effects of elicited descending activity on segmental reflex induced by tonic vibratory stimuli or phasic reflexes, they showed that patients often could augment or inhibit motor activity even when they show no sign of voluntary motor activity. The presence of such "subclinical" function in these cases suggests that even severely injured patients can have surviving axons. Depending on the number of axons, the addition of a small number of

axons may have a relatively large effect on functional recovery.

ROLE OF POTASSIUM IONS IN EVOKED POTENTIAL CHANGES IN ACUTE SPINAL INJURY

Changes in evoked potentials can have many causes besides loss of axons. Action potential conduction depends on ionic gradients across axonal membranes. Membrane potentials and thresholds for action potentials are exquisitely sensitive to extracellular K ionic activity ($[K^+]_e$). For example, an increase of $[K^+]_e$ to 10 mM will block action potential conduction in most neurons. Normally, $[K^+]_e$ is 3 to 4 mM, compared to 90 to 110 mM inside cells. Owing to the large amount of K inside cells, the disruption of even a small proportion of cells and the consequent spilling of their contents into the extracellular space will raise $[K^+]_e$. For example, if we assume that extracellular volume is 20% of total tissue volume, physical disruption of even 5% of cells in the spinal cord will raise $[K^+]_e$

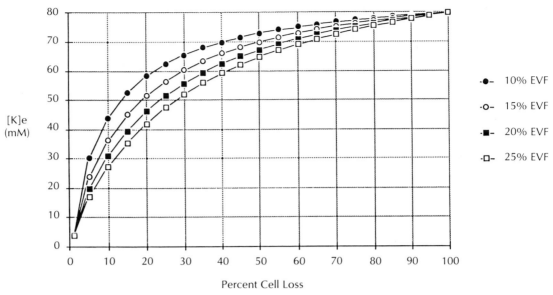

Figure 15-18. Theoretical clearance times of K ions in injured spinal cords, calculated by assuming that extracellular volume is 20% of tissue volume, intracellular K ionic activity is 100 millimolar (mM), and extracellular K ionic activity is 4 mM. The percentage of cell loss refers to the percentage of cells that have equilibrated their contents with extracellular fluids.

to 20 mM. Figure 15-18 shows theoretical calculations for the expected rises of $[K^+]_e$ for increasing percentages of cellular disruption, assuming 10% to 25% extracellular volume fraction.

Using ion-sensitive microelectrodes, we measured $[K^+]_e$ in cat thoracic spinal cords after contusion with a 20-g weight dropped 20 cm in two groups of eight cats.[96] The first group (control) was injured and $[K^+]_e$ levels were recorded in lateral column white matter at the impact site for 4 hours, while blood flow was monitored by hydrogen clearance. The other group was studied in the same way but received paravertebral sympathectomies before injury. Extracellular K ionic activity in both groups rose from 4 mM to 47–54 mM within 5 minutes after impact. Potassium ions cleared from extracellular fluids with a biexponential time course, shown in Figure 15-19. In the control group, $[K^+]_e$ fell with an exponential half-time $(T_{1/2})$ of 38 minutes during the first hour and then 171 minutes during the 2 to 4 hours after

impact. In the sympathectomized group, $T_{1/2}$ values of the two phases were 31 and 120 minutes.

Somatosensory evoked potential conduction across the lesion site depended on $[K^+]_e$ levels, and $[K^+]_e$ clearance depended on blood flow. Contusions immediately abolished SEPs in both groups. However, SEPs recovered at 1 to 2 hours and fell again at 2 to 3 hours in the first group but not the sympathectomized group. Potassium ions gradually returned to 10 mM by 1 to 2 hours, corresponding to the time that SEPs recovered, and did not rise again. Repeated injuries of the spinal cord at 4 hours did not yield a second rise in $[K^+]_e$ in either group, suggesting that the K had left the tissue altogether. The K clearance rate depended on blood flow. The faster the flow, the shorter the $T_{1/2}$ of clearance. In the first group, blood flow in lateral column white matter at the impact site was 13.1 ml/100 g/min before injury and gradually fell over a period of 1 to 2 hours to about 5 ml/100 g/min. Sympathectomy lowered blood pressure

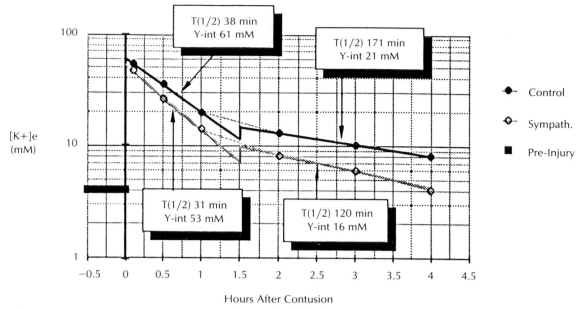

Figure 15-19. Extracellular K ionic activity ([K⁺]e) in spinal cords after a 20 g–20 cm weight drop contusion injury. The data represent mean ion-selective microelectrode-recorded extracellular K ionic activity in the lateral column white matter of cats shortly after injury. Two groups of cats were tested. One group was simply injured (control) and the other group had surgical removal of the paravertebral sympathetic ganglia (Sympath.), which prevents the secondary fall in blood flow at 2 to 3 hours after injury. The K activity rises from a normal level of 4 millimolar (mM) to >50 mM within minutes and then clears out biexponentially with exponential half-times of clearance or T(½) given for each phase.

and reduced spinal cord blood flow to 9.4 ml/100 g/min before injury, but prevented the secondary post-traumatic decline.[95]

The time course of $[K^+]_e$ changes explains the loss of SEP conduction across the impact site. Recovery of SEPs corresponded in timing with the return of $[K^+]_e$ to <10 mM. Since disruption of even 10% of cells at the lesion site will raise $[K^+]_e$ to 20 mM, a level capable of blocking all action potential conduction across the impact site, it is clear that the timing of SEP recovery is a better indicator of tissue damage than the amplitude of initial SEP loss. To estimate the time course of SEP recovery for different injuries, we calculated the time course of K clearances for different initial $[K^+]_e$ rises. If we assume that $[K^+]_e$ of 10 mM blocks action potential conduction, our calculations suggest that 5% disruption of cells in the tissue will result in a loss of SEPs for about 50 minutes. Likewise, 10%, 25%, and 50% disruptions should

block SEP conduction for about 80, 180, and 250 minutes. These estimates suggest that the time course of SEP recovery and not the initial amplitude loss should be the most reliable indicator of tissue damage.

NEUROPHYSIOLOGIC MANIFESTATIONS OF AXONAL DYSFUNCTION

Injured axons conduct slowly, show increased tendency to fatigue during rapid stimulation, and generally have poor safety factors for transmission across injury sites. Injured axons do not conduct high frequency impulses well. Many investigators attribute progressive conduction failure at high frequency stimulation to "fatigue." Prolongations of the refractory period contribute to axonal fatigue. Averaged evoked potentials cannot distinguish between progressive conduction failure during the averaging and overall smaller responses. To study such phenomenon, analysis of individual conducted responses may be necessary.

One approach to assessing axonal dysfunction is to use conditioning stimuli. Sakatani and associates[77] recently assessed action potential conduction in cat dorsal columns after high and low frequency conditioning stimuli. In uninjured spinal cords, delivery of 99 preceding stimuli at 1- and 500-Hz frequencies did not affect the amplitudes of the succeeding 100th responses. Injury to the axons had a differential effect on the responses after low and high frequency conditioning stimuli. Progressive spinal cord compression by 2.5 to 4.5 mm had a greater effect on the high frequency conditioned responses. Response amplitudes conditioned by high frequency stimuli suffered an earlier and greater decline than responses conditioned at 1 Hz. Upon decompression, while both high and low frequency conditioned responses re-

covered gradually, the high frequency responses recovered more slowly (Fig. 15-20). This method is likely to be more sensitive to minor axonal injuries than conventional SEPs.

Another approach was used by Sakatani and associates[77] to analyze individual responses during stimuli trains of different frequencies. Before injury, response amplitudes during repetitive stimulation did not change over a wide stimulation frequency range (10 to 500 Hz). At 1 hour after compression injury, low frequency stimulation (10 Hz) did not affect response amplitudes within the train. Paradoxically, at 33- to 125-Hz stimulation rates, response amplitudes were greater than control (the amplitude of the first action potential in the train). At 100-Hz stimulation rates, response amplitudes initially increased to 134% of controls within several stimuli and then gradually declined to 110% during the remainder of the stimulation.

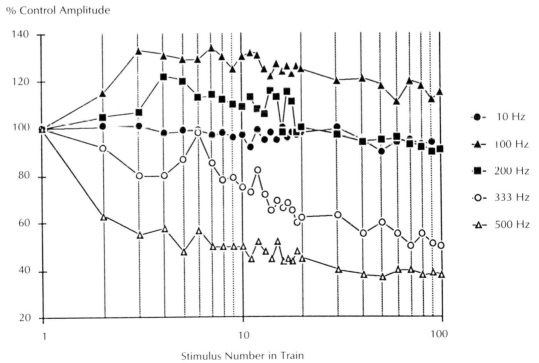

Figure 15-20. The effect of train stimuli on spinal cord responses. Responses were recorded epidurally from the spinal cord dorsum after dorsal root stimulation in a cat 1 hour after the spinal cord was compressed 50% for 5 min. The amplitudes of the responses during trains of 100 stimuli are plotted as a function of the stimulus number in each train. Five stimulus frequencies were tested, over a range of 10 to 500 Hz. Note that low frequency stimulation (10–100 Hz) produced an increase in the amplitude of the dorsal column response, while higher frequency stimulation (333–500 Hz) progressively decreased the amplitudes of the responses.

At 333- to 500-Hz frequencies, response amplitudes and conduction velocities declined significantly during the stimulation. These results suggest that different stimulation frequencies may both enhance and suppress response amplitudes. These effects may be related to extracellular K accumulation. Assessment of individual responses during stimulus trains thus reveals complex mechanisms governing fatigue phenomena in injured spinal axons.

The finding that many axons surviving injury are dysfunctional has several important implications. First, we must discard the simplistic notion that the degree of functional recovery can be equated to the number of surviving axons. Second, the morphologic presence of an axon is not sufficient. We must demonstrate that the axon functions. Third, the observation that many surviving axons may be dysfunctional forces us to revise downward the number of axons that are actually required to support function. For example, as few as 5,000 to 10,000 healthy axons may be sufficient for function. Finally, the finding opens the door to an alternative approach to treating spinal cord injury: improving the function of surviving axons.

DEMYELINATION AS A CAUSE OF AXONAL DYSFUNCTION

Demyelination plays a major role in spinal cord injury. Several observations support this assertion. Blight examined demyelination in cat spinal cords injured with the standard weight drop contusion.[11] Many axons at the lesion site were severely demyelinated. Most of the axons crossing the lesion site remained at least partially demyelinated for weeks after injury. Quantitative morphometric analyses of myelinated axons in spinal-injured animals indicate that demyelination began within 24 hours after contusion and peaked several days later. The mean myelin index (i.e., the ratio of myelin plus axon vs. axon diameter) fell from a normal value of 1.8 to 1.2 by 3 days, and gradually rose to 1.4 by a week. Combined with the massive losses of axons, this finding suggests that the number of functioning axons required to support locomotory recovery in cats is very low indeed.

The time course of remyelination fits well with the pattern of functional recovery that occurs in moderately injured spinal cords. Somatosensory evoked potentials often have very prolonged latencies after spinal cord injury. The onset latencies of cortical SEPs from posterior tibial nerve stimulation may exceed 70 msec, compared to normal latencies of 30 to 35 msec. If and when people or animals recover from spinal cord injury, they usually do so over several weeks with a gradual reduction in the SEP latencies and increases in amplitudes. Such recoveries may be related to remyelination.

The demyelination is probably due to direct trauma to oligodendroglial cells. Myelin draws back in the paranodal region, and the myelin sheath in the internodal region becomes thin. This has two consequences for axonal conduction. First, the drawing back of myelin increases the nodal area and exposes K channels in the paranodal zone. The density of Na channels may decrease in the nodal region. The normally covered K channels may shunt action currents. Together, these will reduce the amount of current available to drive the next node. Second, the capacitance of myelin increases as it grows thinner. Myelin is a material with a high dielectric constant sandwiched between conducting layers of fluid. Just as bringing the plates of a capacitor close together will increase capacitance, decreasing myelin thickness will increase capacitance. Increased capacitance in the internodal regions will blunt the peak currents achieved at the next node.

Blight[9] recorded from axons in spinal cords isolated from cats after injury. He found that a reduced number of axons conducted across the lesion site: only 7% of the axons compared with 61% in uninjured control cords. Of the axons showing conduction across the lesion, 73% could not support conduction when the temperature of the cord was raised to 37°C. Even at room temperature, these axons showed prolonged refractory periods and inability to conduct at high frequencies. Comparing spinal cords of cats that recovered some function after spinal cord injury with those that did not, Blight did not always find that more axons conducted across the lesion site at 25°C. He did find that only 14% of the axons were blocked at body temperatures. These characteristics are typical of the behavior of demyelinated axons.[13, 69]

The temperature sensitivity of conduction in demyelinated axons stems from the effect of temperature on the duration of channel openings. At 25°C, the duration of Na channel activation is more than twice what it is at 37°C. Because the Na channel is open longer, the currents generated at the nodes may become sufficient to overcome the increased capacitance and the shunting effects of demyelination. Cooling spinal cords therefore increases the safety factor for conduction, although the axons may continue to show prolonged refractory periods and inability to sustain high frequency spiking activity. Conversely, heating spinal cords will cause conduction failure. For example, high fevers and hot summer weather can have deleterious effects on the function of patients with spinal cord injury.

IMPROVING AXONAL CONDUCTION: MECHANISMS OF RECOVERY

Several observations indicate that axonal dysfunction contributes to the neurologic deficits in spinal cord injury. During the initial period (2 to 4 hours) after injury, physiologic factors account for much of the deficit in moderately injured spinal cords. For example, although most cats will recover virtually completely from a moderate spinal contusion with a 10-g weight dropped 20 cm onto the thoracic spinal cord, they nevertheless suffer a period of functional loss that can last for days. Axonal conduction can be improved in chronically injured spinal cords by pharmacologic means. 4-Aminopyridine (4-AP) has a remarkable effect on evoked potentials of spinal-injured cats. Figure 15-21 shows an example of vestibulospinal FFRs in a cat at 6 weeks after injury. This cat had no activity in six of eight lower limb muscles in response to free fall. The responses in the two muscles that did have some activity were delayed and quite small. Injection of a placebo (saline) did not change these responses. Within 8 minutes after an intravenous injection of 1 mg/kg of 4-AP, the responses increased dramatically in amplitude and decreased in latency. In the muscles that showed no activity before, large responses with nearly

normal latencies appeared. The effect lasted 4 to 6 hours. Repeated injections tended to produce additive effects.

4-Aminopyridine also increased the general reactivity of the animals, inducing spontaneous micturition in some. Before 4-AP injection, all of the animals had very small or absent vestibulospinal responses. After the injection, the vestibulospinal responses increased significantly (p=0.006). In a majority of the animals, there was no detectable response in the vastus lateralis muscle before 4-AP administration. Robust responses of nearly normal latencies appeared in this muscle in almost all of the animals tested. The effect wore off by 5 hours after injury. Thus, 4-AP not only increased amplitudes of vestibulospinal responses in spinal-injured cats but induced responses in muscles where there were none before and restored existing responses to nearly normal latencies.

The mechanisms of the 4-AP effects on injured spinal cords cannot be attributed solely to the improved conduction in demyelinated or partially demyelinated axons. Blight[12] examined the effects of 4-AP on axonal conduction in isolated cat spinal cords with chronic spinal cord injury. He found that 4-AP improved the latency and amplitude of conducted action potentials in some axons, but not sufficiently to explain the dramatic increases in the FFRs described above. In addition to improving conduction, 4-AP caused axons to respond to electrical stimuli with bursts of action potentials, and increased the amplitude of segmental reflexes. Therefore, 4-AP may be acting on neural structures proximal and distal to the lesion site. This may include lowering the threshold of lumbrosacral neurons, increasing the amount of neurotransmitter release per action potential crossing the lesion site, and increasing the number of action potentials generated per electrical stimulus. If so, other drugs or transplants of neurotransmitter-releasing cells into the lumbrosacral spinal cord may have similar effects and may be used to enhance the excitability of selected neurons.

4-Aminopyridine has been reported to have temporary beneficial effects on neurologic function in patients with demyelination owing to multiple sclerosis. Unfortunately, 4-AP has many effects on the body and central nervous system

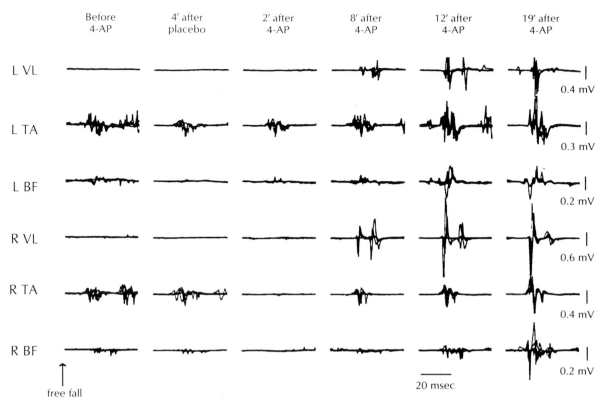

Figure 15-21. Effect of 4-aminopyridine (4-AP) on free fall responses in cats with chronic spinal cord injury. These responses were recorded in a cat at 6 weeks after a thoracic contusion injury. This particular cat had no responses in four of the six muscles tested but had responses in the left and right tibialis anterior (L TA and R TA). Injection of saline (placebo) produced no significant change in the responses. Injection of 4-AP (1 mg/kg) resulted in a dramatic restoration of responses in the left and right vastus lateralis (L VL and R VL) and the left and right biceps femoris (L BF and R BF). In addition, the drug also improved the amplitude and latency of the responses in the L TA and R TA. (The ' symbol = minutes.)

besides improving conduction in injured spinal axons. It raises blood pressure, increases heart rate, enhances epileptogenic foci in the brain, and increases both pre- and postsynaptic excitability owing to the blockade of voltage-sensitive K channels. Owing to its short course of action and these side-effects, 4-AP is probably not an appropriate drug for chronic treatment of spinal conduction deficits associated with demyelination. Nevertheless, 4-AP may be useful for identifying patients who have neurologic deficits attributable to demyelination rather than axon loss. Since future treatments of demyelination will probably involve local administration of drugs or surgical im-

plantation of myelin-producing cells into the injury site, it would be important to show that the patients would indeed benefit from such treatments by using 4-AP as a diagnostic test.

CLINICAL APPLICATION OF EVOKED POTENTIALS

NEUROLOGIC EXAMINATIONS VS. NEUROPHYSIOLOGIC TESTS

Neurophysiologic tests are often compared with neurologic examinations. At the outset, we must dispel the notion that neurophysiologic tests substitute for or replace neurologic examinations. The bottom line for recovery from spinal cord injury is overt and useful function. On the other hand, neurophysiologic studies do provide information that neurologic examinations sometimes cannot. Neurophysiologic tests are extensions of neurologic examinations. Although the stimuli used and the means of documenting responses are different, the principle of activating a response in specific parts of the central nervous system in order to assess the degree of damage remains the same. Finally, like neurologic examinations, there are many pitfalls in neurophysiologic tests. Proper and standard techniques are critical.[46]

Data obtained by neurophysiologic tests differ from neurologic examinations in three fundamental respects. First, because electrical signals can be precisely timed, neurophysiologic tests provide quantitative information, such as axonal conduction velocity, that cannot be readily ascertained by clinical observation. Second, electrical stimulation, as experienced in neurophysiologic tests, elicits a distinctly unnatural form of neuronal activity. The central nervous system does not normally communicate by supramaximal, unitary, and indiscriminate activations of large populations of neurons. Rather, neurons communicate with subtle bursts of delicately timed and spatially distributed excitatory and inhibitory influences. Third, the electrical signals generated by neuronal activity in neurophysiologic tests do not necessarily reflect the intensity or significance of the neuronal activity, as observed in the neurologic examination. Given these differences between neurophysiologic tests and neurologic examinations, the fact that they sometimes contradict each other is not so surprising and does not imply that one or the other gives an inaccurate picture.

Neurophysiologic studies can supplement neurologic examinations. Spinal cord injury typically produces neurologic deficits below a given segmental level associated with an overt fracture in the cervical or thoracic spinal cord. The spinal cord below and above this injury level is usually assumed to be uninjured. Recent neurophysiologic studies have suggested that this assumption should be routinely questioned. Beric and associates[8] studied 130 patients with cervical and tho-

racic spinal cord injuries using lumbrosacral segmental evoked potentials, reflex testing, and urodynamic studies of bladder function. Eighteen of the 130 patients had evidence of lumbrosacral spinal dysfunction that could not be accounted for by the injury. Of these 18 patients, only three had evidence of possible trauma to the lower spine. Beric and associates suggested that these patients suffered an occult injury to the lumbrosacral spinal cord. Neurophysiologically, all 18 patients had abnormally diffuse or absent sacral potentials and a prominent lumbrosacral root potential, which was evoked by peripheral nerve stimulation. Because the lower lesions were masked by the higher lesions, they were not detected until neurophysiologic tests were used. Recognition of occult lesions helps clinicians plan appropriate care of "neuropathic" bladders. Such lesions may also explain the lack of recovery in some moderately injured patients with some sensory and motor preservation below the lesion site.

Function can also be masked by abnormal activity. Dimitrijevic and associates[31] carried out a systematic study of electromyographic responses in a large population of spinal-injured patients. First, they assessed the ability of patients to voluntarily facilitate or inhibit segmental reflexes elicited by peripheral nerve stimulation or vibration stimuli below the lesion site. The results were surprising. A majority of patients with so called "complete" spinal cord injuries were able to alter the segmental reflexes either voluntarily or with descending activity generated by Jendrassik's maneuver. Confirmed recently by Gianutsos and associates,[48] these findings strongly suggest that "subclinical" function may be present in severely spinal-injured patients. Second, they used electromyographic recordings to document the patterns of spasticity in the spinal-injured patients. They found that spasticity was prominent in patients with subclinical residual descending motor influences and usually absent in those who are truly complete. These findings argue against the classic Sherringtonian view that spasticity is a result of disconnection and the consequent excitatory activity of disinhibited neurons in the lumbrosacral spinal cord. The suggestion that spasticity is a product of abnormal subclinical descending activity in the spinal cord opens several interesting possibilities.

SOMATOSENSORY EVOKED POTENTIALS IN SPINAL CORD INJURY

Cortical SEPs have been used extensively to monitor clinical spinal cord injury.[53,74,79] Much ado has been made over discrepancies between neurologic and SEP findings in clinical spinal cord injury. Several reports of false correlations between SEPs and neurologic findings in spinal cord injury have appeared in the literature.[49,52,59,70,88] These reports have emphasized the failure of SEPs to correlate with motor findings. For example, Ginsburg and associates[49] described a patient who suffered significant motor deficits postoperatively but failed to show SEP changes during the operation, concluding with a warning that intraoperative SEPs do not always reflect motor function. Lesser and associates[59] presented a number of cases in which postoperative neurologic deficits were observed in patients with preserved intraoperative SEP. In almost all the cases in which false correlations have been reported, the patients had chronic spinal cord injury, the evoked potentials were small and variable to begin with, and comparisons were made between SEPs and motor findings.

SEPs obtained within 24 hours after spinal cord injury reliably predicted sensory recovery. Between 1980 and 1987, this author studied 500 patients with acute and chronic spinal cord injury,[89,92] comparing median nerve and posterior tibial nerve SEP with neurologic findings. The scoring methods are illustrated in Figures 15-22 and 15-23. Figure 15-24 illustrates the correlations between SEP and neurologic scores. Somatosensory evoked potential obtained on the day of admission correlated better with sensory scores at 6 weeks than with sensory scores obtained on admission. It did not correlate as well with motor findings during the acute phase. In the chronic phase of spinal cord injury (at 6 weeks to 6 months after injury), SEP did not correlate as well with either sensory or motor recovery. Extreme discrepancies between neurologic findings and SEPs are extremely rare. In the past 10 years, there has not been a single case of a patient with no or severely impaired neurologic function and normal SEPs. In addition, not a case has been encountered in which SEPs were absent or severely diminished in a patient with normal sensory function.

The finding that SEPs do not correlate as well with motor function is perhaps not surprising, since SEPs are indeed a test of sensory pathways. The observation that SEPs are less reliable reflections of sensory function during the chronic phase of spinal cord injury, however, raises interesting questions. A majority of these false correlations involved bizarre long latency waves on the SEP that were present in 17% of patients with severe sensory losses. Some cases can be attributed to poor technique. Excluding these two classes of patients, we had a combined false negative and false positive rate of approximately 10% in chronic spinal-injured patients. Approximately one out of 10 patients had either a definite SEP with minimal sensory function in the legs or no SEP in the presence of some sensation in the legs.

Patients with no SEP in either leg on admission had a 95% probability of no clinically detectable sensory function in the legs. The 5% of cases in

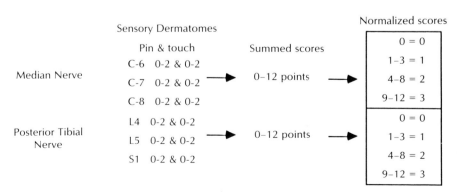

Figure 15-22. Scoring method for sensory recovery. The C-6–C-8 and L-4–S-1 dermatomes were tested for pin and touch sensation (0 = no sensation, 1 = abnormal, 2 = normal). The scores were summed for a total of 12 points and normalized to a scale of 0–3 as shown.

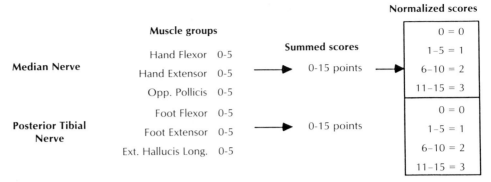

Figure 15-23. Scoring method for motor recovery. The hand flexor, hand extensor, and thumb muscles (Opp. Pollicis) were each scored on the standard clinical scale of 0–5 where 0 represents no movement and 5 is normal movement. These were used for comparison with the median nerve cortical SEP. The foot flexor, foot extensor, and big toe (Ext. Hallucis Long.) were scored in the same way, summed, and normalized for comparison with the posterior tibial cortical SEP.

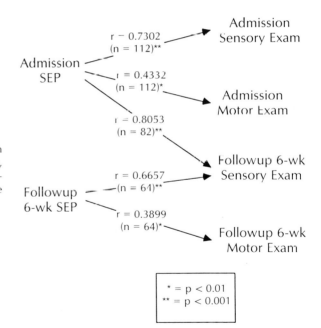

Figure 15-24. Correlations between SEP and neurologic sensory recovery. Admission SEP scores were compared by linear regression with admission sensory, admission motor, followup (6-week) sensory, and followup (6-week) motor examinations. The correlation coefficients are indicated. All the correlations were significant at a p-value of <0.01.

which some function was detected most typically had sensation in dermatomes outside of those innervated by the posterior tibial nerve, the stimulation site in our standard SEP protocol. Patients admitted with a definite SEP in either leg had a 97% probability of having some sensory preservation in the lower limbs. Actually, in several cases

in which the neurologic examination suggested complete sensory loss while SEPs indicated preservation, re-examination of the patient revealed the presence of sensation.

Assessments of SEP changes over a period of time can provide much useful information. An example of the cortical SEPs from a patient with incomplete spinal cord injury is shown in Figure 15-25. This patient was admitted to the hospital with severe quadriparesis and sensory loss. Over a period of several weeks, he gradually recovered function in all four limbs. This case exemplifies many important aspects of cortical SEPs in spinal injured patients, especially those with some sensory or motor preservation below the lesion site. First, SEP evoked from below the lesion level is often so abnormal that waveform components are not recognizable from their latencies. As a result, assessments of SEP changes over time are necessary for interpretation of the significance of SEP findings. Second, evoked potentials wax and wane. Somatosensory evoked potentials activated from below the lesion, as well as SEPs from median nerve stimulation, showed remarkable variations from day to day during the weeks that followed

spinal injury. In some patients with low cervical or thoracic spinal cord lesions, amplitudes of median nerve SEPs may be greater than normal.[89,92]

Neurophysiologic studies have not revolutionized the diagnosis and care of spinal cord injury. Because most spinal cord injury victims are conscious and cooperative, the basic information needed for clinical decisions can be obtained readily from a careful neurologic examination. However, SEPs have proven invaluable for three specialized circumstances. First, some spinal cord injury victims are unconscious from head trauma or drug overdoses. Neurologic examinations are often indecisive, and SEPs can provide critical information for clinical decisions. Second, SEPs can detect malingering or psychiatrically disturbed patients with feigned or hysterical paralysis. Third, SEPs can serve as a check for inadequate

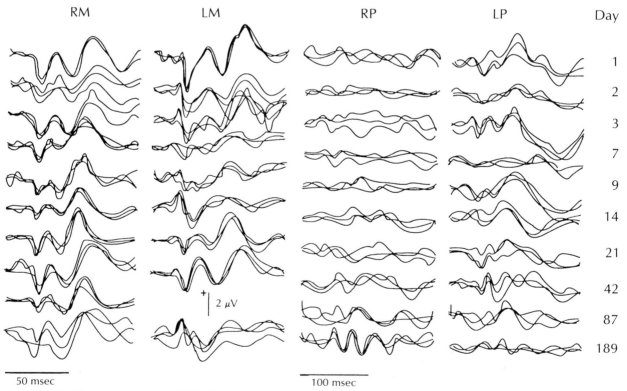

Figure 15-25. Time course of cortical SEP changes in a patient with a C-4–C-5 lesion and incomplete loss of motor and sensory function below the lesion level. One hundred responses were averaged from the scalp after right and left median (RM and LM) and right and left posterior tibialis (RP and LP) stimulation at 2.3 Hz.

neurologic examinations. In the above study, approximately 5% of the patients who were reported on initial examination to have no sensory or motor function below the injury level had some residual SEP. In some of these patients, careful re-examination revealed some sacral sparing or a patch of sensation in the arms or legs that was missed. While these circumstances are individually relatively rare, they combine to justify the use of SEPs in spinal cord injury, especially when questionable neurologic findings have been obtained.

Intraoperative Monitoring with Somatosensory Evoked Potentials

From the outset, many clinicians recognized the potential value of SEPs for monitoring spinal cord function in anesthetized patients undergoing surgical or vascular manipulations of the spinal cord. Cortical SEPs, however, have been severely criticized by many investigators, who have reported high rates of false correlations between SEPs and neurologic function, particularly motor function.[49,52,59,70,88] This has not been the author's experience. Over the past decade, more than 500 patients were studied during intraoperative[93,94] or vascular manipulation of the spinal cord.[7] The author[98] recently analyzed 100 sequential cases monitored intraoperatively at New York University-Bellevue Medical Center from 1985 to 1987. They were separated into four categories:

1. "Unmonitorable"
2. No change
3. Transient change
4. Prolonged changes

Somatosensory evoked potential changes were concluded to be significant only after at least three, and often more, repeated tests over a period of at least 10 minutes. Retrospective analyses with t-tests indicate subjective judgments of SEP amplitude changes in the operating room setting were accurate. Almost all the SEP changes that were felt to be significant turned out to be so at a $p<0.05$ level. Figure 15-26 illustrates the distribution of the cases.

Approximately 20% of the patients tested in the operating room were "unmonitorable." These were patients who, despite having some SEP prior to anesthesia, had absent or very low amplitude (less than 10% of normal) and variable responses after anesthesia. Twenty-five percent showed no significant SEP change, 36% had transient SEP

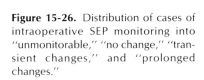

Figure 15-26. Distribution of cases of intraoperative SEP monitoring into "unmonitorable," "no change," "transient changes," and "prolonged changes."

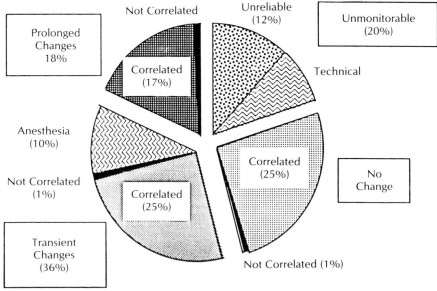

changes that recovered by the end of the operation, and 18% had SEP changes that did not recover to baseline by the end of the operation. There were three cases of false correlations, one in each category other than the "unmonitorable." One patient had small but unchanged SEPs throughout the case and awoke from surgery with neurologic deficits. Another had prolonged neurologic deficits even though his SEPs recovered to baseline by the end of the procedure. The third had improved SEP amplitudes during and after surgery but did not show a corresponding change in neurologic function until several weeks later. The third case is trivial and probably represents limitations of the neurologic examination rather than failure of the SEP.

This limited retrospective study suggests that the rate of false correlations is relatively low, possibly as low as 3%. Several factors probably account for the difference between the author's and others researchers' experiences. First, we carefully distinguished between transient and lasting SEP changes. Second, we were careful not to overinterpret SEPs; patients with small (less than 10% of normal amplitude) and variable SEPs at the beginning of the surgery were excluded. Although there was a relatively high proportion (20%) of so-called "unmonitorable" cases, the reduction in the number of false correlations is well worth this penalty. No information is better than misinformation. Third, we did not use an arbitrary amplitude or latency criterion for judging SEP changes. Instead, the primary criterion was reproducibility of the SEP changes over a period of time usually exceeding 10 minutes. Although a number of investigators have advocated a 50% amplitude decrease as the point at which to take action, we feel that this is too restrictive a definition. Because of the broad range of patients that are monitored intraoperatively, flexible criteria are essential. It is unlikely that any simple rule will apply to all patients. For example, rules should differ depending on whether the patient has an existing lesion, how severe that lesion is, and whether it is acute or chronic.

In many neurosurgical operations, clinical decisions cannot be easily predicated on spinal cord monitoring. For example, in surgery for removal of intraspinal tumors, the clinical goal is often gross total removal. Unlike in angiographic and embolization procedures, in which temporary vascular occlusion is used to test the outcome of a given maneuver, similar provocative tests are not available for surgical manipulations of the spinal cord. Once damage is done with a surgical instrument, SEP monitoring simply documents the change. Thus, although the clinician may learn from the experience, monitoring does not prevent complications from occurring. For example, in a case of an intramedullary tumor removal (Fig. 15-27), loss of cortical SEP to the left posterior tibial nerve occurred early during exposure of the tumor, while cortical SEP to the right posterior tibial nerve diminished with resection of the tumor and gradually recovered by the end of the operation. The patient awoke with dense left hemiplegia and partial sensory losses on the right.

The decision to monitor spinal cord function during surgery should not be made lightly. Monitoring is a time-consuming option that can tie up a trained technician and an expensive instrument for many hours. More important, evoked potential monitoring in the operating room may be deleterious to patients for the following reasons. First, monitoring may slow down operations. The operating room is a hostile environment for neurophysiologic studies. Electrical noise abounds. Setting up the recording and stimulating electrodes, getting good baseline responses, and confirming evoked potential changes take time and can add an hour or more to the surgical procedure and anesthesia time. Second, false alarms may be harmful to patients. Owing to changes in anesthetic levels and technical problems, SEP amplitude changes are commonplace and, more often than not, do not mean damage to the spinal cord. Operations may be interrupted and anesthesia levels changed unnecessarily, and surgeons may even end procedures prematurely because of a false alarm. Third, in patients with existing spinal lesions and abnormal SEP, injury to the spinal cord during the surgical procedure may not be reflected by SEP changes. The surgeon may proceed with a false sense of security and disregard other evidence that the spinal cord is being damaged. While it takes many cases of successful predictions to convince a surgeon to use SEPs, a single false negative will be remembered forever.

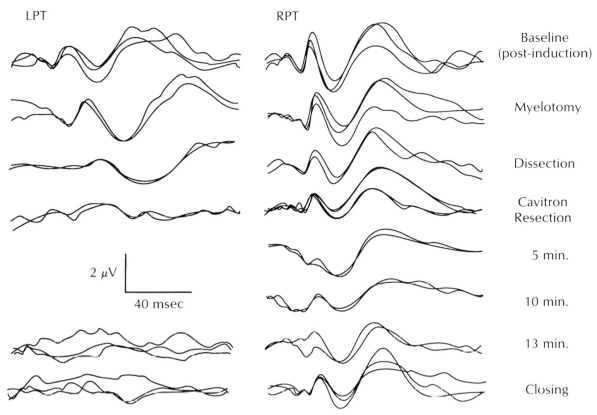

LPT   RPT

Baseline (post-induction)

Myelotomy

Dissection

Cavitron Resection

5 min.

10 min.

13 min.

Closing

2 μV

40 msec

Figure 15-27. Cortical SEP changes during surgical removal of an intramedullary tumor. Each trace represents the average of 100 responses recorded from the scalp after left and right posterior tibialis (LPT and RPT) stimulation. The patient awoke from surgery with a dense left hemiplegia and partial sensory and motor losses on the right.

There are some situations, however, in which spinal cord monitoring has become almost mandatory at the author's institution. One the most dramatic examples of the clinical usefulness of evoked potentials was provided by our experience with monitoring spinal cord angiography and embolization procedures.[7] Before 1981, when spinal cord monitoring was first used in angiographic procedures, the morbidity rate during selective spinal angiography and embolization exceeded 20%. In the 8 years since SEPs were used routinely in such cases, the number of patients that suffered neurologic deficits dropped significantly. Although this reduction is due in part to improvements of embolization techniques, some credit belongs to SEP monitoring. A fall in SEP amplitudes was observed whenever the anterior spinal artery was occluded or injected with high concentrations of contrast material. Because SEP amplitudes did not change with injections of the posterior spinal arteries, we used SEP to identify when contrast was injected into the anterior spinal artery. This greatly shortened the time that the catheter was left in place. Also, before embolization, the vessel was temporarily occluded to check its effect on the SEP. If the occlusion reduced SEP amplitudes, another vessel was chosen. Owing to these two practices, the incidence of postprocedure complication fell from greater than 20% to less than 2%. Although the advent of computerized digital subtraction facilities eliminated the need for SEPs for identifying the anterior spinal artery, most spinal angiography and embolization cases at New York University Medical Center are scheduled around the availability of SEP monitoring because of this experience.

Interventional Neurophysiology

Most neurophysiologic monitoring techniques usually require several minutes to carry out. For example, a reliable cortical SEP can be carried out in the operating room setting within 1 minute using stimulation rates of 2.3 Hz and averaging 100 responses. Confirmation of the finding by repeating the test two or three times and notification of the surgeon would take an additional 5 minutes. A current trend in the evoked potentials field is the development of more sensitive and rapid tests of spinal cord function. The rationale is that surgeons would be able to reverse a given deleterious maneuver if the information were provided quickly enough. Although this may be theoretically true, the emphasis on more sensitive and rapid tests can create problems. Increasing sensitivity of tests will increase the likelihood of false-positive errors. Clinicians quickly tire of false alarms and, at some point, will begin to disregard them with potentially disastrous consequences.

Development of more rapid tests ignores the physiologic bases for evoked potential changes in acute spinal cord injury. Trauma to the spinal cord in the operating room setting is comparable to the contusion model of spinal cord injury in animals. Tissue damage causes a rise in $[K^+]_e$, which will depolarize axons and thereby block action potential conduction. As pointed out above, disruption of as little as 5% of the cells in the tissue can cause $[K^+]_e$ to rise to 20 mM. Recovery of evoked potentials will commence as $[K^+]_e$ returns to <10 mM. Thus, how long an evoked potential is affected by a given action is probably the most important factor to consider when judging the severity of the tissue damage. Since $[K^+]_e$ clearance rates are relatively slow (i.e., with $T_{1/2}$ of 30 minutes of longer), faster tests will not yield information of value.

Faster feedback of information also would be useful only if the onset of injury is sufficiently slow and reversible. In our experience, intraoperative monitoring has had little if any role in many neurosurgical procedures, especially when tissues were being removed from the spinal cord. Evoked potential monitoring did help guide placement of an anterior bone plug and provided warnings of potentially deleterious situations on several occasions, but these were relatively rare. In contrast, evoked potentials has had a major impact on clinical decisions during spinal angiography and embolization procedures. This is because neurophysiologic testing was used to assess the effects of a temporary balloon occlusion prior to injecting emboli into the vessel. This interventional approach to spinal cord monitoring has proven to be very effective.

The use of provocative tests to assess risks of a given procedural step has many attractive features. The provocative test can be applied at a time chosen by the surgeon, and the monitoring can be intensified during the test. Problems with monitoring instrumentation and fluctuations in anesthetic conditions are common in long surgical procedures. Regardless of the speed with which neurophysiologic tests can provide information, lapses in attention and the frequency with which the tests are repeated essentially limit the notification time to 5 minutes. By standardizing the provocative test, specific criteria for action can be developed. The time for decision-making and preparation for appropriate actions can be greatly reduced. Passive monitoring in the operating room is analogous to waiting for horses to escape from the barn. Although faster monitoring techniques may help catch the horses in the act of leaving, the risk is that we may still end up closing the barn door after the horses have left. Interventional neurophysiology reduces this risk.

SUMMARY

Much progress has been made in developing noninvasive techniques to monitor evoked potentials in humans. A decade ago, the significance of evoked potentials recorded from the body surface was very much in question. Clinicians viewed evoked potentials with skepticism. Many of the early studies, for example, emphasized discrepancies between SEPs and neurologic examinations. As more groups gained experience with evoked potentials, however, it has become clear that properly carried out and interpreted evoked potentials are reliable indicators of sensorimotor recovery in spinal cord injury. False correlations with neurologic examinations have been less than 10% when conservative criteria were used to interpret evoked potentials obtained during the acute phase of spinal cord injury. Blatant cases in which evoked potentials have been absent and sensory examinations are normal or vice versa are virtually never seen in institutions with substantial experience with SEPs. Even the electrocardiogram, the most widely accepted physiologic test in clinical use today, probably cannot detect myocardial infarcts with a better accuracy than SEPs predict sensorimotor recovery in spinal cord injury.

One of the most difficult challenges facing researchers today in spinal cord monitoring is the development of rigorous criteria for interpreting evoked potential changes in injury situations. The criteria must be based on a clear understanding of the mechanisms underlying evoked potential changes. Loss of evoked potentials cannot be equated to loss of axons. There are many causes of conduction loss, including demyelination, alterations in excitability of proximal and distal brain structures, and extracellular ionic derangements. Finally, there is a need to develop neurophysiologic approaches that can test the risks of specific surgical maneuvers instead of simply documenting injury to the spinal cord.

REFERENCES

1. Andersson S, Gernandt BE: Ventral root discharge in response to vestibular and proprioceptive stimulation. J Neurophysiol 19:524–543, 1956
2. Barker AT, Freeston IL, Jalinous R, Jarratt JA: Clinical evaluation of conduction time measurements in central motor pathways using magnetic stimulation of human brain. Lancet i:1325–1326, 1986
3. Barker AT, Freeston IL, Jalinous R, Jarratt JA: Motor responses to non-invasive brain stimulation in clinical practice. Electroencephalogr Clin Neurophysiol 61:S70, 1985
4. Barker AT, Jalinous R: Non-invasive magnetic stimulation of human motor cortex. Lancet i:1106–1107, 1985
5. Baskin DS, Simpson RK Jr: Corticomotor and somatosensory evoked potential evaluation of acute spinal cord injury in the rat. Neurosurgery 20:871–877, 1987
6. Berardelli A, Cowan JMA, Day BL et al: The site of facilitation of the response to cortical stimulation during voluntary contraction in man. J Physiol 360:52, 1985
7. Berenstein A, Young W, Ransohoff J et al: Somatosensory evoked potentials (SEP) during spinal angiography and therapeutic transvascular embolization. J Neurosurg 60:777–785, 1983
8. Beric A, Dimitrijevic MR, Light JK: A clinical syndrome of rostral and caudal spinal injury: Neurological, neurophysiological and urodynamic evidence for occult sacral lesion. J Neurol Neurosurg Psychiatry 50:600–606, 1987
9. Blight AR: Axonal physiology of chronic spinal cord injury in the cat: Intracellular recording in vitro. Neuroscience 10:1471–1486, 1983
10. Blight AR: Cellular morphology of chronic spinal cord injury in the cat: Analysis of unmyelinated axons by line sampling. Neuroscience 10:521–543, 1983
11. Blight AR: Delayed demyelination and macrophage invasion: A candidate for "secondary" cell damage in spinal cord injury. Cent Nerv Syst Trauma 2:299–315, 1985
12. Blight AR: Effect of 4-aminopyridine on action potential conduction in myelinated axons of chronically injured spinal cord. Society of Neuroscience [Abstract] 21:15, 1987
13. Blight AR: Effect of 4-aminopyridine on axonal conduction block in chronic spinal cord injury. Brain Res Bull 22:(in press), 1989
14. Blight AR: Motor evoked potentials in CNS Trauma. Cent Nerv Syst Trauma 3:207–214, 1986
15. Blinkov SM, Glezer II: The Human Brain in Figures and Tables: A Quantitative Handbook, pp 53–75. New York, Plenum Press, 1968
16. Brodal A, Pompeiano O, Walberg F: The Vestibular Nuclei and Their Connections: Anatomy and Functional Correlations, pp 193–197. London, Oliver & Boyd, 1962
17. Cohen AR, Young W, Ransohoff J: Intraspinal localization of the somatosensory evoked potential. Neurosurgery 9:157–162, 1981
18. Cracco RQ: Evaluation of conduction in central motor pathways: Techniques, pathophysiology, and clinical interpretation. Neurosurgery 20:199–203, 1987
19. Cracco RQ: Spinal evoked response: Peripheral nerve stimulation in man. Electroencephalogr Clin Neurophysiol 35:379–386, 1973

20. Cracco RQ, Bickford RG: Somatomotor and somatosensory evoked responses. Arch Neurol 18:52–68, 1968

21. Cracco RQ, Cracco JB: Somatosensory evoked potentials in man: Farfield potentials. Electroencephalogr Clin Neurophysiol 41:460–466, 1976

22. Cracco JB, Cracco RQ, Graziani L: Spinal evoked responses in infants and children. Neurology 25:31–36, 1975

23. Dawson GD: Cerebral responses to nerve stimulation in man. Br Med Bull 6:326–329, 1950

24. Desmedt JE: Critical neuromonitoring at spinal and brainstem levels by somatosensory evoked potentials. Cent Nerv Syst Trauma 2:169–186, 1985

25. Desmedt JE: Non-invasive analysis of the spinal cord generators activated by somatosensory input in man: Nearfield and farfield components. Exp Brain Res [Suppl] 9:45–62, 1984

26. Desmedt JE, Cheron G: Spinal and farfield components of human somatosensory evoked potentials to posterior tibial nerve stimulation analyzed with oesophageal derivations and noncephalic reference recording. Electroencephalogr Clin Neurophysiol 56:635–651, 1983

27. Desmedt JE, Nguyen TH: Bit-mapped color imaging of the potential fields of propagated and segmental subcortical components of somatosensory evoked potentials in man. Electroencephalogr Clin Neurophysiol 37:407–410, 1984

28. Dimitrijevic MR: Clinical neurophysiological evaluation of motor and sensory functions in chronic spinal cord injury patients, pp 274–286. In Illis LS (ed): Spinal Cord Dysfunction: Assessment. Oxford, Oxford University Press, 1988

29. Dimitrijevic MR: Neurophysiology in spinal cord injury. Paraplegia 25:205–208, 1987

30. Dimitrijevic MR: Residual motor functions in spinal cord injury, pp 139–155. In Waxman SG (ed): Functional Recovery in Neurological Disease: Advances in Neurology, Vol 47. New York, Raven Press, 1988

31. Dimitrijevic MR, Dimitrijevic M, Faganel J, Sherwood AM: Suprasegmentally induced motor unit activity in paralyzed muscles of patients with established spinal cord injury. Ann Neurol 16:216–221, 1984

32. Dimitrijevic MR, Faganel J: Spasticity: Medical and surgical treatment. Neurology 30:19–27, 1985

33. Dimitrijevic MR, Faganel J, Lehmkuhl LD, Sherwood AM: Motor control in man after partial or complete spinal cord injury. In JE Desmedt (ed): Motor Control Mechanisms in Health and Disease. New York, Raven Press, 1983

34. Dimitrijevic MR, Spencer WA, Trontelj JV, Dimitrijevic MM: Reflex effects of vibration in patients with spinal cord lesion. Neurology 27:1078–1086, 1977

35. Eccles JC, Sasaki K, Strata P: The potential fields generated in the cerebellar cortex by a mossy fiber volley. Exp Brain Res 3:50–80, 1967

36. Eccles JC, Sasaki K, Strata P: The profile of physiological events produced by a parallel fiber volley in the cerebellar cortex. Exp Brain Res 2:18–34, 1966

37. Eidelberg E, Nguyen L, Deza L: Recovery of locomotor function after hemisection of the spinal cord in cats. Brain Res Bull 16:507–515, 1986

38. Eidelberg E, Staten E, Watkins LJ, Smith JS: Treatment of experimental spinal cord injury in ferrets. Surg Neurol 6:243–246, 1976

39. Eidelberg E, Story JL, Walden JG, Meyer BL: Anatomical correlates of return of locomotor function after partial spinal cord lesions in cats. Exp Brain Res 42:81–88, 1981

40. Eidelberg E, Straehley D, Erspamer R: Relationship between residual hindlimb assisted locomotion and surviving axons after incomplete spinal cord injuries. Exp Neurol 56:312–322, 1977

41. Eidelberg E, Walden J, Nguyen L: Locomotor control in macaque monkeys. Brain 104:647–663, 1981

42. Eidelberg E, Yu J: Effects of corticospinal lesions upon treadmill locomotion in cats. Exp Brain Res 43:101–103, 1981

43. Eidelberg E, Yu J: Effects of vestibulospinal lesions upon locomotor function in cats. Brain Res 22:179–183, 1981

44. Erulkar SD, Sprague JM, Whitsel BL et al: Organization of the vestibular projection to the spinal cord of the cat. J Neurophysiol 29:626–664, 1966

45. Evarts EV, Fromm C: The pyramidal tract neuron as summing point in a closed-loop control system in the monkey, pp 56–69. In Desmedt JE (ed): Cerebral Motor Control in Man: Long Loop Mechanisms. Basel, Karger, 1978

46. Fehlings MG, Tator CH, Linden RD, Piper IR: Motor and somatosensory evoked potentials recorded from the rat. Electroencephalogr Clin Neurophysiol 69:65–78, 1988

47. Fehlings MG, Tator CH, Linden RD, Piper IR: Motor evoked potentials recorded from normal and spinal cord-injured rats. Neurosurgery 20:125–130, 1987

48. Gianutsos J, Eberstein A, Ma D et al: A non-inva-

sive technique to assess completeness of spinal cord lesions in humans. Exp Neurol 98:34–40, 1987

49. Ginsburg HH, Shetter AG, Raudzens PA: Postoperative paraplegia with preserved intraoperative somatosensory evoked potentials: Case report. J Neurosurg 62:296–300, 1985

50. Gruner JA, Young W, Decrescito V: The vestibulospinal free fall response: A test of descending function in spinal injured cats. Cent Nerv Syst Trauma 1:139–160, 1984

51. Gualtierotti T, Paterson AS: Electrical stimulation of the unexposed cerebral cortex. J Physiol 125:278–291, 1954

52. Hahn JF, Latchaw JP: Evoked potentials in the operating room. Clin Neurosurg 31:389–403, 1984

53. Homma S, Tamaki T: Fundamental and Clinical Application of Spinal Cord Monitoring. Tokyo, Saikon, 1984

54. Jones SJ, Carter L, Edgar MA et al: Experience of epidural spinal cord monitoring in 410 cases, pp 215–220. In Schramm J, Jones SJ (eds): Spinal Cord Monitoring. New York, Springer-Verlag, 1985

55. Jones SJ, Edgar MA, Ransford AO: Sensory nerve conduction in the human spinal cord: Epidural recordings made during scoliosis surgery. J Neurol Neurosurg Psychiatry 45:446–451, 1982

56. Kakulas BA: Pathomorphological evidence for residual spinal cord functions, pp 163–169. In Eccles JC, Dimitrijevic MR (eds): Recent Achievements in Restorative Neurology: Vol 1. Upper Motor Neurons Functions and Dysfunctions. Karger, Basel, 1985

57. Kakulas BA, Bedbrook GM: Pathology of injuries of the vertebral spinal cord—with emphasis on the microscopic aspects, pp 27–42. In Vinken PJ, Bruyn GW (eds): Handbook of Clinical Neurology, Vol 25. Injuries of the Spine and Spinal Cord, Part I. Amsterdam, North-Holland, 1976

58. Klee M, Rall W: Computed potentials of cortically arranged populations of neurons. J Neurophysiol 40:647–666, 1977

59. Lesser RP, Raudzens P, Lüders H et al: Postoperative neurological deficits may occur despite unchanged intraoperative somatosensory evoked potentials. Ann Neurol 19:22–25, 1986

60. Levy WJ Jr: Clinical experience with motor and cerebellar evoked potential monitoring. Neurosurgery 20:169–182, 1987

61. Levy WJ, McCaffrey M, Hagichi S: Motor evoked potential as a predictor of recovery in chronic spinal cord injury. Neurosurgery 20:138–142, 1987

62. Llinas R, Nicholson C: Analysis of field potentials in the central nervous system, pp 61–84. In Rémond A (ed): Handbook of Electroencephalography and Clinical Neurophysiology, Vol. 2, Part 2B. Amsterdam, Elsevier, 1974

63. Lorente de Nó R: A Study of Nerve Physiology, Part 2. Studies from the Rockefeller Institute, Vol 132. New York, Rockefeller Institute, 1947

64. Maccabee PJ, Levine DB, Pinkhasov EJ et al: Evoked potentials recorded from scalp and spinous processes during spinal column surgery. Electroencephalogr Clin Neurophysiol 56:569–582, 1983

65. Macon JB, Poletti CE: Conducted somatosensory evoked potentials during spinal surgery: Part I. Control conduction velocity measurements. J Neurosurg 57:349–353, 1982

66. Macon JB, Sweet WH, Ojemann RG, Zervas NT: Conducted somatosensory evoked potentials during spinal surgery: Part II. Clinical applications. J Neurosurg 57:354–359, 1982

67. Marsden CD, Merton PA, Morton HB et al: Automatic and voluntary responses to muscle stretch in man, pp 167–177. In Desmedt JE (ed): Cerebral Motor Control in Man: Long Loop Mechanisms. Basel, Karger, 1978

68. Marsden CD, Rothwell JC, Day BL: Long latency automatic responses to muscle stretch in man: Origin and function, pp 509–539. In Desmedt JE (ed): Motor Control Mechanisms in Health and Disease. New York, Raven Press, 1983

69. McDonald WI: Mechanisms of functional loss and recovery in spinal cord damage, pp 23–33. In Symposium on the Outcome of Severe Damage to the Central Nervous System (CIBA Foundation Symposium 34). Amsterdam, Elsevier, 1974

70. McGarry J, Friedgood DL, Woolsey R et al: Somatosensory evoked potentials in spinal cord injuries. Surg Neurol 22:341–343, 1984

71. Merton PA, Hill DK, Morton HB: Scope of a technique for electrical stimulation of human brain, spinal cord and muscle. Lancet i:587–600, 1981

72. Merton PA, Morton HB: Stimulation of the cerebral cortex in the intact human subject. Nature 285:227, 1980

73. Patton HD, Amassian VE: Single-and multiple-unit analysis of cortical stage of pyramidal tract activation. J Neurophysiol 17:345–363, 1954

74. Perot PL Jr: The clinical use of somatosensory evoked potentials in spinal cord injury. Clin Neurosurg 20:367–381, 1973

75. Ramon Y, Cajal S: Degeneration and Regeneration of the Nervous System. London, Oxford University Press, 1928

76. Rothwell JC: The use of motor cortical stimulation to monitor spinal cord function during surgery, pp 287–295. In Illis LS (ed): Spinal Cord Dysfunction: Assessment. Oxford, Oxford University Press, 1988

77. Sakatani K, Ohta T, Shimo-Oku M: Conductivity of dorsal column fibers during experimental spinal cord compression and after decompression at various stimulus frequencies. Cent Nerv Syst Trauma 4:161–180, 1987

78. Sarica Y, Ertekin C: Descending lumbosacral cord potentials (DLCP) evoked by stimulation of the median nerve, pp 43–50. In Schramm J, Jones SJ (eds): Spinal Cord Monitoring. New York, Springer-Verlag, 1985

79. Schramm J, Jones SJ (eds): Spinal Cord Monitoring. New York, Springer-Verlag, 1985

80. Shimoji K, Higashi H, Kano T: Epidural recording of spinal electrogram in man. Electroencephalogr Clin Neurophysiol 30:236–239, 1971

81. Shimoji K, Kano T, Higashi H et al: Evoked spinal electrogram recorded from epidural space in man. J Appl Physiol 33:468–471, 1972

82. Shimoji K, Maruyama Y, Shimizu H et al: Spinal cord monitoring: A review of current techniques and knowledge, pp 16–28. In Schramm J, Jones SJ (eds): Spinal Cord Monitoring. New York, Springer-Verlag, 1985

83. Simpson RK, Baskin DS: Corticomotor evoked potentials in acute and chronic blunt spinal cord injury in the rat: Correlation with neurological outcome and histological damage. Neurosurgery 20:131–137, 1987

84. Thompson PD, Dick JP, Asselman P et al: Examination of motor function in lesions of the spinal cord by stimulation of the motor cortex. Ann Neurol 21:389–396, 1987

85. Willis WD, Coggeshall RE: Sensory Mechanisms of the Spinal Cord, pp 230–238. New York, Plenum Press, 1978

86. Windle WF: Concussion, contusion, and severance of the spinal cord. In Windle WF: The Spinal Cord and Its Reactions to Traumatic Injury. New York, Marcel Dekker, 1980

87. Windle WF, Smart JO, Beers JJ: Residual function after subtotal spinal cord transection in adult cats. Neurology 8:518–521, 1958

88. York DH, Watts C, Raffensberger M et al: Utilization of somatosensory evoked cortical potentials in spinal cord injury. Spine 8:832–839, 1983

89. Young W: Correlation of somatosensory evoked potentials and neurological findings in spinal cord injury, pp 153–165. In Tator CH (ed): Early Management of Acute Spinal Cord Injury. New York, Raven Press, 1982

90. Young W: The interpretation of surface evoked potentials. Trends in Neuroscience 4:277–280, 1981

91. Young W: Recovery mechanisms in spinal cord injury: Implications for regenerative therapy, pp 157–170. In Seil FJ (ed): Neural Regeneration and Transplantation. Frontiers of Clinical Neuroscience, Vol 6. New York, Alan R Liss, 1989

92. Young W: Somatosensory evoked potentials (SEPs) in spinal cord injury, pp 127–142. In Schramm J, Jones SJ (eds): Spinal Cord Monitoring. New York, Springer-Verlag, 1985

93. Young W, Berenstein A: Somatosensory evoked potential monitoring of intraoperative procedures, pp 197–203. In Schramm J, Jones SJ (eds): Spinal Cord Monitoring. New York, Springer-Verlag, 1985

94. Young W, Cohen A, Merkin H et al: Somatosensory evoked potential changes in spinal injury and during intraoperative manipulation. J Am Paraplegia Soc 5:44–48, 1982

95. Young W, Decrescito V, Tomasula JJ: Effect of sympathectomy on spinal cord blood flow autoregulation and posttraumatic ischemia. J Neurosurg 56:706–710, 1982

96. Young W, Koreh I, Yen V, Lindsay A: Effects of sympathectomy on extracellular potassium activity and blood flow in experimental spinal cord contusion. Brain Res 253:105–113, 1982

97. Young W, Meyer P: Neurological and neurophysiological evaluations of spinal cord injury, pp 148–165. In Illis L (ed): Spinal Cord Dysfunction: Assessment. New York, Oxford University Press, 1988

98. Young W, Mollin D: Intraoperative somatosensory evoked potential monitoring of spinal surgery. In Desmedt JE (ed): Neuromonitoring in Surgery, pp 169–173. Basel, Karger, 1989

99. Young W, Ransohoff J: Acute spinal cord injury: Experimental therapy, pathophysiological mechanisms, and recovery of function. In Sherk H (ed): The Cervical Spine, 2nd ed, pp 464–495. Philadelphia, J. B. Lippincott, 1989

100. Young W, Tomasula J, Decrescito V et al: Vestibulospinal monitoring in experimental spinal trauma. J Neurosurg 52:64–72, 1980

16

PHARMACOLOGIC THERAPY OF ACUTE SPINAL CORD INJURY

Wise Young

Several millennia ago, an anonymous Egyptian physician regarded the possibility of recovery from spinal cord injury to be so remote that he recommended withholding water from spinal-injured warriors so that they would die quickly.[42] Recent research, however, suggests acute spinal cord injury may be amenable to pharmacologic therapy given shortly after injury. The hope was first raised by histologic studies suggesting progressive tissue damage in injured spinal cords.

In the past 10 years, laboratory studies have established the sequelae of spinal cord injury in animal models. Blood flow falls in white matter at the injury site, usually 1 to 2 hours after the initial injury. Metabolic changes in the injured cords are reminiscent of ischemia. Many potentially toxic substances are activated and released in injured spinal cords, including free radicals, phospholipases, proteinases, lipid peroxides, and vasoactive eicosanoids. Ionic derangements develop at the injury site. Large amounts of calcium (Ca) enter and precipitate in injured cells, resulting in a profound and prolonged depression of extracellular Ca ionic activity ($[Ca^{2+}]_e$) and progressive Ca accumulation at the lesion site. These observations indicate the presence of a continuing injury response initiated by trauma in the spinal cord.

At least two classes of drugs have been found to alter the progressive tissue damage and improve neurologic outcome in animal spinal cord injury models. These include naloxone, an opiate receptor antagonist, and methylprednisolone, a synthetic corticosteroid. Both of these drugs must be given in large doses, about 10,000 times greater than that required for blocking opiate receptors and activating glucocorticosteroid receptors, respectively. Although the action of naloxone on spinal cord injury is controversial and not well understood, some progress has been made in understanding the mechanisms by which methylprednisolone is beneficial in acute neural injury. Very high doses of methylprednisolone inhibit lipid peroxidation. Lipid peroxidation contributes to the progressive tissue damage in injured spinal cords. Calcium entry into neurons activates phospholipases, releasing arachidonic acid, which is metabolized by lipoxygenase and cyclooxygenase, to prostaglandins, leukotrienes, and free radicals. These eicosanoids are among the most potent vasoactive agents known in biology. Small quantities of these substances will produce pathologic lesions in central nervous tissues that resemble those caused by trauma and ischemia.

The presence of an injury response that leads to progressive tissue damage in injured spinal cords raises an important question. Why do the longest-lived and most critical cells of the body possess such autodestructive tendencies? In this chapter, I will review the rationale of treating acute spinal cord injury in the context of this question. Specifically, I will propose that the injury response is part of a general mechanism that central nervous tissues have evolved to protect themselves against excessive Ca entry.

ACUTE SPINAL CORD INJURY RESPONSE

Allen[4,5] first described the progressive pathologic changes produced by dropping a 20-g weight 20 cm onto exposed spinal cords. Shortly after the contusion, little histologic evidence of tissue damage can be seen at the contusion site except for petechial hemorrhages.[84] However, gross hemorrhagic necrosis develops in gray matter at the impact site within hours. The central hemorrhagic necrotic pattern is a general pattern of injury that has been described from rats to man.[113,114,141] Allen's work was lost for nearly five decades, until several investigators began looking closely at the pathology of injured spinal cords.[21,22,47,59–61,63–65,128,145,173] Their studies showed that rapid endothelial pathology and coagulation in damaged vessels lead to ischemia and progressive tissue damage at the lesion site, suggesting a role of ischemia in spinal cord injury.

Blood flow measurements from contused spinal cords indicated that gray matter blood flow falls rapidly,[62,136,148] while white matter blood flow falls with a delay.[48,139,140,165,168–170,172,175] High-energy metabolites also are rapidly lost, consistent with ischemia.[7–10,38,146,147] The fall in white matter blood flow, however, can vary depending on in-

jury severity. Mild contusions, for example, may elevate white matter blood flow.[120] Autoregulation is disabled at the injury site[167,169] and systemic pressure changes[167,168] may influence post-traumatic spinal blood flow.[150]

Evoked potentials conducting across the injury site correlate with the timing of blood flow changes.[167,168] Somatosensory evoked potentials[160] (SEP) and descending vestibular responses[87,174] are rapidly lost, even after contusions that are not sufficient to produce lasting neurologic deficits in the animals. Evoked potentials begin recovering at 1 to 2 hours. With severe contusions, evoked potentials are lost again and more permanently at 2 to 3 hours. The initial loss of evoked potentials is due to potassium (K) released by traumatized cells.[172] Extracellular K ionic activity ($[K^+]_e$) rises from normal levels of 3 to 4 mM to >54 mM shortly after injury. It recovers to normal in white matter at the lesion by 1 to 2 hours, at the same time evoked responses begin conducting across the injury. The secondary loss of evoked potentials at 2 to 3 hours occurs when white matter blood flow falls to <6 ml/100 g/min.

Although post-traumatic white matter ischemia is worse in more severely injured spinal cords,[48] it is not clear that the fall in blood flow causes further tissue damage. The fall in blood flow may reflect rather than cause secondary injury. In addition, metabolic derangements occur rapidly at the injury site,[8–10] preceding the fall in white matter blood flow. Finally, white matter blood flow falls only by 50% to 60% by 3 hours after injury. Spinal cord white matter normally can tolerate flow losses of this magnitude without permanent damage. Thus, while post-traumatic ischemia correlates with injury severity, a cause–effect relationship has not yet been established.

EXPERIMENTAL TREATMENTS OF ACUTE SPINAL CORD INJURY

The observation of progressive tissue damage in injured spinal cords, even though the causes were not well understood at the beginning, provided the first rationale for seeking acute spinal cord injury treatments. Many treatments have been tried over the past three decades, including hypothermia[2,3] electromagnetic fields,[27-29,152,155] and several classes of drugs given shortly after injury.[157] Different models of spinal cord injury have been used, including the standard weight drop contusion introduced by Allen, compression,[7-11] crush,[88-90,142,151-155] and even ischemia produced by occlusion of the descending thoracic aorta.[70,76,79] A variety of outcome measures have been used for therapeutic efficacy, ranging from blood flow and biochemical measurements to neurophysiologic and locomotory recovery.

The initial studies focused on drugs to manipulate spinal cord blood flow and to prevent ischemia. Antifibrinolytic[47] and vasodilatory[62] agents were among the first tested, and were found to affect spinal blood flow. By 1987, several other drugs that prevent post-traumatic ischemia were reported. These include very high doses of naloxone,[71,170] methylprednisolone,[8,170] thyrotropin-releasing hormone (TRH),[73,74,77] κ opiate receptor blockers,[67,70] Ca channel blockers,[88-90] 21-aminosteroids,[95] and others.[96] Figure 16-1 summarizes the effects of naloxone and methylprednisolone on spinal white matter blood flow at 3 hours after contusion injury.[169,170] White matter spinal cord blood flow is normally 12 to 14 ml/100 g/min[162] and falls to 5 to 6 ml/100 g/min by 3 hours. Naloxone (10 mg/kg) and methylprednisolone (15

mg/kg and 30 mg/kg) prevent this fall. Some drugs that prevent post-traumatic white matter ischemia improve functional recovery. Naloxone[12,67,68,72,82] and methylprednisolone[47,166] were among the first drugs found to have both effects. Thyrotropin-releasing hormone[73] and κ opiate receptor blockers[67] have been reported to have similar effects. In one model, naloxone and methylprednisolone were given 45 minutes after a 20-g–20-cm weight drop contusion of cat thoracic spinal cord.[81,166] Only 17% of untreated spinal-injured cats recovered locomotion. High doses of naloxone (10mg/kg) significantly increased this proportion to 65%, while 1 to 3 mg/kg had no significant effect. About 78% of cats treated with methylprednisolone (15 mg/kg) recovered. Somatosensory evoked potential recovery in the animals showed a similar trend. Combining high-dose naloxone (10 mg/kg) and methylprednisolone (15 mg/kg) significantly increased mortality in spinal-injured cats.

More recent work suggests that the treatment effects are not as robust as originally thought. Some laboratories found no significant effects of high doses of naloxone[91,148,149] or corticosteroids[75] on other injury models. Drug effects apparently differed depending on the injury model. For example, naloxone but not TRH improved functional recovery in a model of spinal cord ischemia.[68,121]

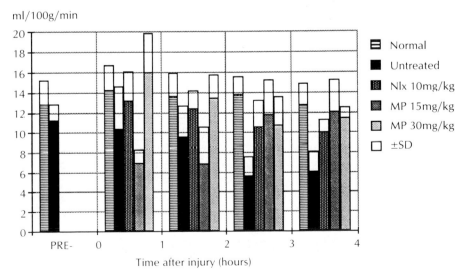

Figure 16-1. Summary of white matter blood flow changes in spinal cords of cats injured with a 20 g–20 cm weight-drop contusion. Five separate experimental series are compared. Normal animals were not injured (n = 6). Untreated were injured and given only saline during the experiment (n = 8). Nlx 10 mg/kg were injured and treated with 10 mg/kg of naloxone at 45 min after injury. MP 15 mg/kg and MP 30 mg/kg were, respectively, given methylprednisolone 15 and 30 mg/kg at 45 min after contusion. The untreated injured cats clearly had a significant fall in blood flow by 2 hours after injury. Naloxone and methylpredisolone both prevented this fall.

Differences in anesthesia, methods of evaluating functional and morphologic outcome, and drug regimens tested may have contributed to discrepancies in therapeutic results.

CLINICAL TRIALS OF NALOXONE AND METHYLPREDNISOLONE

Based on laboratory experiments suggesting that acute spinal cord injury may be treatable, a national multicenter trial was established in 1979. This study, called the National Acute Spinal Cord Injury Study (NASCIS I), was a double-blind randomized clinical trial comparing 1000 mg and 100 mg of methylprednisolone sodium succinate in 300 patients at 10 spinal cord injury centers. Patients admitted within 48 hours of injury were eligible for the trial. Either 100 mg or 1000 mg of methylprednisolone was given intravenously to the patients immediately and then daily for 10 days. The patients were followed up with detailed neurologic examinations for 1 year after injury.

No statistically significant difference was found between the high and low dosage methylprednisolone groups in NASCIS I.[30,31] There was a trend for improvement of motor and sensory scores in both groups.[161] The high dosage group had better scores than the low dosage group at 6 months and 1 year, but the difference turned out to be not statistically significant (p~0.06).

In retrospect, the NASCIS I trial was inadequately designed.[166] First, the drug may have been given too late. All the laboratory studies, with one exception,[71] had tested earlier (less than 1 hour after injury) treatments. No patient in the study received the drug within an hour, the majority were treated 3 hours or more after injury, and some were not treated until 24 to 48 hours. Second, owing to the practice of giving a set amount of the drug irrespective of body weight, the dosages varied. For example, a patient in the high dosage group may have received anywhere from 10 to 15 mg/kg. Third, the dose may have been insufficient. Laboratory experiments suggest that the optimal dose of methylprednisolone is about 30 mg/kg.[36] Fourth, different spinal cord injuries were lumped together, ranging from complete cervical spinal cord injury to incomplete lumbosa-

cral injuries. The responses of such a diverse population to treatment are likely to be quite different. Finally, the trial compared high and low dosage treatments. It did not test treatment against a placebo. Given the lateness of the treatments, the variability of the doses, the possible insufficiency of the dose that was given, and the variety of spinal cord injuries that were lumped together, a barely negative result is not so surprising.

By 1982, laboratory studies suggested that 10 mg/kg doses of naloxone given shortly after injury may be beneficial. Because such doses of naloxone had never been given to patients before, we[81] carried out an initial phase I accelerated dose study, giving 0.1 to 5.4 mg/kg doses of naloxone to 29 spinal-injured patients. Somatosensory evoked potentials were obtained on admission and 6 weeks after spinal cord injury.[160] As shown in Figure 16-2, there was a trend toward better recovery of SEPs with increasing doses of naloxone in this nonrandomized trial. No adverse side-effects were noted with doses up to 5.4 mg/kg. The patients, however, began to complain of flushing sensations at the highest dose. The four patients who were given 5.4 mg/kg all showed some improvement in SEP; one showed dramatic improvement, from an SEP score of 1 to 8.

A second study (NASCIS II) was initiated in 1985. This trial compared spinal-cord injured patients randomly assigned to three groups: placebo (the vehicular solution), naloxone (5.4 mg/kg initial dose and 75% of that dose every hour for 24 hours), and methylprednisolone (30 mg/kg initial dose with 5.4 mg/kg/hour for 24 hours). Patients were treated within 12 hours after spinal cord injury, with an average of 4 to 6 hours. Patients received as much as 10 g of naloxone or 30 g of methylprednisolone over a 24-hour period. The NASCIS II has just been completed, and data analysis will commence when the follow-up studies have been carried out.

OPIATE RECEPTOR MECHANISMS IN NEURAL INJURY

The observation that naloxone has effects on spinal cord blood flow and recovery suggested that

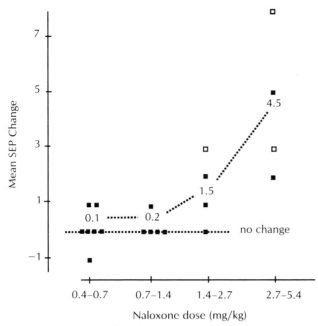

Figure 16-2. Scatterplot of changes in SEP scores in patients with spinal cord injury treated with 0.42 mg/kg to 5.4 mg/kg naloxone. The scores represent the difference in SEP scores between admission and 6 weeks after injury. The posterior tibialis SEP from each leg was scored on a scale of 0–4 where 0 represents no response, 1 is a very small but present response, 2 is small and abnormal in latency, 3 is normal, and 4 is greater than normal. The scores from each leg were summed. Thus, the maximum score difference between admission and followup was 8, i.e. 4 + 4. With an increasing naloxone dose, there appeared to be a trend for greater SEP score differences. The open squares represent patients with some sensory or motor preservation below the lesion level and the solid squares represent patients with none.

The beneficial effects of naloxone on functional recovery in spinal cord injury continues to be debated. However, the advent of naloxone as a potential therapy for spinal cord injury has greatly stimulated researchers. The first quantitative studies of biochemical, morphologic, neurophysiologic, and behavioral outcomes of spinal cord injury were done in response to the excitement associated with the naloxone discovery. Shortly after the first reports that naloxone may be beneficial in spinal cord injury, Hosobuchi and associates[109] suggested its use in stroke. Although the evidence for naloxone effects in cerebral ischemia is quite controversial,[105,117] positive results of naloxone treatment of several ischemia models have been reported.[76,144]

The most striking anomaly in the naloxone results is the huge doses required to affect injured spinal cords. At 10 mg/kg, the dose is 1000 times greater than that necessary to block μ opiate receptors. Generally, 0.5 mg of naloxone (<0.008 mg/kg for a typical 70-kg person) will effectively treat heroin overdose in humans. Naloxone, therefore, may be acting through mechanisms unrelated to blockade of μ opiate receptors. Faden and associates[70] have suggested that the naloxone effects in neural injury are due to blockade of the κ opiate receptor. Naloxone does not bind κ receptors as well as μ receptors, and much larger doses may be required. Faden and associates[68,76–78] reported that the more specific κ antagonists, such as TRH and WIN44,441–3, also have beneficial effects on spinal ischemia models. These findings have not yet been confirmed by other laboratories.

The question of why opiate receptor blockade can protect traumatized spinal cords remains unanswered, since there are no opiate receptors on spinal cord white matter. The site of action of naloxone and TRH in spinal cord injury is not known. It is likely to be acting through some intermediate mechanism. Opiate receptor blockers, however, have been gaining widespread acceptance in the treatment of endotoxic shock and hemorrhagic shock.[69,106,107] Trauma releases glucocorticosteroids, endogenous opioids, catecholamines, serotonin, monokines, lymphokines, and stress-related proteins. High doses of opiate receptor blockers may be acting through an effect on the synthesis

opiate receptors play a role in spinal cord injury. Faden and associates[72] originally attributed the naloxone effects to improvements in systemic pressure. We[170] subsequently argued against this interpretation, finding that the naloxone effects on blood pressure were insufficient to explain the improvement of blood flow. Wallace and Tator[148,149] recently reported that naloxone did not improve cardiac output, spinal cord blood flow, and neurologic outcome after experimental spinal injury in rats. However, they found that raising blood pressure and cardiac output by drugs other than naloxone did improve spinal cord blood flow.[150]

and release of these substances peripherally and centrally. These substances may modulate the spinal cord response to injury.

LIPID PEROXIDATION AND SECONDARY TISSUE DAMAGE

The use of methylprednisolone in spinal cord injury stimulated interest in yet another mechanism of secondary tissue damage: lipid peroxidation. Although methylprednisolone was proposed to act in spinal cord injury as a free radical scavenger more than a decade ago,[47,59,60] the concept did not become popular until several investigators showed that high doses of methylprednisolone (15 to 30 mg/kg) inhibited lipid peroxidation in injured spinal cords.[11,34-36,92-94] In addition, these doses of methylprednisolone reduced metabolic derangements,[38] preserved adenosine triphosphatase activity,[34,35,37] and prevented neurofilament loss in injured spinal cords.[37] Corticosteroids also may directly or indirectly inhibit phospholipase A_2 activity.[102,123] The optimal dose for reducing lipid peroxidation is 30 mg/kg. Doubling the dose to 60 mg/kg aggravated lipid peroxidation. The methylprednisolone effects on blood flow[35,39-41,94,96,97] and gram-negative bacterial sepsis[85] have similar dose–response curves.

Based on these data, Braughler and Hall[36,39] proposed that the therapeutic effects of methylprednisolone on spinal cord injury stemmed not from its glucocorticosteroid activity, but rather from its chemical ability to inhibit lipid peroxidation. This mechanism would explain why such large doses are necessary and why the drug has such a narrow dose–response curve. This proposal provided the rationale for the development of a new family of potent lipid peroxidation inhibitor drugs, called 21-aminosteroids.[95] These drugs have no glucocorticosteroid activity, but are more potent inhibitors of lipid peroxidation than methylprednisolone. Studies are now being carried out with 21-aminosteroid drugs in spinal cord injury models.

Lipid peroxidation has attracted increasing attention recently because it promises to unify many potential causes of secondary tissue damage into a single mechanism. These include the role of Ca, ischemia, membrane breakdown, and the various phenomena that have been found in acutely injured spinal cords. The lipid peroxidation cascade is as follows: Excessive Ca ionic entry[164] disrupts mitochondrial electron transport[54] and diverts electron transport to formation of oxygen and other free radicals.[32] Free radicals attack membrane and enhance phospholipase-mediated breakdown of membranes, releasing lipid peroxides and freeing arachidonic acid.[33] Ubiquitous cycloxygenase enzymes convert free arachidonic acid to prostaglandins and leukotrienes. These substances can cause pathologic and biochemical changes similar to those observed in traumatized or ischemic tissues.[49-53] Figure 16-3 summarizes the lipid peroxidation cascade diagrammatically. Elevated levels of vasoconstrictive prostaglandins and lipid peroxides have been demonstrated in injured spinal cords.[108,110,137] Thus, treatments that prevent lipid peroxidation should affect secondary injury processes on several levels.

The eicosanoids are among the most potent vasoactive agents known.[80,118,129,156] Prostacyclin (PGI_2), an arachidonic metabolite, inhibits platelet aggregation and causes vasodilation.[118] Released by endothelial cells, PGI_2 may cause the hyperemia reported during the early phase of spinal cord injury.[122] Prostacyclin release is modulated by thrombin, bradykinin, histamine, epinephrine, angiotensin II, adenosine triphosphate:diphosphate ratios, acetylcholine, oxygen radicals, serotonin, endotoxin, monokines,[131] lymphokines (interleukin-2), and Ca ions.[80] Endothelial cells also release thromboxane A_2 (TXA_2), a platelet-derived product of arachidonic acid metabolism, but with a delay. Thromboxane A_2 opposes PGI_2 actions, promoting platelet aggregation, thrombosis, and vasoconstriction. It therefore may be responsible for delayed post-traumatic ischemia in white matter. Other arachidonic acid metabolites include leukotrienes, generated by 5-lipoxygenase. Produced by neutrophils, leukotrienes C_4, D_4, and B_4 may contribute to edema by increasing postcapillary venule permeability. Marked increases in TXA_2 and leukotrienes C_4, D_4, and B_4, as well as a decrease in PGI_2, have been reported to occur in injured spinal cords.[58,137]

Lipid peroxidation is therefore an early step in a complicated cascade of biochemical events asso-

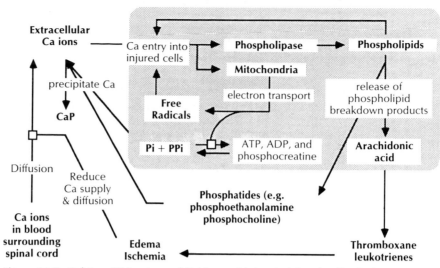

Figure 16-3. Calcium (Ca) entry and lipid peroxidation in injured cells. Ca ions entering the cells activate phospholipases. The phospholipases break down phospholipids, releasing free arachidonic acid and phosphatides, which bind and precipitate Ca ions. In addition, Ca ions will block electron transport in mitochondria, which release free radicals and block the recycling of adenosine disphosphate to adenosine triphosphate. In the meantime, arachidonic acid is metabolized to thromboxane and leukotrienes, which cause edema and ischemia in the tissue, reducing Ca diffusion to the lesion site and slowing the restoration of extracellular Ca activity. (CaP – calcium phosphate; Pi = inorganic phosphate [mono]; PPi = inorganic phosphate [di]; CaP = calcium phosphate.)

ciated with the injury response, many components of which have been shown to occur in injured spinal cords. It potentially ties together many of the biochemical events into a single mechanism. The sequelae of lipid peroxidation is of particular interest because many of the biochemical steps involved can be manipulated by drugs and, in some cases, stopped by several known inhibitors of enzymes. Methylprednisolone may act at the very early stages by preventing lipid peroxidation and thereby slowing the release of free arachidonic acid and the consequent cascade of events. Note that the effect of methylprednisolone on lipid peroxidation may explain its effectiveness as an antiedema agent in brain tumors and toxic shock syndromes.

ROLE OF CALCIUM IN SECONDARY TISSUE DAMAGE

An enormous gradient of Ca normally exists across neuronal membranes. Intracellular Ca ionic activity ($[Ca^{2+}]_i$) is normally <0.1 μM, compared with a normal $[Ca^{2+}]_e$ of >1 mM. Calcium ions should therefore rush into injured neurons. Calcium ions regulate many biologic processes, including transport, secretion, mitosis, and growth. Elevated intracellular Ca ionic activity should disrupt all cellular function. Elevated $[Ca^{2+}]_i$ also activates phospholipases, disrupts mitochondrial electron transport, and interferes with phosphorylation reactions.[32,33] It is little wonder that Ca entry has sometimes been called a final common pathway of cell death.[138]

Using ion-selective microelectrodes, we have demonstrated that $[Ca^{2+}]_e$ falls to <0.01 mM and remains at that level for hours in injured spinal cords.[158,168,169] Therefore, large amounts of Ca must enter cells at the injury site. Application of Ca-containing solutions or Ca iontophores to spinal cords can produce pathologic lesions resembling those caused by trauma or ischemia.[20,23] Calcium deposits have been seen in injured axons at the lesion site of traumatized spinal cords.[24,25] Given the ability of Ca influx to initiate lipid peroxidation and stimulate pathologic prostaglandin production, the initial Ca influx is a likely trigger for the cascade of necrotic biochemical events. The time course of the $[Ca^{2+}]_e$ changes is shown in Figure 16-4.

The magnitude of the fall in $[Ca^{2+}]_e$, however, is much greater than expected. At the lesion center, we[157] found that $[Ca^{2+}]_e$ falls to <0.01 mM within seconds after injury, recovering to 0.1 mM by 4 hours. Assuming, conservatively, that $[Ca^{2+}]_i$ is negligible, that extracellular fluids occupy 15% of the tissue volume, and that $[Ca^{2+}]_e$ is 1.2 mM, complete equilibration of all intracellular fluids with extracellular fluids can be calculated to result in a fall of $[Ca^{2+}]_e$ to no lower than about 0.2 mM. Actually, $[Ca^{2+}]_e$ falls two orders of magnitude lower than this expected level. At the same time that $[Ca^{2+}]_e$ falls, total tissue calcium ($[Ca]_t$) increases.[26,98,171] Within 3 hours after contusion injury, $[Ca]_t$ increases by more than 50%, as shown in Figure 16-5. Since $[Ca]_t$ concentration increases by as much as 1.0 µmol/g of tissue by 3 hours after

injury, the Ca accumulated at the injury site probably represents more than five times the free Ca originally present at the lesion site. Hence Ca ions not only enter cells but appear to be precipitating in large quantities.

Calcium ions probably enter injured cells through many routes, including Ca channels and holes in the membrane. These include three types of channels: the neurotransmitter receptor channel, the voltage-dependent sodium (Na) channel, and the voltage-dependent Ca channels. In addition, Ca may leak into the cells or enter through gross holes in injured cells. Figure 16-6 summarizes the major Ca entry and exit mechanisms. Two mechanisms of Ca efflux are shown: the magnesium–Ca adenosine triphosphatase and Na–Ca carrier exchange. From a therapeutic point of view, the initial Ca entry into injured neurons is difficult to control. Furthermore, since Ca ions are critical for cellular function, drugs that effectively block Ca entry into cells are likely to be pro-

(Text continued on p. 425)

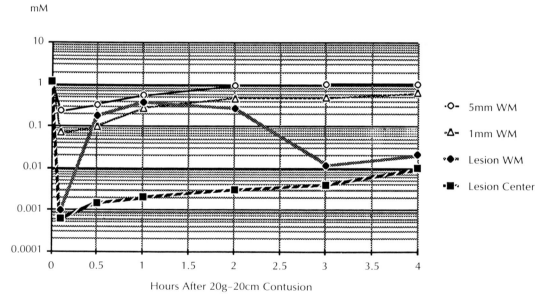

Figure 16-4. Extracellular Ca activity in cat spinal cord after a 20 g–20 cm weight-drop contusion injury. Recordings were made in white matter 5 mm from the lesion (5 mm WM), 1 mm from the lesion (1 mm WM), and at the lesion site (Lesion WM), and in gray matter at the lesion center (Lesion Center). At the lesion center, extracellular Ca activity falls to <0.001 millimolar (mM) recovering slowly to 0.01 mM. In white matter at the lesion site, extracellular Ca also falls to 0.001 mM but recovers to 0.1 mM by 30 to 60 min. It falls again to 0.01 mM at 3 hours when blood flow falls in the white matter.

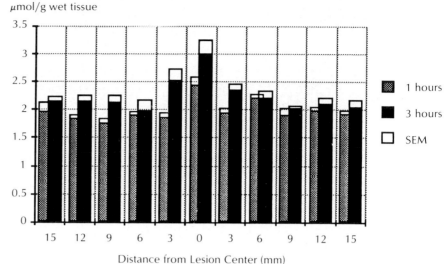

Figure 16-5. Mean total tissue calcium concentrations (μmol/g wet tissue weight) in cat spinal cord at 1 or 3 hours after 20 g–20 cm weight-drop contusion injury. The values represent means of 10 animals for each time point. The spinal cords were sampled in 3-mm pieces, as shown in Figure 16-6. There was a significant rise of tissue Ca by 3 hours after spinal cord contusion. (SEM = standard error of mean.)

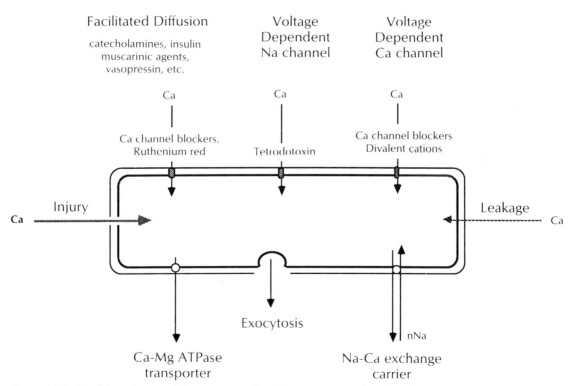

Figure 16-6. Possible pathways of Ca entry into cells. Calcium can enter through at least three types of channels, including excitatory amino acid and other receptor channels, the Na channel, and the voltage-sensitive Ca channels. Calcium can enter the cell through holes made as a result of cell injury and leakage channels. Calcium is removed from cells by two transport mechanisms, the Ca–magnesium adenosine diphosphatase (Ca-Mg ATPase) transporter and the Na–Ca exchange carrier mechanism. In addition, Ca can be extruded from cells by exocytosis.

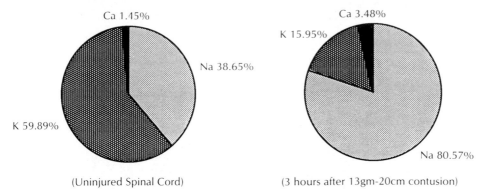

(Uninjured Spinal Cord)   (3 hours after 13gm-20cm contusion)

Figure 16-7. The ionic composition of spinal cord tissues is shown in pie graphs, illustrating the inorganic cation pools before and 3 hours after a severe 13 g–20 cm weight-drop contusion injury. The percentages refer to the proportion of the total ionic pool, i.e. Na + K + Ca. The control data represent averages of measurements made from 48 thoracic spinal cord segments taken from six uninjured cat spinal cords. The injury data (n = 24) come from the lesion site, i.e. 0–3 mm proximal and distal to the lesion center, from 12 untreated injured cords. The most dramatic shift is the replacement of 73% of the K in the tissue by Na.

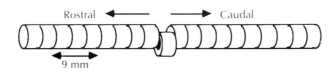

Distribution of Tissue, Water, and Ionic Contents

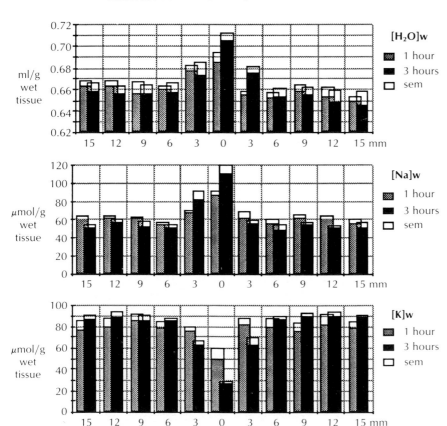

Figure 16-8. Distribution of Na, K, and water shifts in the spinal cord of cats at 1 and 3 hours after a 20 g–20 cm weight-drop contusion injury. The data represent means of 10 animals. The units of concentration are μmol/g wet tissue weight. (SEM = standard error of mean; [K]w = tissue potassium concentration; [Na]w = tissue sodium concentration; [H$_2$O]w = tissue water concentration.)

foundly toxic to the organism. Truly effective Ca channel blockers should be incompatible with life. Calcium channel blockers, however, may improve blood flow at the lesion site.[89,90]

Large derangements of the other ions also occur at the injury site. Figure 16-7 shows the proportions that Na, K, and Ca ions occupy of the tissue inorganic ionic pool. Calcium, which starts out being about 1.5% of the total, increased to nearly 3.5% with 3 hours after injury. The most striking change was the change of tissue K from 60% before injury to less than 16% by 3 hours. Potassium was replaced by Na, which increased from 38% to 80%. Figure 16-8 shows the distribution of total tissue concentrations of Na, K, and water content in spinal cords injured with a 20-g weight dropped 20 cm onto the unsupported spinal cord.

PROTECTION AGAINST EXCESSIVE CALCIUM ENTRY

The findings of progressive tissue damage and, particularly, the roles of lipid peroxidation and Ca in spinal cord injury pose a difficult question. These mechanisms are simply too elaborate to have occurred by accident—lipid peroxidation involves several large families of complex enzymes that are ubiquitously present in all nervous tissues.[163] Given that neurons are among the most critical and longest living cells of the body, that neurons are exquisitely sensitive to Ca, that a sea of Ca ions sits poised to rush into neurons, and that Ca ions can activate lipid peroxidation and the entire cascade of autodestructive mechanisms, the situation presents one of the most intriguing paradoxes in biology. Why are these elaborate autodestructive mechanisms present? Do they serve any purpose? It is inconceivable that this situation evolved without organisms having developed effective mechanisms to protect neurons. A closer look at the Ca changes in spinal cord injury suggests a surprising answer.

Falls in $[Ca^{2+}]_e$ universally accompany central nervous tissue injury, whether the cause is trauma, ischemia, or toxin. In spinal cord injury, $[Ca^{2+}]_e$ falls much lower than expected at the same time that $[Ca]_t$ concentrations increase, suggesting that some substance(s) must be binding and precipitating large amounts of Ca. This substance

must be present in high concentrations, must bind Ca avidly enough to buffer $[Ca^{2+}]_e$ to <0.01 μM, and must be available for many hours after injury in order to keep $[Ca^{2+}]_e$ depressed. One class of substances in nervous tissues meets these criteria: phosphates.[158,159] Phosphates bind Ca avidly.[43,57] Central nervous tissues contain very high concentrations of phosphates. The human spinal cord contains 170 mM of phosphates, which is more than any other biologic substance, with the exception of egg yolk and bacterial particles with high DNA concentrations. Most of the phosphates are in membrane phospholipids. Lipid peroxidation results in release of large amounts of phosphates and phospholipid fragments.

Lowering of $[Ca^{2+}]_e$ is probably the most effective and efficient way of reducing Ca entry into surviving cells.[159] Figure 16-9 summarizes the mechanism by which central nervous tissues may protect cells against excessive Ca entry. Calcium ions enter injured cells through a diversity of

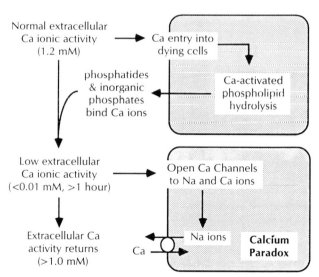

Figure 16-9. Schematic diagram of Ca changes in spinal cord injury. Normal extracellular activity is 1.2 millimolar (mM). Ca enters injured cells, activating phospholipases, which break down membrane phospholipids. The resulting release of phosphatides and inorganic phosphates then binds Ca ions, lowering extracellular Ca ionic activity to <0.01 mM. The exposure to the low levels of extracellular Ca leads to opening of Ca channels to Na and Ca ions. The cells load up with Na ions. Return of extracellular Ca activity leads to a massive influx of Ca into cells, exchanging with Na, i.e. Ca paradox.

channels, initiating lipid peroxidation. The resultant breakdown of membrane phospholipids releases massive amounts of phosphatides and phosphates, which bind Ca ions and temporarily reduce the transmembrane gradient that drives Ca ions into cells. During this time, injured neurons can repair breaks in their membrane, restore their metabolic supplies, and recoup their energies. Cells that are destroyed in this process probably would not survive anyway. The tissue rapidly removes lingering moribund cells that would otherwise consume precious metabolic resources and oxygen. The mechanism is robust and independent of metabolic energy.

Central nervous tissues, therefore, appear to have evolved an elegant and effective mechanism to deal with the problem of excessive Ca entry. By endowing cells with an abundance of Ca-activated phospholipases and lipid peroxidation mechanisms, the organism guarantees complete release of their phosphates into extracellular space. Calcium entry into cells initiates other supporting reactions that hasten the complete destruction of the cells, including the release of free radicals and lysosomal protease enzymes, which will dissolve membranes to expose any hidden phospholipids. It is perhaps not accidental that the spinal cord tissues contain such high concentrations of phosphates. This provides sufficient phosphates to lower $[Ca^{2+}]_e$. In fact, complete release of phosphates from a small percentage of cells in the spinal cord should be more than sufficient to buffer $[Ca^{2+}]_e$ to 1 μM.

CALCIUM PARADOX

The profound and prolonged depression of $[Ca^{2+}]_e$ that occurs in injured spinal cords may have unanticipated side-effects. More than two decades ago, Zimmerman and Hulsmann[176] reported the phenomenon of "calcium paradox" in heart muscles. If an isolated heart is perfused with Ca-free solutions for a period of time and normal Ca-containing solutions are restored, the heart will die. This phenomenon has since been confirmed by many other investigators.[13,100,115,134,135,176] During the Ca-free period, cardiac cells apparently become permeable to Ca and Na. Sodium ions enter the cells in large quantities.[6,45,56,86,132] Upon restoration of normal extracellular Ca, Ca ions rush into the cells through open Ca channels, enhanced by exchange with Na ions leaving the cells.[56,124,132]

The critical levels of $[Ca^{2+}]_e$ that produce Ca paradox in heart are about 10 μM for 30 minutes.[19,111,127] Calcium paradox causes pathologic reactions in heart muscle that are reminiscent of spinal cord injury, including lipid peroxidation,[112] production of eicosanoids,[116] and free radical release.[100,101] A number of drugs that affect free radicals and lipid peroxidation have been reported to help reduce Ca paradox damage to hearts. Hypothermia to 10°C increases the length of time that cardiac cells can be exposed to Ca-free solutions without showing Ca paradox changes.[15,18,83,133] The Ca channel blockers, verapamil,[1,17,66,99,125] diltiazem, and[14] the ionic Ca blockers[16,17,46,55,119,125] reduce the damage produced by Ca paradox. Other treatments include adrenergic blockade,[103,126] reduction of extracellular Na,[44–46] anesthetic agents,[104,143] allopurinol,[126] and chlorpromazine.[130]

All the essential elements of the Ca paradox phenomenon are present in the contused spinal cord.[158] Extracellular Ca ionic activity falls to <0.01 mM [172] and remains depressed for more than 30 minutes. Sodium ions enter cells and accumulate at the lesion site.[165]

To prevent Ca paradox, Ca diffusion to the lesion site from adjacent spinal cord and blood must be reduced. Central nervous tissues appear to offer two ways by which this can be practically achieved. One is restriction of blood flow by vasoconstriction. The other is edema, which decreases the extracellular space through which Ca ions diffuse. Both of these are likely to be mediated by prostaglandins and leukotrienes generated from products of lipid breakdown. Prostaglandins and leukotrienes are among the most potent vasoactive and edema-causing agents known. These two mechanisms will slow down the return of $[Ca^{2+}]_e$. In severe injuries, the release of free radicals and prostaglandins may become excessive. The resultant edema and vasoconstriction may cause further damage to surviving cells. Drugs such as methylprednisolone may be beneficial in such situations. However, oversuppression of lipid peroxidation may lead to rapid restoration of $[Ca^{2+}]_e$ to the tissue and greater tissue damage. This explains the narrow therapeutic range of drugs that have been reported to be beneficial in spinal cord injury.

The occurrence of Ca paradox may explain several puzzling characteristics in spinal cord injury. First, it suggests a reason why drugs like methylprednisolone have such narrow effective dose ranges. The optimal dose of the drug is about 30 mg/kg. Doubling the dose may reverse the beneficial effects and actually result in greater tissue damage. Perhaps this results from overly effective suppression of lipid peroxidation and the failure of the tissue to release sufficient phosphates to depress $[Ca^{2+}]_e$. In fact, 15 mg/kg of methylprednisolone will significantly enhance the recovery of $[Ca^{2+}]_e$ to normal.[172] Second, it provides an evolutionary basis for the elaborate Ca-activated phosphate-release mechanisms in nervous tissues. It may be a general mechanism by which nervous tissues protect themselves against excessive Ca entry and Ca paradox. Third, it may explain why nervous tissues universally respond to injury with a fall in blood flow and edema.

From a therapeutic point of view, the possibility that Ca paradox plays a role in spinal cord injury provides a rationale for use of Ca channel blockers in spinal cord injury. While there is little hope that Ca channel blockers will effectively prevent the initial influx of Ca into neurons after trauma, blockers may be able to reduce secondary entry of Ca into cells through the Ca paradox mechanism.

REFERENCES

1. Alanen KA, Lipasti JA, Tasanne MR, Nevalainen TJ: Effect of verapamil on reperfusion damage and calcium paradox in isolated rat heart. Exp Pathol 25:131–138, 1984
2. Albin MS, White RJ, Acosta-Rua G, Yashon D: Study of functional recovery produced by delayed localized cooling after spinal cord injury in primates. J Neurosurg 29:113–120, 1968
3. Albin MS, White RJ, Yashon D, Harris LS: Effects of localized cooling on spinal cord trauma. J Trauma 9:1000–1008, 1969
4. Allen AR: Remarks on histopathological changes in spinal cord due to impact: An experimental study. J Nerv Ment Dis 41:141–147, 1914
5. Allen AR: Surgery of experimental lesion of spinal cord equivalent to crush injury of fracture dislocation. JAMA 50:941–952, 1911
6. Alto LE, Dhalla NS: Myocardial cation contents during induction of calcium paradox. Am J Physiol 237:713–719, 1979
7. Anderson DK, Means ED, Waters TR: Spinal cord energy metabolism in normal and post laminectomy cats. J Neurosurg 52:387–391, 1980
8. Anderson DK, Means ED, Waters TR, Green BS: Microvascular perfusion and metabolism in injured spinal cord after methylprednisolone treatment. J Neurosurg 56:106–113, 1982
9. Anderson DK, Means ED, Waters TR, Green BS: Spinal cord energy metabolism following compression trauma to the feline spinal cord. J Neurosurg 53:375–80, 1980
10. Anderson DK, Prockop LD, Means ED, Hartley LE: Cerebrospinal fluid lactate and electrolyte levels following experimental spinal cord injury. J Neurosurg 44:715–722, 1976
11. Anderson DK, Saunders RD, Demediuk P et al: Lipid hydrolysis and peroxidation in injured spinal cord: Partial protection with methylprednisolone or vitamin E and selenium. Cent Nerv Syst Trauma 2:257–267, 1985
12. Arias MJ: Treatment of experimental spinal cord injury with TRH, naloxone, and dexamethasone. Surg Neurol 28:335–338, 1987
13. Ashraf M: Oxygen derived radicals related injury in the heart during calcium paradox. Virchows Arch [B] 54:27–37, 1987
14. Ashraf M, Onda M, Hirohata Y, Schwartz A: Therapeutic effect of diltiazem on myocardial cell injury during the calcium paradox. J Mol Cell Cardiol 14:323–327, 1982
15. Baker JE, Bullock GR, Hearse DJ: The temperature dependence of the calcium paradox: Enzymatic, functional, and morphological correlates of cellular injury. J Mol Cell Cardiol 15:393–411, 1983
16. Baker JE, Hearse DJ: Differing potencies and dose-response characteristics in the ability of slow-calcium-channel blockers to reduce enzyme leakage in the calcium paradox. Advances in Myocardiology 6:637–646, 1985
17. Baker JE, Hearse DJ: Slow calcium channel blockers and the calcium paradox: Comparative studies in the rat with seven drugs. J Mol Cell Cardiol 15:475–85, 1983
18. Baker JE, Hearse DJ: The temperature-sensitivity of slow channel calcium blockers in relation to their effect upon the calcium paradox. Eur Heart J 4[Suppl H]:97–103, 1983

19. Baker JE, Kemmenoe BH, Hearse DJ, Bullock GR: Calcium delivery and time: Factors affecting the progression of cellular damage during the calcium paradox in the rat heart. Cardiovasc Res 18:361–370, 1984

20. Balentine JD: Calcium toxicity as a factor in spinal cord injury. Survey and Synthesis of Pathological Research 2:184–193, 1983

21. Balentine JD: Pathology of experimental spinal cord trauma: I. The necrotic lesion as a function of vascular injury. Lab Invest 39:236–253, 1978

22. Balentine JD: Pathology of experimental spinal cord trauma: II. Ultrastructure of axons and myelin. Lab Invest 39:254–255, 1978

23. Balentine JD, Dean D: Calcium-induced spongiform and necrotizing myelopathy. Lab Invest 47:286–295, 1982

24. Balentine JD, Green WB: Ultrastructural pathology of nerve fibers in calcium-induced myelopathy. J Neuropathol Exp Neurol 43:500–510, 1984

25. Balentine JD, Hilton CW: Ultrastructural pathology of axons and myelin in calcium induced myelopathy. J Neuropathol Exp Neurol 39:339–345, 1980

26. Balentine JD, Spector ML: Calcification of axons in experimental spinal cord trauma. Ann Neurol 2:520–523, 1977

27. Borgens RB, Blight AR, McGinnis ME: Behavioral recovery induced by applied electric fields after spinal cord hemisection in guinea pig. Science 238:367–369, 1987

28. Borgens RB, Blight AR, Murphy DJ: Axonal regeneration in spinal cord injury: A perspective and new technique. J Comp Neurol 250:157–167, 1986

29. Borgens RB, Blight AR, Murphy DJ, Stewart LL: Transected dorsal column axons within the guinea pig spinal cord regenerate in the presence of an applied electric field. J Comp Neurol 250:168–180, 1986

30. Bracken MB, Collins WF, Freeman DF et al: Efficacy of methylprednisolone in acute spinal cord injury. JAMA 251:45–52, 1984

31. Bracken MB, Shepard MJ, Hellenbrand KG et al: Methylprednisolone and neurological function 1 year after spinal cord injury. J Neurosurg 63:704–713, 1985

32. Braughler JM, Duncan LA, Chase RL: Interaction of lipid peroxidation and calcium in the pathogenesis of neuronal injury. Cent Nerv Syst Trauma 2:269–283, 1985

33. Braughler JM, Duncan LA, Goodman T: Calcium enhances in vitro free radical-induced damage to brain synaptosomes, mitochondria, and cultured spinal cord neurons. J Neurochem 45:1288–1293, 1985

34. Braughler JM, Hall ED: Acute enhancement of spinal cord synaptosomal (Na+-K+)-ATPase activity in cats following intravenous methylprednisolone. Brain Res 219:464–469, 1981

35. Braughler JM, Hall ED: Correlation of methylprednisolone pharmacokinetics in cat spinal cord with its effect on (Na+-K+)-ATPase, lipid peroxidation and motor neuron function. J Neurosurg 56:838–844, 1981

36. Braughler JM, Hall ED: Current application of "high-dose" steroid therapy for CNS injury: A pharmacological perspective. J Neurosurg 62:806–810, 1985

37. Braughler JM, Hall ED: Effects of multi-dose methylprednisolone sodium succinate administration on injured cat spinal cord neurofilament degradation and energy metabolism. J Neurosurg 61:290–295, 1984

38. Braughler JM, Hall ED: Lactate and pyruvate metabolism in injured cat spinal cord before and after a single large intravenous dose of methylprednisolone. J Neurosurg 59:256–261, 1983

39. Braughler JM, Hall ED: Pharmacokinetics of methylprednisolone in cat plasma and spinal cord following a single intravenous dose of the sodium succinate ester. Drug Metab Dispos 10:551–552, 1982

40. Braughler JM, Hall ED: Uptake and elimination of methylprednisolone from contused cat spinal cord following intravenous injection of the sodium succinate ester. J Neurosurg 58:538–542, 1983

41. Braughler JM, Hall ED, Means ED et al: Evaluation of an intensive methylprednisolone sodium succinate dosing regimen in experimental spinal cord injury. J Neurosurg 67:102–105, 1987

42. Breasted JH: The Edwin Smith Papyrus, Vols I and II. Chicago, University of Chicago Press, 1930

43. Brown WE: Solubilities of phosphates and other sparingly soluble compounds, pp 203–240. In Griffith EJ, Beeton A, Spencer JM, Mitchell DT (eds): Environmental Phosphorus Handbook. New York, John Wiley & Sons, 1971

44. Busselen P: The effect of potassium depolarization on the sodium dependent calcium efflux from goldfish heart ventricles and guinea pig atria. J Physiol 324:309–324, 1982

45. Busselen P: Effects of sodium on the calcium par-

adox in rat hearts. Pflugers Arch 408:458–464, 1987

46. Busselen P: Suppression of cellular injury during the calcium paradox in rat heart by factors which reduce calcium uptake by mitochondria. Pflugers Arch 404:166–171, 1985

47. Campbell JB, DeCrescito V, Tomasula JJ et al: Effect of antifibrinolytic and steroid therapy on contused cords of cats. J Neurosurg 55:726–733, 1974

48. Cawthon DF, Senter HJ, Stewart WB: Comparison of hydrogen clearance and 14C-antipyrine autoradiography in the measurement of spinal cord blood flow after severe impact injury. J Neurosurg 37:591–596, 1980

49. Chan PH, Fishman RA: Brain edema. In Lajtha A (ed): Handbook of Neurochemistry, Vol 10, pp 153–174. New York, Plenum Press, 1985

50. Chan PH, Fishman RA: Brain edema: Induction in cortical slices by polyunsaturated fatty acids. Science 201:358–360, 1980

51. Chan PH, Fishman RA: Transient formation of superoxide radicals in polyunsaturated fatty acids-induced brain swelling. J Neurochem 35:1004–1007, 1980

52. Chan PH, Fishman RA, Caronna J et al: Induction of brain edema following intracerebral injection of arachidonic acid. Ann Neurol 13:625–632, 1983

53. Chan PH, Schmidley JW, Fishman RA, Langar SM: Brain injury edema and vascular permeability changes induced by oxygen-derived free radicals. Neurology 34:315–320, 1984

54. Chance B: The energy-linked reaction of calcium with mitochondria. J Biol Chem 240:2729–2748, 1965

55. Chapman RA, Fozzard HA, Friedlander IR, January CT: Effects of Ca^{2+}/Mg^{2+} removal on aiNa, aiK, and tension in cardiac Purkinje fibers. Am J Physiol 251:C920–C927, 1986

56. Chapman RA, Rodrigo GC, Tunstall J et al: Calcium paradox of the heart: A role for intracellular sodium ions. Am J Physiol 247:H874–H879, 1984

57. Chughtai AR, Marshall R, Nancollas GH: Complexes in calcium phosphate solutions. Journal of Physical Chemistry 72:208–211, 1968

58. Demediuk P, Saunders RD, Anderson DK et al: Membrane lipid changes in laminectomized and traumatized cat spinal cord. Proc Natl Acad Sci USA 82:7071–7075, 1985

59. Demopoulos HB, Flamm ES, Pietronigro DD et al: The free radical pathology and the microcirculation in the major central nervous system disorders. Acta Physiol [Scand] 492:91–119, 1980

60. Demopoulos HB, Flamm ES, Seligman MC et al: Further studies on free radical pathology in the major central nervous system disorders: Effect of very high doses of methylprednisolone on the functional outcome, morphology and chemistry of experimental spinal cord impact injury. Can J Physiol Pharmacol 60:1415–1424, 1981

61. Dohrmann GJ, Wick KM, Bucy PC: Spinal cord blood flow patterns in experimental traumatic paraplegia. J Neurosurg 38:52–58, 1973

62. Dow-Edwards D, DeCrescito V, Tomasula JJ, Flamm ES: Effect of aminophyllin and isoproterenol on spinal cord blood flow after impact injury. J Neurosurg 56:350–358, 1982

63. Ducker TB, Assenmacher DR: Microvascular response to experimental spinal cord trauma. Surgical Forum 20:428–430, 1969

64. Ducker TB, Kindt GW, Kempe LG: Pathological findings in acute spinal cord injury. J Neurosurg 35:700–709, 1971

65. Ducker TB, Perot PL: Spinal cord oxygen and blood flow in trauma. Surgical Forum 22:413–415, 1971

66. Eichelberg D, Peters R, Schmutzler W: Recognition of the "calcium paradox" and the effects of verapamil and gallopamil in human adenoidal mast cells. Agents Actions 14:410–413, 1984

67. Faden AI: Opiate antagonists and thyrotropin-releasing hormone: II. Potential role in the treatment of central nervous system injury. JAMA 252:1452–1454, 1984

68. Faden AI, Hallenbeck JM, Brown CQ: Treatment of experimental stroke: Comparison of naloxone and thyrotropic releasing hormone. Neurology (New York) 32:1083–1087, 1982

69. Faden AI, Holaday JW: Opiate antagonists: A role in treatment of hypovolemic shock. Science 205:317–318, 1979

70. Faden AI, Jacobs TP: Opiate antagonist WIN 44,441–3 stereospecifically improves neurologic recovery after ischemic spinal injury. Neurology 35:1311–1315, 1985

71. Faden AI, Jacobs TP, Holaday JW: Comparison of early and late naloxone treatment in experimental spinal injury. Neurology (NY) 32:677–681, 1982

72. Faden AI, Jacobs TP, Holaday JW: Opiate antagonist improves neurologic recovery after spinal injury. Science 211:493–494, 1980

73. Faden AI, Jacobs TP, Holaday JW: Thyrotropin

releasing hormone improves neurologic recovery after spinal trauma in cats. N Engl J Med 305:1063–1067, 1981

74. Faden AI, Jacobs TP, Mougey E, Holaday JW: Endorphins in experimental spinal injury: Therapeutic effect of naloxone. Ann Neurol 10:326–332, 1981

75. Faden AI, Jacobs TP, Patrick DH, Smith MT: Megadose corticosteroid therapy following experimental traumatic spinal injury. J Neurosurg 60:712–717, 1984

76. Faden AI, Jacobs TP, Smith GP et al: Neuropeptides in spinal cord injury: Comparative experimental models. Peptides 4:631–634, 1983

77. Faden AI, Jacobs TP, Smith MT: Comparison of thyrotropin-releasing hormone (TRH), naloxone, and dexamethasone treatments in experimental spinal injury. Neurology 33:673–678, 1983

78. Faden AI, Jacobs TP, Smith MT: Thyrotropin-releasing hormone in experimental spinal injury: Dose response and late treatment. Neurology 34:1280–1284, 1984

79. Faden AI, Jacobs TP, Zivin JA: Naloxone but not a delta antagonist improves neurological recovery after spinal stroke in the rabbit. Life Sci 33[Suppl 1]:707–710, 1983

80. Feuerstein G, Feuerstein N, Hallenbeck J: Cellular and humoral interactions in acute microvascular injury: A pivotal role for the endothelial cell. Crit Care Med 8:99–118, 1987

81. Flamm ES, Young W, Collins WF et al: A phase I trial of naloxone treatment in acute spinal cord injury. J Neurosurg 63:390–397, 1985

82. Flamm ES, Young W, Demopoulos HB et al: Experimental spinal cord injury: Treatment with naloxone. Neurosurgery 10:227–231, 1982

83. Ganote CE, Sims MA: Parallel temperature dependence of contracture-associated enzyme release due to anoxia, 2,4-dinitrophenol (DNP), or caffeine and the calcium paradox. Am J Physiol 116:94–106, 1984

84. Goodkin R, Campbell JB: Sequential pathological changes in spinal cord injury. Surgical Forum 20:430–432, 1969

85. Greisman SE: Experimental gram-negative bacterial sepsis: Optimal methylprednisolone requirements for prevention of mortality not preventable by antibiotics alone (41455). Proc Soc Exp Biol Med 170:436–442, 1982

86. Grinwald PM: Calcium uptake during post-ischemic perfusion in the isolated rat heart: Influence of extracellular sodium. J Mol Cell Cardiol 14:359–365, 1982

87. Gruner JA, Young W, DeCrescito V: The vestibulospinal free fall response: A test of descending function in spinal injured cats. Cent Nerv Syst Trauma 1:139–160, 1984

88. Guha A, Tator CH, Endrenyi L, Piper I: Decompression of the spinal cord improves recovery after acute experimental spinal cord compression injury. Paraplegia 25:324–339, 1987

89. Guha A, Tator CH, Piper I: Effect of a calcium channel blocker on posttraumatic spinal cord blood flow. J Neurosurg 66:423–430, 1987

90. Guha A, Tator CH, Piper I: Increase in rat spinal cord blood flow with the calcium channel blocker, nimodipine. J Neurosurg 63:250–259, 1985

91. Haghighi SS, Chehrazi B: Effect of naloxone in experimental acute spinal cord injury. Neurosurgery 20:385–388, 1987

92. Hall ED: Glucocorticoid effects on central nervous excitability and synaptic transmission. Int Rev Neurobiol 23:165–195, 1982

93. Hall ED, Braughler JM: Acute effects of intravenous glucocorticoid pretreatment on the in vitro peroxidation of cat spinal cord tissue. Exp Neurol 72:321–324, 1981

94. Hall ED, Braughler JM: Effects of methylprednisolone on spinal cord lipid peroxidation and (Na+-K+)-ATPase activity: dose response analysis during the first hour after contusion injury in the cat. J Neurosurg 57:247–253, 1982

95. Hall ED, McCall JM, Chase RL et al: A nonglucocorticoid steroid analog of methylprednisolone duplicates its high-dose pharmacology in models of central nervous system trauma and neuronal membrane damage. J Pharmacol Exp Ther 242:137–142, 1987

96. Hall ED, Wolf DL: A pharmacological analysis of the pathophysiological mechanisms of posttraumatic spinal cord ischemia. J Neurosurg 64:951–961, 1986

97. Hall ED, Wolf DL, Braughler JM: Effects of a single large dose of methylprednisolone sodium succinate on experimental posttraumatic spinal cord ischemia: Dose-response and time-action analysis. J Neurosurg 61:124–130, 1984

98. Happel RD, Smith KP, Banik ML et al: Ca²⁺ accumulation in experimental spinal cord trauma. Brain Res 211:476–479, 1981

99. Hearse DJ, Baker JE: Verapamil and the calcium paradox: A reaffirmation. J Mol Cell Cardiol 13:1087–1090, 1981

100. Hearse DJ, Humphrey SM, Bullock GR: The oxygen paradox and the calcium paradox. J Mol Cell Cardiol 10:641–668, 1978

101. Hess ML, Manson NH: Molecular oxygen: Friend and foe. The role of the oxygen free radical system in the calcium paradox, the oxygen paradox and ischemia/reperfusion injury. J Mol Cell Cardiol 16:969–985, 1984

102. Hirata F, Schiffman E, Venkatasubramanian K et al: A phospholipase A_2 inhibitory protein in rabbit neutrophils induced by glucocorticoids. Proc Natl Acad Sci USA 77:2533–2536, 1980

103. Hirata M, Fukui H, Shimamoto N: Inhibition by reserpine of myocardial damage due to calcium paradox in isolated guinea pig hearts. Jpn J Pharmacol 36:114–117, 1984

104. Hoka S, Bosnjak ZJ, Kampine JP: Halothane inhibits calcium accumulation following myocardial ischemia and calcium paradox in guinea pig hearts. Anesthesiology 67:197–202, 1987

105. Holaday JW, D'Amato RJ: Naloxone or TRH fails to improve neurological deficits in gerbil models of "stroke." Life Sci 31:385–392, 1982

106. Holaday JW, Faden AI: Naloxone acts at central opiate receptors to reverse hypotension, hypothermia and hypoventilation in spinal shock. Brain Res 189:295–299, 1980

107. Holaday JW, Faden AI: Naloxone reversal of endotoxin hypotension suggests role of endorphins in shock. Nature 275:450–451, 1978

108. Horrocks LA, Demediuk P, Saunders RD et al: The degradation of phospholipids, formation of metabolites of arachidonic acid, and demyelination following experimental spinal cord injury. Cent Nerv Syst Trauma 2:115–120, 1985

109. Hosobuchi Y, Baskin OS, Woo SK: Reversal of induced ischemic neurologic deficit in gerbils by the opiate antagonist naloxone. Science 215:69–71, 1982

110. Hsu CY, Halushka PV, Hogan EL et al: Alterations of thromboxane and prostacyclin levels in experimental spinal cord injury. Neurology 35:1003–1009, 1985

111. Hunt WG, Willis RJ: Calcium exposure required for full expression of injury in the calcium paradox. Biochem Biophys Res Commun 126:901–904, 1985

112. Julicher RH, Sterrenberg L, Koomen JM et al: Evidence for lipid peroxidation during the calcium paradox in vitamin E-deficient rat heart. Naunyn-Schmiedebergs Archiv Pharmacol 326:87–89, 1984

113. Kakulas BA, Bedbrook GM: A correlative clinicopathological study of spinal cord injury. Proceedings of the Australian Association of Neurology 6:123–132, 1969

114. Kakulas BA, Bedbrook GM: Pathology of injuries of the vertebral spinal cord—with emphasis on the microscopic aspects. In Vinken PJ, Bruyn GW: Handbook of Clinical Neurology, Vol 25: Injuries of the Spine and Spinal Cord, Part I, pp 27–42. Amsterdam, North-Holland, 1976

115. Kanaide H, Meno H, Nakamura M: Metabolic and physical changes during calcium paradox induced in the rat heart. Br J Exp Pathol 68:319–330, 1987

116. Karmazyn M: Calcium paradox-evoked release of prostacyclin and immunoreactive leukotriene C4 from rat and guinea-pig hearts: Evidence that endogenous prostaglandins inhibit leukotriene biosynthesis. J Mol Cell Cardiol 19:221–230, 1987

117. Kastin AJ, Nissen C, Olson RD: Failure of MIF-1 or naloxone to reverse ischemia-induced neurological deficits in gerbils. Pharmacol Biochem Behav 17:1083–1085, 1982

118. Kontos HA, Wei EP, Ellis EF et al: Prostaglandins in physiological and in certain pathological responses of the cerebral circulation. Fed Proc 40:2326–2330, 1981

119. Koomen JM, Schevers JA, Noordhoek J, Zimmerman AN: Magnesium and the calcium paradox: The occurrence of "spasmodic contractions" during Ca^{2+}-Mg^{2+}-free perfusion of isolated rat heart. Basic Res Cardiol 78:227–238, 1983

120. Lohse DC, Senter HJ, Kauer JS: Spinal cord blood flow in experimental transient paraplegia. J Neurosurg 52:335–345, 1980

121. Long JB, Martinez Arizala A, Petras JM, Holaday JW: Endogenous opioids in spinal cord injury: A critical evaluation. Cent Nerv Syst Trauma 3:295–316, 1986

122. McIntire TM, Zimmerman GA, Satoh K et al: Cultured endothelial cells synthesize both platelet activating factor and prostacyclin in response to histamine, bradykinin and adenosine triphosphate. J Clin Invest 76:271, 1985

123. Metz R, Giebler C, Forster W: Evidence for a direct inhibitory effect of glucocorticoids on the activity of phospholipase A_2 as a further possible mechanism of some actions of steroid anti-inflammatory drugs. Pharmacol Res Commun 12:817–827, 1980

124. Nayler WG, Perry SE, Elz JS, Daly MJ: Calcium, sodium, and the calcium paradox. Circ Res 55:227–237, 1984

125. Oksendal AN, Jynge P: Myocardial protection by micromolar manganese in the calcium paradox and additive effects of verapamil. Basic Res Cardiol 81:581–593, 1986

126. Oksendal AN, Jynge P: Tissue protection by adrenergic blockade in the calcium paradox? Basic Res Cardiol 82:138–145, 1987

127. Oksendal AN, Jynge P, Sellevold OF et al: The calcium paradox phenomenon: A flow rate and volume response study of calcium-free perfusion. J Mol Cell Cardiol 17:959–972, 1985

128. Osterholm JL: The pathophysiological response in spinal cord injury. J Neurosurg 40:5–33, 1974

129. Pickard JD: Role of prostaglandins and arachidonic acid derivatives in the coupling of cerebral blood flow to cerebral metabolism. J Cereb Blood Flow Metab. 1:361–384, 1981

130. Rabkin SW: Effect of chlorpromazine on myocardial damage in the calcium paradox. J Cardiovasc Pharmacol 9:486–492, 1987

131. Rossi V, Brevario F, Ghezzi P et al: Prostacyclin synthesis induced in vascular cells by interleukin 1. Science 229:174–176, 1985

132. Ruano-Arroyo G, Gerstenbluth G, Lakatta EG: "Calcium paradox" in heart is modulated by cell sodium during the calcium-free period. J Mol Cell Cardiol 16:783–793, 1984

133. Rudge MF, Duncan CJ: Comparative studies on the calcium paradox in cardiac muscle: The effect of temperature on the different phases. Comp Biochem Physiol [A] 79:393–398, 1984

134. Ruigrok TJ: Possible mechanisms involved in the development of the calcium paradox. Gen Physiol Biophys 4:155–165, 1985

135. Ruigrok TJC, Burgerdijk FJA, Zimmerman ANE: The calcium paradox: A reaffirmation. European Journal of Cardiology 3:59–63, 1975

136. Sandler AN, Tator CH: Review of the effects of spinal cord trauma on vessels and blood flow in the spinal cord. J Neurosurg 45:638–646, 1976

137. Saunders RD, Dugan LL, Demediuk P et al: Effects of methylprednisolone and the combination of alpha-tocopherol and selenium on arachidonic acid metabolism and lipid peroxidation in traumatized spinal cord tissue. J Neurochem 49:24–31, 1987

138. Schanne, FA, Kane AB, Young EE, Farber JL: Calcium dependence of toxic cell death: A common pathway. Science 206:700–702, 1979

139. Senter HJ, Venes JL: Altered blood flow and secondary injury in experimental spinal cord trauma. J Neurosurg 49:569–578, 1978

140. Senter HJ, Venes JL: Loss of autoregulation and posttraumatic ischemia following experimental spinal cord trauma. J Neurosurg 50:198–206, 1979

141. Spiller WG: A microscopic study of the spinal cord in two cases of Pott's disease. Bulletin of the Johns Hopkins Hospital 9:125–133, 1898

142. Tator CH, Rivlin AS, Lewis AJ, Schmoll B: Effect of acute spinal cord injury on axonal counts in the pyramidal tract of rats. J Neurosurg 61:118–123, 1984

143. Tunstall J, Busselen P, Rodrigo GC, Chapman RA: Pathways for the movements of ions during calcium-free perfusion and the induction of the "calcium paradox." J Mol Cell Cardiol 18:241–254, 1986

144. Turner DM, Kassell NF, Sasaki T et al: High dose naloxone produces cerebral vasodilation. Neurosurgery 15:192–197, 1984

145. Wagner F, Taslitz N, White RJ, Yashon D: Vascular phenomenon in the normal and traumatized spinal cord. Anat Rec 163:281, 1969

146. Walker JG, Yates RR, O'Neill JJ, Yashon D: Canine spinal cord energy state after experimental trauma. J Neurochem 29:929–932, 1977

147. Walker JG, Yates RR, Yashon D: Regional canine spinal cord energy state after experimental trauma. J Neurochem 33:397–401, 1979

148. Wallace CM, Tator CH: Failure of naloxone to improve spinal cord blood flow and cardiac output after spinal cord injury. Neurosurgery 18:428–432, 1986

149. Wallace CM, Tator CH: Spinal cord blood flow measured with microspheres following spinal cord injury in the rat. Can J Neurol Sci 13:91–96, 1986

150. Wallace CM, Tator CH: Successful improvement of blood pressure, cardiac output, and spinal cord blood flow after experimental spinal cord injury. Neurosurgery 20:710–715, 1987

151. Wallace CM, Tator CH, Frazee P: Relationship between posttraumatic ischemia and hemorrhage in the injured rat spinal cord as shown by collodial carbon angiography. Neurosurgery 18:433–439, 1986

152. Wallace MC, Tator CH, Gentles WM: Failure of blood transfusion or naloxone to improve clinical recovery after experimental spinal cord injury. Surg Neurol 28:269–276, 1987

153. Wallace MC, Tator CH, Lewis AJ: Chronic regenerative changes in the spinal cord after cord compression injury in rats. Surg Neurol 27:209–219, 1987

154. Wallace MC, Tator CH, Lewis AJ: Failure of blood transfusion or naloxone to improve clinical recovery after experimental spinal cord injury. Neurosurgery 19:489–494, 1986

155. Wallace MC, Tator CH, Piper I: Recovery of spi-

nal cord function induced by direct current stimulation of the injured rat spinal cord. Neurosurgery 20:787–884, 1987

156. Wolfe LS: Eicosanoids: Prostaglandins, thromboxanes, leukotrienes, and other derivatives of carbon-20 unsaturated fatty acids. J Neurochem 38:1–14, 1982

157. Young W: Blood flow, metabolic and neurophysiological mechanisms in spinal cord injury, pp 463–473. In Becker D, Povlishock JT (eds): Central Nervous System Trauma Status Report 1985. Bethesda, Maryland, National Institutes of Health, NINCDS, 1985

158. Young W: Calcium paradox in neural injury: A hypothesis. Cent Nerv Syst Trauma 3:235–251, 1986

159. Young W: Cellular defenses against excessive Ca entry in brain and spinal cord injury, pp 71–98. In Cerra FB, Shoemaker WC (eds): Critical Care: State of the Art, Vol 8. Fullerton, CA, Society of Critical Care Medicine, 1987

160. Young W: Correlation of somatosensory evoked potentials and neurological findings in clinical spinal cord injury, pp 153–166. In Tator CH (ed): Early Management of Cervical Spinal Injury. New York, Raven Press, 1981

161. Young W: Goals of regeneration in the spinal cord. In Seil FJ (ed): Neural Regeneration Research for the Clinician. New York, Alan R Liss, 1988

162. Young W: Hydrogen clearance measurement of blood flow: A review of technique and polarographic principles. Stroke 11:552–564, 1980

163. Young W: The post-injury responses in trauma and ischemia: Secondary injury or protective mechanisms. Cent Nerv Syst Trauma 4:27–52, 1987

164. Young W: Role of calcium in spinal cord injury. Cent Nerv Syst Trauma 2:109–114, 1985

165. Young W, DeCrescito V: Sodium ionic changes in injured spinal cords: Mechanisms of edema (abstract). Proceedings of the Society of Neuroscience 16:267, 1986

166. Young W, DeCrescito V, Flamm ES et al: Pharmacological treatments of acute spinal cord injury: A review of naloxone and methylprednisolone. Clin Neurosurg 34:675–697, 1988

167. Young W, DeCrescito V, Tomasula J, Ho V: The role of the sympathetic nervous system in pressor responses induced by spinal injury. J Neurosurg 52:473–481, 1980

168. Young W, DeCrescito V, Tomasula JJ: Effect of sympathectomy on spinal cord blood flow autoregulation and posttraumatic ischemia. J Neurosurg 56:706–710, 1982

169. Young W, Flamm ES: Effect of high dose corticosteroid therapy on blood flow, evoked potentials, and extracellular calcium in experimental spinal injury. J Neurosurg 57:667–673, 1982

170. Young W, Flamm ES, Demopoulos HB et al: Effect of naloxone on posttraumatic ischemia in experimental spinal contusion. J Neurosurg 55:209–219, 1981

171. Young W, Koreh I: Potassium and calcium changes in injured spinal cords. Brain Res 365:42–53, 1986

172. Young W, Koreh I, Yen V, Lindsay A: Effects of sympathectomy on extracellular potassium activity and blood flow in experimental spinal cord contusion. Brain Res 253:105–113, 1982

173. Young W, Ransohoff J: Acute spinal cord injury: Experimental therapy, pathophysiology mechanisms, and recovery of function. In Sherk H (ed): The Cervical Spine, 2nd ed, pp 464–495. Philadelphia, J.B. Lippincott, 1989

174. Young W, Tomasula JJ, DeCrescito V et al: Vestibulospinal monitoring in experimental spinal trauma. J Neurosurg 52:64–72, 1980

175. Young W, Yen V, Blight A: Extracellular calcium activity in experimental spinal cord contusion. Brain Res 253:115–123, 1982

176. Zimmerman ANE, Hulsmann WC: Paradoxical influence of calcium ions on the permeability of the cell membranes in the isolated rat heart. Nature 211:646–647, 1966

17

CLINICAL PHYSIOLOGIC CONSIDERATIONS AND ANESTHETIC MANAGEMENT OF PATIENTS WITH SPINAL CORD INJURY

Richard M. Sommer

Sanford M. Miller

Levon M. Capan

The potentially devastating effect of spinal cord injury on the victim's quality of life makes this type of trauma a special concern for physicians who care for injured patients. Integrated neural activity is carried from the brain to the rest of the body via the spinal cord. Interruption of this flow of information causes paralysis, sensory deficits, and, ultimately, reduced ability to maintain an independent existence.

The pathophysiologic impairments caused by spinal cord injury affect the cardiovascular, respiratory, gastrointestinal, genitourinary, neurologic, and musculoskeletal systems. The extent of these changes is related to the severity of the neurologic injury.

This chapter will elucidate the physiologic effects of acute and chronic spine and spinal cord injury. The anesthetic management of patients with these injuries will also be discussed.

NEUROLOGIC INJURY

Although penetrating injuries occur, most spinal cord damage is the result of blunt trauma. Neurologic deficits usually result from vascular insufficiency produced by pressure on the spinal cord. Experimental work has demonstrated that impact trauma results in mechanical destruction and hemorrhage, decreased perfusion, tissue hypoxia, edema, and, ultimately, necrosis of neural elements. It has been observed that inhibition of axoplasmic transport begins within 2 hours of injury and marked blockade is present at 4 hours. Axoplasmic function is completely inhibited within 6 hours following severe trauma.[2]

Animal studies have revealed the following histologic changes. Seconds after cord trauma, flame-shaped hemorrhages appear in the gray matter and pia arachnoid. White matter hemorrhage develops from 10 minutes to 4 hours after injury. These effects result from microcirculatory disturbance and lead to irreversible cystic degeneration and neurolysis.[27] Necrosis begins within 24 hours, and after this time recovery cannot occur.[61,88]

Since neurons within the central nervous system do not regenerate, the neurologic outcome depends on the magnitude of the initial insult and the success of early resuscitation. Animal experiments in which spinal cord hypothermia, hypertonic agents such as mannitol, glucocorticoids, hyperbaric oxygen, perfusion-maintaining vasopressors, ε-aminocaproic acid, dimethyl sulfoxide, and naloxone have been employed have demonstrated some favorable results. However, none of these has proven to have beneficial effects in humans.[2,12,15,39,40]

Neurologic injury after trauma may be complete or incomplete. Incomplete lesions are those in which function is preserved more than one level below the injury. The presence of sacral sparing, distal motor or sensory function, and somatosensory evoked potentials indicate incomplete injuries. Complete injuries are those in which no sign of distal neurologic function exists. Complete lesions may be reversible or irreversible. No neurologic recovery will occur if complete neurologic injury persists after the period of spinal shock.[60,115] A complete lesion implies a total interruption of communication across the injury even though the cord has not been physically transected.

The pharmacologic approach to neural preservation after injury has no proven benefit in humans. One treatment modality that may have value in cases of impingement on the spinal cord by vertebral displacement is early realignment and decompression of the cord. In some cases this has resulted in complete neurologic recovery even from complete quadriplegia.[18] Nevertheless, the best predictor of ultimate neurologic outcome is the severity of the initial insult to the spinal cord.[121]

Neurologic function has been shown to deteriorate in 4.9% of patients with spinal cord injury during hospital care as a complication of operative intervention, skeletal traction, halo application, or Stryker frame rotation.[82] Airway management must be added to the list of potential hazards. Physicians caring for these patients must always bear in mind the possibility of extending neuro-logic injury when any manipulation is performed, especially when managing the airway.

PULMONARY COMPLICATIONS

VENTILATORY INSUFFICIENCY

The reported mortality from respiratory complications in cervical spine injured patients ranges from 7% to 78%.[20,41] The most common pulmonary pathology is atelectasis and pneumonia. Risk factors include increased age and reduced vital capacity.[100] A variety of mechanisms may predispose the patient to these complications. Brain injury, shock, alcohol intoxication, and recent intake of licit or illicit drugs can cause central respiratory depression either directly or indirectly, by interfering with brainstem perfusion. Hypoventilation and accumulation of tracheobronchial secretions may then set the stage for atelectasis and pneumonia. Airway obstruction may be caused by a foreign body, soft-tissue trauma, hematoma, hemorrhage, laryngotracheal injury, or facial trauma. Chest injuries such as rib fractures, hemothorax, and pneumothorax may cause ventilatory failure.[112]

The ventilatory embarrassment caused specifically by spinal injury results from paralysis of the abdominal and intercostal muscles and the diaphragm, which is innervated from C-3 to C-5. Thus, complete injuries above C-3 denervate the diaphragm and all of the other major respiratory muscles. Cervical cord lesions at or below C-5 permit at least some degree of voluntary diaphragmatic control. Spinal cord injuries below T-12 cause little or no respiratory embarrassment. However, as the level of injury ascends, the abdominal and intercostal muscles' contribution to breathing is reduced and eventually lost. These muscles stabilize the rib cage and abdominal wall during inspiration, thus increasing the efficiency of diaphragmatic contraction. In addition, the abdominal and intercostal muscles are critical for forced expiration and coughing.[125] Patients with high thoracic and low cervical cord injuries are therefore at risk for pneumonia due to reduced ability to forcefully exhale, cough, and remove secretions. Quadriplegic patients without diaphragmatic paralysis or injury have a decrease in total lung capacity, vital capacity, expiratory reserve volume, and functional residual capacity. The FEV_1/FVC ratio is normal, but the maximum midexpiratory flow rate is reduced 40% and the peak expiratory flow rate is reduced 53% (Table 17-1).[41,56,84]

Diaphragmatic paralysis is usually bilateral in spinal cord injury. However, unilateral paralysis may result from ascending cord edema, nerve root injury, or unilateral intramedullary injury. If the neural elements are not destroyed the opportunity for recovery exists.[21] Low hemicervical injury at C-7 causes paradoxical movement of the hemithorax and has been mistaken for flail chest because of loss of the stabilizing effect of the rib cage on the affected side.[64]

Pulmonary function in patients with complete cervical cord injury improves during the first 5 months following injury. Vital capacity doubles by 3 months and expiratory flow rate increases with it. This increase is thought to be caused by the return of abdominal and intercostal muscle tension, which improves the effectiveness of diaphragmatic contraction.[74] Pulmonary perfusion and ventilation studies demonstrate normal pulmonary perfusion, although areas of ventilation/perfusion abnormality are present. Ventilatory exchange of administered radioisotopes is prolonged; this is thought to be due to loss of the coordinated intercostal and abdominal muscle contribution to normal tidal breathing.[59]

Ventilatory deterioration may occur in quadriplegics during the early postinjury period because

of extension of spinal cord edema to higher cervical spinal segments and the resultant impairment of diaphragmatic movement. Should this process extend to the anterolateral portion of the spinal cord at levels between C-2 and C-4, sleep apnea may occur. Unless the patient breathes voluntarily or ventilatory support is provided, he will die. The risk of this catastrophic event is greatest in the first 5 days following injury.[44,97]

The best way to monitor ventilatory function is with arterial oxygen and carbon dioxide analysis. Airway control with an endotracheal tube and ventilatory management with positive pressure ventilation should be considered when mild hypoxemia and hypercarbia develop, since compensatory mechanisms are impaired, especially in patients with cervical cord injuries.

The optimal position for spontaneous respiration in the quadriplegic patient is supine. In the supine position the diaphragm moves cephalad during exhalation because of the pressure of the abdominal contents, allowing for adequate diaphragmatic excursion during inhalation. In the upright position, the diaphragmatic contraction is less efficient because of its flatter shape.[7]

DEEP VENOUS THROMBOSIS AND PULMONARY EMBOLISM

The development of deep venous thrombosis is associated with Virchow's triad of decreased blood flow, a hypercoagulable state, and vessel wall lesions. Deep venous thrombosis develops in 14% to 100% of spinal cord injured patients who do not receive prophylaxis.[91] A study of 500 spinal cord injured patients reported 66 cases of thromboembolism, 15 of which were fatal, within the first 2 weeks after injury. Indeed, pulmonary embolism may occur within 24 hours of development of deep venous thrombosis, and pulmonary emboli have been reported from 4 to 85 days after trauma.[35,45,46]

Therefore, it is critical that spinal cord injured patients receive preventive treatment during the first 90 days after injury. Low dose heparin, external pneumatic calf compression, dextran, and graduated compression with elastic stockings are all effective for deep venous thrombosis prophylaxis.[23,108] External calf compression alone, and

Table 17-1. Effect of Low Cervical Spinal Cord Injury on Lung Mechanics

PULMONARY PARAMETER	PARAMETER REDUCTION
Total lung capacity	26%
Vital capacity	49%
Expiratory reserve volume	64%
Functional residual capacity	21%
FEV_1/FVC	No change
Maximum midexpiratory flow	40%
Peak expiratory flow	53%

FEV_1/FVC = Forced expiratory volume in one second/forced vital capacity.
(From Forner JV: Lung volumes and mechanics of breathing in tetraplegics. Paraplegia 18:258, 1980)

external calf compression in combination with aspirin and dipyridamole are valuable techniques for reducing deep venous thrombosis.[50]

Heparin is usually administered in doses of 5000 units, subcutaneously, twice daily. This schedule results in a significant reduction in pulmonary embolism. Even greater protection may be afforded by use of an adjusted-dose schedule, maintaining the activated partial thromboplastin time at 1.5 times control. However, this technique not only requires much higher quantities of heparin, a mean of 13,200 units per dose, but is also associated with bleeding in 24% of patients.[49]

Placement of a Kim-ray–Greenfield filter in the inferior vena cava is indicated in patients with deep venous thrombosis and pulmonary embolism in the following circumstances:[63]

1. Hemorrhage or pulmonary embolism while receiving heparin
2. Contraindication to heparin, recent major trauma, or recent neurologic surgery
3. Extensive deep venous thrombosis with loosely attached thrombi in the inferior vena cava or iliac veins

CARDIOVASCULAR EFFECTS OF SPINAL CORD TRAUMA

Spinal shock, usually manifested by hypotension and bradycardia, and pulmonary edema are the major early cardiovascular complications in patients who suffer high spinal cord injury.[87] However, the immediate reaction to direct compression of the spinal cord in animals is sympathetic activation, hypertension, and bradycardia.[44,55] This response is not seen in the clinical setting, probably because it is short-lived and vital signs are usually not taken until long after the sympathetic response ends.

IMMEDIATE HEMODYNAMIC REACTION TO TRAUMA

Thoracic spinal cord compression causes a pressor response lasting 3 to 4 minutes, which is mediated by α-adrenergic receptors. The subsequent hypotension is due to reduced α-adrenergic output and

responds to sympathomimetic agents.[4,99] Continuity of the spinal cord from the area of trauma to the thoracic level must exist prior to the injury, otherwise no pressor response occurs. Cats that had spinal cord transection at T-1 and subsequently underwent cervical cord compression demonstrated no pressor response.[34]

Greenhoot and Mauck demonstrated that the initial response to cervical cord compression in dogs was tachycardia and hypertension. Subsequently, a variety of abnormal cardiac rhythms, including sinus pauses, multifocal atrial beats, nodal escape beats, ventricular premature contractions, and ventricular tachycardia, were noted.[51] Atropine and vagal section prevented the bradycardic response, and propranolol abolished tachycardic activity. The authors concluded that the initial response to cord compression in dogs was sympathetic activation and subsequent reflex parasympathetic activity.

Evans and associates found that thoracic spinal cord compression in monkeys resulted in immediate pressor and bradycardic responses and that bradycardia preceded the hypertension. The bradycardia could be prevented with atropine; arrhythmias that developed 90 seconds after injury could be prevented by propranolol. They concluded that the arrhythmias were mediated by both vagal and sympathetic mechanisms. Spinal afferents to the medulla caused the initial bradycardia. Efferent sympathetic activity from the spinal cord caused vasoconstriction, tachycardia, arrhythmias, hypertension, and increased myocardial contractility.[38] The effects of sympathetic stimulation, increased myocardial work, and life-threatening malignant arrhythmias may lead to sudden death or myocardial ischemia and infarction.[51]

SPINAL SHOCK

The signs of spinal shock, hypotension, bradycardia, increased vascular capacitance, flaccid paralysis, areflexia, poikilothermy, and fecal and urinary retention persist up to 8 weeks after injury.[1] Severe bradycardia is a potentially major complication of high spinal cord injury. Thoracic and lumbar spinal cord injury rarely cause bradycardia. Lehmann and associates found that all patients with severe cervical cord injury had persistent bradycardia, while 6 of 17 with mild cervical injury and only 3 of 23 patients with thoracolumbar injury had bradycardia. In addition, hypotension, supraventricular arrhythmia, and cardiac arrest were more common in patients with cervical injury. The frequency of bradyarrhythmias peaked on day 4; arrhythmias in all patients resolved spontaneously by 2 to 6 weeks after injury. The mechanism of bradycardia is thought to be vagal activity in the absence of compensatory high thoracic sympathetic tone.[76]

Winslow and associates found that 22 of 83 patients with traumatic quadriplegia had significant bradycardia and that patients with bradycardia accounted for 66% of those who died in their study. Other factors, such as an older population, coexistent disease, and more complicated injuries, probably were contributory factors in the increased mortality.[127] Prophylaxis with atropine 0.4 to 0.6 mg intravenously is beneficial in reducing the risk of this complication. Long-term vagolytic therapy with propanthaline bromide 7.5 to 30 mg orally four times a day and pacemaker placement were also beneficial in reducing episodes of bradycardia.[127]

Tibbs and associates studied myocardial blood flow in dogs and demonstrated that cervical spinal cord transection causes decreased myocardial blood flow due to hypotension. Although myocardial ischemia was not demonstrated in the dog study, the implication for humans is that spinal shock in patients with pre-existing coronary artery disease may increase the risk of myocardial ischemia.[118]

Patients with spinal cord injury are sensitive to intravenous volume loading, drugs, and anesthetics. In a study of 22 acutely quadriplegic patients undergoing surgery, dehydration was present in many and six had left ventricular dysfunction, which was thought to be caused by the early pressor response and not by pre-existing ischemic cardiomyopathy. Hemodynamic management consisted of pulmonary artery catheterization, volume loading to a pulmonary capillary wedge pressure of 18 mm Hg, and inotropic support for the treatment of cardiogenic shock.[80]

Effective and accurate hemodynamic management requires complete knowledge of the cardio-vascular status: preload, afterload, heart rate and rhythm, and cardiac output. Therefore, during the period of shock, pulmonary artery catheterization is desirable in order to define the hemodynamic status and direct therapy.[1,120] Severe bradycardia caused by vagal dominance is treated with vagolytic drugs (atropine), β-adrenergic agonists (isoproterenol, epinephrine), or cardiac pacing. Reduced preload is treated with fluid infusion, reduced afterload is managed with vasoconstrictors, and depressed myocardial contractility is managed with inotropic agents. It is important to recognize that the etiology of shock in spinal cord injured patients is not necessarily reduced vascular resistance; hypovolemia, bradycardia, sepsis, and poor ventricular function may be causative or contributory.[80] Measurement of urine output and colloid oncotic pressure is useful for monitoring renal perfusion and preventing pulmonary edema.[1]

PULMONARY EDEMA

Pulmonary edema has been demonstrated at central venous pressures that are lower than control values in spinal cord injured dogs.[16] Pulmonary edema may develop in cervical cord injured patients with normal pulmonary artery and pulmonary capillary wedge pressures.[95,117,129] The term "neurogenic pulmonary edema" is used to describe the protein-rich edema fluid found in some patients with brain or spinal cord injury. The mechanism that has been proposed to explain the development of this type of edema is as follows: At the time of injury the initial pressor response causes a severe elevation of pulmonary vascular pressures, which in turn produces hydrostatic pulmonary edema, loss of capillary integrity, and, ultimately, exudation of protein-rich fluid.[75,117,129] In addition, since these patients are frequently hypotensive they may receive a large fluid challenge in order to maintain systemic blood pressure. When spinal shock resolves, the fluid volume returned to the heart and lungs increases. The heart may fail; when this is combined with reduced capillary integrity, pulmonary edema develops.[87] The left ventricle may be especially prone to failure because of the stress it undergoes in the immediate postinjury period.[55,80]

AUTONOMIC HYPERREFLEXIA

When the period of spinal shock ends, 2 to 6 weeks after the injury, reflexes reappear. Violent muscle spasms and autonomic hyperreflexia may be precipitated by cutaneous, visceral, and proprioceptive stimuli.[8] The symptoms associated with hyperreflexia—nasal obstruction, facial tingling, headache, shortness of breath, nausea, and blurred vision—are caused by acute, severe hypertension. Bradycardia, arrhythmias, sweating, cutis anserina (goose flesh), cutaneous vasodilation above and pallor below the injury level, and occasionally loss of consciousness and seizures may also result from autonomic hyperreflexia. Retinal, cerebral, and subarachnoid hemorrhage, myocardial strain, and pulmonary edema may follow the most severe reactions.[62,66,83,104,130] Patients with spinal cord injury above T-6 have a 48% to 85% chance of developing autonomic hyperreflexia, while those with lower lesions are able to compensate for vasoconstriction below the injury with vasodilation at higher levels.[77,104]

The pathophysiologic mechanism of autonomic hyperreflexia is as follows: Afferent impulses enter the spinal cord and cause uninhibited reflex outflow over the entire sympathetic chain below the injury level (Fig. 17-1). Vasoconstriction and hypertension induce reflex bradycardia via baroreceptor and vagal pathways.[43,66,104] Prevention and treatment is accomplished with ganglionic blockers, α-adrenergic blockers, catecholamine depleters, vasodilators, or general and regional anesthetics.[33,57,70,98]

Surgery, especially within the pelvis and lower abdomen, performed without anesthesia is asso-

MECHANISM OF AUTONOMIC HYPERREFLEXIA

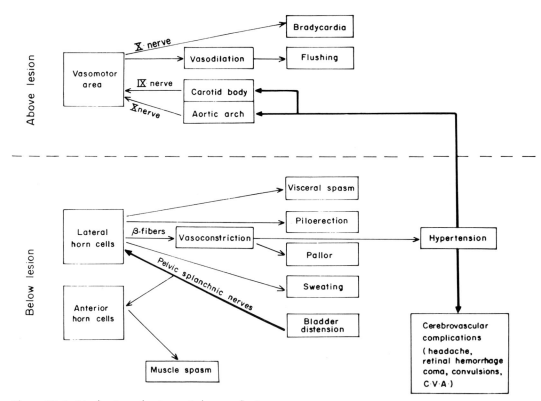

Figure 17-1. Mechanism of autonomic hyperreflexia.

ciated with a high incidence of autonomic hyperreflexia. Both general and regional anesthetics are valuable in preventing this response.[3,8,71,104] Topical anesthesia for procedures such as cystoscopy is not sufficient to prevent the response to bladder distension.[104] Spinal anesthesia is more reliable in preventing autonomic hyperreflexia than epidural block. This may be a result of the difficulty in assessing the adequacy of anesthesia when motor and sensory function are abnormal. The anesthesiologist is more certain that the anesthetic agent has been injected into the proper compartment with spinal anesthesia than with epidural because proper needle position is confirmed by aspirating cerebrospinal fluid.[8,17,71,104]

AIRWAY MANAGEMENT

The acutely traumatized patient may require tracheal intubation in order to establish an airway for surgery, relieve obstruction, treat ventilatory failure, provide a conduit for pulmonary toilet, prevent aspiration of gastric contents, or allow for hyperventilation of the patient with increased intracranial pressure. Patients with thoracic cord injury do not present special problems for tracheal intubation, but those with diagnosed or suspected cervical spine injury and instability may be at risk for extension of injury during airway manipulation. In addition, a probable full stomach; head, mouth, or neck trauma; vagal reflexes; and hypoxia and hypercarbia make airway management especially difficult.

Patients with cervical spine instability are at risk of exacerbation of the injury when the usual maneuvers for securing the airway are performed before the neck is stabilized.[6,81] The best emergency stabilization of the spine is achieved with a combination of sandbags, backboard, Philadelphia collar, and tape (Figs. 17-2, 17-3, 17-4).[44,94] Another useful technique is to have assistants immobilize the neck by traction on the head and chest during airway maneuvers. This technique is helpful, but it may not completely eliminate neck motion during direct laryngoscopy; therefore, neural injury may still occur.[81]

Quadriplegic patients are at risk for aspiration of gastric contents.[44,79] Agents that decrease gastric acidity and volume, such as metoclopramide,[26,103]

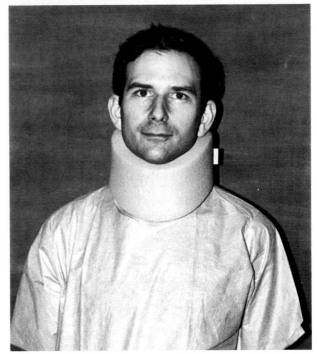

Figure 17-2. Soft collar applied to patient's neck. Minimal support is achieved with this device.

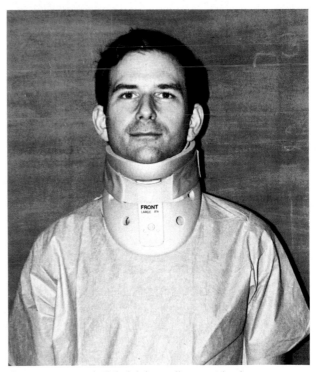

Figure 17-3. Hard Philadelphia collar provides better support than the soft collar, but it is not sufficient to prevent movement during laryngoscopy.

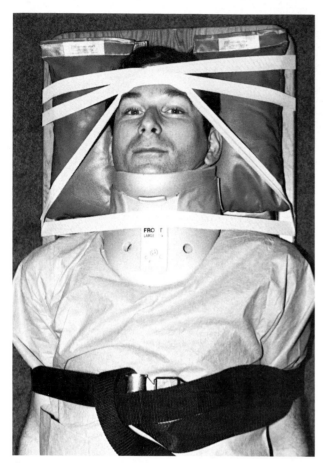

Figure 17-4. Hard collar with sandbags on both sides of the head and tape across the patient holding him to the rigid spinal board.

tribute to bradycardia, one should be certain the patient is well oxygenated prior to intubation.[29,44]

Some authors have suggested that patients with cervical spine injury should be intubated under general anesthesia and muscle relaxation.[30] Although this approach provides greater comfort to the patient than an awake–sedated technique, it may be associated with difficulty in visualizing the vocal cords by direct laryngoscopy. If the head and neck are immobilized, the patient cannot assume the sniffing position, which involves flexion of the lower cervical spine and extension at the atlanto-occipital joint.[32] Endotracheal intubation is facilitated by this position because it aligns the tracheal, pharyngeal, and oral axes. Difficulty in exposing the larynx leads to repeated efforts at intubation, which sets the stage for pulmonary aspiration in the presence of a full stomach, a frequent occurrence in spinal injured patients. Also, the pressure of the laryngoscope may cause extension of the injury in anesthetized patients whose relaxed perivertebral muscles can no longer prevent vertebral movement.[81]

The use of direct laryngoscopy in the spontaneously breathing patient has advantages. Ventilation is preserved and visualization of the larynx need not be as good, since intubation is facilitated by observation or auscultation of air movement through the larynx. The amount of pressure required with laryngoscopy can, therefore, be reduced. In addition, vertebral movement during laryngoscopy is limited, at least to some extent, by the residual perivertebral muscle tone. Nevertheless, this technique is not as safe as one that produces no pressure on the neck (Fig. 17-5).

The most favorable technique for elective intubation is the fiberoptic-guided approach.[86,90,124] Since this technique does not require the patient to be in the sniffing position, the risk of extending neural injury is substantially reduced. Patient comfort may be achieved by administration of sedatives, topical anesthesia, and superior laryngeal nerve blockade. However, one should be aware that anesthesia of the larynx and trachea, while improving patient comfort, also increases the risk of aspiration of blood, secretions, and gastric contents.[123] Although this technique is the method of choice, it may be unsuccessful if the optics are obscured by blood and secretions.

sodium bicitrate,[22,42,103] ranitidine,[25,58,89,126] and cimetidine,[24,29,42,58,89,116] may reduce the risk of this complication. Mechanically removing stomach contents with nasogastric suction is also useful. However, none of these measures is reliable in the immediate postinjury period. Only a cuffed endotracheal tube can assure prevention of aspiration.

In the absence of a sympathetic response, severe vagal reflexes may accompany tracheal intubation or suctioning, resulting in marked bradycardia and hypotension. Prior to airway manipulation, atropine sulfate, 0.4 to 0.8 mg in adults or 0.025 mg/kg in children, is useful in preventing this response. In addition, since hypoxia may con-

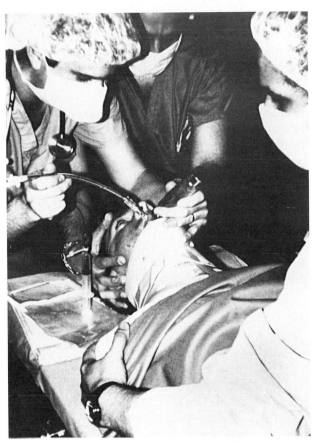

Figure 17-5. Direct laryngoscopy with manual in-line traction applied to prevent head and neck motion. Several assistants are required for this technique.

Another useful intubation technique is jet ventilation with oxygen, using a 14-gauge angiocath inserted through the cricothyroid membrane, while the patient is under anesthesia with intravenous agents. Fiberoptic intubation may then be performed orally or nasally.[65,92,111,114]

Blind nasal intubation is not the approach of choice, but on occasion it may prove useful. Since the stability of the head and neck must be maintained, one cannot employ the neck flexion maneuver to assist intubation if the tube does not easily enter the trachea.

Retrograde, guidewire-facilitated tracheal intubation is a useful approach when intubating patients with cervical spine instability.[67,73,96,119] This may be combined with use of the fiberoptic bron-

choscope. The guidewire is recovered from the mouth and passed through the suction port of the bronchoscope, which may then be easily inserted into the trachea. The advantages of both bronchoscope and guidewire are thus utilized.[101]

While the previously mentioned techniques are useful in elective circumstances when time is not crucial, they are not, by themselves, appropriate for the apneic patient. The apneic patient must first be ventilated with bag, mask, and oxygen to achieve adequate oxygenation. The neck is stabilized, and either gentle direct laryngoscopy with tracheal intubation, or cricothyrotomy is performed. Blind intubation is not possible in the presence of apnea.[11,14,106,107,110,111]

The general principles of airway management for patients with suspected or confirmed cervical spine instability are, therefore: prevent neck motion, oxygenate, prevent vagal reflexes, and prepare for a difficult tracheal intubation by having trained personnel and sufficient equipment available to treat any emergencies that may arise.

Positioning after tracheal intubation is as important as the actual intubation procedure. Movement of the neck during positioning may produce damage to the spinal cord. The patient must be positioned with extreme caution, with one member of the team applying axial traction to the neck at all times. The patient is kept awake, though lightly sedated, to permit evaluation of neurologic function after completion of positioning. When an operation is performed in the prone position the patient is asked to maintain his neck in a rigid posture prior to turning. The entire body should be moved to the operating table as a rigid unit.

UROLOGIC COMPLICATIONS

Renal failure remains a common late cause of death in patients with spinal cord injury,[9] although the mortality rate has been declining since the early 1950s, when 43% of deaths in spinal cord injured patients were caused by this complication. According to the most recent data, only 3% to 15% of paraplegics die of uremia. The major etiology of renal failure is chronic pyelonephritis and reflux nephropathy caused by improper bladder function. Renal amyloidosis, resulting from chronic decubitus ulcers and sepsis, may also produce renal failure in spinal injured patients.[78]

Under normal circumstances the urinary tract is protected from bacterial infection by the urethral mucosa; the length of the male urethra; complete bladder emptying, which washes out contaminating organisms; surface mucopolysaccharides, which prevent bacterial adherence; complement activity; leukocytic phagocytosis; immunoglobulin production; and prostatic antibacterial secretion in males. Spinal cord injured patients are prone to urinary tract infections, asymptomatic bacteriuria, catheter-associated infection, and pyelonephritis due to incomplete bladder emptying. The result of these infections is nephron damage, formation of infected calculi, renal or perinephric abscess, and urosepsis.[5]

Normal bladder filling requires accommodation to an increasing volume of urine at low intravesical pressure with appropriate sensation, closure of the bladder outlet at rest and during increases in intra-abdominal pressure, and absence of involuntary bladder contractions. In order for the bladder to empty properly there must be coordinated and adequate contraction of the bladder musculature with concomitant lowering of resistance of the sphincters and no anatomic obstruction.[9] Normal coordinated bladder function thus requires an intact neuraxis from the pons to the conus medullaris and uninterrupted neural connections with the bladder.

During the stage of spinal shock, suppression of autonomic activity produces a noncontractile and areflexic bladder. However, the smooth and perhaps the striated sphincters of the bladder continue to function. The result is urinary retention, which requires catheter drainage. When spinal shock resolves, detrusor hyperreflexia with striated sphincter dyssynergia can be demonstrated urodynamically and fluoroscopically; the results indicate bladder contraction, smooth sphincter relaxation, and obstruction at the striated sphincter. The dangers of elevated intravesical pressures are incomplete bladder emptying, bladder wall thickening (trabeculation) and blockage of the ureterovesical junction, hydrone-

phrosis, infection, and stone formation. Thus, in the early stages of injury the bladder is flaccid and its outlet is contracted. The resulting urinary retention must be treated by catheterization. Once the requirement for continuous drainage for monitoring urine output ends, frequent intermittent catheterization with complete drainage should be instituted. Indwelling Foley catheterization is undesirable because it increases the incidence of colonization and infection of the urinary tract.[5]

Provided distal spinal cord function is preserved, detrusor muscle function eventually returns. This results in involuntary voiding due to reflex activity; however, bladder emptying is incomplete. Lesions of the spinal cord close to the conus medullaris lead to detrusor areflexia, competent but nonrelaxing smooth sphincter, and a striated sphincter that retains tone but is not under voluntary control. This usually results in a high compliance bladder, but occasionally a low compliance bladder develops.[9]

The upper urinary tract sequelae of bladder obstruction can be avoided by preventing distension of the bladder by catheterizing frequently, decreasing bladder hyperactivity, increasing bladder capacity, and decreasing outlet resistance so that leakage can occur at a pressure lower than 40 cm of water.[9]

Pharmacologic agents that block parasympathetic-mediated bladder contraction, such as propantheline bromide (Pro-Banthine), oxybutynin chloride (Ditropan), and flavoxate hydrochloride (Urispas), may be useful. The striated muscle relaxants, baclofen and diazepam, reduce striated sphincter tone and promote bladder emptying. Transurethral sphincterotomy in patients with lesions above T-6 has been shown to significantly reduce intravesical and urethral pressure, and thus decrease the incidence of autonomic dysreflexia.[10]

Patients with spinal cord injury require frequent urinary tract surveillance, which should include an intravenous pyelogram, voiding cystourethrogram, urodynamics, and urine culture. Urinary tract infection and colonization require antimicrobial therapy; the source of the infection should be determined.[5,78] Prophylactic use of antimicrobials has been reported by some to be beneficial in preventing infection, but controversy on this topic exists.[78]

The risk of renal stone formation in spinal cord injured patients is estimated to be 8% in the first 8 years after injury. Risk factors for renal stones are male sex, neurologically complete lesions, and concomitant history of bladder stones. Calculi usually develop within the first 3 months after injury.[28] The composition of the stones in 98% of cases is calcium phosphate (apatite) and magnesium ammonium phosphate (struvite).[19]

Contamination by urea-splitting bacteria promotes ammonia, bicarbonate, and carbonate formation as well as increased urine alkalinity, which increases the potential for precipitation and formation of bladder calculi. Acetohydroxamic acid appears to be beneficial in preventing infection-induced urinary stones due to its inhibitory effect on urease.[52]

Renal calculi must be removed in order to prevent infection and loss of renal function. Delayed therapy may cause morbidity in 20% of patients with renal stones.[17] Extracorporeal shock wave lithotripsy, endourologic stone extraction (percutaneous stone removal or urethroscopy), and open surgical therapy each have a role in the current management of renal calculi.[72]

GASTROINTESTINAL COMPLICATIONS

According to one study, gastrointestinal complications are seen in 11% of patients with spinal cord injury. Ileus, gastric dilatation, peptic ulcer disease, and pancreatitis may complicate the acute phase of injury. In the chronic paraplegic, gastrointestinal problems include fecal impaction, peptic ulcer disease, superior mesenteric artery syndrome, hepatitis, amyloidosis, diverticulosis, and hiatal hernia with gastroesophageal reflux. The frequency of gastrointestinal problems depends on the level of injury. They are seen in 14% of quadriplegics, 11% of patients with high thoracic injuries, and about 5% of patients with low thoracic or lumbar injuries. Gastrointestinal complications are caused by loss of sympathetic activity

after injury. Unchecked parasympathetic activity results in enhanced glandular secretion and relaxation of gastric sphincters and the ileocecal valve.[48]

Gastrointestinal bleeding is seen in approximately 5% of cases, and is usually caused by duodenal or gastric ulceration. The use of large doses of steroids does not increase the risk of ulceration and bleeding provided that prophylaxis is given in the form of histamine-receptor blockade or antacids. The use of high doses of heparin significantly increases the risk of bleeding.[37] The risk factors for hemorrhage in the gastrointestinal tract are complete spinal cord injury, high level (especially cervical) injury, and concomitant organ system failure.[37,68,113,122]

The development of post-traumatic acalculous cholecystitis has been reported. Hypotension, sepsis, biliary stasis, and subsequent cystic duct obstruction are probably the underlying mechanisms of this complication. The diagnosis may be very difficult to make in the paraplegic patient since he may be completely asymptomatic. Fever, leukocytosis, increased bilirubin and alkaline phosphatase, and food intolerance should increase clinical suspicion and suggest the need for definitive diagnostic measures.[13]

ANESTHETIC CONSIDERATIONS

The choice of anesthetic, monitoring, and airway management techniques depends on the severity of the patient's physiologic derangement. Patients may require intensive therapy throughout the operative period. Muscle relaxant selection is based on the potential of hyperkalemic response to depolarizing agents. Finally, the conduct of anesthesia must take into account the special requirements of evoked potential monitoring, when that is used.

MUSCLE RELAXANTS[53]

Cardiac arrest from rapid development of hyperkalemia may occur after succinylcholine administration in the presence of denervation, extensive muscle damage, spinal cord injury, burns, motor neuron damage, or tetanus. In all of these conditions there is a substantially increased sensitivity to the effects of both acetylcholine and succinylcholine.

Following injury, acetylcholine receptors proliferate over the entire muscle membrane. This is in contrast to the normal circumstance, in which the receptor is located exclusively at the neuromuscular junction. Normally, depolarization results in a small flux of potassium across the muscle cell membrane. Injured or denervated muscle may undergo a potassium flux 33 to 44 times normal in response to succinylcholine depolarization. The released potassium then enters the circulation and may produce cardiac asystole. The amount of potassium released can be reduced by administering nondepolarizing relaxants in doses that produce complete paralysis. Under such circumstances there is certainly no need to give a depolarizing muscle relaxant.

The hyperkalemic response to succinylcholine begins 5 to 15 days following trauma and lasts 6 months or longer in patients with upper motor neuron injuries. The most conservative approach is to avoid depolarizing relaxants once injury has occurred. None of the nondepolarizing relaxants produce hyperkalemia, and all of them can be used safely.

GENERAL ANESTHESIA

Once the airway management and muscle relaxant issues are settled, the choice of anesthetic technique must be considered. If orthopedic surgery or neurosurgery is being performed, and monitoring of the nervous system, particularly the spinal cord, is desired, the anesthetic must be one that does not interfere with the monitoring.

During spinal surgery spinal cord function may be compromised by either direct compression of neural elements or reduced spinal cord blood flow. Such compromise must be recognized before permanent injury occurs. The wake-up test and monitoring of somatosensory evoked responses have been used to achieve this goal.

Patients undergoing spinal surgery in which intraoperative neurologic evaluation will be performed by the wake-up test should be told preoperatively that they will be awakened and asked to move their hands and feet during surgery. Hand movement serves as a control to determine if the patient is indeed awake; if the hands move but the feet do not, a neurologic deficit is present and manipulation of the spine may have created the deficit. Attempts must be made to relieve spinal cord compression or improve cord blood flow. The wake-up test requires the use of an anesthetic that is easily reversible within a short period of time.

Dorgan and associates reported their experience with 102 scoliosis operations.[31] Premedication was morphine sulfate 0.2 mg/kg and atropine 0.01 mg/kg intramuscularly. Anesthetic induction consisted of thiopental 5 mg/kg, and tracheal intubation was facilitated by curare 1 mg/kg. Maintenance anesthesia was provided with nitrous oxide 67%, oxygen 33%, and morphine sulfate 0.1 mg/kg. Potent volatile anesthetics were not employed and no additional relaxant was given. After the orthopedic manipulation the nitrous oxide was discontinued. Patients were called by their first name and asked to move their hands and feet. Approximately 5 minutes were required for patients to wake up. If patients failed to respond within this time, relaxant and opiate reversal agents were employed. In general, patients were cooperative, but weak from the residual sedative and relaxant effects. Once the test was complete the patients were reanesthetized. In this study, four patients awoke with new neurologic deficits. In three cases neural recovery was effected by partial release of the distracting force. The other patient had immediate rod removal but still had a neurologic deficit postoperatively.

Although the wake-up test has been used successfully, it has several disadvantages. In general, the test can be conducted only once during each operation because after it is completed, the patient is reanesthetized with a benzodiazepine in order to reduce recall. The consequence is that subsequent wake-ups are difficult or impossible to perform. In addition, if compromise of spinal cord function occurs after the test, the functional impairment would go unnoticed until the patient's recovery from anesthesia.

Continuous intraoperative monitoring of somatosensory evoked potentials (SEPs) overcomes these limitations and does not require patient awakening. Noninvasive electrophysiologic assessment of neural structures that are at risk during surgery provides information about sensory nerves and pathways within the spinal cord. As in the wake-up test, if deterioration of sensory evoked responses occurs intraoperatively associated with surgical manipulation, a corrective maneuver is employed to decrease compression of the spinal cord or improve spinal cord perfusion.

In order to monitor the nervous system with somatosensory evoked responses, a structure amenable to monitoring must be at risk. In the case of sensory evoked responses, the motor pathways are not monitored. Equipment and personnel must be available to perform the monitoring. Sites for stimulation and recording of responses must be available. The possibility of intervening to improve function when deterioration in response to spinal manipulation is detected should be available.[54]

Engler and associates reported their experience with 55 patients who underwent Harrington rod placement while SEPs were monitored. No patient awakened postoperatively with a neurologic deficit and there was no need for a wake-up test. The monitoring technique required that potent inhalation agents be avoided since they adversely affect the evoked response. Instead, nitrous oxide, fentanyl, thiopental, and muscle relaxant were used to induce and maintain anesthesia.[36]

Hypothermia, hypoxia, hypocarbia and hypercarbia, hypoglycemia, reduction in cerebral blood flow, severe anemia, and anesthetics can cause reduction in amplitude and increase in latency of the SEP.[54,102] The impact of these deviations can be so severe that monitoring may be impossible. The challenge for the anesthesiologist is to choose an anesthetic technique that maintains homeostasis and has the smallest impact on the SEP.

The effect of anesthetics on the cortical, subcortical, and spinal cord response to peripheral nerve stimulation has been studied in normal patients. McPherson and associates found that anesthetic induction with fentanyl 25 μg/kg and thiopental 0.5 to 1.0 mg/kg resulted in increased latency but no amplitude change in the SEP. Addition of 50% nitrous oxide, or isoflurane or enflurane up to 1%, caused decreased amplitude of the SEP in the upper extremity; nitrous oxide caused the largest SEP decrement. Stimulation of the lower extremity revealed that the cortical evoked response was not influenced by these concentrations of isoflurane and enflurane. However, nitrous oxide decreased the SEP response.[85]

Pathak and associates observed that patients receiving 60% nitrous oxide to which 0.5, 0.75, and 1.0 minimum alveolar concentration (MAC) of halothane, enflurane, or isoflurane was added had a graded, dose-dependent decrease in the evoked response, manifested by reduced amplitude.[93] Wolfe and Drummond evaluated sensory evoked responses when 60% nitrous oxide was administered with isoflurane 0.5, 1.0, and 1.5 MAC, and compared this with isoflurane 1.0 and 1.5 MAC alone. They observed that nitrous oxide with isoflurane severely reduced the evoked cortical response and that removing nitrous oxide doubled the response. In addition, they found that the subcortical response was not significantly altered by changing nitrous oxide and isoflurane concentrations.[128] Sebel and associates found that enflurane and halothane, administered in concentrations that ranged from 0.5% to 2.0%, caused increased latency and decreased amplitude of the cortical evoked response. However, like Wolfe and Drummond, they found that the subcortical response was substantially less affected by these inhalation anesthetics.[105]

The effect of several intravenous anesthetics on the somatosensory evoked response has also been studied. Induction of anesthesia with thiopental or midazolam results in no change in the SEP. Addition of fentanyl, 10 μg/kg, to midazolam causes no change in the SEP, but this dose of fentanyl added to thiopental has a depressant effect on amplitude. The addition of nitrous oxide to these anesthetics results in depression of the SEP. The only anesthetic induction agent that has been shown to increase the SEP is etomidate.[69,109]

It is clear from these data that most anesthetics have a negative impact on SEPs. The best approach is to provide an anesthetic in which fairly constant depth is maintained and to avoid the combination of potent anesthetic vapors and nitrous oxide. In addition, since the brainstem evoked response appears to be well preserved, one may consider monitoring it instead of the cortical SEP (Fig. 17-6).

In selecting an anesthetic technique for patients undergoing spinal surgery one must consider the following issues:

1. Airway management
2. Cardiovascular derangements such as spinal shock and autonomic hyperreflexia
3. Pulmonary complications such as pneumonia and pulmonary edema
4. Risk of a hyperkalemic response to depolarizing muscle relaxants
5. Risk of aspiration of gastric contents
6. Intraoperative neurologic monitoring

No particular anesthetic technique has been shown to improve outcome in this patient popula-

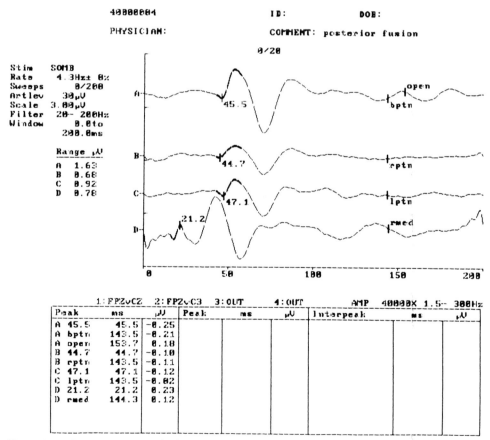

Figure 17-6. Somatosensory evoked potential monitoring during lumbar posterior fusion surgery. The x axis is time in milliseconds and the y axis is voltage. Near field scalp recordings were made using FPZ vs. CZ and FPZ vs. C3 leads. Curve A is the response to bilateral posterior tibial stimulation; curve B is the response to right posterior tibial stimulation; curve C is the response to left posterior tibial stimulation; curve D is the response to right median nerve stimulation. Recordings were made during general anesthesia.

tion. Therefore, the anesthesiologist must choose an approach that takes into account all of the problems presented by the patient. The goal is to maintain or improve physiologic status, relieve pain, prevent complications, and provide optimal conditions for surgery.

REFERENCES

1. Albin MS: Acute cervical spinal injury. Crit Care Clin 1:267, 1985
2. Albin MS, White RJ: Epidemiology, physiopathology, and experimental therapeutics of acute spinal cord injury. Crit Care Clin 3:441, 1987
3. Alderson JD, Thomas DG: The use of halothane anaesthesia to control autonomic hyperreflexia during transurethral surgery in spinal cord injured patients. Paraplegia 13:183, 1975
4. Alexander S, Kerr FWL: Blood pressure responses in acute compression of the spinal cord. J Neurosurg 21:485, 1964
5. Anderson RU: Urologic complications in spinal cord-injured patients. Urology 32 [Suppl 3]:31, 1988
6. Aprahamian C, Thompson BM, Finger WA, Darin JC: Experimental cervical spine injury model: Evaluation of airway management and splinting techniques. Ann Emerg Med 13:584, 1984
7. Babinski MF: Anesthetic considerations in the patient with acute spinal cord injury. Crit Care Clin 3:619, 1987
8. Barker I, Alderson J, Lydon M, Franks CI: Cardiovascular effects of spinal subarachnoid anesthesia: A study in patients with chronic spinal cord injuries. Anaesthesia 40:533, 1985
9. Barrett DM, Wein AJ: Voiding function: Relevant anatomy, physiology, pharmacology, p 863. In Gillenwater JY, Grayhack JT, Howards SS, Duckett JW (eds): Adult and Pediatric Urology. Chicago, Yearbook Medical Publishers, 1987
10. Barton CH, Khonsari F, Vaziri ND et al: The effect of modified transurethral sphincterotomy on autonomic dysreflexia. J Urol 135:83, 1986
11. Boyd AD: Tracheostomy and cricothyrotomy, p 32. In Worth M (ed): Principles and Practice of Trauma Care. Baltimore, Williams & Wilkins, 1982
12. Bracken MB, Shepard MJ, Hellenbrand KG, Collins WF: Methylprednisolone and neurological function 1 year after spinal cord injury. J Neurosurg 63:704, 1985
13. Branch CL Jr, Albertson DA, Kelly DL: Post-traumatic acalculous cholecystitis on a neurosurgical service. Neurosurgery 12:98, 1983
14. Brantigan CO, Grow JB: Cricothyroidotomy: Elective use in respiratory problems requiring tracheostomy. J Thorac Cardiovasc Surg 71:72, 1976
15. Braughler JM, Hall ED: Current application of "high dose" steroid therapy for CNS injury: A pharmacological perspective. J Neurosurg 62:806, 1985
16. Brisman R, Kovach RM, Johnson DO et al: Pulmonary edema in acute transection of the spinal cord. Surg Gynecol Obstet 139:363, 1974
17. Broecker BH, Hranowsky N, Hackler RH: Low spinal anesthesia for the prevention of autonomic dysreflexia in the spinal cord injured patient. J Urol 122:366, 1979
18. Brunnette DD, Rockswold GL: Neurologic recovery following rapid spinal realignment for complete cervical spinal cord injury. J Trauma 27:445, 1987
19. Burr RG: Urinary calculi composition in patients with spinal cord lesions. Arch Phys Med Rehabil 59:84, 1978
20. Carter RE: Respiratory aspects of spinal cord injury management. Paraplegia 25:262, 1987
21. Carter RE: Unilateral diaphragmatic paralysis in spinal cord injured patients. Paraplegia 18:267, 1980
22. Chen CT, Toung TJK, Haupt HM et al: Evaluation of the efficacy of Alka-Seltzer effervescent in gastric acid neutralization. Anesth Analg 63:325, 1984
23. Consensus Conference: Prevention of venous thrombosis and pulmonary embolism. JAMA 256:744, 1986
24. Coombs DW, Hooper D, Pageau M: Emergency cimetidine prophylaxis against acid aspiration. Ann Emerg Med 11:252, 1982
25. Dammann HG, Muller P, Simon B: Parenteral ranitidine: Onset and duration of action. Br J Anaesth 54:1235, 1982
26. Davies JAH, Howells TH: Management of anesthesia for the full stomach case in the casualty department. J Postgrad Med [July Suppl] 58, 1973
27. De La Torre JC: Spinal cord injury: A review of basic and applied research. Spine 6:315, 1981
28. DeVivo MJ, Fine PR, Cutter GR, Maetz HM: The risk of renal calculi in spinal cord injury patients. J Urol 131:857, 1984
29. Doble G, Jordan J, Williams JG: Cimetidine in the prevention of the pulmonary acid aspiration

(Mendelson's) syndrome. Br J Anaesth 51:967, 1979

30. Doolan LA, O'Brien JF: Safe intubation in cervical spine injury. Anaesth Intensive Care 13:319, 1985

31. Dorgan JC, Abbott TR, Bentley G: Intra-operative awakening to monitor spinal cord function during scoliosis surgery: Description of the technique and report of four cases. J Bone Joint Surg [Br] 66:716, 1984

32. Dripps RD, Eckenhoff JE, Vandam LD: Introduction to Anesthesia: The Principles of Safe Practice, 6th ed, p 180. Philadelphia, WB Saunders 1982

33. Dykstra DD, Sidi AA, Anderson LC: The effect of nifedipine on cystoscopy-induced autonomic hyperreflexia in patients with high spinal cord injuries. J Urol 138:1155, 1987

34. Eidelberg EE: Cardiovascular response to experimental spinal cord compression. J Neurosurg 38:326, 1973

35. El Masri WS, Silver JR: Prophylactic anticoagulant therapy in patients with spinal cord injury. Paraplegia 19:334, 1981

36. Engler GL, Spielholtz NI, Bernhard WN et al: Somatosensory evoked potentials during Harrington instrumentation for scoliosis. J Bone Joint Surg [Am] 60:528, 1978

37. Epstein N, Hood DC, Ransohoff J: Gastrointestinal bleeding in patients with spinal cord trauma: Effects of steroids, cimetidine and mini-dose heparin. J Neurosurg 54:16, 1981

38. Evans DE, Kobrine AL, Rizzoli HV: Cardiac arrhythmias accompanying acute compression of the spinal cord. J Neurosurg 52:52, 1980

39. Faden AI: New pharmacologic approaches to spinal cord injury: Opiate antagonists and thyrotropin releasing hormone. Cent Nerv Syst Trauma 2:5, 1985

40. Flamm ES, Young W, Collins WF et al: A phase I trial of naloxone treatment in acute spinal cord injury. J Neurosurg 63:390, 1985

41. Forner JV: Lung volumes and mechanics of breathing in tetraplegics. Paraplegia 18:258, 1980

42. Foulkes E, Jenkins LC: A comparative evaluation of cimetidine and sodium citrate to decrease gastric acidity: Effectiveness at the time of induction of anaesthesia. Can Anaesth Soc J 28:29, 1981

43. Frankel HL, Mathias CJ: Cardiovascular aspects of autonomic dysreflexia since Guttmann and Whiteridge. Paraplegia 17:46, 1979

44. Fraser A, Edmonds-Seal J: Spinal cord injuries. Anaesthesia 37:1084, 1982

45. Frisbie JH, Sarkarati M, Sharma GVRK, Rossier AB: Venous thrombosis and pulmonary embolism occurring at close intervals in spinal cord injury patients. Paraplegia 21:270, 1983

46. Frisbie JH, Sasahara AA: Low dose heparin prophylaxis for deep venous thrombosis in acute spinal cord injury patients: A controlled study. Paraplegia 19:343, 1981

47. Gardner BP, Parsons KF, Soni BM, Krishnan KR: The management of upper urinary tract calculi in spinal cord damaged patients. Paraplegia 23:371, 1985

48. Gore RM, Mintzer RA, Calenoff L: Gastrointestinal complications of spinal cord injury. Spine 6:538, 1981

49. Green D, Lee MY, Ito VY et al: Fixed vs adjusted-dose heparin in the prophylaxis of thromboembolism in spinal cord injury. JAMA 260:1255, 1988

50. Green D, Rossi EC, Yao JST et al: Deep vein thrombosis in spinal cord injury: Effect of prophylaxis with calf compression, aspirin, and dipyridamole. Paraplegia 20:227, 1982

51. Greenhoot JH, Mauck HP: The effect of cervical cord injury on cardiac rhythm and conduction. Am Heart J 83:659, 1972

52. Griffith DP, Khonsari F, Skurnick JH, James KE: A randomized trial of acetohydroxamic acid for the treatment and prevention of infection-induced urinary stones in spinal cord injury patients. J Urol 140:318, 1988

53. Gronert GA, Theye RA: Pathophysiology of hyperkalemia induced by succinylcholine. Anesthesiology 43:89, 1975

54. Grundy BL: Evoked potential monitoring, p 345. In Blitt CD (ed): Monitoring in Anesthesia and Critical Care Medicine. New York, Churchill Livingstone, 1985

55. Guha A, Tator CH: Acute cardiovascular effects of experimental spinal cord injury. J Trauma 28:481, 1988

56. Haas F, Axen K, Pineda H et al: Temporal pulmonary function changes in cervical cord injury. Arch Phys Med Rehabil 66:139, 1985

57. Hall PA, Young JV: Autonomic hyperreflexia in spinal cord injured patients: Trigger mechanism—dressing changes of pressure sores. J Trauma 23:1074, 1983

58. Harris PW, Morison DH, Dunn GL et al: Intramuscular cimetidine and ranitidine as prophylaxis against gastric acid aspiration syndrome—A randomized double-blind study. Can Anaesth Soc J 31:599, 1984

59. Hiraizumi Y, Fujimaki E, Hishida T et al: Regional

lung perfusion and ventilation with radioisotopes in cervical cord-injured patients. Clin Nucl Med 11:352, 1986

60. Holdsworth F: Fractures, dislocations and fracture-dislocations of the spine: A review paper. J Bone Joint Surg [Am] 52:1534, 1970

61. Iizuka H, Yamamoto H, Iwasaki Y et al: Evolution of tissue damage in compressive spinal cord injury in rats. J Neurosurg 66:595, 1987

62. Jane MJ, Freehafer AA, Hazel C et al: Autonomic dysreflexia: A cause of morbidity and mortality in orthopedic patients with spinal cord injury. Clin Orthop 169:151, 1982

63. Jarrell BE, Posuniak E, Roberts J et al: A new method of management using the Kim-Ray Greenfield filter for deep venous thrombosis and pulmonary embolism in spinal cord injury. Surg Gynecol Obstet 157:316, 1983

64. Jasper N, Kruger M, Ectors P, Sergysels R: Unilateral chest wall paradoxical motion mimicking a flail chest in a patient with hemilateral C7 spinal injury. Intensive Care Med 12:396, 1986

65. Jorden RC, Moore EE, Marx JA, Honigman B: A comparison of PTV and endotracheal ventilation in an acute trauma model. J Trauma 25:978, 1985

66. Kiker JD, Woodside JR, Jelinek GE: Neurogenic pulmonary edema associated with autonomic dysreflexia. J Urol 128:1038, 1982

67. King HK, Wang LF, Khan AK, Woolen DJ: Translaryngeal guided intubation for difficult intubation. Crit Care Med 15:869, 1987

68. Kiwerski J: Bleeding from alimentary canal during the management of spinal cord injury patients. Paraplegia 24:92, 1986

69. Koht A, Shutz W, Schmidt G et al: Effects of etomidate, midazolam, and thiopental on median nerve somatosensory evoked potentials and the additive effects of fentanyl and nitrous oxide. Anesth Analg 67:435, 1988

70. Kurnick NB: Autonomic hyperreflexia and its control in patients with spinal cord lesions. Ann Intern Med 44:678, 1956

71. Lambert DH, Deane RS, Mazuzan JE: Anesthesia and the control of blood pressure in patients with spinal cord injury. Anesth Analg 61:344, 1982

72. Lazare JN, Saltzman B, Sotolongo J: Extracorporeal shock wave lithotripsy treatment of spinal cord injured patients. J Urol 140:266, 1988

73. Lechman MJ, Donahoo JS, MacVaugh H: Endotracheal intubation using percutaneous retrograde guidewire insertion followed by antegrade fiberoptic bronchoscopy. Crit Care Med 14:589, 1986

74. Ledsome JR, Sharp JM: Pulmonary function in acute cervical cord injury. Am Rev Respir Dis 124:41, 1981

75. Lee DS, Kobrine A: Neurogenic pulmonary edema associated with ruptured spinal cord arteriovenous malformation. Neurosurgery 12:691, 1983

76. Lehmann KG, Lane JG, Piepmeier JM, Batsford WP: Cardiovascular abnormalities accompanying acute spinal cord injury in humans: Incidence, time course and severity. J Am Coll Cardiol 10:46, 1987

77. Lindan R, Joiner E, Freehafer AA, Hazel C: Incidence and clinical features of autonomic dysreflexia in patients with spinal cord injury. Paraplegia 18:285, 1980

78. Lloyd LK: New trends in urologic management of spinal cord patients. Cent Nerv Syst Trauma 3:3, 1986

79. Luce JM: Medical management of spinal cord injury. Crit Care Med 13:126, 1985

80. MacKenzie CF, Shin B, Krishnaprasad D et al: Assessment of cardiac and respiratory function during surgery on patients with acute quadriplegia. J Neurosurg 62:843, 1985

81. Majernick TG, Bieniek R, Houston JB, Hughes HG: Cervical spine movement during orotracheal intubation. Ann Emerg Med 15:417, 1986

82. Marshall LF, Knowlton S, Garfin SR et al: Deterioration following spinal cord injury: A multicenter study. J Neurosurg 66:400, 1987

83. McGregor JA: Autonomic hyperreflexia: A mortal danger for spinal cord damaged women in labor. Am J Obstet Gynecol 151:330, 1985

84. McMichan JC, Michel L, Westbrook PR: Pulmonary dysfunction following traumatic quadriplegia. JAMA 243:528, 1980

85. McPherson RW, Mahla M, Johnson R, Traystman RJ: Effects of enflurane, isoflurane, and nitrous oxide on somatosensory evoked potentials during fentanyl anesthesia. Anesthesiology 62:626, 1985

86. Messeter KH, Petterson KI: Endotracheal intubation with the fibreoptic bronchoscope. Anaesthesia 35:294, 1980

87. Meyer GA, Berman IR, Doty DB et al: Hemodynamic responses to acute quadriplegia with or without chest trauma. J Neurosurg 34:168, 1971

88. Meyer PA Jr, Rosen JS, Hamilton BB et al: Fracture dislocation of the cervical spine: Transportation, assessment, and immediate management. In American Academy of Orthopedic Surgeons (ed): Instructional Course Lectures. St. Louis, CV Mosby, 1976

89. Morison DH, Dunn GL, Fargas-Babjak AM et al: A double-blind comparison of cimetidine and ranitidine as prophylaxis against gastric aspiration syndrome. Anesth Analg 61:988, 1982

90. Mulder JS, Wallace DH, Woolhouse FM: The use of the fiberoptic bronchoscope to facilitate endotracheal intubation following head and neck trauma. J Trauma 15:638, 1975

91. Myllynen P, Kammonen M, Rokkanen P et al: Deep venous thrombosis and pulmonary embolism in patients with acute spinal cord injury: A comparison with nonparalyzed patients immobilized due to spinal fractures. J Trauma 25:541, 1985

92. Neff CC, Pfister RC, Sonnenberg EV: Percutaneous transtracheal ventilation: Experimental and practical aspects. J Trauma 23:84, 1983

93. Pathak KS, Ammandio M, Kalamchi A et al: Effects of halothane, enflurane and isoflurane on somatosensory evoked potentials during nitrous oxide anesthesia. Anesthesiology 66:753, 1987

94. Podolsky S, Baraff LJ, Simon RR et al: Efficacy of cervical spine immobilization methods. J Trauma 23:461, 1983

95. Poe RH, Reisman JL, Rodenhouse TG: Pulmonary edema in cervical spinal cord injury. J Trauma 18:71, 1978

96. Powell WF, Ozdil T: A translaryngeal guide for tracheal intubation. Anesth Analg 46:231, 1967

97. Quimby CW, Williams RN, Greifenstein FE: Anesthetic problems of the acute quadriplegic patient. Anesth Analg 52:333, 1973

98. Raeder JC, Grisvold SE: Perioperative autonomic hyperreflexia in high spinal cord lesions: A case report. Acta Anaesthesiol Scand 30:672, 1986

99. Rawe SE, Perot PL: Pressor response resulting from experimental contusion injury to the spinal cord. J Neurosurg 50:58, 1979

100. Reines HD, Harris RC: Pulmonary complications of acute spinal cord injuries. Neurosurgery 21:193, 1987

101. Riou B, Barriot P, Bodenan P, Viars P: Retrograde tracheal intubation in trauma patients. Anesthesiology 67:A130, 1987

102. Russ W, Sticher J, Scheld H, Hempelmann G: Effects of hypothermia on somatosensory evoked responses in man. Br J Anaesth 59:1484, 1987

103. Schmidt JF, Jorgensen BC: The effect of metoclopramide on gastric contents after preoperative ingestion of sodium citrate. Anesth Analg 63:841, 1984

104. Schonwald G, Fish KJ, Perkash I: Cardiovascular complications during anesthesia in chronic spinal cord injured patients. Anesthesiology 55:550, 1981

105. Sebel PS, Erwin CW, Neville WK: Effects of halothane and enflurane on far and near field somatosensory evoked potentials. Br J Anaesth 59:1492, 1987

106. Simon RR, Brenner BE: Emergency cricothyroidotomy in the patient with massive neck swelling: Part 1. Anatomical aspects. Crit Care Med 11:114, 1983

107. Simon RR, Brenner BE, Rosen MA: Emergency cricothyroidotomy in the patient with massive neck swelling: Part 2. Clinical aspects. Crit Care Med 11:119, 1983

108. Skillman SS, Collins REC, Coe NP et al: Prevention of deep vein thrombosis in neurosurgical patients: A controlled, randomized trial of external pneumatic compression boots. Surgery 83:354, 1978

109. Sloan TB, Ronai AK, Toleikis JR, Koht A: Improvement of intraoperative somatosensory evoked potentials by etomidate. Anesth Analg 67:582, 1988

110. Smith RB: Transtracheal ventilation during anesthesia. Anesth Analg 53:225, 1974

111. Smith RB, Myers EN, Sherman H: Transtracheal ventilation in pediatric patients. Br J Anaesth 46:313, 1974

112. Soderstrom CA, Brumback RJ: Early care of the patient with cervical spine injury. Orthop Clin North Am 17:3, 1986

113. Soderstrom CA, Ducker TB: Increased susceptibility of patients with cervical cord lesions to peptic gastrointestinal complications. J Trauma 25:1030, 1985

114. Spoerel WE, Narayan PS, Singh NP: Transtracheal ventilation. Br J Anaesth 43:932, 1971

115. Stauffer ES: Fractures and dislocations of the spine: Part I. The cervical spine. In Rockwood CA, Green DP (eds): Fractures in Adults. Philadelphia, JB Lippincott, 1984

116. Strain JD, Moore EE, Markovchick VJ, Van Duzer-Moore S: Cimetidine for the prophylaxis of potential gastric acid aspiration pneumonitis in trauma patients. J Trauma 21:49, 1981

117. Theodore J, Robin E: Speculations on neurogenic pulmonary edema. Am Rev Respir Dis 113:405, 1976

118. Tibbs PA, Young B, Todd EP et al: Studies of experimental spinal cord transection: Part IV. Effects of cervical spinal cord transection on myocardial blood flow in anesthetized dogs. J Neurosurg 52:197, 1980

119. Tobias R: Increased success with retrograde guide for endotracheal intubation. Anesth Analg 62:366, 1983

120. Troll GF, Dohrmann GJ: Anesthesia of the spinal cord injured patient: Cardiovascular problems and their management. Paraplegia 13:162, 1975

121. Wagner FC Jr, Chehrazi B: Early decompression and neurological outcome in acute cervical spinal cord injuries. J Neurosurg 56:699, 1982

122. Walters K, Silver JR: Gastrointestinal bleeding in patients with acute spinal cord injuries. Int Rehabil Med 8:44, 1986

123. Walts LF: Anesthesia of the larynx in a patient with a full stomach. JAMA 192:705, 1965

124. Wang JF, Reeves JG, Gutierrez FA: Awake fiberoptic laryngoscopic tracheal intubation for anterior cervical spinal fusion in patient with cervical cord trauma. Int Surg 64:69, 1979

125. Whitelaw WA: The respiratory pump, p 51. In Guenter CA, Welch MH (eds): Pulmonary Medicine. Philadelphia, JB Lippincott, 1982

126. Williams JG: H_2 receptor antagonists and anaesthesia. Can Anaesth Soc J 30:264, 1983

127. Winslow EBJ, Lesch M, Talano JV, Meyer PR Jr: Spinal cord injuries associated with cardiopulmonary complications. Spine 11:809, 1986

128. Wolfe DE, Drummond JC: Differential effects of isoflurane/nitrous oxide on posterior tibial somatosensory evoked responses of cortical and subcortical origin. Anesth Analg 67:852, 1988

129. Wray NP, Nicotra MB: Pathogenesis of neurogenic pulmonary edema. Am Rev Respir Dis 118:783, 1978

130. Yarkony GM, Katz RT, Wu YC: Seizures secondary to autonomic dysreflexia. Arch Phys Med Rehabil 67:834, 1986

18

PATHOLOGY OF SPINAL CORD TRAUMA

Kurt Jellinger

The spinal cord is protected from injury by the complex bony structure forming the spinal canal. Except in the cervical region, a considerable degree of force is needed to damage the cord. In general, spinal cord injury is the result of a short mechanical stress or impact to which the cord and its covering are subjected at the time of the trauma. The degree of damage to the cord depends on the nature and dynamics of the traumatic force and on the level at which the spine and cord received the injury. Traumatic lesions of the spinal cord are classified as resulting from:

1. Direct violence, or injury to the cord by sharp or penetrating means, as in stab wounds and injury from penetrating missiles
2. Indirect violence, due to mechanical impacts transmitted to the cord with or without injury (fracture, fracture-dislocation, or subluxation) of the spine
3. A combination of direct and indirect violence, as in wounds with high-velocity missiles or fracture-dislocations resulting from blunt force in which the cord or its coverings are lacerated or pierced by dislocated bony fragments, causing penetrating injury

High-velocity missiles that pass at speed through the spinal column, even without touching either the dura mater or the spinal cord, may cause extensive damage at the level of impact or several spinal cord segments from impact via indirect lesions. In general, sharp or direct violence results in *penetrating* or open injuries, and indirect or blunt force results in *closed* or nonpenetrating injuries. As in craniocerebral trauma, this separation depends on the integrity of the dura, although in spinal trauma secondary infections are much less frequent than in open brain injuries. According to the pathogenesis, the resulting lesions are classified as:

1. Primary (direct) traumatic lesions due to direct mechanical damage inflicted at the time of the trauma and observable either immediately or with in a few minutes after injury
2. Secondary traumatic or reactive lesions developing from nontraumatic but injury-related factors (e.g., edema, ischemia, circulation disorders, biochemical disorders, and other post-traumatic reactions)
3. Late sequelae of both primary and secondary traumatic effects: scar formation, secondary degeneration, or regenerative phenomena
4. Late complications and delayed progressive disorders (myelopathies) arising at various intervals after injury

The pathology of human spinal injuries, including birth and infantile cord injuries[31,79,120,168] and delayed post-traumatic myelopathies,[15,51,75,160] has been extensively reviewed in a number of sources.[12,39,69,75,81–83,89,103,107,155,185] The aim of this chapter is to present an overview of the principal mechanisms and neuropathologic features of spinal trauma in humans and to discuss clinical implications. Experimental spinal cord trauma will not be addressed.

PENETRATING CORD INJURIES

The spinal cord may be directly injured with or without serious damage to the spine by stab wounds from knives and other penetrating objects, high- and low-velocity missiles, or by displaced bone fragments after blunt spinal trauma. The incidence of penetrating cord injuries, in which the dura mater and meninges are slit, ranges from 5% to 10% in civilian injuries[75] and from 65% to 85% in warfare casualties.[89,177] In general, the injury to the spine is less severe than to the cord, which may be directly damaged without obvious injury to the spine by stabs or tiny fragments of high-velocity missiles that pass between the vertebral laminae.

The extent and shape of cord damage depends on the size, velocity, and direction of impact of the penetrating object. Bodies with a small diameter produce small and localized, well-defined stabs or puncture wounds with little or no bleeding and inconspicuous external wounds, which may remain unrecognized clinically or even at autopsy. Larger objects with higher velocities, and displaced bone fragments usually cause irregularly shaped wounds or lacerations. The damage to the cord is usually circumscribed and most severe at the level of the penetrating violence; it may range from small superficial defects or localized stabs or punctures to incomplete or total cord transection or complete disruption of the cord with dural tears, as is seen after extreme hyperextension of the cervical spine in adults[72] or obstetrical trauma.[159] Remote lesions, including edema, necrosis, or hemorrhage, may be found anywhere in the cord.[75,89]

Missile injuries of the cord include:[88,189]

1. Perforating wounds, in which the missile transverses the spinal canal or cord and leaves it through an exit wound, causing tearing of the dura and total or subtotal transection of the cord over several segments, with little bleeding and only slight bruising of tissues (Fig. 18-1)
2. Penetrating wounds, in which the missile enters the spinal canal and remains in it, either extradurally or within the cord. There may be laceration of the meninges, spinal

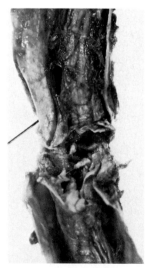

Figure 18-1. Gunshot wound with subtotal transection of spinal cord.

vessels, or cord tissue, with extraspinal bleeding, which usually does not compress the cord. In rare cases, small fragments of shells or bone that have pierced the dura may be included in the spinal canal without damaging the cord.

3. Depressed wounds or ricochet injury of the cord, in which missiles ricochet outside of the spinal canal, with or without piercing the dura, causing direct or indirect damage to the cord. After tangential shot wounds, even if the bullet does not enter the spinal canal, there may be laceration of the meninges and spinal vessels and incomplete destruction of the cord.[75]

4. Compression or laceration of the cord by displaced bone fragments or due to blast effects. In these injuries the cord often escapes direct damage. High-velocity missiles passing through the vertebral bodies or spine, even without touching the dura or spinal cord, may cause extensive damage at the level of the impact and extending over some distance above and below (Fig. 18-2) due to contusion and a variety of mechanical effects.[68,75,103]

5. Secondary lesions and remote injuries in various parts of the cord. These have been reported in cases of spinal concussion resulting from gunshot wounds or bursting of high-explosive shells without damage to the spine or any external wounds.[49,89] They are possibly results of remote circulatory disorders.

Stab wounds resulting from a penetrating knife or other sharp instrument most often affect the cervical and upper thoracic region. They produce well-defined lesions ranging from small wounds to hemisection of the cord (which results in Brown-Séquard syndrome[28]) or even complete transection. Because the vertebral laminae protect the spinal cord on the dorsal surface, stab wounds usually enter slightly laterally or dorsolaterally to the midline. The severance of cord tissue is therefore greater on one side than the other, and the posterior columns are involved more severely than the ventrolateral columns. The lesion is local and, unless complicated by vascular injury, is lim-

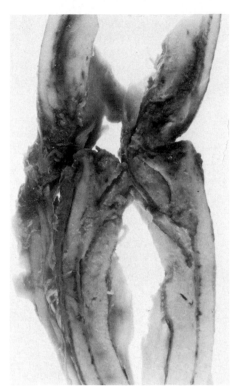

Figure 18-2. Gunshot wound of the upper cervical spine, with transection at C-3–C-4 and central hemorrhage ascending to C-1; patient survived 5 days.

ited to the level of the wound, with surrounding hemorrhage and edema (Fig. 18-3). There may be additional epidural, subdural, and intramedullary hemorrhage or laceration.[88]

Spinal wounds in *blunt injuries*, with complete disruption of the occipito-atlantal joints, complete transection of the lower brain stem or upper cervical cord, tearing of the dura, and unilateral or bilateral disruption of the vertebral arteries, have been reported after extreme hyperextension (retroflexion) of the cervical spine followed by sudden death,[67,72,188] in birth injury during breech extraction,[160,168] and in some cases of severe fracture of the cervical spine (Fig. 18-4). Complete disruption of the lower thoracic cord may be survived for long periods.[83] Even in total transection of the cord, the dura is rarely completely torn across; the ends of the cord are often kept in approximation by the dural sheath.

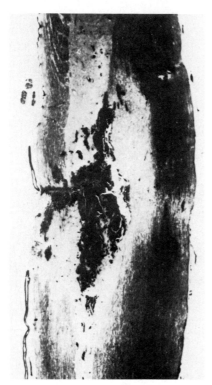

Figure 18-3. Fresh stab wound from penetrating knife, with local hemorrhage and perifocal edema (Woelcke's myelin stain).

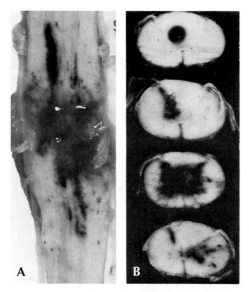

Figure 18-4. (A) Hemorrhagic necrosis (transection) of spinal cord at C-5 and (B) fusiform central hemorrhage ascending to C-1, with fracture of the spine following a striking accident by a crane bucket; patient survived 4 days.

The gross changes and histopathology of penetrating cord wounds depend on the type of injury and the time that has elapsed since the trauma. As in cerebral wounds, three stages of tissue reaction are distinguished:[68,89,157]

1. Early phase of necrosis, covering the changes during the first 2 to 3 days
2. Intermediate stage of resorption and organization within the first week
3. Late stage of repair and scar formation

The early changes of spinal cord wounds are disintegration of nervous tissue, its coverings, and vessels. Stab wounds are clearly delimited in the case of partial and total transection, whereas missile wounds are more ragged and destructive. The dura and meninges may be slit or torn; the edges of torn dura tend to rejoin except in severe disruption, while the margins of the cord wounds are often separated in the initial stage. Bleeding into the wound canal, often seen in brain damage, is rare in the cord. Cross section of the wound canal shows three different zones:[125,154,157]

1. The central "debris" zone or stab canal, with total destruction of tissue and hemorrhages, that is, with irreversible changes of all elements undergoing liquefaction necrosis
2. The intermediate "squashed" or indirect but irreversibly damaged zone, with vacuolation of the tissue and hemorrhage also undergoing liquefaction
3. An outer zone of "reversible" tissue swelling or peritraumatic edema, with plasma exudation and progressive astroglial swelling

The light microscopic features and time sequence of traumatic lesions have been confirmed by ultrastructural studies of experimental stab wounds in the spinal cord.[43,93] Edema in noninfectious stab wounds is already present 4 minutes after injury, and within 30 minutes to 2 hours strikingly increases in severity and extent. Edema, astroglial swelling, and spread of fluid in the extracellular spaces further increase for 12 hours following trauma. They later regress, but are still demonstrable for up to 8 days.[113,154] In the early stages, the extracellular spaces contain nonproteinaceous fluid, while in later stages breakdown of the blood–brain barrier causes plasma exudation due to membrane dysfunction, hypercalcemia, and ischemia.[12] Axonal swelling and myelin disruption are seen several hours to 4 days after injury in the peritraumatic area.[12,42,154]

After the immediate post-traumatic period, the necrotic tissue undergoes resorption and organization by proliferation of microglia and phagocytes, causing more rapid resorption of blood in the spinal cord than in the brain.[89] Due to progressive glial and mesenchymal proliferation and peripheral vascularization, about 8 to 10 days after injury the wound is surrounded by highly vascularized granulation tissue, which gradually replaces the central dissoluted areas. Organization also starts from the meninges, and the damaged parts of the cord are later replaced by a gliomesenchymal or connective tissue scar, the formation of which starts about 3 to 4 weeks after trauma. At the site of destruction there is local cicatrization, consisting largely of connective tissue and adherent, grossly thickened meninges, and dura containing hemosiderin deposits. Collagenous thickening of the meninges is usually most intensive at the site of injury, but may extend several segments above or below. The arachnoid may become thickened and opaque, and may adhere to either dura or spinal cord. It may contain irregular cavities filled with cerebrospinal fluid, causing "adhesive arachoiditis,"[96a,103] which compresses the cord.

Following transection of the cord there may be complete dehiscence with a gap between the disruptured ends (see Fig. 18-1). The cord segments are surrounded by thickened meninges and show adherence to the dura and thinning to the point of dehiscence.[83] There is obliteration of the subarachnoid space due to fibrosis, and replacement of cord tissue by gliocollagenous scar, in which nerve root proliferation is conspicuous. Foreign bodies, such as retained bullets, splinters, or bone fragments, are surrounded by connective tissue with foreign body reaction.

Infections, serious complications of any kind of penetrating wound, are rare in spinal injury as compared to open brain trauma.[47,177] They include:

1. Epidural and subdural empyema, extremely rare complications of spinal injuries that may or may not be associated with leptomeningitis[89]
2. Purulent leptomeningitis, the incidence of which in World Wars I and II ranged from 5% to 20%.[89,103] It is usually limited to the level of penetrating injury (Fig. 18-5), and rarely extends over the total length of the cord. It extremely rarely may spread to the basal cisterns.
3. Spinal cord infection adjacent to the wound canal accompanied by severe edema. Diffuse post-traumatic myelitis and spinal cord abscess are extremely rare complications of penetrating trauma.[89]

CLOSED CORD INJURIES

In civil life, closed injuries are the most frequent traumatic lesions of the spine and spinal cord. They are the results of both blunt forces transmitted to the cord and penetrating violences that do not pierce the dura mater or spinal canal. They may be caused by road accidents, industrial accidents, diving into shallow water, falls, and accidents in sports and games. Traumatic damage to

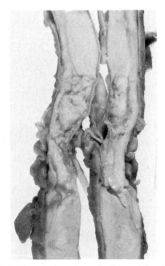

Figure 18-5. Spinal purulent meningitis with old softening of cord after gunshot injury of neck; patient survived 6 weeks.

the neural elements occurs with or without bony and soft-tissue injuries such as subluxations and fracture-dislocations of the spine. Often there is concurrent injury to both the spine and spinal cord, although the level of the injuries may not coincide. The type and extent of spinal cord lesions are based on the biomechanics of spinal injury,[136] according to which closed cord trauma may be classified as:

1. Indirect cord injury, due to blunt trauma to the cord without space-consuming damage to the spine, that is, without considerable displacement of the bony alignment and disks. This occurs when the impact causes a comparatively small-load cross section of the spine, for example, in longitudinal shearing and distraction, flexion, rotation or rotation–flexion, and posteroanterior acceleration.
2. Direct cord injury, due to blunt or penetrating forces causing space-occupying bony or ligamentous damage, fracture-dislocation or subluxation resulting in compression or contusion of the cord, or both, for example, in crush injuries

In general, the cord lesion is rarely confined to the point of impact to the spine, but may spread over many segments above or below. This spread is due to both primary and secondary traumatic changes. In about 15% of closed cord injuries, lesions are seen at multiple levels.[108]

Due to the anatomic and biomechanical conditions of the human spine, the cervical region and thoracolumbar junction are the most frequent sites of traumatic damage.[60,103] Cervical spine injuries are particularly devastating and often cause death. In a series of 100 autopsy cases, cervical cord damage was the cause of death for two-thirds of the patients, and accounted for three-fourths of the cases with short survival.[83] About 60% of acute fatal cervical injuries are associated with traumatic craniocerebral lesions. They often involve the upper cervical cord,[38,67,99,151] while fracture-dislocations and subluxations of the cervical spine are most common at the level of the C-5–C-6 vertebrae.[23,68] Thoracic fractures are less common than cervical, and in these the lower tho-

racic levels are more likely to be involved. Low thoracic injuries are typically caused by crushing or extreme flexion of the spine in falls or road or mining accidents. Upper thoracic spine trauma may show second-level injury.[137] Lesions of the lumbar spine can damage the conus or compress the cauda equina.

BIOMECHANICS OF SPINAL INJURY

Most of the existing knowledge of the biomechanics of spinal injury is based on studies of the adult spine.[136] Often, the mechanisms of neural injury can be deduced from the associated bony and soft-tissue injuries,[120] although these can be missing, and there may be little relationship between the types of deforming forces to the spine and the spine's radiologic appearance and resultant neurologic deficit.[9] In contrast to the movable head, the spinal cord is rarely submitted to acceleration and translation injuries. Hyperflexion, dorsiflexion (hyperextension) with or without rotation, vertical compression and longitudinal distraction, and rotation are the most familiar mechanisms by which the spine and cord can be damaged. Often more than one mechanism is involved in cord injuries.

According to the physical forces acting at the moment of impact the following major types of neuronal injury in spinal trauma are distinguished:[12,75,120]

1. Flexion and deflexion (ventroflexion and dorsiflexion) injuries
2. Vertical compression and longitudinal distraction trauma
3. Rotation injuries
4. Injuries with combined mechanisms

FLEXION AND DEFLEXION INJURIES

Flexion and deflexion injuries are produced either by ventroflexion (anterohyperflexion) or by retroflexion or dorsiflexion forces, and frequently involve the cervical spine. They result in disk protrusion, tears of the interspinous, anterior, or posterior common ligaments, or annulus fibrosus of one or more intervertebral disks with or without bony fracture-dislocation and subluxation. Spinal cord damage is produced by compression, transverse or longitudinal shear, torsion, and rotation forces, among which transverse and longitudinal forces appear to be the most important.[94,134,136] Experimental studies of the cervical spine in flexion and extension show sectioning of ligaments from anterior to posterior and vice versa with small increment motion followed by sudden disruption of motion segments.[121]

Flexion injuries of the cervical spine may or may not be associated with cord lesions. In minor degrees of ventrohyperflexion, dislocation of the cervical spine without considerable reduction of the anteroposterior diameter of the spinal canal ("hyperflexion sprain" or subluxation) produces hardly any cord lesion unless the cervical spine is pathologically stiff.[23,123] Sudden and extreme hyperflexion of the cervical spine in a forward direction, usually resulting in tears of the posterior ligament (hyperflexion sprain) and disk protrusion without bony fracture (flexion subluxation), is often associated with severe local damage to the cord, particularly central necrosis and hemorrhage (Figs. 18-6, 18-7). Cord damage is caused by a "pincers mechanism," compressing the cord between the posterior part of the inferior vertebra and the posterior arch of the dislocated upper vertebra,[123] and a "thrust effect," due to axial tension and shearing stresses, causing central necrosis and damage to the posterior columns.[26,149]

Extreme hyperflexion and flexion subluxation of the cervical spine in children, usually with normal radiography (no vertebral fracture or deformity), is often associated with complete cord transection and severe anatomic cord damage.[32,120] This is due to the increased physiologic mobility and susceptibility of the pediatric cervical spine to flexion–extension injuries.[24,168] Since the upper cervical segments in children show the greatest physiologic mobility, flexion subluxation trauma most often involves the upper cervical cord.[52,120,122] Extreme anterohyperflexion of the neck in infants due to occipital blows, diving, or child abuse may cause acute fatal hemorrhage and tears in the central parts of the upper cervical cord and lower medulla without damage to the occipitospinal articulations or spine (see Fig. 18-7), whereas in children older than 8 years, similar to adults, both

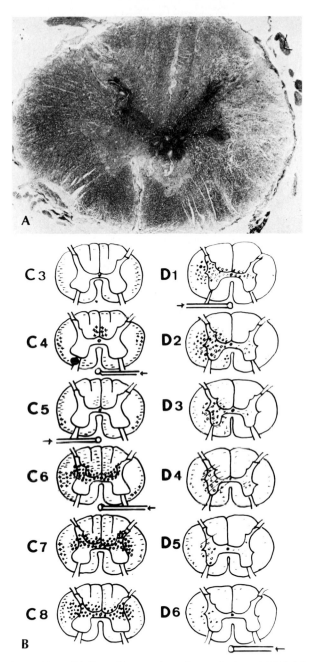

Figure 18-6. (*A*) Central hemorrhage in cervical cord (C-7) following anteflexion injury of neck due to drunken fall on the occiput without vertebral fracture; patient survived 2 days. (*B*) Diagram of cord lesions.

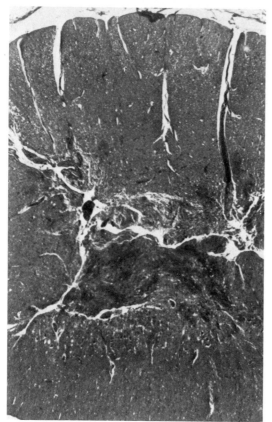

Figure 18-7. Central hemorrhage of the C-1–C-2 level following extreme hyperflexion injury of neck in child abuse; patient survived 2 days.

flexion and extension forces are more likely to injure the lower cord segments.[120] While ventroflexion injuries of the odontoid are rarely complicated by lethal cord damage,[107] a postmortem radiologic series of fatal traffic accidents with 21% neck lesions, particularly at the upper cervical level, included a large number of hyperflexion injuries in adult pedestrians, most notably at the occipito-atlantal junction.[4]

Hyperextension or, more correct, *retroflexion injuries* are due to lateral and backward retroflexion or dorsiflexion of the head and cervical spine resulting from facial or frontal trauma (e.g., a fall or blow on the forehead or diving into shallow water). They are often associated with bony dislocation, ventral fracture-dislocation, avulsion of ar-

ticular processes, or disruption and displacement of intervertebral disks, which result in central cord lesions (Figs. 18-8, 18-9, 18-10). Pure retroflexion due to skull traction results in fracture of the neural arches or pedicles, but rarely in cord damage.[60]

In the rather frequent retroflexion injury of the cervical spine, with or without rotation, separation between the vertebral body and the adjacent lower intervertebral disk results in dislocation or ventral fracture-dislocation, disruption and displacement of the disc, rupture of the anterior longitudinal ligament, and dislodging of the posterior ligament from the vertebral body. These mechanisms reduce the anteroposterior diameter of the spinal canal and "squeeze" the cord by a "pincers mechanism," causing central cord destruction.[24,123,153]

Hemorrhage and necrosis that mainly affect the central portion of the spinal cord are due to both pincers action and extremely high axial tension and tearing of nervous tissue directed in a cranial

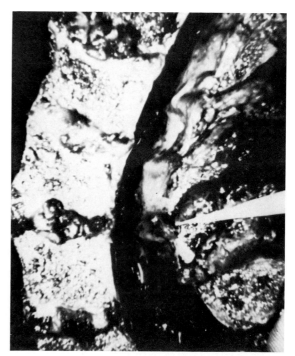

Figure 18-8. Fracture of cervical spine following hyperextension injury with bulging disk in subject with cervical spondylosis.

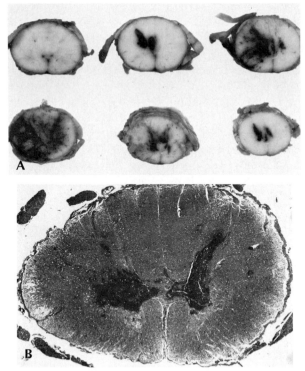

Figure 18-9. (*A*) Central hemorrhage of cervical cord following hyperextension (dorsiflexion) injury of neck (*B*) with "butterfly" hemorrhage in central gray matter, patient survived 2 days.

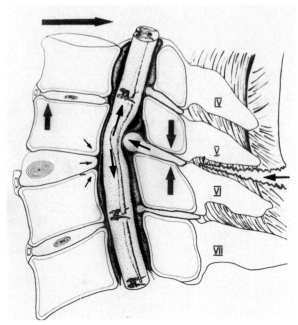

Figure 18-10. Schematic biomechanics of forces acting on cervical spine and cord during hyperextension (dorsiflexion) injury of the neck.

and caudal direction (see Fig. 18-10). Disruption of ligamentous structures of the cervical spine is produced by rotational forces in addition to anteflexion or retroflexion.[26,136] Marar[102] suggested a combination of retroflexion and backward shearing forces. Hyperextension is maximum at the C-5–C-6 junction, and injury to the cord most likely occurs in this area.[23,144]

Retroflexion causes significant cord damage in both children and adults, particularly in patients with cervical spondylosis due to tearing of intervertebral disks and angulation and crush of the already narrowed cord.[83,181] Injury to the cord that is caused by both direct mechanical stresses and additional ischemia ranges from small butterflylike focal intramedullary hemorrhages or hemorrhagic necrosis in the gray matter to extensive crushing of the total cord (Figs. 18-11, 18-12; see

Fig. 18-9). Traumatic damage may extend over several spinal cord segments and may be complicated by spinal cord infarction due to compression, kinking (Fig. 18-13) or thrombosis of vertebral arteries,[52,59,66,69,91,141,146,147,150,152] or compression of a radicular tributary (see Fig. 18-12). Compression of cord vessels is rare.

Retroflexion injuries of the neck and head that result in fracture or dislocation of the odontoid are caused by forces acting in a vertical direction (e.g., a direct blow, a fall on the head, or being thrown through car windshield). In such injuries the fractured process may be driven into the upper cervical cord, leading to immediate death[67,107] or acute tetraplegia.[71] Severe retroflexion injury may result in laceration of the craniocervical junction with complete transection of the upper cervical spine and cord[38,72] or lower medulla.[188]

VERTICAL COMPRESSION AND LONGITUDINAL DISTRACTION INJURIES

Compression and longitudinal distraction injuries, which are caused mainly by vertical (cephalad–

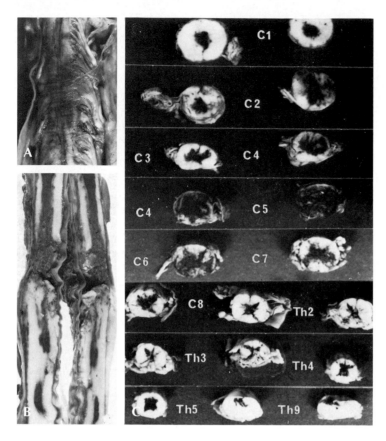

Figure 18-11. Destruction of the cord at C-7 with little local subarachnoid bleeding (*A*) and a fusiform central hemorrhage (*B*) extending to the medulla and thoracic cord (*C*). This man was found dead with a fractured cervical spine.

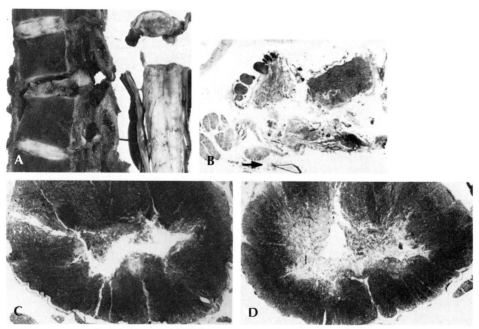

Figure 18-12. (*A*) Necrosis of cervical cord at C-7 due to fracture-dislocation with disk disruption following a dive into shallow water. (*B*) Compression of radicular artery and damage to anterior root at C-7 (*C, D*) with biconical fusiform central ischemic necrosis at C-5 to T-1.

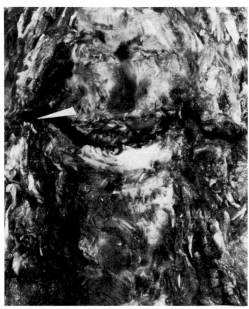

Figure 18-13. Tear at C-5–C-6 intervertebral disk following hyperextension injury of the neck with kinking of the left vertebral artery embedded in a blood clot (*arrow*). (Courtesy Dr. J. T. Hughes)

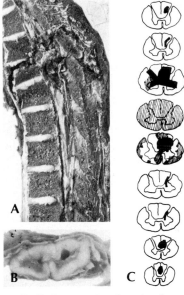

Figure 18-14. (*A, B*) Compression–bursting fracture of C-7 with displacement of the vertebral body causing compression of cord. (*C*) Diagram of cord lesion extending from C-5 to T-4.

caudal) stress to the vertebral column due to falls on the head, buttocks, or neck, car accidents, and so on, result in either fracture of the end-plates and flattening of the vertebral body or, when the acceleration impact and force magnitude exceed their structural tolerance but do not rupture the ligamentous complex, bursting of the nucleus or intervertebral disk. The majority of these injuries occur at the thoracolumbar junction (T-12 to L-2 levels)—the most movable part of the thoracolumbar spine, in the lower cervical column (Fig. 18-14), and, less often, at the thoracic level. They are associated with anterior or, more often, posterior displacement of bony fragments, that is, protrusion of the compressed vertebral body into the transverse plane or acute retropulsion of a ruptured disk,[48] which compresses the spinal cord (see Figs. 18-8, 18-14). The degree of damage to the cord varies greatly. Because the space between it and the bony canal is greater at the thoracic than at the cervical level, the cord is less constantly damaged, and its injury is often incomplete. In severe cases, however, there may be complete or almost total destruction of the neural tissue at the level of the lesion.

Autopsy and surgical findings of constricted and elongated segments in the cervical and thoracic cord following violent forces in infants suggests that longitudinal distraction, rather than flexion or extension–compression, is the mechanism involved.[30,54] During a forceful breech extraction the spinal cord can be ruptured by longitudinal distraction along with its investing dura and leptomeninges, whereas the vertebral column will remain completely intact.[56,97,168] Due to the physiologic susceptibility of the neonatal and infant spine to traction and shearing forces, damage occurs more readily to the cord than to bony structures. The more elastic the spine, the more serious the cord lesions will be with longitudinal distraction.[120]

ROTATION INJURIES

Rotation injuries, which may involve all parts of the vertebral body, its articulations, pedicles, and the ligamentous complex, result in unilateral or bilateral dislocation or stable or unstable fracture-dislocation due to interlocking of the bodies and destruction of the intervertebral disks. In rotational fracture-dislocations, which are most common in the thoracolumbar junction and upper lumbar spine, the effects on the cord are due more to compression and less to the sudden jar at the time of accident. This type of injury is almost invariably associated with severe damage to the cord and roots in the conus–cauda region.[68,75]

COMBINED INJURIES

Combined mechanisms occur in a large number of spine and spinal cord injuries, particularly in the cervical region, which shows the highest incidence of dislocations, followed by the lower thoracic region. Pure flexion or extension forces do not produce ligamentous rupture, dislocation, or fracture-dislocation. For these to occur, rotation forces must also be present at the time of the accident.[136] Frequently associated lesions, including lacerated ligaments, tearing of disks, and various types of cord and root lesions, result from a variable combination of physical forces. The most important combinations will be discussed here.[75]

Flexion–rotation injuries produce unstable fracture-dislocation with rupture of the posterior ligament, separation of the spinous processes, and fracture or dislocation of the lower articular processes of the upper vertebra. Injuries of this type result in either unilateral or bilateral facet dislocation and fracture-dislocation. The unilateral type is always associated with rupture of the corresponding joint capsule and supraspinous and interspinous ligaments[18]. Bilateral facet dislocation and fracture-dislocation commonly produces rupture of the posterior ligament, supraspinous and interspinous ligaments, and ligamentum flavum, and often shows compression or crushing of the cord.[136,179]

Retroflexion–rotation injuries of the neck produce rupture of the anterior longitudinal ligament or posterior subluxation or dislocation of the superior vertebral body, often resulting in compression (pinching) of the cord. When cervical spondylosis is present, minor trauma may produce subluxation without rupture of the anterior longitudinal liga-

ment.[24] Similar injuries affect the lower thoracic and lumbar spine less frequently.[136]

Ventroflexion and dorsiflexion plus rotation, compression, and tearing of the cervical spine occurs in posteroanterior acceleration injury of the neck, commonly referred to as *whiplash injury.* In angular acceleration of the head and neck,[172] severe rotation and translational acceleration trauma of the head create excessive distortion of the spine, leading to damage of the neck soft tissue and muscles, anterior and posterior ligament, nerve roots, and disks, with or without damage to the cord.[44,107,109] The severity and incidence of these injuries is related to the motion of the head and spine during acceleration. In fatal cases of craniospinal injury, which typically result from traffic accidents in which the person dies immediately, there is a marked tendency for the spine and cord to be damaged in the upper or lower cervical regions.[38,107] In some of these combined injuries, usually caused by impact to the forehead and face, a combination of dorsiflexion and distortion of the spine, with or without rotation, results in fracture-dislocation or dislocation of the lower cervical column and disruption of ligaments and disks with anteroposterior compression of the cord (see Fig. 18-12).

Similar complex mechanisms include ventroflexion and dorsiflexion of the neck with rotation or distorsion occurring in swimming, gymnastic, and traffic accidents, and cervicomedullary injuries with or without osseous or ligamentous damage occurring in football. These injuries are usually complicated by hemorrhages or central destruction of the upper cervical cord.[100,130,150] Comparable or less severe damage that involved the cervical region and lower parts of the cord was observed in experimental whiplash injury[116] and rotational acceleration of the head in which acceleration peaks of 40,000 radians/sec with a duration of 5 msec also produced cerebral contusions.[172]

In whiplash injury to the head and neck following posteroanterior acceleration of the whole body, generally produced by a rear-end car collision, the severity of damage to the head, cervical spine, and associated tissues is related to the velocity of the impact and the movement of the head and spine during acceleration. Movement is characterized by ultra-rapid oscillations of the head, forward and backward.[105,117] According to mathematical models,[109,118] initial flexion of the head is accompanied by high acceleration levels. The degree of flexion appears to decrease with increasing car seat stiffness. The force and bending movements most likely to cause injury were found to reach a maximum during retroflexion. Their greatest amplitude was in the lower cervical region, where they may produce tearing of the disks.[45] Whiplash injury often occurs without fracture or dislocation of the cervical spine. It may be associated with hemorrhage into the neck soft tissue and muscles,[44,65] but only rarely results in anatomic damage to the cervical cord and roots with irreversible neurologic deficits.[45]

Other combined injuries with extreme dorsiflexion and ventroflexion of the neck with rotation, compression, distorsion, tension, and tearing forces (e.g., in diving accidents), with or without damage to the lower cervical spine and ligamentous rupture, are often associated with severe compression of the lower cervical cord (Fig. 18-15).

TYPES OF SPINAL CORD LESIONS

The extent of the damage to the spinal cord, roots, coverings, and vasculature following nonpenetrating injuries depends on the type, degree, and site of action of the physical events at the moment of trauma as well as the mechanisms of injury, while their morphologic appearance depends on the period of survival. According to their relationship to the site of injury and to the presumed pathogenesis, the pathologic changes are separated into three major groups:[75,89,107]

1. The *main damage*, situated at the level of or adjacent to the site of injury, represents the local consequence of physical trauma. It has its largest transverse extent at the site of the maximum load of violence to the spine and cord, and may extend several segments above or below the point of bruising. The main damage includes laceration of the meninges; extradural, subdural, and subarachnoid hemorrhage; and damage to the cord ranging from petechial hemorrhage and edema to extensive hemorrhage, necrosis, or compression lesions. It may be accompanied by damage to spinal roots and vasculature, leading to secondary ischemic cord lesions.

2. *Neighboring lesions*, occurring in the areas adjacent to the main damage, include hemorrhages, ischemic or hemorrhagic necroses, central areas of cone-shaped or cylindrical necrosis (often extending a considerable distance above and below the initial point of injury), and edema progressing in both transverse and longitudinal directions with formation of focal vacuolar or spongy lesions, particularly in the peripheral white matter. These lesions, considered to be chiefly of secondary traumatic origin, occur after latent periods and result from a complex variety of noxious factors.

3. *Remote lesions*, without direct local relationship to the primary site of injury and commonly without apparent local damage to the spine and cord, include central hemorrhage

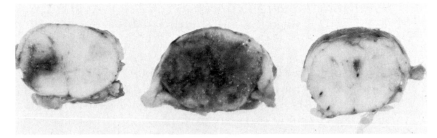

Figure 18-15. Hemorrhagic necrosis of entire cord at the C-4 level with fracture-dislocation in a diving accident. (Courtesy of Dr. R. Lindenberg)

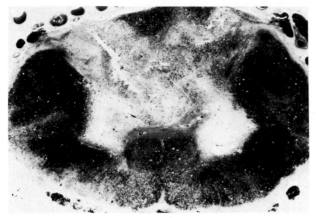

Figure 18-16. Late stage of central liquefaction necrosis in posterior columns of low thoracic cord ("remote lesion").

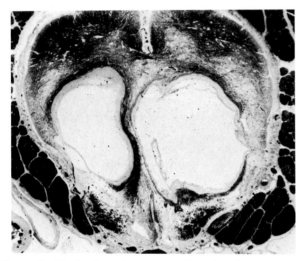

Figure 18-17. Cystic cavities in sacral cord with progressive clinical symptoms 15 years following fracture of the thoracic spine.

or cylindrical necrosis that often extends over several segments and later gives rise to cystic lesions or isolated necrotic foci (Figs. 18-16, 18-17). Most remote lesions are considered to be results of secondary or posttraumatic circulation disorders.[49,76,89] Depending on the period of survival, the pathologic lesions can be categorized as early or acute, intermediate, and late

changes, the character and chronological consequences of which are similar to those in penetrating injuries.[12,68,75,89,107] It has been implied that, except for petechial hemorrhage (Fig. 18-18), the human spinal cord may show no significant macroscopic or histopathologic changes until 6 to 24 hours after trauma.[75,83] Therefore, there is a considerable latent period between the moment of injury and the necrosis in the traumatized area of the spinal cord. This has been confirmed in several trauma models.[11,12,43,119]

EXTRAMEDULLAR HEMORRHAGES

Traumatic epidural and subdural bleeding is rather uncommon in adults and almost never causes cord compression;[89,107,184] however, such hemorrhages are more common in the absence of significant spinal injury.[29,76,106] Among 94 fatal spinal injuries, Holzer and Kloss[67] saw 3.6% epidural, 4.3% subdural, and 7.5% combined subdural and epidural hemorrhages. Klaue[89] found 2.3% subdural hematomas among 130 autopsies of spinal injuries from World War II. Extensive extradural and subarachnoid hemorrhage was common in the acute fatal spinal injuries reported by Kakulas and Bedbrook.[83] Extradural spinal bleeds are also frequent in birth injuries and perinatal distress.[34,168,167]

Traumatic spinal epidural hematoma is of less clinical importance than spontaneous extradural hemorrhage, although mild trauma has been considered a precipitating factor in some such cases.[29,76] Epidural hematoma was found in 0.5% to 1.4% of spinal injuries with vertebral fractures.[50,187] Davis and associates[38] noted spinal extradural hemorrhage associated with spinal fracture only in nine of 180 cases, some of them causing compression damage to the spinal cord (Fig. 18-19, 18-20).[69,75] Spinal epidural hemorrhage was also reported after minor trauma or microtrauma in the absence of bony damage with slowly progressive cord lesions.[29,104]

Spinal subdural hematoma following major injury in adults is rare, except when associated with thrombocytopenia or other bleeding disorders.[76] Only three of Klaue's[89] 130 autopsy cases of spinal

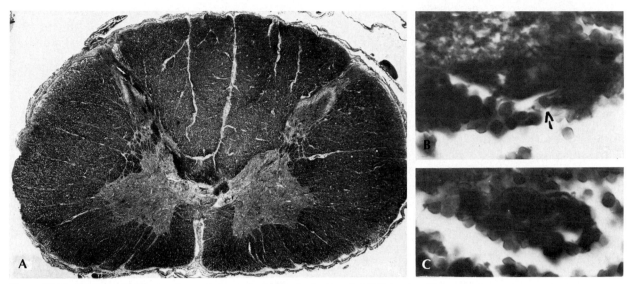

Figure 18-18. (*A*) Petechial hemorrhages in posterior horn of spinal cord at C-5 due to phleborrhexis (*arrow*) (*B, C*) following neck injury; patient survived 18 hours.

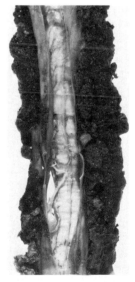

Figure 18-19. Extensive extradural spinal hemorrhage due to acute lethal fracture of the neck from a fall down an elevator shaft. (Courtesy of Dr. R. Lindenberg)

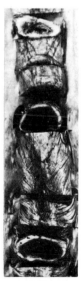

Figure 18-20. True hematomyelia due to rupture of intramedullary arteriovenous malformation (AVM).

injuries had extensive spinal subdural hematomas, and none of these caused cord compression. In rare cases, chronic spinal subdural hemorrhage was seen following very minor trauma, causing progressive cord compression.[161,191] Spinal subdural hematoma often occurs following birth injury and is considered an important factor in perinatal paraplegia.[167] Obstetric trauma may cause both subdural and epidural spinal hematomas.

Spinal subarachnoid hemorrhage as a result of severe injury to the spinal axis is very rare in comparison to intracranial traumatic subarachnoid bleedings,[89,107] except in patients with bleeding disorders and in the perinatal period.[22,34] Hemorrhage to the upper cervical pioarachnoid, however, is not infrequently seen in acute fatal craniocerebral and craniospinal injuries.[38,83,95] Spinal contusions are usually associated with small local subarachnoid hemorrhages beneath the area of impact, with a slight tendency toward further increase.[12,75] In experimental spinal cord injury, pioarachnoidal hemorrhage is first observed at the area of impact. It surrounds the cord within 30 minutes, with no further increase for up to 4 hours after injury.[175] Mild trauma may be a precipitating factor of intrathecal hemorrhages resulting from spinal angiomas and other vascular malformations or tumors.[76,77]

CONCUSSION OF THE SPINAL CORD

Spinal cord concussion, a reversible disturbance of spinal cord function caused by sudden jarring of the spine, implies functional disorders for which the histopathology is unknown. Similar to cerebral concussion, this condition is attributed to a variety of conditions and pathogenic factors.[75] Based on experimental data, it has been related to transitory changes of nerve cells and axons, and of microcirculation and vascular permeability, as seen in transitory traumatic paraplegia.[41-43,175] Similar transitory extravasation of labeled serum proteins in the brainstem and upper cervical cord has been observed in experimental percussion–concussion due to sudden mechanical loading of the brain of some milliseconds.[135] Neuronal or metabolic changes with axonal damage have been related to sudden and short-lasting pressure changes and tissue deformity, causing axonal reactions without anatomic residual lesions.[128,129] In humans, however, the pathogenic mechanisms of spinal cord concussion are still poorly understood.

COMPRESSION OF THE SPINAL CORD

A sudden or permanent reduction of between 30% to almost 50% of the anteroposterior diameter of the spinal canal is generally tolerated before the cord suffers from compression damage.[70,143] Compression of the cord may result from fracture-dislocation or dislocation of vertebrae by more than one third of their diameter, or by bony or cartilaginous protrusions, hernial disks, dislocated slivers of bone, exostoses, or spondylotic bars. In stable fracture-dislocations the vertebrae may return to their normal position; however, in unstable fractures the damaged vertebrae are still capable of moving and may intensify damage to the cord. Because many of the lesions are unstable or restorable by adequate treatment, bony or cartilaginous compression that may cause serious damage to the cord at the time of injury frequently are not detected at autopsy.[68,83,89,185]

Compression of the cord rarely occurs from extensive extramedullary hemorrhage. Damage to the cervical cord often results from acute or transitory compression in flexion–extension traumas due to pinching or squeezing mechanisms. Damage to the cord in fracture-dislocation of the thoracic and lumbar spine is more often due to permanent compression than to the sudden jar of the accident. Because the space within the spinal canal is greater at the thoracolumbar level than in the cervical region, the lower parts of cord are less permanently damaged and the lesions are often incomplete. Vertical compression fracture of the low thoracic spine only rarely produces permanent compression of the cord. Despite spontaneous or therapeutic restoration of the bony alignment, compression of the cord may result from sheared-off bony spicules occasionally unrecognized on radiographs or computed tomographic scans (Fig. 18-21).

The pathologic findings of spinal cord compression are necrosis, hemorrhages, and edema, the severity and extent of which greatly depend on the

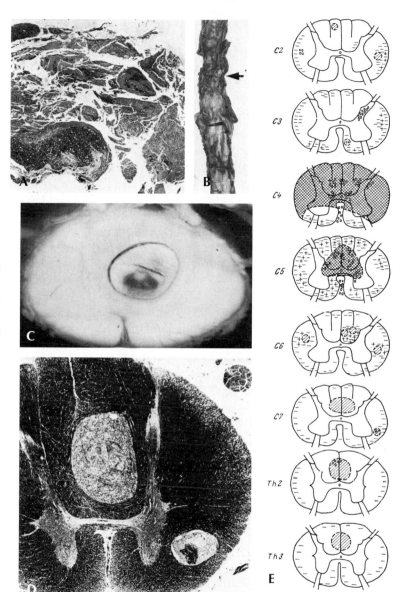

Figure 18-21. (*A*) Compression of cervical cord at C-4 level due to unrecognized bony spicule (*B, arrow*) in fracture-disclocation at C-4 after a drunken fall; patient survived 4 days. (*C, D*) Multisegmental fusiform central necrosis in posterior columns and small necrotic focus in ventrolateral white matter. (*E*) Diagram of spinal cord lesions.

intensity and course of compression.[12,43,75,164,165] Grossly, the cord appears narrow and constricted, with edematous swelling above and below. Local changes at the site of compression range from edema, hemorrhage, and necrosis or tissue disintegration spreading from the central gray matter to the periphery, and from the level of compression rostrally and caudally, to almost complete transverse necrosis. They are often associated with central cone-shaped cylindrical necroses in the ventral portion of the posterior funiculi or extending upward and downward over some distance in other parts of the white matter (see Fig. 18-21), with spongy necroses or vacuolating foci in the marginal white matter, or with ischemic infarctions of adjacent segments resulting from microcirculation disorders or compression of radicular or spinal cord vessels (see Figs. 18-12, 18-21).

With longer survival, the acute changes subside and are gradually replaced after several days by demyelination, degradation, and reparative changes, leading to the formation of cystic cavities or glial or gliocollagenous scars, which replace the necrotic areas. After survival periods of months or years, at the level of the fracture-dislocation there is a dense fibrous scar with adjacent meninges and partial obliteration of the subarachnoid space. The cord becomes thinned and sclerotic or partially or completely demyelinated with anterior root degeneration (Fig. 18-22), or is converted into a fibrous or gliotic band, with cysts present in both the thickened pia-arachnoid and the spinal cord.

From experimental models of mechanical cord compression with impact trauma causing either reversible or irreversible neurologic deficits, a composite of pathogenic factors producing cord injury has been discussed.[7,12,43,164,165] In addition to mechanical deformation and distortion of axons and other tissue elements due to pressure and axial tension, depression of metabolic rate and ischemia due to microcirculation disorders, vasospasm or vascular compression, and shifts in electrolytes appear to be important for the development of edema and tissue necrosis, although many of the underlying mechanisms need to be further elucidated.

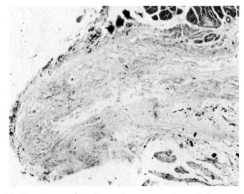

Figure 18-22. Demyelination of cross section of the conus and anterior roots following compression fracture at the T-11 level; patient survived 2 months.

CONTUSION OF THE SPINAL CORD

Contusion includes all traumatic changes of the cord and its coverings resulting from indirect (blunt) violence. This violence is transmitted to the cord in nondisruptive crush injuries that do not display the continuing compression and reversible dysfunctions characteristic of concussion. The underlying pathologic changes range in severity from minimal petechial hemorrhages and axonal lesions to extensive crushing in which the cord is pulped, or almost complete transverse necrosis. Complete tears are rare. The pathology of the lesions is similar to that of cerebral contusions, and is graded in three stages:[68,75,89,107]

Early (acute) stage of hemorrhage and necrosis
Intermediate stage of resorption and organization
Final or defective stage

EARLY STAGE

Early pathologic changes are hemorrhage and necrosis in the central gray matter at the site of impact, progressing to the adjacent white matter. In acute fatal cases surviving less than 6 to 24 hours, conspicuous changes, other than petechial hemorrhages in the central gray matter, are unusual or absent (see Figs. 18-6, 18-18). Grossly, the cord at the site of impact may be flattened, with transverse grooving, or soft and swollen, of bluish-red discoloration. The pia-arachnoid is hemorrhagic, but usually intact (see Fig. 18-11). On section, there are small hemorrhagic foci in the gray matter. These are often confined to its central parts, but may involve one or both posterior horns or the whole gray matter (Fig. 18-23; see Fig. 18-15). The limits between gray and white matter have usually disappeared. Disruption of the pia-arachnoid with extrusion of cord substance or complete tears is rare even with massive fracture-dislocation. The lesion is rarely of a single transverse type, involving only one or two segments at the site of impact (see Fig. 18-15). It often extends in a tapering fashion for some distance above and below the maximum lesion (see Figs. 18-9, 18-11,

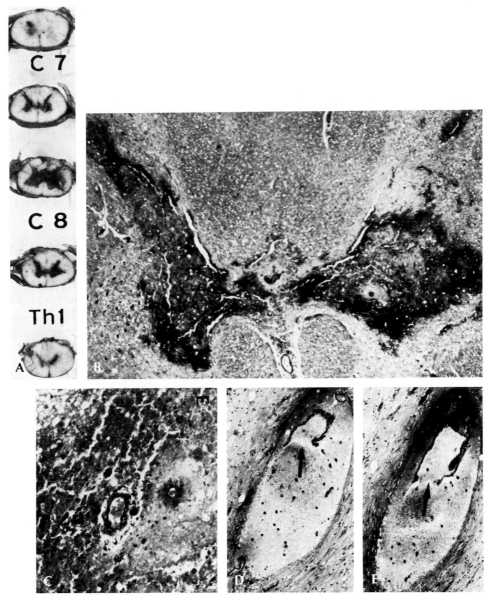

Figure 18-23. (*A, B*) Butterflylike hemorrhage due to coalescent hemorrhages in central gray matter following hyperextension injury; patient survived 2 days. (*C, D*) Rupture of small vessels (*arrows*). Fibrinoid necrosis and (*E*) thrombosis of small vessels in necrotic cord area.

18-23). In a recent magnetic resonance imaging series five of 19 patients with acute cord injury showed hemorrhagic foci.[92]

Histologically, the early stage shows small hemorrhages, primarily situated in the ventral part of the posterior horn and around the central canal (see Fig. 18-18). They result from initial extravasation of erythrocytes around thin vessels. Rhexic bleeding originating from traumatic tears of small intramedullary vessels has been observed in early fatal cases (see Fig. 18-23).[75,89,107,184,185]

The vulnerability of the central gray matter may be due to both local structures and the different vascularization of the gray and white matter. It is believed that the earliest changes in spinal cord contusion are disruption of axons and capillary endothelial cell junctions in the central gray matter. This demonstrates the high and uniform density of the microvasculature.[170] Disruption of small vessels in the central gray matter near the central canal could be caused by mechanisms similar to the "central cavitation effect," which results in periventricular and subependymal hemorrhages in craniocerebral trauma.[171] In addition, longitudinal and transverse tearing, stretching, rotational, and combined forces may be active. These forces may also cause tears and hemorrhages in the spinal roots of the injured segments.[75,95,107]

Initial leakage of erythrocytes is followed by capillary and venous engorgement, coalescence of disseminated them, and extension of microhemorrhages into most of the gray matter, which becomes edematous and necrotic. As early as 2 to 4 hours after trauma there is considerable vascular congestion, edema, and damage to the vessel walls, with leakage of protein-rich edema fluid (vasogenic edema) into the adjacent tissue. Additional confluent hemorrhages arise from rupture of congested intramedullary venules. This has been demonstrated on serial sections (see Figs. 18-18, 8-23).

In crushed areas there is often fibrinoid necrosis, endothelial swelling with occasional obliteration, occlusion, and thrombosis of small intramedullary vessels (see Fig. 18-23) and pial veins. Occlusion of arteries with recent fibrin thrombi was observed in the meninges and spinal cord within 24 hours after injury.[185] The central area of the crushed cord also includes a zone of mechanically damaged nervous tissue, with disruption of cell membranes and axons undergoing liquefaction necrosis with dissolution and disintegration. In severe trauma producing complete segmental necrosis at the site of injury, the central lesion involves large parts of gray matter within a few hours after trauma. Chromatolysis, neuronal death, disruption, and swelling of axons and myelin are demonstrable. By 8 to 24 hours there is centrifugal progression of both necrosis and hemorrhages from the gray to the adjacent white matter and to the periphery of the cord, and from the impact area rostrally and caudally. The lesions are accompanied by considerable edema, which also tends to progress in both centrifugal and longitudinal directions, causing vacuolation of the white matter with swelling and disintegration of axons and myelin (Fig. 18-24). Finally, the whole cross section of the cord is involved, becoming round and tense. Within its coverings the subarachnoid and subdural spaces are obliterated. In persons who survive the first 24 hours, cellular reactions become obvious. Areas of gross injury experience hemorrhagic necrosis with leukocytic infiltrates, followed by mobilization of macrophages, which introduce resorption and degradation of damaged tissues.

Although hemorrhage and hemorrhagic necrosis are sometimes confined to the site of impact, the bleeding often extends as a fusiform mass for some distance above and below the level of injury. *Traumatic hematomyelia*, a term introduced by Ollivier[115] and Cruveilhier,[36] refers to this collection of blood within the cord, ranging in extent from small coalescent hemorrhages to solid intramedullary clots of blood extending longitudinally over several segments, usually in the ventral part of the posterior columns next to the central canal (see Figs. 18-9, 18-11, 18-23). Marburg[103] differentiated four groups of hemorrhagic cord lesions following trauma:

1. Multiple small hemorrhages of petechial type due to diapedesis
2. Large primary traumatic tubular or fusiform hemorrhage resulting from ruptured vessels

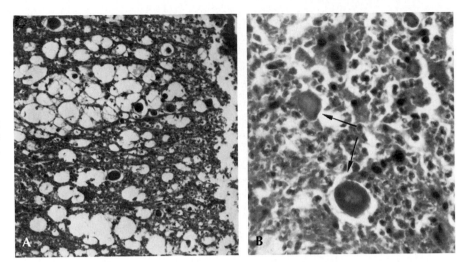

Figure 18-24. (*A, B*) Peritraumatic edema with spongy changes of white matter and axonal swellings (*arrows*).

3. Secondary bleeding into adjacent tissue due to reactive venorhexis and microcirculation disorders
4. Hemorrhagic necrosis ("red malacia") resulting from both primary mechanical and secondary lesions

Although Oppenheim[118a] and others have claimed that about 90% of all cases of hematomyelia are of traumatic origin, solid fusiform hematoma is considered to be a rare event following spinal injury,[75,89,103,185] seen in only 0.8% of one autopsy series.[40] However, it is a frequent complication of spinal vascular malformations (see Fig. 18-20)[77] and other disorders.[85,96]

Central hemorrhagic necrosis of the gray matter, with variable longitudinal extension, is the most common and characteristic type of cord lesion in human and experimental spinal cord trauma. It is to be distinguished from other types of central cord necrosis. *Central spinal cord infarction* with or without hemorrhages may occur at the site of impact and extend as a fusiform lesion for some distance above and below the level of injury (Fig. 18-25). It is attributed to spinal cord circulation disorders related to trauma, for example, com-

pression, kinking or thrombosis of vertebral arteries after hyperextension injury of the neck,[3,52,59,68,141,150] compression or occlusion of radicular tributaries or spinal cord vessels—only rarely confirmed at autopsy,[75,77,185] or otherwise compromised blood flow in the central spinal cord areas.[148]

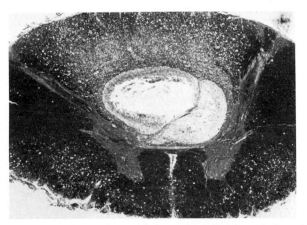

Figure 18-25. Bilateral central cystic necrosis of cervical cord following hyperextension injury of the neck; patient survived 6 months.

Central fusiform necrosis, usually confined to the ventral portions of the posterior columns next to the central canal, is a frequent lesion in spinal injury and cord compression (Fig. 18-26; see Figs. 18-16, 18-17, 18-21, 18-25). It extends above or below the site of trauma or resembles a remote lesion without local relation to the original crushing. The early changes are edema, axonal swelling, and myelin breakdown associated with congestion and fibrinoid necrosis of small vessels, plasmatic exudation, and some hemorrhage (Fig. 18-27). Fusiform lesions later undergo progressive liquefaction with little degradation and gliomesenchymal reaction, finally resulting in large cylindrical cysts or cavities filled with creamy debris or clear fluid (see Fig. 18-16), referred to as "cysts with necrotic contents."[89,103] These fusiform necroses, which are also seen in a variety of spinal cord lesions (e.g., compression, myelitis, and infarction) are rarely found in acute fatal spinal injury. More often, after 3 to 4 days survival,[69,75,89,107] they have been attributed to either primary mechanical disruption of axons in the posterior columns due to compression and tearing forces[107] or microcirculation disorders and loss of perfusion through arteries[13] or venous drainage disorders.[76,75,148]

Experimental trauma models using various mechanisms of spinal cord injury have confirmed

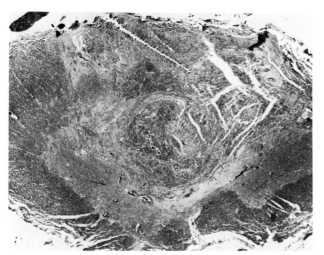

Figure 18-26. Central necrosis in ventral part of posterior columns at C-6 following a car accident, with fracture-dislocation at C-3–C-4; patient survived 6 days.

the pathologic sequential evolutionary development of lesions in humans.[11,12,43,84,119] In severe experimental injury, hemorrhage and necrosis involve the central gray matter as early as 5 to 30 minutes following trauma. They then spread to the periphery of the impact site, being initially complete in the gray matter by 4 hours and producing necrosis of the entire cross section of the cord, including white matter, after only 8 to 24 hours. The lesions show progression from the impact site rostrally and caudally at about 18 hours after injury, and usually result in a fusiform zone of necrosis involving the complete cross-sectional area of the cord and tapering off above and below in a conical manner, the tapering portions of the necrotic lesions being longer than the area of maximum necrosis (see Fig. 18-27). This configuration of cord necrosis is similar to that found in human spinal injuries and in spinal cord necrosis attributable to spinal cord vascular disease.[11,12,74,148]

Light and electron microscopic studies have shown that the earliest tissue damage is mechanical, with disruption of tissue membranes, tearing of axons, and disruption of intramedullary blood vessels causing petechial hemorrhages and alterations of the blood–cord barrier.[11-13,21,43,84,148] Hemorrhages, fibrinoid necrosis, and disruption of major and small vessels and of endothelial cell junctions are observed immediately after impact. These are followed by increased pinocytotic activity of endothelial cells and an increase of extracellular space, shown ultrastructurally as early as 15 minutes after trauma.[41,58]

Traumatic hemorrhages due to vascular disruption are followed by secondary bleeds due to stasis and perfusion disorders. These lesions usually antedate the evolution of parenchymal necrosis and ischemia with neuronal and myelinic disintegration seen at 2 to 4 hours after injury. Perivascular edema and necrosis are first seen at the site of injury, and subsequently progress in a radial and longitudinal direction. About 24 hours after injury the damaged cord is composed of hemorrhagic necrosis with only a small rim of intact white matter. At the necrotic margins, leukocytes are present, and edema or demyelination develop further.

The nature and time course of progressive hemorrhagic necrosis of the spinal cord after injury in humans has generally been confirmed in experi-

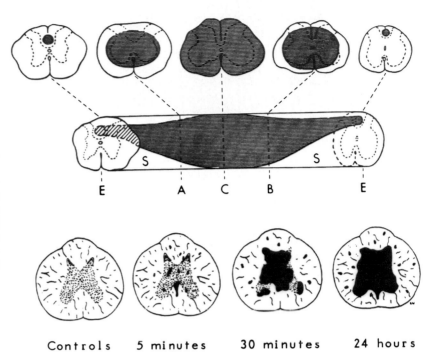

Figure 18-27. (A) Biconical configuration of experimental spinal cord injury with maximum necrosis of entire cross section (C). There is extension above and below (A, B) with tapering ends (E) in the posterior columns. (Adapted from Balentine JD: Pathology of experimental spinal cord trauma: I. The necrotic lesion as a function of vascular injury Lab Invest 39:236–253, 1978); (B) Evolution of necrosis and hemorrhage at the level of experimental trauma. (Adapted from Dohrmann GJ, Wick KM, Bucy PC: Spinal cord blood flow patterns in experimental traumatic paraplegia. J Neurosurg 38:52–58, 1973)

mental animals. It is suggested that the very early damage is mechanical, but that this is aggravated by a composite of various factors, including ischemia, energy dysfunctions and edema due to microcirculation, and biochemical disorders (e.g., electrolyte shifts, free radical generation, neuromediator changes, and calcium toxicity). The exact effectiveness of the multifactoral mechanisms in both experimental and human spinal cord injury, documented by a considerable latent period between the moment of impact and the full development of necrosis in the traumatized area and adjoining regions, however, awaits further elucidation.

INTERMEDIATE STAGE

Intermediate pathologic changes differ from those in the early and late stages. At about 24 to 48 hours after injury, the transverse progression of the acute hemorrhagic necrosis becomes maximal and complete. Longitudinal spread of necrosis and edema may continue for 3 to 6 days after trauma. Within 2 to 3 weeks the acute changes are gradu-

ally replaced by resorption and a reparative phase that may continue for up to several months or years.

The edema largely subsides and the small hemorrhages are absorbed during the first 1 to 2 weeks following trauma, leaving only a few iron-pigment or hemosiderin-laden phagocytes. The pleomorphic leukocytes of the early reaction are replaced by lymphocytes and macrophages, which invade the margins of the necrotic area. There is progressive destruction of myelin with partial or complete demyelination of the damaged segment and adjoining areas (Figs. 18-28 to 18-33; see Fig 18-22). Lipid phagocytes invade the necrotic areas and are frequently clustered around small vessels. In grossly damaged areas there are countless closely apposed phagocytes; where the damage is slight, as in margins of the injury, scattered phagocytes are found.

The development of reactive astrocytic gliosis in any particular part of the lesion depends on the degree of tissue damage: where this is mild, reactive astrocytosis starts at about 24 to 36 hours after injury. In severely damaged areas, however,

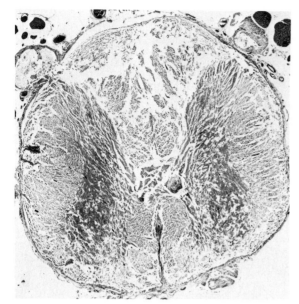

Figure 18-28. Demyelination of whole cross section of lumbar cord following gunshot fracture of the thoracic spine; patient survived 4 weeks.

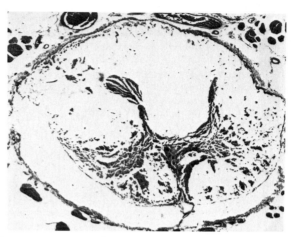

Figure 18-29. Cystic destruction of midthoracic cord following fracture-dislocation; patient survived 6 weeks.

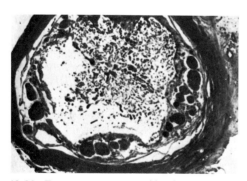

Figure 18-30. Transverse necrosis of lumbar cord with meningeal fibrosis after compression fracture; patient survived 2 months.

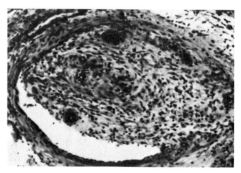

Figure 18-31. Post-traumatic vasopathy with intimal proliferation of anterior spinal artery 4 weeks after low thoracic vertebral fracture.

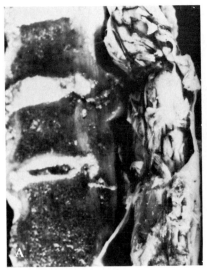
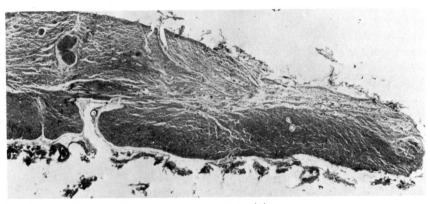

Figure 18-32. (*A*) Chronic delayed cervical myelopathy 12 years after hyperextension injury of the neck with progressive paraplegia. *A* shows fusion of cervical vertebrae with spondylotic ridge narrowing the spinal canal. (*B*) There is grooving and flattening of the cord at C-4 with demyelination of posterolateral areas. Small intramedullary neuroma in the posterior fissure is seen (*arrow*).

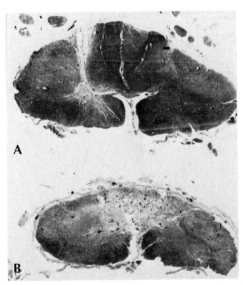

Figure 18-33. Delayed myelopathy following traumatic atlanto-axial dislocation. Degeneration of posterior columns with small intramedullary neuromas and unilateral cystic degeneration of gray matter are seen (myelin stain).

where the astroglia is damaged along with the nervous parenchyma, organization is by proliferating mesenchymal elements originating from leptomeninges and vessels.

Where there is progressive cystic transformation of the central necrotic areas or of almost the entire spinal cord, only small areas of marginal white matter are preserved (see Figs. 18-30, 18-32). The resolving area is surrounded by a highly vascularized granulation tissue, which replaces the defect in a centripetal direction. Vascular proliferation may occur, particularly in the preserved areas of the gray matter and in the anterior fissure, progressing to the central areas,[103] but vascular proliferation may be missing. Other vascular changes, for example, intimal proliferation and obliterative angiopathy (see Figs. 18-22, 18-32, 18-33), have been seen as early as 4 weeks after injury,[76,103,184] and may cause secondary ischemic infarction at sites remote from the original site of injury.

Cavitating necroses and focal lacunar lesions found in areas adjacent to the contusion undergo liquefaction and are transformed into cysts surrounded by gliomesenchymal scars (see Fig. 18-16). Many of the surviving axons bordering the lesions are swollen, and remaining neurons show central chromatolysis (axonal reaction), which may persist for up to 3 years.[68] At some time after injury, secondary degeneration of the long fiber tracts and of spinal roots starts, the latter usually more severely involving the anterior roots.

FINAL OR DEFECTIVE STAGE

As time progresses, the pathologic picture gradually changes, and the damaged parts of the cord are replaced by scar formation. After survival periods of 5 years and more, at the level of an old fracture-dislocation, a dense fibrous scar is formed by fusion of the thickened periosteum with the dura mater. The arachnoid is thickened and discolored from residual hemorrhage, and the subarachnoid space is partially obliterated. The cord is constricted with atrophy, loss of parenchyma, or cystic dissolution, and shows obscured architectural markings.[10,79,83,89,103,183,184]

In persons surving months or years following nondisruptive cord injury, the cord is tapered to a narrow band surrounded by a thickened mantle of fibrotic meninges or a massive duromeningeal scar adhering to the cord. The cord shows local defects or extensive cystic destruction, or is largely replaced by connective tissue with numerous cavities (Figs. 18-34, 18-35, 18-36). Remnants of nervous tissue and gliotic islands may be seen within the fibrous scar (see Fig. 18-32).

After total disruption or complete loss of spinal cord substance, the cord is replaced by fibrous scar tissue and there is loss of continuity between the two ends of the divided cord,[83] although a total gap between the disrupted ends of the cord is rare. There may be loss of normal structures with demyelination or cystic cavitations (see Figs. 18-34, 18-35, 18-36), or replacement of most of the cross section by a large cavity formed by highly vascularized fibrous tissue and surrounded by thickened meninges (see Figs. 18-32, 18-33). The less damaged regions of the cord and a zone above and below the main damage always show intense

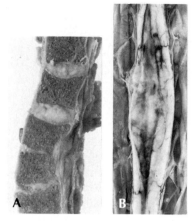

Figure 18-34. Late stages of spinal injury. (*A*) Fusion of cervical vertebrae and (*B*) anterior aspect of damaged cord with dura opened, 5 years after a fall from a window.

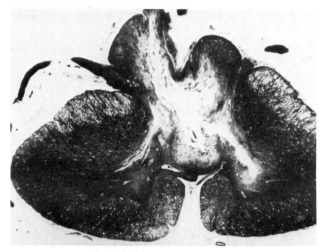

Figure 18-35. Central cystic necrosis in C-5 following neck fracture; patient survived 2 years.

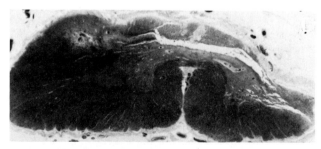

Figure 18-36. Cystic cavitating scar in posterior–posterolateral columns and gray matter of cervical cord 15 years after fracture-dislocation of C-2–C-3 (myelin stain).

gliosis. Signs of active degradation with numerous phagocytes can be seen after survival periods of 5 years and more,[83,103] whereas iron or hemosiderin from bleedings are usually absent. Regenerative phenomena are frequently seen in these traumatic scars. The spinal roots are thinned and demyelinated, and often firmly surrounded by meningeal scars.

In some patients with tetraparesis who survived neck injury without bony damage, cord lesions are limited to small gliotic foci and small cysts in central gray matter, with or without degeneration of the lateral or posterior columns (see Fig. 18-25), suggesting residues of central cervical cord injury.[10,75,186]

Cephalad or caudad from the level of traumatic injury, patchy areas of demyelination and gliosis or cystic cavities with necrotic or fluid contents surrounded by gliomesenchymal scars can be present, particularly in the ventral part of the posterior columns, representing residues of central fusiform necrosis (see Figs. 18-16, 18-34, 18-35, 18-36). Above and below the level of traumatic cord injury, there is Wallerian degeneration of the ascending and descending fiber tracts.

Nonspecific and nonprogressive changes of spinal vasculature in late stages after injury include organization and recanalization of occluded pial and intramedullary vessels, obliterative angiopathy with endothelial proliferation, splitting of the internal elastic lamina, and fibrotic thickening of intramedullary (see Figs. 18-31, 18-33) and pial vessels.[75,76,185] These late vascular changes, referred to as "post-traumatic vasopathy,"[103] may contribute to delayed ischemic cord lesions.

POST-TRAUMATIC MYELOPATHIES

Delayed post-traumatic changes of the spinal cord include early and late types of post-traumatic myelopathies. These may result from chronic biomechanical irritation, arachnopathy, vascular disorders, progressive intramedullary cyst formation, or combinations of pathogenic factors. Acute or progressive delayed myelopathies may occur following neck injuries with incompletely reduced or unstable fracture-dislocations of the cervical spine that are due to compression and tearing of the

ventral and dorsal aspects of the cord or repeated contact pressure.[24,123] Another type of progressive myelopathy is associated with central cyst formation, which clinically produces a syringomyelia syndrome that develops at various intervals after spinal injuries at various levels.[15]

Morphologic data are available on several types of myelopathy:

1. Post-traumatic cystic myelopathy (post-traumatic syringomyelia)
2. Delayed myelopathy following injury to the craniocervical junction
3. Late myelopathy of the lower cervical cord related to spondylosis
4. Delayed myelopathy associated with post-traumatic arachnopathy

POST-TRAUMATIC CYSTIC MYELOPATHY

Post-traumatic syringomyelia, post-traumatic cystic myelopathy, and post-traumatic spinal cord cysts are terms used to describe cystic cavities within the spinal cord seen at or extending cephalad or caudad from the level of traumatic injury.[15,46,51,90,110,114,160,173] Post-traumatic syringomyelia was found in 2.3% of paraplegics.[15] With respect to pathomorphology and pathogenesis, four types of intramedullary cavities, often extending over many segments, are distinguished in late stages of spinal injury:[75]

1. Sequelae of central hemorrhagic necrosis at the site of injury
2. Ischemic infarction (myelomalacia) related to spinal injury
3. Central liquefaction cysts or cavitation in posterior columns
4. Hematomyelia due to hemorrhage into preexisting syringomyelia

Central hemorrhagic necrosis, a frequent type of traumatic lesion at the site of injury and in adjacent regions, undergoes dissolution or liquefaction with subsequent peripheral organization. The resulting cavity involves the central gray and adjoining white matter (see Fig. 18-35). It may be confined to the dorsolateral quadrant of the cord, and can be unilateral or bilateral (see Fig. 18-36).

The first example was that of Bastian,[17] who reported a small cavitation in the gray matter on one side in a patient surviving traumatic tetraplegia for 6 months. The cavity, which is later surrounded by a gliomesenchymal scar or a thick collagenous lining, often shows its maximum diameter in the cervical cord. It may extend over many segments above and below the site of injury, and usually has no connection with the subarachnoid space.[15] Cavities may be multiple, or separated or crossed by glial ridges or collagenous fibers, or may replace the whole cord, which is reduced to a small rim of tissue surrounded by grossly thickened dura–arachnoid.[75,83]

Myelomalacic cysts, confined to the central gray matter with unilateral or bilateral cavitation of the anterior horns or total gray substance (see Fig. 18-25), are located at the site of injury or at a distance from it. The fusiform lesion may extend over several segments. In quality and distribution it resembles that of spinal cord infarction due to vascular disease in humans and experimental animals.[15,48,74,76,148] Impairment of vascular supply following spinal cord injury with thrombosis, occlusion, obstruction, or compression of radicular, extramedullary, and intramedullary arteries has been confirmed by selective angiography and autopsy.[75,76,184]

Central fluid-filled cysts located in the anterior parts of the posterior columns and dorsal horns, and often extending over many segments, are the most frequent substrate of "post-traumatic syringomyelia" demonstrated at autopsy,[15,46,90] at surgery,[15,114,138] or using neuroimaging methods.[33,51,132,160] These multisegmental, fluid-filled cysts are lined by glia or collagen and are separated from a central canal (see Figs. 18-16, 18-17, 18-25, 18-26). They can be crossed by glial bridges. Double cysts may be separated by nervous tissue.

All known cases of central fluid-filled cysts had cavities extending from the level of injury over some or many segments, occasionally from the lower thoracic level to the upper cervical cord or low medulla.[15,77] They lack any recognizable connection with the subarachnoid space, the central canal, or the fourth ventricle, and never show extension to the anterior horns or anterior columns. The cavities contain fluid that may be under pressure and may act as a space-occupying lesion or that may be propagated during any maneuvers that increase pressure in the subarachnoid space and thus may produce progressive neurologic deficits.[15,51]

Whatever the cause of cyst formation, pathologic studies and the high protein and cellular content of the fluid in most cavities suggest that they originate from liquefaction of necrotic cord tissue rather than from production of cerebrospinal fluid-equivalent fluid by gliotic tissue or migration of cerebrospinal fluid. The morphology and localization of these fluid-filled cavities suggest that they develop from fusiform cysts with necrotic contents,[103] which extend into the nontraumatized regions of the cord many years after the original injury and may be propagated by changes of intraspinal venous pressure.[15,182] Similar cysts are found in compressive cervical myelopathy.[80] The morphology of these lesions differs from that of idiopathic syringomyelia, although rare cases of the latter following mild trauma have been seen.[15]

A rare form of post-traumatic cystic myelopathy may result from acute hemorrhage into a pre-existing syringomyelia.[57,184] In this type, cavities are extensive, and involve almost the entire length of the cord; their walls are formed of glial tissue with numerous capillaries. Trauma, although often minimal, is thought to precipitate the acute exacerbation of "Gower's syringal hemorrhage."[124]

OTHER DELAYED POST-TRAUMATIC MYELOPATHIES

Traumatic damage to the *craniocervical junction*, with fracture of the odontoid process of the dens due to traffic or sports accidents or falls from heights, is associated in about 25% of cases with severe neurologic deficits. In acute fatal cases it is complicated by compression, traction, or disruption of the upper cervical cord from the medulla.[10,107] Craniocervical junction injuries can be complicated by delayed acute fatal spinal cord compression due to an unstable dislocation of the odontoid process occurring weeks to years after a primarily noncomplicated injury.[71,87,150] Chronic delayed myelopathy, a rare complication of fracture-dislocation of the odontoid, is similar in its clinicopathologic appearance to that associated with developmental anomalies of the craniocervical junction.[37,174]

Of 30 clinically reported cases, only seven have been studied at autopsy.[78] There is considerable narrowing of the sagittal diameter of the upper cervical canal, with indentation due to luxation and pseudarthrosis of the atlas; a dural scar and thickened pia-arachnoid; flattening and compression of the upper cervical cord, showing demyelination or diffuse necrosis; and glial scar formation in large parts or even the whole cross section of the cord (see Fig. 18-33). Fibrosis of intramedullary vessels, but no compression or occlusion of the vertebral and spinal arteries, has been seen. Spinal cord damage is attributed to recurrent compression due to critical reduction of the anteroposterior diameter of the spinal canal and to repeated biomechanical stresses on the cord due factors such as hyperextension, angulation, torsion, and tension with neck movements, complicated by hypertrophic arachnopathy and circulation disorders related to chronic biomechanical stresses.[75,78]

Delayed myelopathy following hyperextension and hyperflexion injury of the lower cervical spine

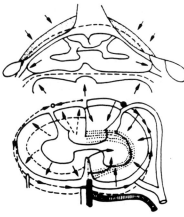

Figure 18-38. Cross section of cervical cord with arterial supply and venous drainage at lower right. (Adapted from Jellinger K: Morfologia e patogenes; delle mielorizopatie cervical; da spondilartros; In Testa C (ed): Mielorizopatie Cervical; Spondilartros, pp 35–64. Verona, Edizone Libreria Cortina, 1983)

has been observed in elderly patients, often with traumatic fusion of the cervical vertebrae superimposed by spondylotic changes and osteophytes.[123,152] As in spondylotic myelopathy, there is considerable narrowing of the sagittal diameter of the spinal canal with indentation, transverse grooving, and damage to the spinal cord ranging from pure deformity and flattening to subtotal transverse damage or central cystic necrosis with Wallerian tract degeneration.[6,68,69,80] There may be marginal demyelination or damage to the posterolateral parts of the cervical cord (see Fig. 18-32), with demyelination of the spinal roots and fibrosis of the radicular and intramedullary vessels. Progressive spinal cord damage in this condition is attributed to intermittent compression and combined biomechanical and circulatory disorders due to axial tension and distortion forces on both the cord and its vasculature. This is schematically summarized in Figures 18-37 and 18-38. The composite of various pathogenic factors appears to be similar to those suggested for cervical spondylotic myelopathies.[25,26,55,68,69,73,74,123]

Myelopathy due to *chronic arachnopathy* (adhesive spinal meningopathy) is a late complication of spinal injuries that is rare as compared with its incidence after intrathecal instillation of chemical

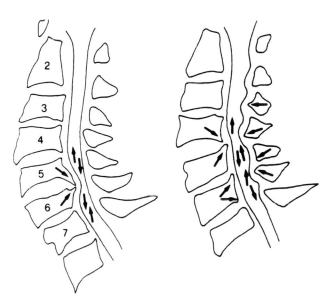

Figure 18-37. Scheme of biomechanical factors acting on the cervical cord and its vasculature during movements of the cervical spine.

agents, spinal anesthesia, or myelography.[68,69,183] Post-traumatic arachnopathy mainly involves the cervical cord, and less often the lower cord regions and cauda equina. It is associated with marginal demyelination, diffuse or focal lesions with gliosis, infarction or cystic necrosis of central parts of the cord, and pathologic changes of small arachnoid or perimedullary arteries without considerable involvement of intramedullary vessels.[75]

These lesions are attributed to direct pressure or chronic permeability disorders of the pia-glia and to microcirculation disorders of the marginal spinal cord vasculature. Besides marginal cord lesions in the supply areas of small perimedullary arteries, there may be damage to central parts of the cord supplied by intramedullary vessels.

The morphologic features of this type of myelopathy are similar to those found in chronic meningitis, meningovascular syphilis, or other chronic perimedullary processes.[69,112,148]

NEONATAL AND INFANTILE SPINAL CORD TRAUMA

Although birth injuries of the vertebral column are comparatively rare,[111,120,127] spinal cord lesions are frequently encountered in newborn infants[5]; however, spinal cord injury is uncommon from infancy to 15 years of age.[120] In an unselected series of fetal and neonatal autopsies in which a complete neuropathologic examination was performed, injury to the spinal cord and its coverings were observed in 10% to 33% of the cases.[34,167,168] Fractures of the spinal column were found in only 1% of the cases.[111]

The mechanism involved in intrapartum spinal cord injury is generally thought to involve longitudinal traction of the neonatal spine during breech extraction and subsequent rupture of the cord.[27,21,56] Because of the extreme elasticity of the fibrocartilagineous spine and its investing soft tissues, the resulting cord lesion is often present without radiographic or post mortem evidence of dislocation or fracture.[1,31,111] The incidence of breech delivery with cord injury in older series ranged from 38% to 75%,[35,126,159] but improvement of obstetrical management and care have considerably reduced the incidence of spinal trauma at birth.[5,31,86,139a] According to Towbin,[67] however, cord injury still appears to be a causal factor in about 10% of neonatal deaths. In addition to traumatic breech delivery, spinal injuries also occur after cephalic presentation and fetal malposition.[98] The anatomic findings in acute fetal spinal injury in the neonatal and perinatal period include the following: meningeal lesions with dural tears and extradural and extraspinal hemorrhage; cord lesions with lacerations, hemorrhages, necrosis, and edema; spinal root damage with tears, avulsion, and perineural bleeds.

Epidural hemorrhage is the most frequent lesion in spinal injury in both premature and term infants, most commonly along the posterior aspect of the cervical and upper thoracic cord, but may also involve the entire length of the spinal canal. Extradural hemorrhage is not necessarily lethal, and may occur without other spinal damage, but is often associated with various lesions to the cord, roots, and meninges, including subdural and subarachnoid spinal bleeds. Large epidural hematomas may cause displacement or compression of the cord.

Cord lesions in neonatal trauma include deep laceration, distortion, and rare complete disruption of the cord at the craniocervical junction or at deeper levels.[159,169] In most cases, nontransectional cord injury features focal hemorrhage, hemorrhagic necrosis, vascular congestion, and edema, which particularly affects the central gray matter. The most common sites of birth injury are the low cervical region and the cervicothoracic junction; traumatic damage to the low thoracic and lumbar cord is rare.[86,127,139a,167] The dura mater and spinal nerve roots may be torn. Perivertebral soft-tissue lesions, simultaneous cord and brain stem injury, and intramural laceration and thrombosis of the vertebral arteries have been reported.[191]

Spinal cord injury may occur during intrauterine life as a result of malposition with extreme hyperextension of the head and neck,[63] during labor as the fetus is compressed and forced down the birth canal, and during the final extraction of the fetus. Most intrapartum cord injuries without bony damage are due to longitudinal traction (elongation) or extreme ventral and lateral flexion. Forceful longitudinal traction during the second stage of labor, particularly when combined with flexion, retroflexion, or torsion in the vertebral axis, is generally thought to be the most important mechanism of neonatal spinal cord and brain stem injury.[5,56,167] Facilitating factors are premature birth and abnormalities of the uterus and placenta.

The trauma may occur in breech delivery, with forceps traction in cephalic deliveries, and after fetal malposition. Whereas in cephalic presentations the upper cervical cord is most often damaged, in traumatic breech delivery or extraction, all parts of the neuraxis are involved, with less common injury to the upper cervical cord.[5,15] Flexion of the spine increases the traction of the cord, particularly in the cervical region, and may sharply reduce the diameter of the bony canal. The cord, undergoing buckling distortion, is subject to direct compression injury with or without vertebral subluxation, the latter often escaping detection. In breech and transverse extraction, longitudinal stretching and compression result in damage to the cord, particularly when there is additional lateral traction.[68] In breech delivery, when the head is held tightly by uterine contraction, the entire spinal column can be stretched to the extent of rupture of the meninges and even the cord, with frequent extraspinal and intramedullary hemorrhage. Due to the extreme elasticity of the neonatal spine, permitting motions impossible

to the adult vertebral column without fracture or dislocation, the resulting damage involves the cord more readily than the bony structures. The resulting injuries to the cord and brain stem may be lethal or may be survived for variable periods, with severe deficits.

While the pathology of acute neonatal trauma to the spine and cord has been systematically studied, there are a limited number of postmortem observations of the late stages or sequelae of these injuries.[5,56,79,139a,159,178] The character and development of lesions do not differ significantly from those in adults. In general, there is severe destruction of the cord, rarely reaching total disruption, with focal connective tissue scars and adherent, grossly thickened meninges with some hemosiderin deposits (Figs. 18-39, 18-40) and occasional arachnoid cysts. Remnants of nervous tissue may be seen within the fibrous scars. Vascular lesions with occlusion of intramedullary or pial vessels and the anterior spinal artery at the level of injury (see Fig. 18-40) may result in ischemic infarction of the gray matter in caudal segments. In cervical cord trauma the lesion may extend to the central portions of the thoracic or lumbar cord.[79] Damage to lower cord areas due to vascular lesions, or spinal root damage due to epidural bleeding or meningeal scars (arachnopathy) may be responsible for the lack of development of spasticity following ini-

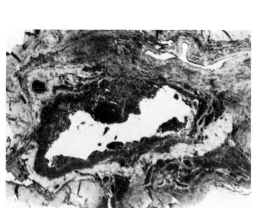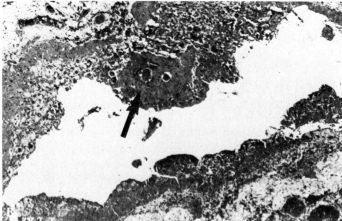

Figure 18-39. (*A, B*) Cervical injury at breech delivery; infant survived 7 weeks. Cystic destruction at C-7 with a duromeningeal scar is seen in *A*. *B* shows preserved nervous tissue islands (*arrow*) within fibrotic scar.

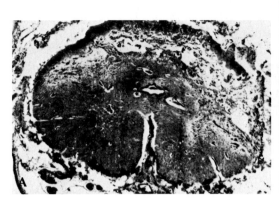
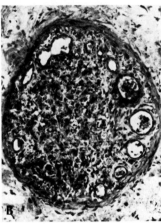

Figure 18-40. Low thoracic injury after manual extraction; neonate survived 3 weeks. (*A*) Incomplete necrosis at the T-7 level. (*B*) Organized and partially recanalized occlusion of the anterior spinal artery at the T-7 level (van Gieson stain).

tial flaccid paraplegia in infants due to neonatal cord injury.[5,167]

Spinal injury is uncommon from infancy to the age of 16 years, although cervical cord trauma has been reported in battered child syndrome,[163] and has been considered a causal mechanism in some cases of unexplained death in infants.[169] The incidence of pediatric spinal cord trauma among all spinal cord injuries has been reported as anywhere from 0.65% to 9.4%.[120] Although many children with spinal cord trauma have associated spinal injuries,[61] traumatic myelopathy often occurs without evidence of fracture or dislocation. This is due to age-related anatomic and biomechanical peculiarities of the vertebral column in infants and young children, rendering the pediatric spine exceedingly vulnerable to deforming forces.[32,120] Since most of the age-related changes in anatomy and biomechanics occur in the upper cervical segment, it is much more frequently involved than the lower cord regions.

The mechanisms of cord injury, which often cause transient subluxation without bone injury, include hyperextension, flexion, repetitive flexion–extension, longitudinal distraction, combined mechanisms, and direct crush injury.[120] The neurologic lesions encountered in children include complete or severe incomplete transection and central cord syndromes, which are related to the central cord necrosis seen in adult hyperextension injury.[75,83,153] Flexion injury is a frequent mecha-

nism in pediatric spinal cord trauma inducing central or complete cord necrosis.[120] Repetitive flexion–hyperflexion injury in child abuse causes severe central cord syndrome,[163] with acute fatal hemorrhage and tears in the central parts of the upper cervical cord and lower medulla without spinal fracture-dislocation (see Fig. 18-7).

TRAUMATIC LESIONS OF SPINAL ROOTS

While traumatic rupture of the intradural parts of cervical spinal roots is well known to clinicians and neuroradiologists,[101,145,162,180] there is little mention of lesions of spinal roots or sensory ganglia in postmortem series of craniospinal or spinal injuries.[75,95,103,107,158] Hemorrhages in the dorsal roots, and particularly in their entry zones, are frequent findings in acute cervical cord injury, and have been particularly observed in dorsiflexion trauma of the neck (Fig. 18-41). Hemorrhage and rupture of the posterior roots mainly occur next to or at the root entry zone and may be associated with subarachnoid hemorrhage or damage to the cord in this particular area. Disruption of the dorsal roots is attributed to tearing forces, which may also cause hemorrhage or necrosis in Lissauer's marginal zone and in the posterior horns.[139] Tearing of the anterior roots with hemorrhage at their exit (see Fig. 18-41) appears to be less frequent. Hemorrhage into the posterior roots and sensory

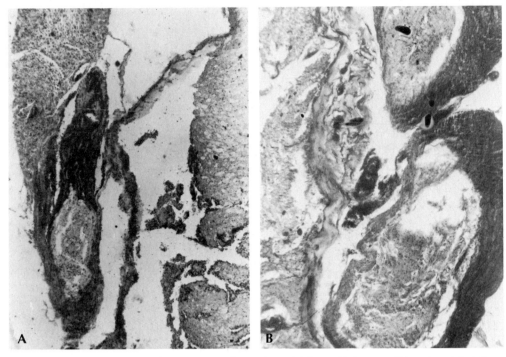

Figure 18-41. (*A, B*) Traumatic damage to spinal roots in neck injury with fracture-dislocation at C-4–5 and central hemorrhagic cord necrosis after fall; patient survived 3 days. *A* shows hemorrhage and tearing of anterior spinal root at exit. *B* shows necrosis of posterior root near the entry zone.

ganglia of the cervical cord without fracture of the spine or pia-arachnoid bleeding around the cord were reported in fatal head injuries.[158] Hemorrhage into the anterior and posterior cervical spinal roots accompanied by pia-arachnoid and intramedullary bleeding were seen after fatal flexion–extension (whiplash) trauma[95] and in acute dorsiflexion injuries of the neck, associated with central cord lesions.[75,107]

On serial sections, Mayer and associates[107] demonstrated rupture of small radicular vessels that were probably small veins accompanying the spinal roots transversing the dura. Rupture and tearing of small radicular veins and rhexic hemorrhage into the spinal roots are attributed to dislocation of the vertebral column against the dural sac and spinal cord in dorsiflexion. This may also cause tearing of the roots before transversing the dura. Intradural rupture of cervical spinal roots and avulsion of the brachial plexus are typical results

of extreme tearing and traction of the forearms in motorcycle injuries.[101,145,180] Rupture and avulsion usually occur at the low cervical level or cervicothoracic junction and may be combined with spinal cord damage.[166] In late stages of such injuries large neuromas are observed at the site of the disrupted anterior cervical roots (Fig. 18-42).

REGENERATION PHENOMENA

The problem of repair processes in the spinal cord following compression and transection in humans and animals has been the subject of many studies.[53,131,142,176,183] Severed axons and tracts in the central nervous system of adult mammals, in general, do not regenerate after injury.[19] Peripheral nerves regenerate vigorously after injury, usually while in contact with Schwann cells or other glia, but even in the peripheral nervous system, little is

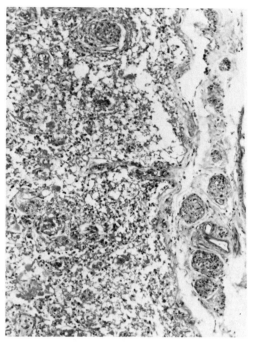

Figure 18-42. Large neuroma in anterior root at C-6 after disruption of brachial plexus and cervical roots in motorcycle accident; patient survived 3 years.

cells and bundles of axons with or without peripheral-type myelin fibers, which resemble traumatic neuromas seen after peripheral nerve damage. These changes have been observed following spinal cord trauma, compression, and infarction, and in multiple sclerosis and other conditions.[53,68,69,75,83a,183,186] In a systemic histologic study of spinal cords in a series of cases of traumatic paraplegia surviving between 12 months and 32 years, Wolman[183,186] found regenerating fibers in and near the damaged segments both above and below the site of maximum damage. The bundles of regenerating fibers are seen in four main locations:

1. In the thickened pia-arachnoid on the posterior or posterolateral aspect of the damaged cord adjacent to the posterior root entry zone (see Figs. 18-32, 18-33)
2. In the thickened pia-arachnoid or its vessels in the anterior fissure or on the anterolateral aspect of the cord near the site of attachment of the anterior nerve roots (see Fig. 18-43)

known about the factors required for regeneration. It is widely believed, on the basis of grafting experiments, that the success of axonal regeneration depends on the environment that surrounds the injured axon.[2,8,16]

Peripheral nervous system elements, in particular Schwann cells and peripheral-type myelin, have been described frequently as components of regenerative processes in the central nervous system and particularly in the spinal cord following compression, destructive processes, and trauma.[64,68,69,73,75,183,186] The occurrence of Schwann cells and peripheral-type myelin within the spinal cord has been described frequently in various experimental conditions.[53,93] Heterotopic regeneration of peripheral nerve fibers into the subarachnoid space has been observed, mainly concentrated around marginal blood vessels.[133] It has been suggested that the astrocytic glial membrana limitans prevents Schwann cells from entering into central nervous system tissue.[20,62]

In the human spinal cord, regenerative phenomena usually occur as proliferating Schwann

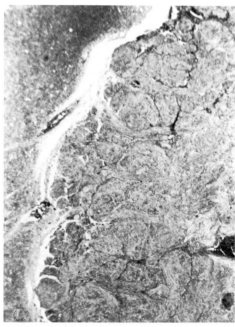

Figure 18-43. Small neuromatous regenerates around pial vessels and in lateral marginal zone 19 years after cord injury.

3. Within the spinal cord, which is replaced by numerous bundles of myelinated or unmyelinated axons accompanied or separated by dense fibrous scars or a loosely arranged fibroglial meshwork. It surrounded by a dense glial layer around the periphery of the cord remnants. Occasional nerve bundles accompany or are adherent to intramedullary blood vessels; some are in perivascular spaces.

4. In the cord, where compact arrangements of axons surround the walls of large cystic cavities above or below the maximum damage. Most of the bundles of regenerated nerve fibers consist of whorls containing collagen, Schwann cells, and axons without or with myelin of the peripheral type.[53]

These structures, which represent nonspecific regenerative responses to injury, are to be distinguished from true neoplasms or microdysplasias, that is, neurofibromas or schwannomas.[83a,140] Whether the regenerated axons seen in many cases of cord injury with long survival have any functional significance is still unresolved. In the reported human cases with extensive neuroma formation, however, there was no evidence of any appreciable clinical improvement or functional recovery.[183,186] Hence, in general, structural restitution by regenerating intraspinal axons is poor.[131]

REFERENCES

1. Abrams IF, Bresnan MJ, Zuckerman JE et al: Spinal cord injuries secondary to hyperextension of the head in breech presentation. Obstet Gynecol 41:369-378, 1973
2. Aguayo AJ: Axonal regeneration from injured neurons in the adult mammalian central nervous system, pp 457-484. In Cotman CW (ed): Synaptic Plasticity and Remodelling. London, Guilford Press, 1985
3. Ahmann PA, Schmith SA, Schwartz JF et al: Spinal cord infarction due to minor trauma in children. Neurology 25:301-307, 1975
4. Alker GJ, Young O, Leslie EV et al: Postmortem radiology of head and neck injuries in fatal traffic accidents. Radiology 114:611-617, 1975
5. Allen JF: Birth injuries of the spinal cord. In Vinken PJ, Bruyn GW (eds): Handbook of Clinical Neurology, Vol 25. Amsterdam, North Holland Publishing Co, 1976
6. Al-Mefti O, Harkey LH, Middleton TH et al: Myelopathic cervical spondylotic lesions demonstrated by magnetic resonance imaging. J Neurosurg 68:217-222, 1988
7. Anderson MJ, Schutt AH: Spinal injury in children: A review of 156 cases seen from 1950 through 1978. Mayo Clin Proc 55:499-504, 1980
8. Anderson PM, Turmaine M: Peripheral nerve regeneration through grafts of living and freeze-dried CNS tissue. Neuropathol Appl Neurobiol 12:389-399, 1986
9. Atlas SW, Regenbogen V, Rogers LF, Kwang SF: The radiographic characterization of burst fractures of the spine. AJR 147:572-582, 1986
10. Bahlmann H, Ossenkopp G: Spätschicksal nach Rückenmarksverletzung. Z Neurol 204:87-94, 1973
11. Balentine JD: Hypotheses in spinal cord trauma research. In Becker DP, Povlishock JT (eds): CNS Trauma Status Report, Vol. 31. 455-461, 1985
12. Balentine JD: Impact injuries of the spine and spinal cord. In Leestma JE (ed): Forensic Neuropathology. New York, Raven Press, 1988
13. Balentine JD: Pathology of experimental spinal cord trauma: I. The necrotic lesion as a function of vascular injury. Lab Invest 39:236-253, 1978
14. Barnes R: Paraplegia in cervical spine injuries. J Bone Joint Surg [Br] 30:234-244, 1948
15. Barnett HJM, Jousse AT: Posttraumatic syringomyelia (cystic myelopathy). In Vinken PJ, Bruyn GW (eds): Handbook of Clinical Neurology, Vol 26. Amsterdam, North Holland Publishing Co, 113-157, 1976
16. Barron KD: Axon reaction and central nervous system regeneration, pp 3-36. In Seie FJ (ed): Nerve, Organ and Tissue Regeneration: Research Perspectives. New York, Academic Press, 1983
17. Bastian HC: On a case of concussion-lesion with extensive secondary degeneration of the spinal cord. Proc Roy Med-Chir Soc London 50:499, 1867
18. Beatson TR: Fractures and dislocations of the cervical spine. J Bone Joint Surg [Br] 45:21-35, 1963
19. Berry M: Regeneration of axons in the central nervous system. In Navaratnam V, Harrison RI (eds): Progress in Anatomy, Vol 3, 213-233. London, Oxford University Press, 1983
20. Blakemore WF: Invasion of Schwann cells into the spinal cord of the rat following injections of lysolecithin. Neuropathol Appl Neurobiol 2:21-39, 1976

21. Blight AR: Delayed demyelination and macrophage invasion in seary damage in spinal cord injury. Cent Nerv Syst Trauma 2:254-266, 1985

22. Bouzarth WF, Futterman P: Delayed traumatic spinal subarachnoid hemorrhage. JAMA 265:880-882, 1968

23. Braakman R: Injuries of cervical spine with neurological symptoms. In Vinken PJ, Bruyn GW (eds): Handbook of Clinical Neurology, Vol 25. Amsterdam, North Holland Publishing Co, 1976

24. Braakman R, Penning L: Injuries of the Cervical Spine. Amsterdam, Excerpta Medica, 1971

25. Brain WR, Wilkinson M: Cervical spondylosis and other disorders of the cervical spine. Philadelphia, WB Saunders, 1967

26. Breig A, El Nadi AF: Biomechanics of the cervical spinal cord: Relief of contact on and overstretching of the spinal cord. Acta Radiol [Diagn] 4:602-624, 1966

27. Bresnan MA: Neurologic birth injuries. Postgrad Med J 49:202-206, 1971

28. Brown-Sequard CE: Lectures on the physiology and pathology of the nervous system and on the treatment of organic nervous affections. Lancet 2:593, 659, 755, 821, 1869

29. Bruyn GW, Bosma NJ: Spinal extradural hematoma. In Vinken PJ, Bruyn GW (eds): Handbook of Clinical Neurology, Vol 26, pp 1-31. Amsterdam, North Holland Publishing Co, 1976

30. Burke DC: Traumatic spinal paralysis in children. Paraplegia 10:1-14, 1974

31. Byers RK: Spinal cord injuries during birth. Dev Med Child Neurol 17:103-110, 1975

32. Cheshire DJE: The pediatric syndrome of traumatic myelopathy without demonstrable vertebral injury. Paraplegia 15:74-87, 1977

33. Cohen WA, Young W, DeCrescito V et al: Posttraumatic syrinx formation: Experimental study. ANJR 6:823-827, 1985

34. Coutelle C: Über Wlutungen in den Wirbelkanal bei Neugeborenen und Säuglingen. Wiss Z Humboldt Univ Berlin 17:548-549, 1969

35. Crothers B, Putnam MC: Obstetrical injuries of the spinal cord. Medicine 6:41-126, 1927

36. Cruveilhier J: Pathologische Anatomie: I. Die Krankheiten des Gehirns und des Rückenmarks. Bearb BA Kähler. Leipzig I. Voss 1841

37. Dastur DK, Wadia NH, Desai AD, Singh G: Medullospinal compression due to atlanto-occipital dislocation and sudden hematomyelia during compression. Brain 88:897-924, 1965

38. Davis D, Bohlman H, Walker AE et al: The pathological findings in fatal craniospinal injuries. J Neurosurg 34:603-613, 1971

39. Davison C: General pathological considerations in injuries of the spinal cord. In Brock S (ed): Injuries of the Brain and Spinal Cord, pp 495-522. London, Cassell & Co, 1960

40. De la Torre JC: Spinal cord injury: Review of basic and applied research. Spine 6:315-335, 1981

41. Dohrmann GJ, Wagner FC, Bucy PC: Transitory traumatic paraplegia: An electron microscopic study in monkey. J Neurosurg 35:263-271, 1971

42. Dohrmann GJ, Wick KM, Bucy PC: Spinal cord blood flow patterns in experimental traumatic paraplegia. J Neurosurg 38:52-58, 1973

43. Ducker TB: Experimental injury of the spinal cord. In: Vinken PJ, Bruyn GW (eds): Handbook of Clinical Neurology, Vol 25, pp 9-26. Amsterdam, North Holland Publishing Co, 1976

44. Emminger E: Pathologisch-anatomische Befunde bei frischer Halswirbelsäulenverletzung. Verh Dtsch Ges Orthop 54:282-293, 1968

45. Erdmann H: Schleuderverletzung der Halswirbelsäule: Die Wirbelsäule in Forschung und Praxis, Vol 56. Stuttgart, Hippokrates, 1973

46. Feigin I, Ogata J: Schwann cells and peripheral myelin within human central nervous tissue. J Neuropathol Exp Neurol 30:603-611, 1971

47. Foerster O: Die traumatischen Läsionen des Rückenmarks auf grund der kriegserfahrungen. In Bumke O, Foerster O (eds): Handbuch der Neurologie, pp 1721-1927, supplement. Teil, Berlin, Springer, 1929

48. Fried LC, Aparicio O: Experimental ischemia of the spinal cord: Histologic studies after anterior spinal artery occlusion. Neurology 23:289-293, 1973

49. Gagel O: Die Fernschädigung des Rückenmarks bei einem Trauma der Halswirbelsäule. Zschr Ges Neurol 174:670-680, 1942

50. Gauthier G: L'hématome extradural rachidien sans fracture de la colonne. Psychiatr Neurol (Basel) 146:149-175, 1963

51. Gebarski SS, Maynard FW, Gabrielsen TO et al: Posttraumatic progressive myelopathy: Clinical and radiologic correlation employing MR imaging, delayed CT metrizamide myelography, and intraoperative sonography. Radiology 157:379-386, 1985

52. Gilles FH, Bin H, Sotrel A: Infantile atlantooccipital instability. Am J Dis Child 133:30-37, 1979

53. Gilmore SA, Sims TJ: The role of Schwann cells in the repair of glial cell deficits in the spinal cord. In Das GD, Wallace RB (eds): Neural Transplantation and Regeneration, pp 245-269. New York, Springer, 1986

54. Glasauer FE, Cares H: Biomechanical features of traumatic paraplegia in infancy. J Trauma 13:166-170, 1973

55. Gooding MR, Wilson CB, Hoff JT: Experimental cervical myelopathy. J Neurosurg 43:9-17, 1975

56. Gordon N, Marsden B: Spinal cord injury at birth. Neuropediatrics 2:112-118, 1970

57. Gowers WR: Lectures on diseases of the nervous system. Lecture VIII, 2nd series, p 250. London, J&A Churchill, 1904

58. Griffiths IR, McCulloch MC: Nerve fibers in spinal cord impact injuries. J Neurol Sci 58:335-349, 1983

59. Gutmann G: Arteria vertebralis. Berlin, Springer, 1985

60. Guttmann L: Spinal Cord Injuries, 2nd ed. London, Blackwell Scientific Publications, 1976.

61. Hadley MN, Zabramski JM, Browner CM et al: Pediatric spinal trauma: Review of 122 cases of spinal cord and vertebral column injuries. J Neurosurg 68:1824, 1988

62. Hall SM, Kent AP: The response of regenerating peripheral neurites to a grafted optic nerve. J Neurocytol 16:317-331, 1987

63. Hallström B, Sallmader U: Prevention of spinal cord injury in hyperextension of the fetal head. JAMA 204:107-110, 1968

64. Hardman JM: Cerebrospinal trauma. In Davis RL, Robertson DM (eds): Textbook of Neuropathology, p 447. Baltimore, Williams & Wilkins, 1985

65. Hinz P: Die Verletzungen der Halswirbelsäule durch Schleuderung und Abknickung, pp 1-69. Stuttgart, Hippokrates, 1972

66. Hinz P, Tamaska L: Arteria vertebralis und Schleuderverletzungen der Wirbelsäule. Arch Orthop Trauma Surg 64:268-277, 1968

67. Holzer FJ, Kloss K: Tödliche Wirbelsäulenverletzungen. Wien Klin Wochenschr 74:125-129, 1962

68. Hughes JT: Disease of the spine and spinal cord. In Adams JH, Corsellis JAN, Duchen LW (eds): Greenfield's Neuropathology, 4th ed, pp 779-812. London, Edward Arnold & Co, 1984

69. Hughes JT: Pathology of the Spinal Cord. London, Lloyd-Duke 1978

70. Hukuda S, Wilson CB: Experimental cervical myelopathy. J Neurosurg 37:631-652, 1972

71. Jahna H: Brüche des dens epistrophei. Mschr Unfallh 68:99-148, 1961

72. Jarosch K, Hinz P: Hinterhauptsabriß von der halswirbelsäule. Mschr Unfallh 72:89-99, 1969

73. Jellinger K: Morfologia e patogenesi delle mielorizopatie cervicali da spondilartrosi. In Testa C (ed): Mielorizopatie Cervicali Spondilartrosiche, pp 35-64. Verona, Edizione Libreria Cortina, 1983

74. Jellinger K: Morphologie und Pathogenese spinaler Durchblutungsstörungen. Nervenarzt 51:65-77, 1980

75. Jellinger K: Neuropathology of cord injuries. In Vinken PJ, Bruyn GW (eds): Handbook of Clinical Neurology, Vol 25, pp 43-123. Amsterdam, North Holland Publishing Co, 1976

76. Jellinger K: Traumatic vascular disease of the spinal cord. In Vinken PJ, Bruyn GW (eds): Handbook of Clinical Neurology, Vol 12, pp 556-630. Amsterdam, North Holland Elsevier Publishing Co, 1972

77. Jellinger K: Vascular malformations of CNS. Neurosurg Rev 9:177-216, 1986

78. Jellinger K, Lunglmayer G, Vass K: Progressive Spätmyelopathie nach Luxationsfraktur des Dens epistrophei. Dtsch Z Nervenheilk 190:107-135, 1967

79. Jellinger K, Schwingshackel A: Birth injury of the spinal cord. Neuropediatrics 4:111-123, 1973

80. Jinkins JR, Bashir R, Al-Mefti O et al: Cystic necrosis of the spinal cord in compressive cervical myelopathy. AJR 147:767-776, 1986

81. Kakulas BA: Pathology of spinal injuries. Cent Nerv Syst Trauma 1:117-129, 1984

82. Kakulas BA, Bedbrook GM: A correlative clinicopathologic study of spinal cord injury. Proceedings of the Australian Association of Neurologists 6:123-132, 1984

83. Kakulas BA, Bedbrook GM: Pathology of injuries of the vertebral column with emphasis on the macroscopic aspect. In Vinken PJ, Bruyn GW: Handbook of Clinical Neurology, Vol 25, pp 27-42. Amsterdam, North Holland Publishing Co, 1976

83a. Kamiya M, Hashizime Y: Pathological studies of aberrant peripheral nerve bundles of spinal cords. Acta Neuropathol 79:18–22, 1989

84. Kapadia SI: Ultrastructural alterations in blood vessels of the white matter after experimental spinal cord trauma. J Neurosurg 61:539-544, 1984

85. Kawakami Y, Mair GP: Haematomyelia associated with anticoagulant therapy, an intramedullary ependymoma and Schwann cells. Acta Neuropathol 26:253-258, 1973

86. Keuth U: Geburtstraumatische Schädigungen. In Handbuch der Kinderheilk, Vol I/2, p 126. Berlin, Springer, 1971

87. Kienböck R: Über Verletzungen im Bereich der ersten Halswirbel und Formen der Kopfverrenkung. Fortschritte a/d Gebiet Röntgenstrahlen 25:95-150, 1918

88. Kirkpatrick E: Missile injuries of the spine and spinal cord. In Leestma JE (ed): Forensic Neuropathology. New York, Raven Press, 1988

89. Klaue R: Beitrag zur pathologischen Anatomie der Verletzungen des Rückenmarks mit besonderer Berücksichtigung der Rückenmarkskontusion. Arch Psychiat Nervenkr 180:206-270, 1948

90. Klawans HL: Delayed traumatic syringomyelia. Diseases of the Nervous System 29:525-528, 1968

91. Krauland W, Kugler B: Verletzungen der A. vertebralis: Eine histologische Studie, pp 73-89. In Gutmann G (ed): Arteria vertebralis. Berlin, Springer, 1985

92. Kulkarni VM, McArdle CB, Kopanicky D et al: Acute spinal cord injury: MR imaging at 15 T. Radiology 164:837-844, 1987

93. Lampert PW, Cressman M: Axonal regeneration in the dorsal columns of the spinal cord of rats. Lab Invest 13:825-834, 1964

94. Lausberg G: Chirurgische therapie Traumatischer Rückenmarkschäden. In Hopf HC, Poeck K, Schliack H (eds): Neurologie in Praxis und Klinik, Vol 1, pp 3.95-3.101. Stuttgart, Georg Thieme Verlag,1983

95. Leichsenring F: Pathologisch-anatomische Befunde in der Halswirbelsäulenregion bei verstorbenen Patienten mit Schleudertraumen. Dtsch Med Wochenschr 89:1469-1475, 1964

96. Leramo OB, Rewcastle NB: Rupture of central canal with multisegmental haematomyelia. J Neurol Sci 54:89-97, 1982

96a. Lesoin F, Rousseau M, Thomas CE: Posttraumatic spinal arachnoid cysts. Acta Neurochirurgica (Wien) 70:227–234, 1984

97. Leventhal HR: Birth injuries of the spinal cord. J Pediatr 56:447-453, 1960

98. Lindberg U, Hagberg B, Olsson Y, Sourander P: Injury of the spinal cord at birth. Acta Paediatr Scand 64:546-550, 1975

99. Lindenberg R: Trauma of meninges and brain. In Minckler J (ed): Pathology of the Nervous System, Vol 2, pp 1705-1765. New York, McGraw-Hill, 1971

100. Liss L: Fatal cervical cord injury in a swimmer. Neurology 15:675-677, 1965

101. Malin JP, Sinn M: Läsionen des Plexus brachialis. In Hopf HC, Poeck K, Schliack H (eds): Neurologie in Praxis und Klinik, Vol 3, pp 2.65-2.70. Stuttgart, Georg Thieme Verlag, 1986

102. Marar BC: Hyperextension injuries of the cervical spine. The pathogenesis of damage to the spinal cord J Bone Jt Surgg 56A:1655-1662, 1974

103. Marburg O: Die traumatischen Erkrankungen des Gehirns und Rückenmarks. In Bumke O, Foerster O (eds): Handbuch der Neurologie, Vol 11, Part I, pp 1-177. Berlin, Springer, 1936

104. Markham HW, Lynge HN, Stahlman GE: The syndrome of spontaneous spinal epidural hemorrhage. J Neurosurg 26:334-342, 1967

105. Martinez JL, Garcia DJ: A model for whiplash. J Biomech 1:23-32, 1968

106. Mattle H, Sieb JP, Rohner M, Mumenthaler M: Nontraumatic spinal epidural and subdural hematomas. J Neurol 37:1351-1356, 1987

107. Mayer ET, Peters G: Pathologische Anatomie der Rückenmarksverletzungen. In Kessel A, Guttmann E, Maurer A (eds): Neuro-Traumatologie mit Einschluß der Grenzgebiete, Vol 2, pp 39-61. München, Urban & Schwarzenberg, 1970

108. McCormick WF: Trauma. In Rosenberg RN, Schochet SS (eds): The Clinical Neurosciences: Neuropathology, Vol 3, p 241. New York, Churchill Livingstone, 1983

109. McKenzie JA, Williams JF: The dynamic behavior of the head and cervical spine during whiplash. J Biomech 4:477-490, 1971

110. McLean DR, Miller JDR, Allen PBR, Ezzeddin SA: Posttraumatic syringomyelia. J Neurosurg 39:485-492, 1973

111. Müller KM, Löbker U: Perinatale kindliche Rückenmarksverletzungen. Zentralbl Allg Pathol 114:209-219, 1971

112. Nakano I, Mannen T, Mizutani T et al: Peripheral white matter lesions in the spinal cord with changes in small arachnoid arteries in system lupus erythematosus. Acta Neuropathol 1988 (in press)

113. Noack W, Wolff JR, Güldner FH, Moritz A: Über die akuten Veränderungen im Parietalkortex der Ratte nach spitzen Traumen. Acta Neuropathol 19:249-264, 1971

114. Nurick S, Russell JA, Deck MDF: Cystic degeneration of the spinal cord following spinal cord injury. Brain 93:211-222, 1970

115. Ollivier GP: Über das Rückenmark und seine Krankheiten Leipzig. L. Voss, 1824

116. Ommaya AK, Faas F, Yarnell P: Whiplash injury and brain damage: An experimental study. JAMA 204:285-289, 1968

117. Ommaya AK, Hirsch AE: Tolerances for cerebral concussion from head impact and whiplash in primates. J Biomech 4:13-21, 1971

118. Orne D, Liu YK: A mathematical model of spinal response to impact. J Biomech 4:49-71, 1971

119. Osterholm JL: The pathophysiology of spinal cord trauma. Springfield, IL, Charles C Thomas, 1978

120. Pang D, Wilberger JE: Spinal cord injury without radiographic abnormalities in children. J Neurosurg 57:114-129, 1982

121. Panjabi MM, White AA, Johnson RM: Cervical spine mechanisms as a function of transection components. J Biomech 8:327-336, 1975

122. Papadasiliou V: Traumatic subluxation of the cervical spine during childhood. Orthop Clin North Am 9:945-954, 1978

123. Penning L: Functional pathology of the cervical spine. Amsterdam, Excerpta Medica, 1968

124. Perot F, Feindel W, Lloyd-Smith D: Hematomyelia as a complication of syringomyelia. J Neurosurg 25:447-451, 1966

125. Peters G: Die gedeckten Rückenmarksverletzungen. In Lubarsch O, Henke F, Rössle R (eds): Handbuch der Speziellen Pathologischen Anatomie und Histologie, Vol 13, pp 126-141. Berlin, Springer, 1955

126. Pierson RN: Spinal and cranial injuries of the baby in breech deliveries. Surg Gynecol Obstet 37: 802-815, 1923

127. Potter EL: Pathology of the Fetus and Infant. Chicago, Year Book Medical Publishers, 1961

128. Povlishock JT: Traumatically induced axonal damage without concomitant change in focally related neuronal somata and dendrites. Acta Neuropathol 70:53-59, 1986

129. Povlishock JT, Becker DP, Miller JD et al: The morphologic substrates of concussion. Acta Neuropathol 47:1-11, 1979

130. Pribilla O: Über eine tödliche Verletzung der Halswirbelsäule beim Bodenturnen. Mschr Unfallheilk 65:143-148, 1962

131. Puchala E, Windle WF: The possibility of structural and functional restitution after spinal cord injury. Exp Neurol 55:1-42, 1977

132. Quencer RM, Green BA, Eismond FJ: Post-traumatic spinal cord cysts: Clinical features and characteristics with metrizamied CT. Radiology 146:415-423, 1983

133. Raine CS: Heterotopic regeneration of peripheral nerve fibers into the subarachnoid space. J Neurocytol 11:109-118, 1982

134. Raynor RB, Kingman AF: Cervical spine injuries. J Trauma 8:597-604, 1968

135. Rinder L, Olsson Y: Studies on vascular permeability changes in experimental brain concussion. Acta Neuropathol 11:183-200, 1968

136. Roaf R: Biomechanics of injuries of the spinal column. In Vinken PJ, Bruyn GW (eds): Handbook of Clinical Neurology, Vol 25. Amsterdam, North Holland Publishing Co, 1976

137. Rogers LF, Thayer C, Weinberg PE, Kim KS: Acute injuries of the upper thoracic spine associated with paraplegia. AJR 134:67, 1980

138. Rossier AB, Werner E, Wildi E, Berney J: Contribution to the study of late cervical syringomyelia syndromes after dorsal or lumbar traumatic paraplegia. J Neurol Neurosurg Psychiatry 31:99-107, 1968

139. Röttgen P: Über traumatische intradurale Wurzelabrisse. Nervenarzt 23:348-349, 1952

139a. Rudiger KD, Wockel W: Morphologische Spätbefunde nach gerburtstraumatischer Rückenmarksläsion. Schweiz. Medizinische Woschenschrift 102:545–548, 1972

140. Russell DS, Rubinstein LJ: Pathology of the Tumours of the Central Nervous System, 5th ed, pp 538–539. London, Edward Arnold & Co, 1989

141. Saternus S, Burtscheidt FG: Zur Topographie der Verletzungen der A. vertebralis. In Gutmann G (ed): Arteria vertebralis, pp 61-72. Berlin, Springer, 1985

142. Scaravilli F, Duchen LW: Regeneration in the CNS. In Glynn LE (ed): Handbook of Inflammation, Vol 3, pp 383-392. Amsterdam, Elsevier-North Holland Biomed Press, 1981

143. Scarff JE: Injuries of the vertebral column and spinal cord. In Brock S (ed): Injuries of the Brain and Spinal Cord and Their Coverings, 4th ed, pp 530-589. London, Cassell & Co, 1960

144. Scher AT: Diversity of radiological features in hyperextension injury of the cervical spine. S Afr Med J 58:27-30, 1980

145. Schliack H: Lähmungen peripherer Nerven, Plexus und Spinalwurzeln. In Bock HE (ed): Klinik der Gegenwart. München, Urban & Schwarzenberg, 1974

146. Schmitt HP: Risken und Komplikationen der Manualtherapie der Wirbelsäule aus neuropathologischer Sicht. Nervenarzt 59:32-35, 1988

147. Schmitt HP: Rupturen und Thrombosen der Arteria vertebralis nachgedeckten mechanischen insulten. Schweiz Arch Neurol Psychiatr 110:363, 1976

148. Schneider H: Kreislaufstörungen und Gefäßprozeße des Rückenmarks. In Doerr W, Seifert G (eds): Spezielle Pathologische Anatomie, Vol 13/1, pp 511-649. Berlin, Springer, 1980

149. Schneider RC, Cherry G, Pantek H: The syndrome of acute central cervical spinal cord injury. J Neurosurg 11:546-577, 1951

150. Schneider RC, Gosch HH, Norrell H et al: Vascu-

lar insufficiency and differential distortion of brain and cord caused by cervico-medullary football injuries. J Neurosurg 33:363-375, 1970

151. Schneider RC, McGillicuddy JE: Concomitant craniocerebral and spinal trauma with special reference to the cervicomedullary region. In Vinken PJ, Bruyn GW (ed): Handbook of Clinical Neurology, Vol 24, pp 141-177. Amsterdam, North Holland Elsevier Publishing Co, 1976

152. Schneider RC, Schemm GW: Vertebral artery insufficiency in acute and chronic spinal trauma. J Neurosurg 18:348-360, 1961

153. Schneider RC, Thomson JM, Bebin J: The syndrome of acute central cervical spinal cord injury. J Neurol Neurosurg Psychiatr 21:216, 1958

154. Schröder JM, Wechsler W: Ödem und Nekrose in der grauen und weissen Substanz beim experimentellen Hirntrauma. Acta Neuropathol 5:82-111, 1965

155. Shenkin HA, Horn RC, Grant FC: Lesions of the spinal epidural space producing cord compression. Arch Surg 51:125-146, 1945

156. Shulman ST, Madden JD, Esterly M et al: Transection of the spinal cord: A rare obstetrical complication of cephalic delivery. Arch Dis Child 46:291-297, 1971

157. Spatz H: Gehirnpathologie im Kriege: Von den Hirnwunden. Zentralbl Neurochir 6:162-212, 1941

158. Spicer EJF, Strich SJ: Hemorrhages in posterior-root ganglia in patients dying from head injuries. Lancet II:1389-1391, 1967

159. Stern WE, Rand RW: Birth injuries to the spinal cord. Am J Obstet Gynecol 78:498-512, 1959

160. Stevens JM, Olney JS, Kendall BE: Post-traumatic cystic and non-cystic myelopathy. Neuroradiology 27:48-56, 1985

161. Stewart DH Jr, Watkins ES: Spinal cord compression by chronic subdural hematoma. J Neurosurg 31:80-82, 1969

162. Sunderland S: Avulsion of spinal nerve roots. In Vinken PJ, Bruyn GW (eds): Handbook of Clinical Neurology, Vol. 26. Amsterdam, North Holland Publishing Co, 1976

163. Swischuk LE: Spine and spinal cord trauma in the battered child syndrome. Radiology 92:733-738, 1969

164. Tarlov IM: Acute spinal cord compression paralysis. J Neurosurg 36:10-20, 1972

165. Tarlov IM: Spinal Cord Compression. Springfield, IL, Charles C Thomas, 1957

166. Tillmann B, Engel H: Klinische und pathologisch-anatomische Spätbefunde nach Wurzelausrissen des Armplexus. Fortschr Neurol Psychiatr 42:28-37, 1974

167. Towbin A: CNS damage in the fetus and newborn infant. Am J Dis Child 119:529-542, 1970

168. Towbin A: Spinal cord and brainstem injury at birth. Arch Pathol Lab Med 77:620-632, 1964

169. Towbin A: Spinal injury related to the syndrome of sudden death ("crib-death") in infants. Am J Clin Pathol 49:562-567, 1969

170. Turnbull IM: Blood supply of the spinal cord. In Vinken PJ, Bruyn GW (eds): Handbook of Clinical Neurology, Vol 19, pp 478-491. Amsterdam, North Holland Publishing Co, 1975

171. Unterharnscheidt F: Die traumatischen Hirnschäden: Mechanogenese, Pathomorphologie und Klinik. Z Rechtsmed 71:153-221, 1972

172. Unterharnscheidt F, Higgins LS: Traumatic lesions of brain and spinal cord due to non-deforming angular acceleration of the head. Texas Reports on Biology and Medicine 27:127-166, 1969

173. Vernon JD, Chir B, Silver JR, Ohry A: Posttraumatic syringomyelia. Paraplegia 20:339-364, 1982

174. Wadia NH: Myelopathy complicating congenital atlanto-axial dislocation. Brain 90:449-473, 1965

175. Wagner EC Jr, Dohrmann GJ, Bucy PC: Histopathology of transitory traumatic paraplegia in the monkey. J Neurosurg 35:272-276, 1971

176. Waksman SG (ed): Functional Recovery in Neurological Diseases. Advances in Neurology, Vol 47. New York, Raven Press, 1988

177. Wannamaker GT: Spinal cord injuries. J Neurosurg 11:517-524, 1954

178. Weber M, Noetzel H, Beckmann R: Beitrag zur geburtstraumatisch bedingten Rückenmarksschädigung. Med Welt 25:947-952, 1974

179. Weller RO, Swash M, McLellan DL, Scholtz CL: Clinical Neuropathology, pp 96-101. Berlin, Springer, 1983

180. Wiedenmann O: Neurologische Störungen als Folge von Ausriβverletzungen des Plexus brachialis im Vergleich zu den Befunden des positiven Myelogramms. Z Orthop 97:67-78, 1963

181. Wilkinson M: Pathology. In Brain WR, Wilkinson M (eds): Cervical Spondylosis, pp 98-123. London, William Heinemann, 1967

182. Williams B, Terry AF, Jones F, McSweeney T: Syringomyelia as a sequel of traumatic paraplegia. Paraplegia 19:67-80, 1981

183. Wolman L: Axon regeneration after spinal cord injury. Paraplegia 4:175-184, 1966

184. Wolman L: The disturbances of circulation in traumatic paraplegia in acute and late stages. Paraplegia 2:231-236, 1965

185. Wolman L: The neuropathology of traumatic paraplegia. Paraplegia 2:233-251, 1964

186. Wolman L: Post-traumatic regeneration of nerve fibers in human spinal cord and its relationship to intramedullary neuroma. Pathol Bacteriol 94: 123-129, 1967

187. Wortis S, Sharp L: Fractures of the spine. JAMA 117:1585-1591, 1941

188. Wuermling HB, Struck G: Hirnstammrisse bei Verkehrsunfall. Beitr Gerichtl Med 23:297-302, 1965

189. Yashon D: Missile injuries of the spinal cord. In Vinken PJ, Bruyn GW (eds): Handbook of Clinical Neurology, Vol 26. Amsterdam, North Holland Publishing Co, 1976

190. Yates PO: Birth trauma to the vertebral arteries. Arch Dis Child 33:436–441, 1959

191. Zilkha A, Nicoletti JM: Acute spinal subdural hematoma. J Neurosurg 41:627-630, 1974

SPECIAL CONSIDERATIONS

19

DIAGNOSIS AND TREATMENT OF PATHOLOGIC SPINAL FRACTURES SECONDARY TO METASTATIC DISEASE

Thomas J. Errico

John P. Kostuik

Management of pathologic spinal fractures secondary to metastatic disease is one of the most challenging aspects of orthopedic surgery. These pathologic injuries differ drastically from traumatic injuries in several major ways. Traumatic injuries to the spine usually occur in young healthy individuals, whereas metastatic disease typically occurs in an older age group. Similarly, traumatic injuries usually affect individuals without major underlying medical illness. Metastatic disease often occurs in elderly individuals who have other noncancerous illnesses or are further debilitated by their malignancy or by treatment modalities for their malignancy. Traumatic injuries usually fall into specific fracture patterns secondary to the biomechanics of the injury. On the other hand, pathologic fractures of metastatic disease assume a wide spectrum of patterns based on the location of the original metastatic nidus, the local biologic aggressiveness of the tumor, and the aggregate response of the lesion to treatment modalities previously used. Furthermore, management techniques in metastatic disease, as opposed to traumatic injuries, may take advantage of the reduced life expectancy of this patient population.

INCIDENCE OF METASTASES TO THE SPINE

The musculoskeletal system is the third most common site for distant metastases for neoplastic disease; the liver and lung are the most common sites.[28] The spinal column, as well as the long bones, is a frequent site of musculoskeletal metastases.[5,20]

Clinically it is apparent that, due to the development of effective chemotherapeutic regimens, patients are now presenting with skeletal lesions with less overall involvement of visceral structures; thus they can be expected to have a longer survival rate. Patients may live for many years with multiple metastatic lesions to bone.[22] It is therefore crucial that effective management techniques be available to control pain, minimize deformity, and prevent loss of neurologic function secondary to neural compression.

PATHOPHYSIOLOGY

Metastatic disease of the spinal column commonly disseminates via a hematogenous route,[45] often through Batson's plexus (Fig. 19-1).[2,3] The well-vascularized cancellous portion of the posterior vertebral body is the most common initial site. As the lesion expands locally, there may be destruction of the pedicles and spreading from the bone

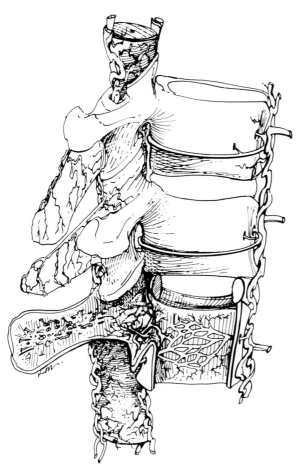

Figure 19-1. Batson's plexus, by which hematogenous spread of metastatic disease to the spine may occur.

into the epidural space. This can result in compression of the neural structures either by direct extension of the tumor or by pathologic collapse of the vertebral body. Evidence of cord compression was demonstrated by Barron and associates in 5% of 704 autopsies of patients with systemic cancer. This rose to 10% in carcinoma of the prostate and 14% in multiple myeloma.[1]

Although much less common, metastasis to the spine may also occur by apparent direct extension, as is seen in lesions of the upper lumbar spine by hypernephroma or lesions at the cervicothoracic junction secondary to apical lung lesions.

CLINICAL MANIFESTATIONS

Unless systemic treatment arrests the progress of initially asymptomatic foci, clinical manifestations become apparent as the lesion grows and destroys increasing proportions of the vertebral segment. Pain is the most common early sign.[31] The pain is secondary to the expansile nature of the lesion in the bone, pathologic fracture, or a combination resulting in "segmental spinal instability."[47] The pain may be localized to a specific area of the spinal column or, more commonly, may be diffuse, in a referred pain distribution. Complaints of radicular symptoms are commonly seen not only in the cervical and lumbar regions, but also presenting as trunk–girdle radiation with thoracic and thoracolumbar lesions.[24] These symptoms may help to localize the lesion, but the differential diagnoses of routine disk pathology, herpetic neuropathies, or polyradicular plexus lesions must be considered.

In order to establish the diagnosis, early complaints of pain in a patient with known neoplastic disease should be carefully evaluated. Often the nature of the pain, rather than the location and intensity, is more helpful to the clinician.[21] While cancer patients experience routine aches and pains, certainly a persistent dull pain not relieved by rest and often worse at night bears diagnostic investigation.

The threat of neurologic compromise is a key factor in the prompt recognition and treatment of metastatic disease of the spine. Neurologic dysfunction may present in a slow progressive form or with a sudden rapid onset. The rate of progression will depend on the location of the compressive lesion, the biologic aggressiveness of the specific tumor involved, and the pathomechanics of the compression. The time from onset to maximum neurologic deficit may be hours or days. Barron and associates reported that 30% of the patients in their series developed paraplegia within a week. The rapidity of onset may also change suddenly, with a slow progressive paraparesis developing overnight into complete paraplegia.[1]

Sensory findings in patients with the slow onset of symptoms may be vague and misleading as to the exact location of the lesion.[1] There may be associated complaints of vague dysesthesias. Ataxic gait disturbances may be secondary to cord compression and must be differentiated from an intracranial lesion.

End-stage cancer patients whose walking ability is slowly deteriorating may be suffering from a slowly enlarging mass with epidural compression of the cauda equina. This mild progressive lower extremity dysfunction may be confused with an overall general debilitation. At the opposite end of the spectrum, an aggressive destructive lesion of the upper thoracic spine may cause pathologic collapse of one or more vertebrae and result in rapid-onset paraparesis or complete paraplegia.

Bladder and bowel dysfunction often parallels the course of motor and sensory dysfunction, and may occur slowly in an insidious fashion or rapidly when accompanying paraparesis or paraplegia. Often the initial complaint is of hesitancy or urgency. This may be followed by retention and overflow. In an elderly male patient these symptoms may be mistakenly attributed to benign prostatic hypertrophy.

DIAGNOSTIC STUDIES

ROUTINE RADIOGRAPHY

Metastatic lesions of the spine, as with other areas of bony involvement, may present in either a lytic or blastic form. While prostatic cancers are most commonly associated with blastic metastases, lesions secondary to breast carcinomas may also be blastic or may present with a mixed lytic–blastic lesion.

It is important to keep in mind that before a destructive lesion is apparent on routine radiographs approximately 30% to 50% of the bone must be destroyed.[21] Therefore, early in the course of the disease process the only radiographic finding may be a localized area of osteopenia (Fig. 19-2). As progressive destruction occurs from its usual site in the posterior aspect of the vertebral body, involvement of the pedicle is often manifested by absence of one pedicle, as seen on the anteroposterior radiograph projection. This has commonly been referred to as the "winking owl" sign (Fig. 19-3).[32]

With diffuse involvement of the entire vertebral body (Fig. 19-4), pathologic fracture or fracture-dislocation may result. In this instance a previously lytic vertebral body may now appear blastic because the remaining bone is compressed, giving the appearance of increased density.

OTHER RADIOGRAPHIC PROCEDURES

Bone Scans

At present, technetium 99m bone scanning is the most sensitive diagnostic aid available for the detection of bony metastases, with a reported accuracy of 95% to 97%.[4,8] This represents a significant advantage in terms of sensitivity over routine radiographs. It is important to bear in mind, however, that false positives secondary to degenerative arthritis, infection, and traumatic lesions may occur. An important false negative occurs with a rapidly progressive lesion with little to no reactive new bone formation, as in lesions of multiple myeloma or rapidly progressive carcinomas.

Computed Tomography

The use of computed tomography (CT) in metastatic disease of the spine closely parallels the advances made in CT scanning for degenerative disease of the spine. Computed tomography provides a safe, rapid, and noninvasive means of obtaining high resolution images of the spine that clearly demarcate the limits of bony lesions and their soft-tissue extensions. Enhancement with intravenous contrast material may further delineate the borders between abnormal and uninvolved re-

(*Text continued on p. 504*)

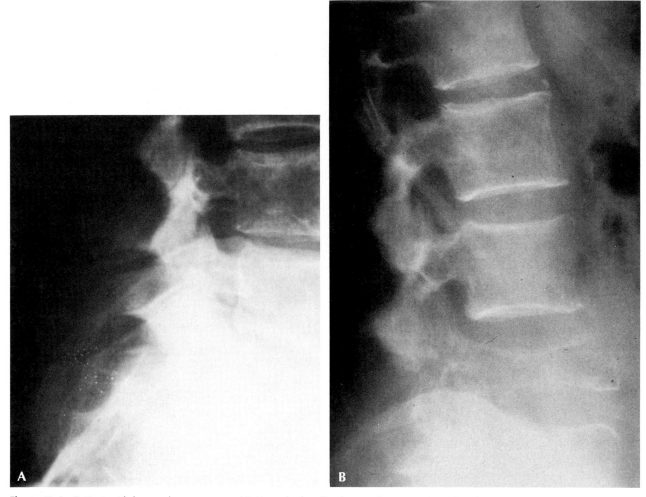

Figure 19-2. Patient with known breast cancer. (*A*) Note the localized area of osteopenia within the body of L-4. (*B*) Despite radiotherapy the lesion went on to collapse secondary to lack of structural support within the destroyed body.

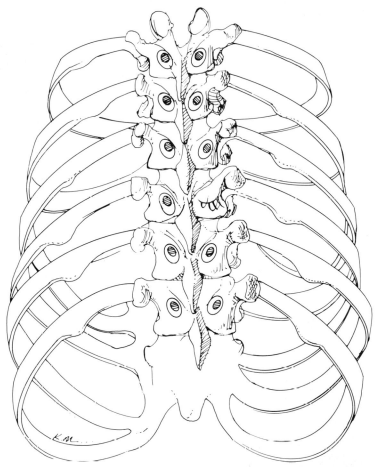

Figure 19-3. The "winking owl" sign is often the earliest radiologic clue to vertebral body involvement in metastatic disease.

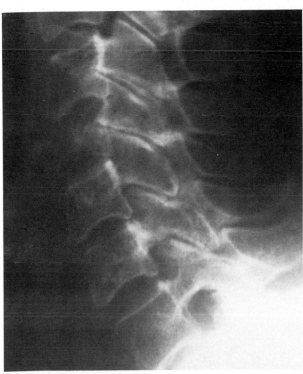

Figure 19-4. Complete involvement of the vertebral body of C-4 in a patient with breast cancer.

gions (Fig. 19-5). Computed tomography may also be helpful in differentiating a diffuse osteopenic region or infectious lesions from frank tumor destruction.

Computed Tomography–Myelography

Myelography is useful in cases of metastatic disease of the spine with neurologic impairment. While the area of bony destruction is readily apparent after routine radiographs and CT scanning, these modalities do not clearly define the degree of epidural spread up and down the canal or the occurrence of skip epidural lesions. When a complete block is present dye must be introduced both above and below the lesion to completely verify the upper and lower extent of the lesion.[1]

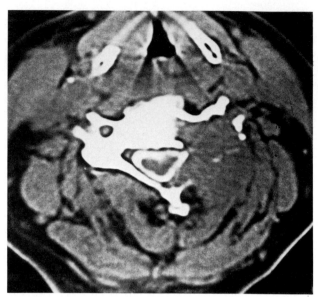

Figure 19-6. Destructive lesion of C-6 secondary to metastatic breast cancer—CT–myelogram. The myelographic dye clearly demarcates the relationship of the destructive lesion emanating from the left pedicle and the dural tube.

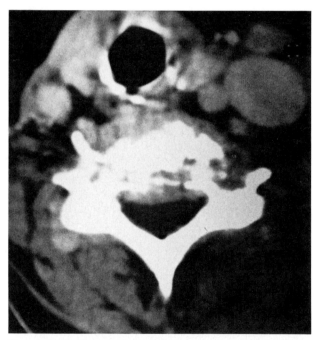

Figure 19-5. Neurologically normal patient with metastatic breast carcinoma to C-6—CT with intravenous contrast material. The pickup by the tumor cells of intravenous contrast material clearly delineates the extent of tumor encroachment into the spinal canal.

The use of CT shortly after myelography often yields the most accurate relationship between the bone lesion and the neural structures (Fig. 19-6).

Magnetic Resonance Imaging

Magnetic resonance imaging has in many instances supplanted myelography, even in cases of profound neurologic dysfunction. It is not only helpful in establishing the presence of metastatic foci in the spine, but, more importantly, documents their relationship to the neural tissue (Fig. 19-7).

Magnetic resonance imaging has advantages over CT–myelography in cases of complete block in which, in order to determine the upper extent of an epidural lesion, dye must be introduced through a second portal above the lesion. Magnetic resonance imaging quite clearly delineates the entire area of epidural compression. A relative disadvantage, however, of this method is the necessity to image the entire spine to detect poten-

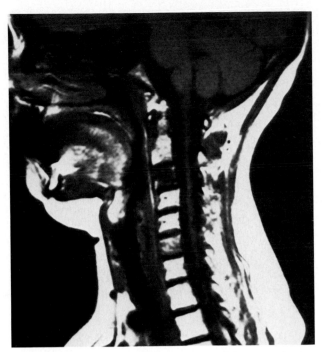

Figure 19-7. Magnetic resonance imaging of the cervical spine in a patient with involvement of C-3 and C-6 reveals the absence of neural compression at the involved levels.

tial areas of "distant" epidural metastasis, as opposed to merely fluoroscoping the spine quickly after introduction of myelographic contrast material.

Interventional Angiography

When there is suspicion of a hypervascular lesion, the state of vascularity is best assessed by selective angiography of the spinal segments involved. This is particularly important in preoperative investigation of highly vascular lesions such as hypernephroma or thyroid metastases, or for embolic palliative treatment. Preoperative selective arterial embolization within 24 to 48 hours of the surgical procedure can greatly diminish the intraoperative blood loss with hypervascular lesions (Fig. 19-8).

BIOPSY

While the above radiographic procedures may all help to establish the presence and extent of metastatic disease, the only definitive method of confirming this in a vertebral segment is by biopsy. This may be performed by either open or closed techniques.

Closed vertebral biopsy may be safely performed with the use of a variety of specialized needles.[12,39] The procedure may be performed through a posterolateral approach under radiographic control or under biplane fluoroscopic control. Computed tomographic-guided needle aspiration and biopsy techniques using CT to verify the precise location of the biopsy site are also in use (see Fig. 19-5). If closed techniques are not successful, open techniques will usually yield the positive diagnosis.

TREATMENT

The goals of treatment in pathologic fractures secondary to metastatic disease are relief of pain, restoration of stability, and maintenance or restoration of neurologic function. In the vast majority of patients these may be achieved with conservative measures, including appropriate chemotherapeutic regimens or radiotherapy. Generally speaking, surgical intervention should be reserved for cases in which conservative measures have little chance of succeeding or have already failed.

Decisions with regard to nonoperative or operative management should be based on:

1. Specific tumor types and predicted sensitivity to treatment
2. Assessment of spinal stability
3. Presence or absence of neurologic deficit
4. Rapidity of the onset of neurologic signs

SPECIFIC TUMOR TYPES AND PREDICTED SENSITIVITY TO TREATMENT

Cancers of the breast, lung, kidney, prostate, and thyroid and melanoma are all tumors that fre-

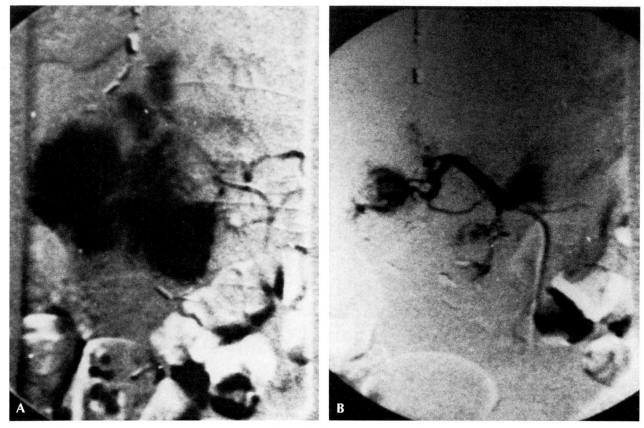

Figure 19-8. Metastatic hypernephroma to the body of L-1. (*A*) Selective arteriography shows the diffuse vascularity of the lesion. (*B*) Note the decreased vascular flow following preoperative embolization.

quently metastasize to bone. Obviously, the underlying tumor type and its known response to treatment greatly determines the necessity for surgical intervention. In one series of patients with breast cancer who had metastasis to the spine, only 26 of 2467 patients required any form of surgical intervention.[10] Unfortunately, some metastatic lesions, such as hypernephroma and melanoma, have poor responses to treatment. In such cases surgical measures are employed more frequently.

ASSESSMENT OF SPINAL STABILITY

Assessment of spinal stability is difficult in metastatic destructive lesions. While traumatic frac-

tures of the spine result in reproducible fracture patterns based on the pathomechanics of the forces applied to the spine, tumor destruction varies according to the basic biologic aggressiveness of the lesion and the tumor's response to treatment. The instability associated with a pathologic fracture secondary to metastatic disease is a dynamic process; it continually increases if tumor growth continues unchecked.

Instability of the spinal column is caused by bony destruction and a relative ligamentous laxity. The precise etiology of bony destruction by tumor is not yet clearly elucidated. It is evident that the tumor cells activate both osteoclasts and osteoblasts. In lytic lesions the osteoclastic response predominates; the reverse occurs in blastic lesions. These processes leave the ligamentous structures intact; however, their bony insertions may be missing. A relative ligamentous laxity results, due to shortening of the spinal column because of destruction of the vertebral bodies or to lack of bony ligamentous insertions. This apparent ligamentous laxity, however, may be restored to normal if the original height of the individual vertebral bodies can be restored. This is in counterdistinction to acute traumatic processes, in which bony destruction is usually accompanied by true ligamentous disruption.

Stability of the spine is best assessed by integrating the information obtained from the history, physical examination, plain radiographs, and CT and by noting the location of the lesion. Radiographically, use of the three-column (anterior, middle, and posterior) concept of spinal stability allows a systematic approach to assessing instability patterns.

The usual site of hematogenous spread of metastatic foci is the cancellous bone of the vertebral body in the area of the pedicle. The lesion grows outward from its original focus, causing increasing destruction. Thus, the usual pattern is initial unilateral destruction of the middle spinal column (Fig. 19-9A), although any pattern may occur. Further destruction may progress to involve the entire anterior and middle columns (Fig. 19-9B). When tumor destruction spreads posteriorly through the pedicles to the neural arches all three columns of the spine can be involved (Fig. 19-9C).

Metastatic spread from its primary focus usually develops in a haphazard fashion; it commonly involves the entire anterior and the remainder of the middle column. Virtually any pattern of destruction is possible, and de novo metastatic foci may yield numerous noncontiguous lesions within the same vertebral body. The resultant instability depends on the specific columns affected.

Assessment of plain radiographs offers a general overview of the extent of vertebral column destruction. Computed tomography accurately depicts the extent of destruction within each of the three columns. Assessment of stability can be determined by the number of columns involved. Lesions that involve only one column are stable lesions. Stability can be preserved, provided conservative measures are available to check the dynamic spread of destruction. Lesions with two-column involvement should be considered unstable. Tumors with great sensitivity to conservative treatment modalities, such as breast carcinomas, may "heal" into a stable configuration, but until such time they should be treated as unstable conditions. Unless neurologic indications demand immediate surgical intervention, conservative therapy and short-term bracing should be considered in these patients. Three-column involvement is a markedly unstable situation. Even with very "sensitive" tumor types, these lesions will probably require a stabilization procedure and possibly anterior and posterior surgery.

Stability may be restored to destroyed segments of the spine if tumor growth can be halted by either chemotherapy or radiation. External support with bracing may be used for 2 to 3 months while healing occurs. If these conservative measures fail, however, restoration of stability will be best accomplished by surgical reconstruction or reinforcement of the columns involved. In patients with an anticipated life expectancy of less than 1 year, this is often accomplished by techniques employing methyl methacrylate. The use of methyl methacrylate will provide instantaneous stability and allow rapid mobilization of the patient. Subsequent irradiation, if necessary, in levels clinically used today will not affect the structural integrity of the cement.[37]

Patients with a life expectancy of greater than 1 year may be better served by techniques that utilize fusion. An exception to this is the extremely unstable situation of three-column destruction in which both anterior and posterior procedures are planned. With prolonged life expectancy in this situation, methyl methacrylate may be used either anteriorly or posteriorly, provided that the bony fusion extends over the same or greater levels.

NEUROLOGIC DEFICITS

In metastatic disease with limited life expectancy, the preservation of neurologic function is of utmost importance to the patient as well as those who provide care for the patient. The results in the literature regarding return of neurologic function, whether through radiation therapy, laminectomy, or both, have shown limited suc-

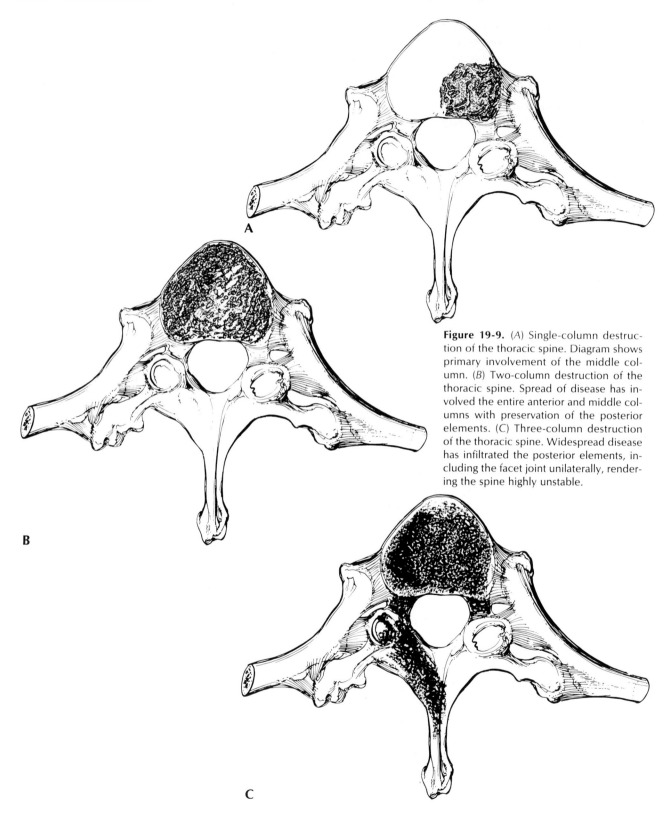

Figure 19-9. (A) Single-column destruction of the thoracic spine. Diagram shows primary involvement of the middle column. (B) Two-column destruction of the thoracic spine. Spread of disease has involved the entire anterior and middle columns with preservation of the posterior elements. (C) Three-column destruction of the thoracic spine. Widespread disease has infiltrated the posterior elements, including the facet joint unilaterally, rendering the spine highly unstable.

cess.[34,35,53] Livingston and Perrin, in 1978, reviewed the results of 100 extensive laminectomies for neurologic deficits in metastatic disease. They defined "satisfactory" recovery as the ability to walk, urinary continence, and survival of 6 months or longer. They considered satisfactory results to have been achieved in 40 of the 100 laminectomy patients. This, however, included 29 preoperative ambulators.[31] Gilbert and associates, also in 1978, compared the results of radiotherapy alone in 170 patients to the results of laminectomy followed by radiotherapy in 65 patients. Success was defined as ambulation after treatment. The treatment group included preoperative ambulators and nonambulatory patients. Ambulation was preserved in 46% with laminectomy and radiotherapy, as compared to 49% of those with radiotherapy alone.[22,23] These results are certainly consistent with other reports of clinical neurologic improvement in 20% to 40% of patients after decompressive laminectomy.[6,10,11,24,36,38,44,50,52]

The majority of metastatic lesions to the spine with cord involvement cause anterior epidural compression.[33] Doppman and associates concluded, by means of an angiographic study in rhesus monkeys, that an anterior epidural mass larger than 4 mm in diameter could not be adequately decompressed by laminectomy.[14] Since the majority of metastatic tumor compression is anterior it is not surprising that a comparison between laminectomy followed by radiotherapy and radiotherapy alone would not find significant differences.

The most important factors in deciding treatment for patients with neurologic deficits are:

1. Response to high-dose steroids
2. Anticipated radiosensitivity of the metastatic tumor
3. Rapidity of onset and the amount of neurologic deficit
4. Stability of the vertebral column
5. Location of the dural compression (i.e. anterior, posterior or circumferential)

In cases of progressive neurologic deficits, the use of high-dose steroids often stabilizes the neurologic picture enough to allow a thorough evaluation of the above factors. Patients with slowly pro-

gressive neurologic deficits secondary to a radiosensitive tumor and a stable spine can be safely treated with radiotherapy. However, even with a slowly progressive lesion, extensive tumor destruction, creating an unstable spine, may result in progressive neurologic dysfunction despite radiotherapy. With the rapid onset of progressive neurologic loss, patients are better treated with decompressive procedures followed by stabilization.

When decompressive procedures are warranted they should be preceded by a careful assessment of the location of the compression. Past results of laminectomy and inability to remove the anterior tumor have led to the increasing use of anterior decompressive procedures associated with stabilization techniques. These will be outlined later.

STABILIZATION OF THE CERVICAL SPINE

Metastatic disease of the cervical spine may present anywhere on a spectrum from mild insidious onset of pain to dramatic onset with an acute "chin on chest" deformity (Fig. 19-10). When instability exists or decompressive procedures are indicated stabilization should be performed. Many authors have recommended stabilization procedures for treatment of malignant lesions of the cervical spine.[7,9,15,17,18,26,30,41]

ANTERIOR PROCEDURES

Replacement of destroyed vertebral bodies in the anterior cervical spine has been accomplished using various constructs, including iliac crest, fibular struts, tibial struts, methyl methacrylate, and methyl methacrylate reinforced with various types of metal.[7,9,15,17,18,26,30,40–42] Wang and associates performed biomechanical testing on 11 different anterior cervical spine constructs ranging from a simple cement plug to combined anterior and posterior fixation. It was apparent that most fixation constructs failed to regain the structural strength of the normal spine under extension loads. Even complex rigid anterior fixation devices using plates and screws failed in extension by inferior screw pullout from the bone. They further concluded that anterior and posterior fixation did

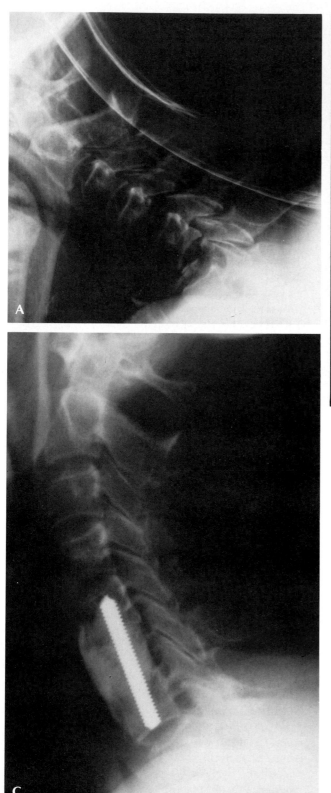

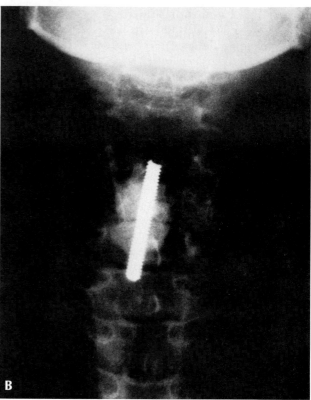

Figure 19-10. "Chin on chest" deformity. (*A*) This 59-year-old woman with known metastatic lung carcinoma was undergoing radiotherapy to the lower cervical spine for involvement of C-6. She walked into radiotherapy complaining of severe pain in the neck and an inability to lift her chin from her chest. This lateral view demonstrates the complete collapse of the body of C-6 with the inferior end-plate of C-5 almost resting on C-7. (*B, C*) Postoperative anteroposterior and lateral views demonstrate restoration of normal cervical alignment. A 3/16th-inch threaded Steinmann's pin is embedded into the bodies of C-5 and C-7 with a plug of methyl methacrylate cement substituting for the body of C-6. Note that the restoration of vertebral height allows the posterior facet joints to realign normally.

not improve strength, although it did increase the fixation rigidity.[49]

In the clinical situation, although not without failures, a wide variety of cervical constructs using either bone grafting, cement, or cement reinforced with metal have provided satisfactory results.[9,16,18,27,30,41] Because of the obvious weakness of constructs to extension loading, it is critical to key the vertebral substitute well into the bodies above and below to prevent anterior dislodgement. With cement constructs, a threaded pin or small one third tubular plate driven up into the vertebral body above and below will help to prevent dislodgement (Fig. 19-11). Care is taken to avoid compression of the dura with the cement. An interpositional layer of Gelfoam sponge is used between the construct and the dura. During the polymerization phase the wound is irrigated with cold saline.

If the posterior elements are intact, then anterior replacement alone will suffice. Otherwise, a supplemental posterior procedure is performed (Fig. 19-12). Fielding and associates recommended that in supplemental posterior fusions in which local anterior reoccurrence was probable, the fusion should include two levels above and below the anterior graft.[18]

POSTERIOR PROCEDURES

Posterior techniques may be used alone when confronted mainly with posterior column destruction. A wide variety of techniques have been used, including spinous process wiring, facet wiring, sublaminar wiring, and application of wire mesh and cement.[9,16,18,25,30,41] The choice between bone grafting and the use of methyl methacrylate is based on the life expectancy of the patient. When methyl methacrylate fusion is chosen, the posterior elements should be wired together with conventional techniques; the cement is then carefully molded to the spine. If the dura is exposed, care is taken to avoid injury. When the longevity of the patient is in doubt, a combination of cement stabilization and bony fusion may be performed. Clark and associates used a technique employing both cement and bone graft. The cement is placed over underlying iliac corticocancellous bone graft to help ensure rigidity until the fusion has consolidated.[9]

STABILIZATION OF THE THORACIC AND LUMBAR SPINE

As in the cervical region, stability must be assessed by means of the three-column concept. Since most metastases start in the vertebral bodies, some compromise of the anterior and middle column is invariably present.

ANTERIOR PROCEDURES

Posterior laminectomy procedures further destabilize the spine and generally fail to debulk much of the anterior focus of tumor mass. Furthermore, patients who have already had previous radiotherapy to their backs have increased risk for poor wound healing and dehiscence following posterior procedures. In order to avoid problems associated with posterior wounds, and in an attempt to improve upon the mediocre results of neurologic recovery following laminectomy, various anterior decompressive and stabilization techniques have been developed. Many authors have described the use of anterior vertebrectomy and vertebral substitution for metastatic disease of the thoracic and lumbar spine.[27,30,43,47,48,51]

Harrington has successfully used a technique of embedding double Harrington rods and hooks into the anterolateral aspect of the vertebral bodies to reduce pathologic fracture-dislocations. This is performed in conjunction with decompression of the spinal canal and methyl methacrylate substitution of the vertebral body. He has recently reported excellent spinal restoration in 72 of 75 patients, associated with complete resolution or improvement of neurologic function in 69%.[26]

A similar method using a different surgical construct was introduced by Sundaresan and associates to replace vertebral bodies anteriorly with methyl methacrylate and to decompress the spinal canal. Their construct embedded two smooth Kirschner wires into vertebral segments above and below the defects left after vertebrectomy. Methyl methacrylate was then used to fill the gap; the Kirschner wires were incorporated to prevent dislodgement. They reported preservation of ambulation in 78 of 101 patients. More impressive, however, was the 70% improvement in patients who were nonambulators prior to treatment. This represents an improvement rate twice that gener-

(Text continued on p. 516)

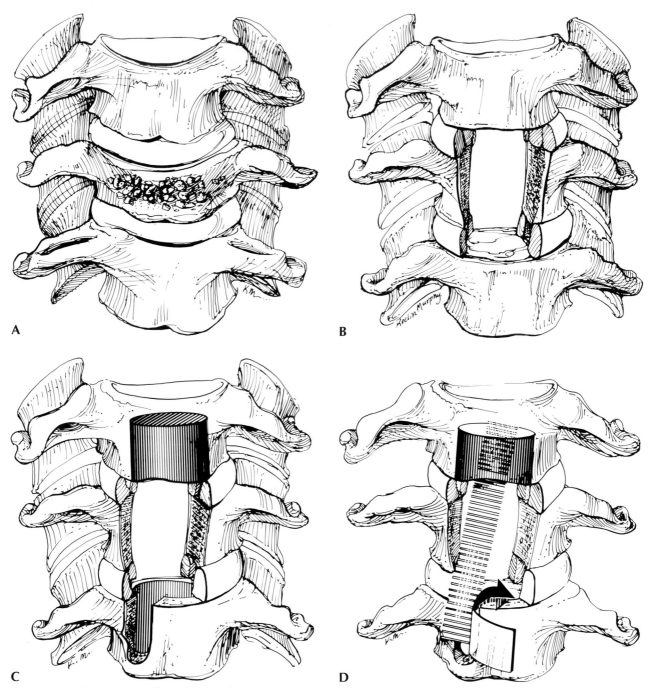

A

B

C

D

Figure 19-11. Anterior cervical procedure with a cement construct. (*A*) Diagrammatically shown are three cervical vertebrae as the surgeon would see them through an anterior approach to the spine. The central vertebra has been destroyed by tumor. (*B*) A near complete vertebral body resection is performed, including the disks and end-plates of the vertebra above and below. Decompression of the canal is performed as dictated by neurologic compression. (*C*) In order to insert a metallic rod, a trough is made in the anterior aspect of the body below, eccentrically off the midline. The cancellous bone of the vertebral bodies is excavated through the end-plates by means of curettes or an angled drill. (*D*) Either a heavy Steinmann's pin cut to length or a small AO semitubular plate is inserted up into the body above and then downward through the trough into the vertebral body below.

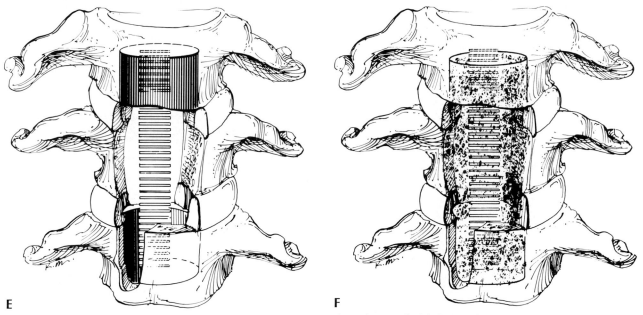

E   **F**

Figure 19-11. Continued (*E*) The rod is centralized, moving it away from the trough. (*F*) Cement is then added to the construct. If the canal has been opened an interpositional layer of gelfoam is placed to protect the dura. In order to get a better cement fill the rod can be temporarily removed while a small amount of cement is packed gently into the posterior aspect of the space. The rod is then reinserted and cement is packed anterior to the rod, filling the trough flush to the level of the adjacent vertebral bodies.

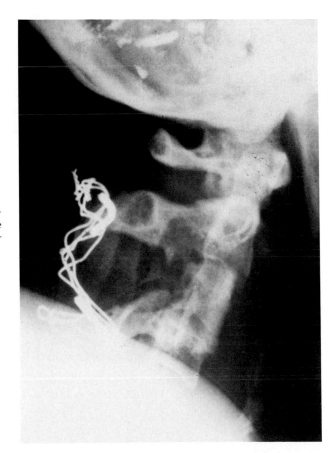

Figure 19-12. Demonstration of anterior cervical fusion combined with posterior wiring and onlay of methyl methacrylate cement. Patient had destruction of both anterior and posterior elements by multiple myeloma.

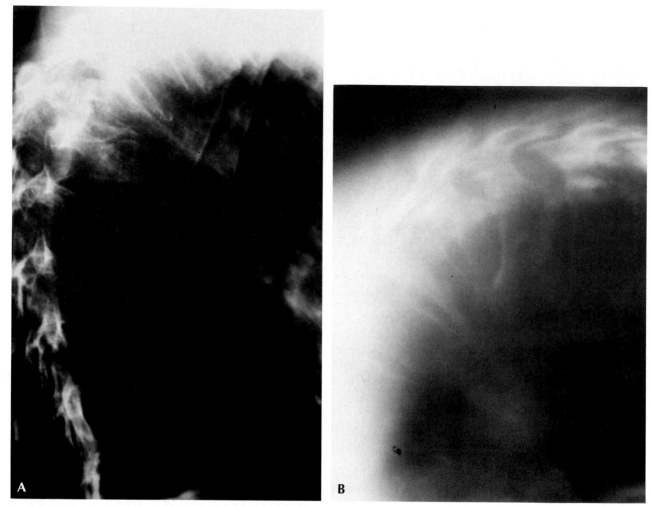

Figure 19-13. (A) Pathologic collapse of two upper thoracic vertebrae secondary to previously un-diagnosed lymphoma in a 73-year-old woman who presented to the emergency room with the acute onset of severe paraparesis. (B) Tomograms more clearly demonstrate the acute kyphotic deformity over the region of the two collapsed thoracic vertebrae.

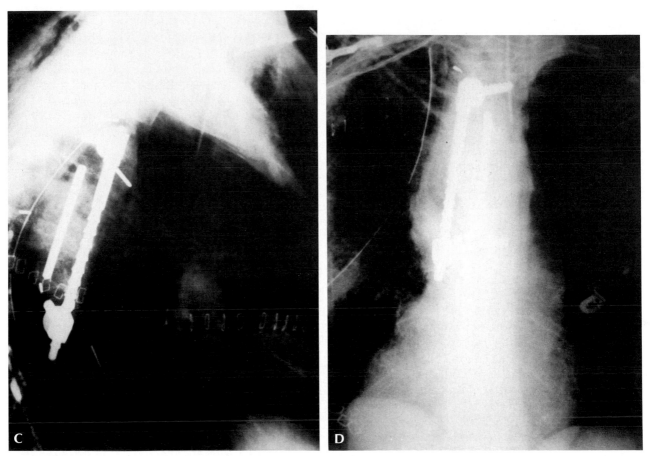

Figure 19-13. Continued. (*C, D*) Anterior Kostuik–Harrington instrumentation was used to correct the kyphotic deformity. A threaded Steinmann's pin was inserted into the body above and below. Cement was used as a vertebral substitute.

ally reported for nonambulatory patients undergoing radiotherapy.[47]

Depending on the specific clinical setting, a variety of anterior stabilization techniques may be used following anterior decompressive surgery. When a significant kyphotic deformity exists, the anterior Kostuik–Harrington system may be used to restore anatomic alignment of the spine (Fig. 19-13). When patients have relatively long life expectancies, many surgeons are reluctant to employ cement. For single or double vertebral body replacement, anterior Kostuik–Harrington instrumentation has been used in conjunction with a bicortical iliac strut graft to obtain a solid anterior arthrodesis (Fig. 19-14).[29] With life expectancy of less than 1 year, cement replacement of the body may be performed (Fig. 19-15).

When there is no severe associated kyphotic deformity and life expectancy is less than 1 year, simple vertebrectomy and replacement of the vertebral body with a methyl methacrylate construct should suffice. After canal decompression and tumor removal, two or three stacked heavy-threaded rods or Harrington rods are wedged into bodies above and below, followed by application of methyl methacrylate cement (Fig. 19-16).[30] Alternatively, a method of vertebral body replacement using a combination of methyl methacrylate cement and Silastic, with (Fig. 19-17) or without (Fig. 19-18) a metallic internal fixation, can be used. A 72% rate of significant neurologic improvement was noted after anterior decompressions using these techniques,[30] which is comparable to other reports.[27,47]

Anterior replacement alone will not, however, suffice in all situations. Sundaresan reported the need for additional posterior stabilization in 10 of his 101 patients.[47] When all three spinal columns are destroyed by tumor, the anterior procedure will need to be supplemented by posterior instrumentation, either staged or performed simultaneously (Fig. 19-19).

POSTERIOR SEGMENTAL INSTRUMENTATION

Carefully selected patients may benefit from posterior segmental instrumentation using either Harrington–Luque,[30] Luque rodding,[13,19] or even Cotrel–Dubousset techniques (Fig. 19-20). The advantages of segmental fixation are obvious in the soft osteoporotic bone of most cancer patients. The technique allows multiple levels to be spanned when dealing with patients with lesions in multiple levels of the thoracic and lumbar spine. The application of methyl methacrylate incorporating not only the rods, but the individual wires or hooks at each level, allows rapid mobilization of the patients without brace or corset (see Fig. 19-12). The relief of pain in these patients is often dramatic and rewarding.

The disadvantages to posterior segmental instrumentation are:

1. Posterior decompression must be relied on to relieve anterior dural compression in many cases.
2. If a long decompression is necessary, a large laminectomy leaves no segmental fixation at multiple levels.
3. One must often operate through irradiated skin, which has poor healing qualities.
4. There is a risk of passing sublaminar wires or hooks into the neural canal, which may already be compromised by epidural tumor spread.

These techniques may, however, offer a viable solution to the patient with multiple-level involvement and significant pain that interferes with quality of life. Although the literature is limited, at present it appears that spanning the involved segment for three levels above and below should suffice. The use of double 1.22-mm (16-gauge) wire at each level with 3/16-inch rods has also been suggested.[19] If Cotrel–Dubousset instrumentation is to be used, hook configuration patterns should be spaced to allow for fixation two to three levels above and below the affected area.

If a posterior technique is selected for use as either a single-stage or part of a two-stage procedure, caution should be used in patients who have had previous radiation because of their increased risk of infection.[46] Wound breakdown around a long posterior instrumentation is a difficult complication to manage. Deep nonabsorbable suture materials should be used for wound closure, as irradiated fascial structures may delay healing past

(Text continued on p. 524)

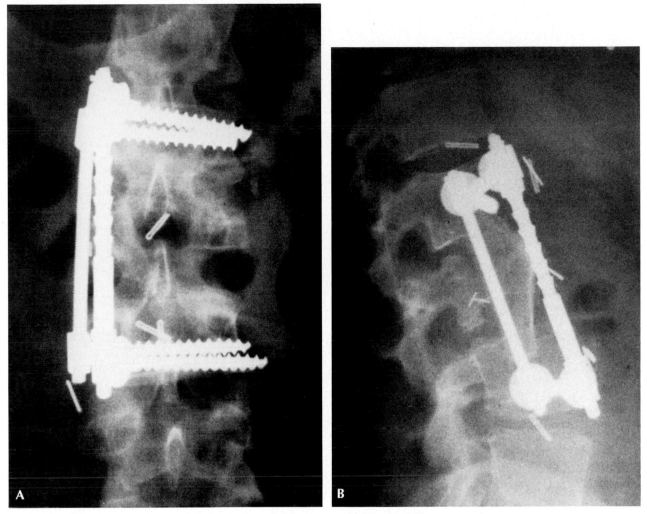

Figure 19-14. (*A, B*) Anterior Kostuik–Harrington instrumentation and a bicortical iliac strut graft replace the L-2 vertebral body in a 62-year-old man with unusual metastatic breast carcinoma.

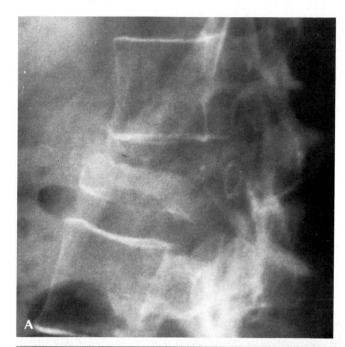

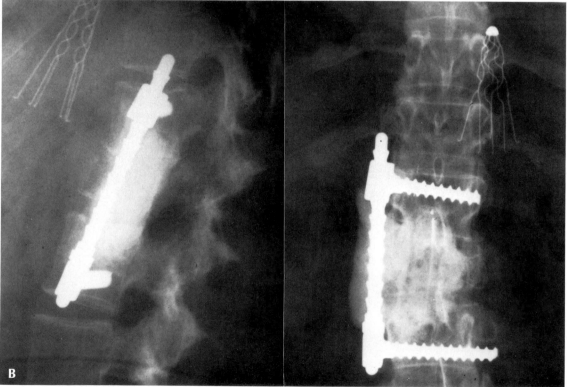

Figure 19-15. End-stage breast cancer. (*A*) Note the significant collapse of the L-1 vertebral body. (*B*) Because of the limited life expectancy in this patient the vertebral segment was replaced with a cement replacement technique.

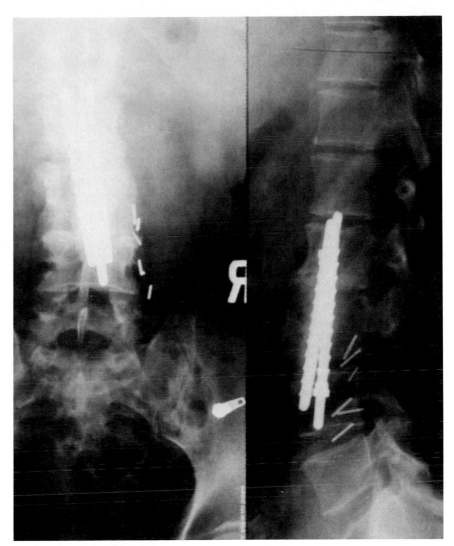

Figure 19-16. Postoperative radiographs of a patient following vertebrectomy of L-3 and canal decompression of a metastatic lung carcinoma. Harrington rods were inserted from L-2 to L-4 and methyl methacrylate cement was used to substitute for the vertebral body.

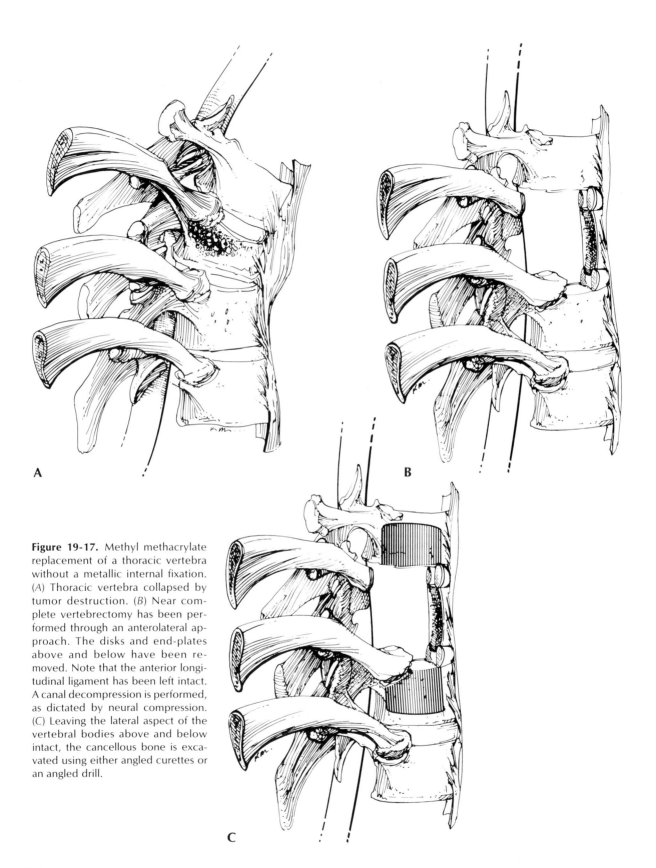

Figure 19-17. Methyl methacrylate replacement of a thoracic vertebra without a metallic internal fixation. (A) Thoracic vertebra collapsed by tumor destruction. (B) Near complete vertebrectomy has been performed through an anterolateral approach. The disks and end-plates above and below have been removed. Note that the anterior longitudinal ligament has been left intact. A canal decompression is performed, as dictated by neural compression. (C) Leaving the lateral aspect of the vertebral bodies above and below intact, the cancellous bone is excavated using either angled curettes or an angled drill.

A

B

C

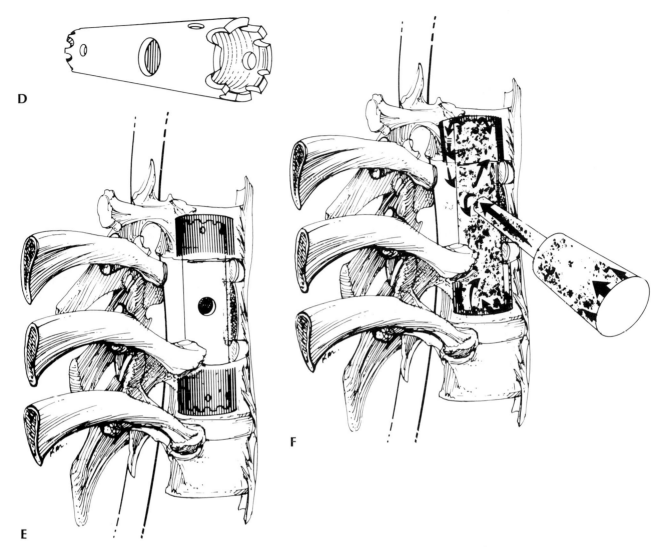

Figure 19-17. Continued. (*D*) A Silastic tube of appropriate diameter is fashioned to fit into the vertebral body above as well as below. A hole is made with a rongeur in the lateral portion of the tube to accept a syringe filled with methyl methacrylate in a highly liquid phase. (*E*) The cement is "pressurized" into the tube until it is seen to exude out of the bodies above and below. Care is taken to avoid migration of the cement into the spinal canal. (*F*) Finally, cement is packed all around the tube, avoiding the spinal canal, until it is flush with the lateral aspects of the vertebral bodies above and below.

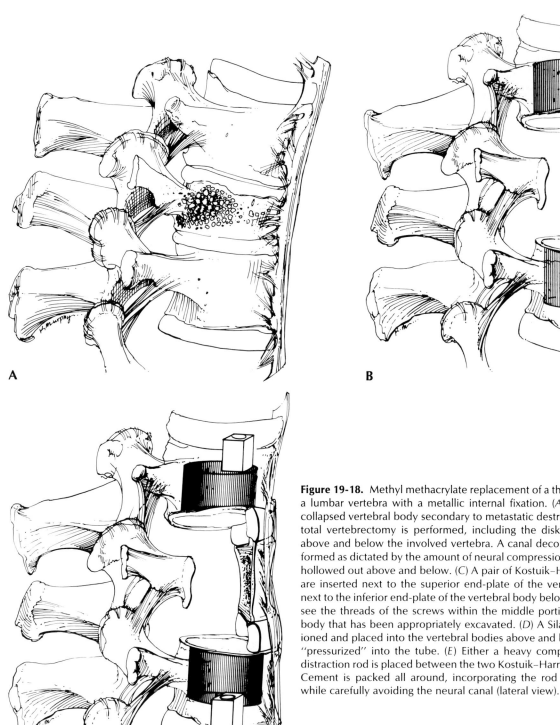

A

B

C = Lateral view

Figure 19-18. Methyl methacrylate replacement of a thoracolumbar and a lumbar vertebra with a metallic internal fixation. (*A*) Lateral view of collapsed vertebral body secondary to metastatic destruction. (*B*) A near total vertebrectomy is performed, including the disks and end-plates above and below the involved vertebra. A canal decompression is performed as dictated by the amount of neural compression. The bodies are hollowed out above and below. (*C*) A pair of Kostuik–Harrington screws are inserted next to the superior end-plate of the vertebra above and next to the inferior end-plate of the vertebral body below. Often one can see the threads of the screws within the middle portion of a vertebral body that has been appropriately excavated. (*D*) A Silastic tube is fashioned and placed into the vertebral bodies above and below. Cement is "pressurized" into the tube. (*E*) Either a heavy compression rod or a distraction rod is placed between the two Kostuik–Harrington screws. (*F*) Cement is packed all around, incorporating the rod into the cement while carefully avoiding the neural canal (lateral view).

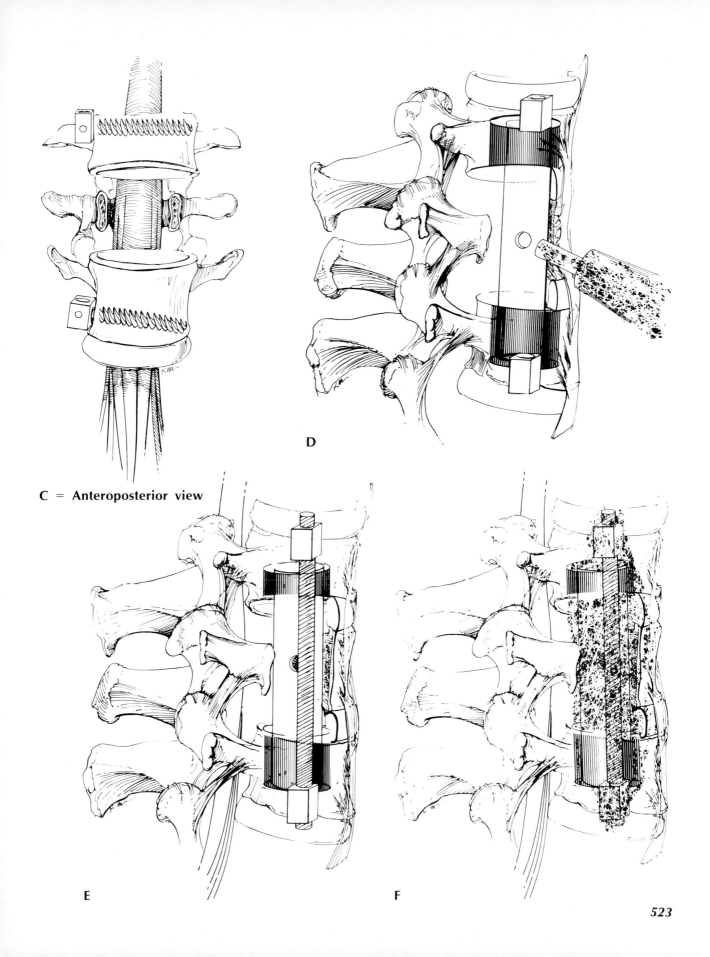

C = Anteroposterior view

D

E

F

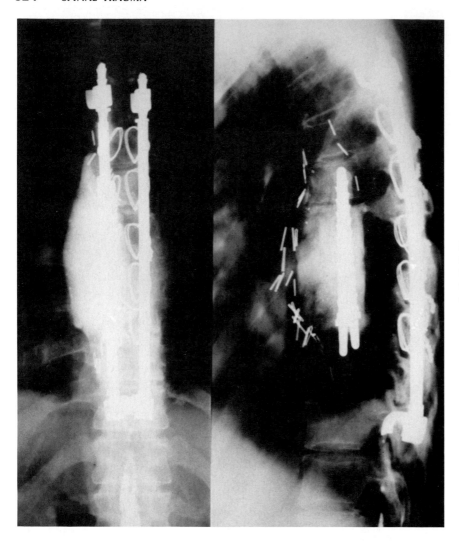

Figure 19-19. Radiographs following anterior and posterior stabilization of a metastatic lesion of hypernephoma that had caused extensive destruction of all three spinal columns.

the lifetime of synthetic absorbable suture materials. Preoperative plastic surgery consultation should be considered regarding mobilization of muscle layers at the time of surgery or possible use of tissue expanders preoperatively to provide extra coverage.

SUMMARY

Involvement with patients with metastatic disease is an increasing aspect of orthopedic surgery due to advances in longevity achieved over the last decade. The treatment of spinal metastases de-

mands comprehensive evaluation and decision making on the part of the orthopedic surgeon. By far, the vast majority of cases can adequately be managed with the conservative measures outlined. The results with anterior decompression and stabilization, however, have proven to yield better results with regard to neurologic recovery than either radiotherapy or laminectomy and radiotherapy.

Decision making is crucial, as no single technique will best solve each clinical dilemma. The rational application of the principles and techniques outlined above can dramatically enhance the quality of life for this patient population.

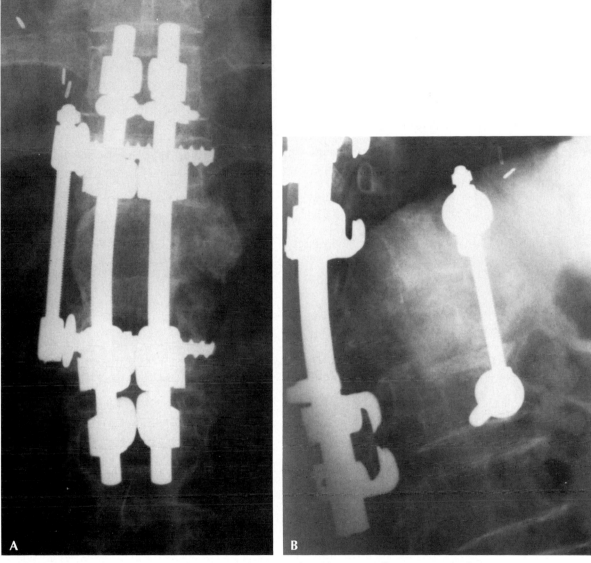

Figure 19-20. (*A, B*) Radiographs of a patient with metastatic thyroid cancer. Following angiography and selected embolization she had anterior resection of the tumor. Because of a good long-term prognosis an allograft was used instead of cement. A single Kostuik–Harrington rod was used for internal fixation. Three-column destruction had been demonstrated and therefore a second-stage posterior stabilization with Cotrel–Dubousset instrumentation was performed.

REFERENCES

1. Baron KD, Hirano A, Araki S, Ferry RD: Experiences with metastatic neoplasms involving the spinal cord. Neurology 9:91, 1959

2. Batson OV: The function of the vertebral veins and their role in the spread of metastases. Ann Surg 112:138-149, 1940

3. Batson OV: The vertebral vein system. AJR 78:195-212, 1957

4. Blair RJ, McAfee JG: Radiological detection of skeletal metastases: Radiographs versus scan. International Journal of Oncology 1:1201-1205, 1976

5. Boland PJ, Lane JM, Sundaresan N: Metastatic disease of the spine. Clin Orthop 169:95-102, 1982

6. Brice J, McKissock W: Surgical treatment of malignant extradural spinal tumors. Br Med J, 1:1341-1344, 1965

7. Chadduck WM, Boop WC Jr: Acrylic stabilization of the cervical spine for neoplastic disease: Evolution of a technique for vertebral body replacement. Neurosurgery 13:23-29, 1983

8. Citron DL, Bessent RG, Greig WR: A comparison of the sensitivity and accuracy of the 99Tcm-phosphate bone scan and skeletal radiograph in the diagnosis of bone metastases. Clin Radiol, 28:107-117, 1972

9. Clark CR, Keggi KJ, Panjabi MM: Methylmethacrylate stabilization of the cervical spine. J Bone Joint Surg [Am] 66:40-46, 1984

10. Cobb CD, Leavens ME, Eckles N: Indications for non-operative treatment of spinal cord compression due to breast cancer. J Neurosurg 47:653-658, 1977

11. Constans JP, De Divitiis E, Donzelli R et al: Spinal metastases with neurologic manifestations: Review of 600 cases. J Neurosurg 59:111-118, 1983

12. Craig FS: Vertebral body biopsy. J Bone Joint Surg [Am] 38:93-102, 1956

13. DeWald RL, Bridwell KH, Prodromas C, Rodts MF: Reconstructive spinal surgery as palliation for metastatic malignancies of the spine. Spine 10:21-26, 1985

14. Doppman JL, Girton M: Angiographic study of the effect of laminectomy in the presence of acute anterior epidural masses. J Neurosurg 45:653-658, 1977

15. Dunn EJ: The role of methylmethacrylate in the stabilization and replacement of tumors of the cervical spine: A project of the Cervical Spine Research Society. Spine 2:15-24, 1977

16. Dunn EJ, Davidson RI, Anas PP: Tumors involving the cervical spine: Diagnosis and management. In Bailey RW, Sherk HH, Dunn EJ et al (eds): The Cervical Spine, pp 477-495. Philadelphia, JB Lippincott, 1983

17. Fidler MW: pathologic fractures of the cervical spine: Palliative surgical treatment. J Bone Joint Surg [Br] 67:352-357, 1985

18. Fielding JW, Pyle RN Jr, Fietti VG: Anterior cervical vertebral body resection and bone-grafting for benign and malignant tumors: A survey under the auspices of the Cervical Spine Research Society. J Bone Joint Surg [Am] 61:251-253, 1979

19. Flatley TJ, Anderson MH, Anast GT: Spinal instability due to malignant disease: Treatment by segmental spinal stabilization. J Bone Joint Surg [Am] 66:47-52, 1984

20. Fournasier VL, Horne JG: Metastases to the vertebral column. Cancer 36:590-594, 1975

21. Francis KC, Hutter RP: Neoplasms of the spine in the aged. Clin Orthop 26:54-66, 1963

22. Gilbert HA, Kagan R: Evaluation of radiation therapy for bone metastases: Pain relief and quality of life. AJR 129:1095, 1977

23. Gilbert RW, Kim JH, Posner JB: Epidural spinal cord compression from metastatic tumor: Diagnosis and treatment. Ann Neurol 3:40-51, 1978

24. Hall AJ, MacKay NS: The results of laminectomy for compression of the cord or cauda equina by extradural malignant tumor. J Bone Joint Surg [Br] 55:497, 1973

25. Hansebout RR, Blomquist GA Jr: Acrylic spinal fusion: A 20 year clinical series and technical note. J Neurosurg 53:606-612, 1980

26. Harrington KD: Anterior decompression and stabilization of the spine for spinal cord compression from metastatic malignancy: 92 operations for 77 patients. Presented at the annual meeting of the American Academy of Orthopaedic Surgeons, Las Vegas, Nevada. January 27, 1985

27. Harrington KD: The use of methylmethacrylate for vertebral body replacement and anterior stabilization of pathologic fracture-dislocation of the spine due to metastatic malignant disease. J Bone Joint Surg [Am] 63:36-46, 1981

28. Jaffe WL: Tumors and Tumorous Conditions of the Bones and Joints. Philadelphia, Lea & Febiger, 1958

29. Kostuik JP: Anterior fixation for fractures of the thoracic and lumbar spine with or without neurologic involvement. Clin Orthop 189:116-124, 1984

30. Kostuik JP, Errico TJ, Gleason TG, Errico CC: Spinal stabilization of vertebral column tumors. Spine 13:250-256, 1988

31. Livingston KE, Perrin RG: The neurosurgical management of spinal metastases causing cord and cauda equina compression. J Neurosurg 49:839-843, 1978

32. MacNab I: Backache. Baltimore, Williams & Wilkins, 1977

33. Martin NS, Williamson J: The role of surgery in the treatment of malignant tumors of the spine. J Bone Joint Surg [Br] 52:227-237, 1970

34. Millburn L, Hibbs GG, Hendrickson FR: Treatment of spinal cord compression from metastatic carcinoma: Review of the literature and presentation of a new method of treatment. Cancer 21:447-452, 1968

35. Mones RJ, Dozier D, Berrett A: Analysis of medical treatment of malignant extradural spinal cord tumors. Cancer 19:1842-1853, 1966

36. Mullan J, Evan JP: Neoplastic disease of the spinal extradural space. Arch Surg 74:900-907, 1957

37. Murray JA, Bruels MC, Lindberg RD: Irradiation of polymethylmethacrylate: In vitro gamma radiation effect. J Bone Joint Surg [Am] 56:311-312, 1974

38. Nather A, Kamal Bose: The results of decompression of cord or cauda equina compression from metastatic extradural tumors. Clin Orthop 169:103-108, 1982

39. Ottolenghi CE: Aspiration biopsy of the spine: Technique and results in 1078 cases. J Bone Joint Surg [Am] 49:1479, 1967

40. Panjabi MM, Goel VK, Clark CR et al: Biomechanical study of cervical spine stabilization with methylmethacrylate. Spine 10:198-203, 1985

41. Raycroft JF, Hockman RP, Southwick WD: Metastatic tumors involving the cervical vertebrae: Surgical palliation. J Bone Joint Surg [Am] 60:763-768, 1978

42. Scoville WB, Palmer AH, Samra K, Chong G.: The use of acrylic plastic for vertebral replacement or fixation in metastatic disease of the spine. J Neurosurg 27:274-279, 1967

43. Siegal T, Tiqva R, Siegal T: Vertebral body resection for epidural compression by malignant tumors. J Bone Joint Surg [Am] 67:375-382, 1985

44. Smith R: An evaluation of surgical treatment for spinal cord compression due to metastatic carcinoma. J Neurol Neurosurg Psychiatry 28:152-157, 1965

45. Springfield DS: Mechanisms of metastasis. Clin Orthop 169:15-19, 1982

46. Sundaresan N, Galicich JH, Lane JM: Harrington rod stabilization for pathologic fractures of the spine. J Neurosurg 60:282-286, 1984

47. Sundaresan N, Galicich JH, Lane JM et al: Treatment of neoplastic epidural cord compression by vertebral body resection and stabilization. J Neurosurg 63:676-684, 1985

48. Turner PL, Prince HG, Webb JK, Sokal MPJW: Surgery for malignant extradural tumors of the spine. J Bone Joint Surg [Br] 70:451-455, 1988

49. Wang GJ, Lewish GD, Reger SI et al: Comparative strengths of various anterior cement fixations of the cervical spine. Spine 7:717-721, 1983

50. White WA, Patterson RII Jr, Bergland RM: Role of surgery in the treatment of spinal cord compression by metastatic neoplasm. Cancer 27:558-561, 1971

51. Winter RB: Anterior spinal cord decompression and spine stabilization for metastatic disease: A case report. Spine 7:70-72, 1982

52. Wright RL: Malignant tumors in the spinal extradural space: Results of surgical treatment. Ann Surg 157:227-231, 1963

53. Young RF, Post EM, King GA: Treatment of spinal epidural metastases. Randomized prospective comparison of laminectomy and radiotherapy. J Neurosurg 53:741-748, 1980

20

PATHOLOGIC SPINAL FRACTURES DUE TO INFECTIONS

Kent M. Patrick

Infection involving the spinal column often alters the integrity of the spine through the destruction of bone, disk, and cartilage. This structural disruption, combined with the normal forces of gravity and muscle tension on the spine, can lead to vertebral collapse and the development of kyphotic deformity. When bone is involved and collapse or deformity is present, the fractures can be considered pathologic. The deformity may be so mild as to go relatively unnoticed or may be severe enough to result in paraplegia.

Although a host of microorganisms—pyogenic, nonpyogenic, and fungal—can infect the spinal column, worldwide, the most common organism is tuberculosis. In this chapter we will look at tuberculosis as well as pyogenic and fungal osteomyelitis of the spine. To aid in diagnosis and treatment, we will take particular note of the similarities and differences between tuberculous and nontuberculous infections.

TUBERCULOSIS OF THE SPINE

HISTORY AND INCIDENCE

Tuberculosis of the spine has been noted in Egyptian mummies dating from 3000 BC.[17] Pott's disease, as tuberculosis of the spine is often called, was described by Sir Percivall Pott in the 1800s.[65] At the turn of the century tuberculosis was the leading cause of death in Western society.[48]

Tuberculosis of the spine is currently a less common problem in the developed countries of the world, where a higher standard of living has allowed better medical care, nutrition, and housing. However, tuberculosis remains a problem for Asia, Africa, Mexico, and Central and South America, as well as inner city areas within the United States. As peoples from these parts of the world migrate to the developed nations, we can expect to see an increase in the number of cases reported. There will also be an increase in the

529

numbers of cases seen in the indigenous population as this organism is reintroduced to people who have no immunity from previous exposure. This may not have a profound effect on the majority of the people, but will become an important consideration for the increasing homeless populations and those immunosuppressed through illness or drug therapy (e.g., persons infected with the human immunodeficiency virus, those with immunosuppressed cancer, and transplant patients).

In spite of significant advances in the surgical and chemotherapeutic approaches to this disease, 30,000 cases of tuberculosis were documented in the United States alone in 1977, with a 10% fatality rate.[48] Between 1971 and 1977, the incidence per 100,000 population in the United States dropped from 15.8% to 13.9%.[10] The Centers for Disease Control (CDC) issue an annual summary of notifiable diseases. In this summary 22,436 cases of tuberculosis were reported in 1988.[10a] Although this malady has been present for thousands of years, it has yet to be eliminated.

SITE

Unlike pyogenic osteomyelitis, tuberculosis frequently involves the spine. Hodgson reported a 58.7% involvement of the spine in his analysis of 1000 consecutive cases of bone and joint tuberculosis.[33] As compared with nontuberculous osteomyelitis, in tuberculosis the spine is involved in 1% to 5% of cases.[45,68,77] Spinal involvement with tuberculosis has been described for all levels of the spine, from C-1 to the sacral segments. The major site of infection is the vertebral body at the thoracolumbar junction. L-1 was the most commonly involved vertebra of the 587 spinal tuberculosis patients in Hodgson's series.[33] His cases showed a bell-shaped curve with an even drop in cases from L-1 proximally and distally. This pattern can best be explained according to the etiology of spinal tuberculosis.

AGE AND SEX

In tuberculous spinal osteomyelitis, males generally outnumber females, although both sexes are equally susceptible. This is in contrast to pyogenic spinal osteomyelitis, in which males clearly outnumber females. This difference will be discussed in the section on pyogenic infections.

In less developed countries where overcrowding and poor nutrition exist, children are the most susceptible; consequently, the disease is more prevalent in children. In more developed countries, the disease affects adults more often. This will most likely be the case in the United States for new cases of tuberculosis, where the majority of the population has not been previously exposed and has had no chance to develop resistance. The increasing numbers of undernourished and poorly housed children in the United States, however, may too be at great risk.

ETIOLOGY

Involvement of the spine with mycobacterium tuberculosis is primarily through spread from infected abdominal or pelvic organs at the level of the spine. The kidney is a major site of tuberculosis involvement. Seeding of the spine is thought to occur proximally and distally through Batson's venous plexus and lymphatic channels.[4,5] A pulmonary infection can also lead to a spinal focus through spread of the bacilli to the abdominal or pelvic organs and from hematogenous spread to the hip joint, where venous drainage ultimately mingles with the pelvic veins and Batson's plexus. The venous pathway also explains the existence of multiple spinal foci.[33]

PATHOGENESIS

The site of the spinal focus is generally the vertebral body on either side of the vertebral disk. Involvement of the posterior elements or transverse process is rare. Once established, the organism sets off a characteristic cascade of events. The first stage is the granulation tissue phase. This is the "pre-pus" phase described by Hodgson.[33] It consists of an inflammatory reaction with Langhans' giant cells, epithelioid cells, and some small inflammatory cells. Early in the course of the disease, these changes are noted in connection with the small veins. There is rapid spread along the veins, with resultant thrombosis, cellular edema, and tissue necrosis. This progresses to form a paravertebral or cold abscess made up of necrotic tissue, granulation tissue, caseous matter, and necrotic bone. This represents the second stage in the pathogenesis of tuberculous vertebral osteomyelitis.

The paravertebral abscess is the classic finding in active spinal tuberculosis. The importance of this was not appreciated until 1940, when Swett, Bennett, and Street pointed out that patients with an abscess had clinical disease and those without an abscess had no active disease.[74] Hodgson noted failure to diagnose an abscess infrequently; failure of diagnosis was usually associated with lumbar disease, in which diagnosis of an abscess is difficult with plain radiographs.[33] Newer, more sophisticated studies such as magnetic resonance imaging, computed tomography, and ultrasound may help eliminate these missed abscesses (Fig. 20-1).

The infectious process gradually enlarges as more tissue is destroyed. The contents of the abscess differ with the age of the process. Early in its evolution, the pus is a green-yellow fluid with small fragments of bone, cartilaginous end-plate, and granulation tissue, as well as inflammatory cells. With further time, the pus thickens to a toothpastelike material that is both whiter and thicker. Still later, it can become caseous and even solid, with an off-white color. Calcification within the abscess may occur even later.

As the abscess enlarges during the early phases, the periosteum is lifted off the adjacent vertebrae and further necrosis of bone occurs. The vertebral body is rendered helpless to the spreading infection. The involved avascular vertebrae may be destroyed or sequestrated. The sequestra may be small or quite large; these segments of dead bone may be prone to pathologic fractures.[33] The larger sequestered fragments may be pushed posteriorly into the spinal canal, causing neurologic compromise in the form of pressure paraplegia, which differs from that seen with kyphosis secondary to bone collapse. The former occurs more acutely and the latter more slowly.

The intervertebral disk is predominantly an avascular structure, and tends not to be directly involved in the infection. Often the disk becomes detached from the vertebral end-plates, and the annulus fibrosus detaches from the vertebral bodies through the periosteum. The disk can eventually float free in an abscess cavity. The disk, like sequestrated bone, can be retropulsed into the spinal canal.

Granulation tissue makes up the abscess wall and, when in contact with the dura mater, can cause pachymeningitis. In and of itself this is not a problem, but if and when healing occurs, this granulation tissue can turn into a dense fibrous tissue that may strangulate the cord. This may progress to a late-onset paraplegia that is irreversible. It may be recognized early in its clinical course by sensory changes.

Enlargement of the active abscess may cause the body to attempt to spontaneously expel the abscess cavity through the formation of the classic prevertebral, paravertebral, or psoas abscesses. These may drain spontaneously or may require surgical intervention.

The body's attempt at spontaneous drainage can affect many other organs, since the abscess lies

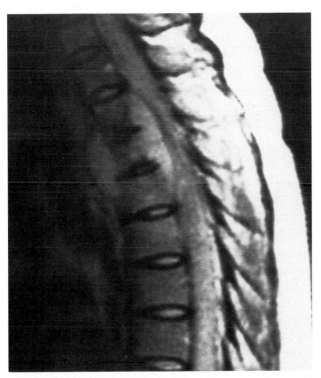

Figure 20-1. Active pulmonary tuberculosis in a 39-year-old woman. Magnetic resonance imaging of the thoracic spine obtained for minor complaints revealed a large pre- and paravertebral abscess. Despite the obvious cord compression she was neurologically normal.

deep within the body. The abscess can penetrate the trachea, esophagus, vena cava, bronchus, lung, pleura, pericardium, mediastinum, aorta, liver, kidney, ureter, abdominal cavity intestine, urinary bladder, vagina, and rectum.[33] The lung is the most commonly involved organ. Fang, Ong, and Hodgson reported 10% of 327 consecutive cases of thoracic spinal tuberculosis with lung penetrations.[23]

In cervical spine involvement, abscesses may occur in the retropharyngeal region, leading to anterior displacement of the pharynx, larynx, trachea, and esophagus. This may cause Millar's asthma, a condition first described by Millar in the 1800s in patients with cervicodorsal tuberculosis complicated by cyanosis, suffocation, and death due to airway compromise.[41] More commonly, the abscess tracts laterally behind the strong prevertebral fascia to exit in the posterior triangle of the neck, producing a sinus. Rupture of the abscess into the pharynx has also been described.

Kyphosis develops in patients with spinal tuberculosis for a number of reasons. The first and most obvious is that with involvement of the vertebral bodies there is bony destruction, with loss of mechanical integrity of the spine. The combined effects of gravity and muscle forces lead to spinal collapse. Without involvement of the posterior elements, as is the case in the majority of tuberculosis cases, all the destruction tends to be anterior; thus, the collapse leads to kyphosis (Fig. 20-2). The more vertebrae involved, the greater the shortening of the anterior column and the greater the instability and kyphosis. This is compounded in growing children, who also experience the loss of the anterior vertebral growth plates (Fig. 20-3). As in congenital kyphosis, the posterior elements maintain their growth potential, causing a progressive deformity. Even in cases in which there is a spontaneous fusion of the posterior elements, kyphosis can progress due to the thinness of the spontaneous fusion and the persisting growth posteriorly.[63] Compensatory lordosis can occur proximal and distal to the kyphosis.

Lateral deviation of the spine can occur early in the evolution of tuberculosis of the spine. This tends to happen in the lower thoracic or upper lumbar spine, where the infection can be traced to

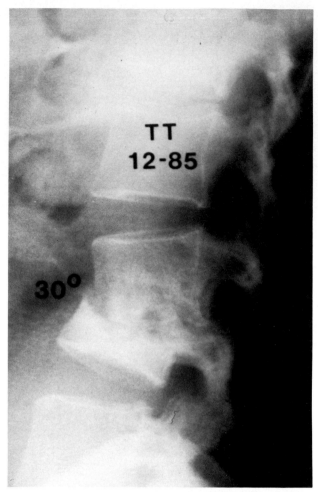

Figure 20-2. Increasing low back pain and kyphotic deformity of the upper lumbar spine in this 25-year-old woman was proven with biopsy to be due to a tuberculous lesion.

the kidney on the involved side. There is early unilateral destruction of the vertebral body.

Revascularization is an important part of the healing phase. It can occur with control of the disease by the body's defenses or with medical intervention. Revascularization in the bony spinal column can be seen on radiographs as radiodense or ivory vertebrae. Cleveland and Bosworth[12] described this as "avascular necrosis." Revascularized areas will eventually return to a normal appearance.

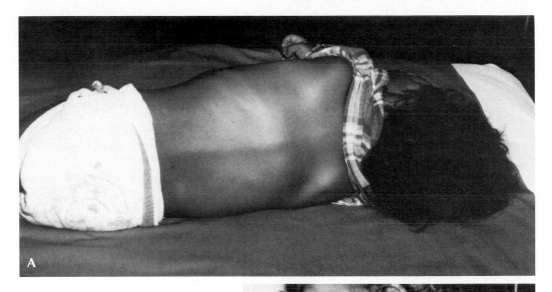

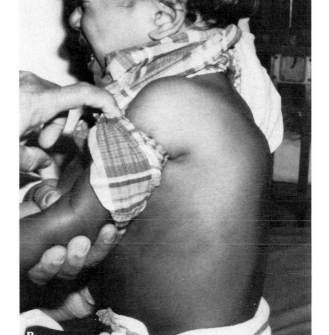

Figure 20-3. (*A, B*) There is obvious gibbus deformity in this infant as a result of a tuberculous lesion.

With healing, the involved segment can go on to spontaneous fusion through a fibrous or bony ankylosis. Even with healing, tiny pockets of live bacteria may remain dormant for years, only to be reactivated at some later date through decreased resistance brought on by increasing age, disease, or steroids.[79]

PARALYSIS

Paralysis can result from spinal tuberculosis in a number of ways. The compressive form of paraplegia is seen with progressive kyphotic deformity, in which the products of infection, including sequestrated disk and bone along with granulation tissue and pus, are retropulsed against the dura mater and cord. This is usually reversible by adequate anterior decompression and stabilization. The speed and extent of reversibility appear to be related to the amount of pressure and its duration.

In the acute stages of spinal tuberculosis, it is possible for the tubercle bacilli to penetrate the dura and invade the motor component of the cord. This "cord penetration," described by Hodgson and associates,[34] tends to be irreversible. It is distinguished clinically by severe lower limb spasticity and clonus.

Late paralysis of healing can occur through fibrosis, as in pachymeningitis, or secondary to progressive kyphosis with severe late angulation.

O'Brian studied neurologic complications associated with spinal tuberculosis. He found that the highest incidence of neurologic involvement was at T-10, even though the greatest number of cases of spinal tuberculosis involved L-1. He concluded that a statistically higher incidence of paraplegia at T-10 in tuberculous infection of the spine with kyphosis is associated with the critical cord:canal ratio occurring at that level, rather than with the vascular supply of the cord through the artery of Adamkiewicz.[63]

In 1988, Hsu, Cheng, and Leong reported on Pott's paraplegia of late onset.[39] They studied 22 patients with a mean age of 18 years, who presented after initial symptoms. Of the 14 patients with active disease, in 12 patients paralysis was caused by activity at the internal kyphus, and in two paralysis was caused by a soft healing bony ridge. The remaining eight patients with healed disease had hard bony ridges compressing the cord.

CLINICAL PRESENTATION

The patient with acute disease may present with back or neck pain, depending on the site of involvement. A history of malaise, night sweats, low-grade fever, loss of appetite with or without weight loss, and easy fatigability may be present. In conjunction with neck or back pain, there may be complaints of referred or radicular pain to the shoulders and upper extremities or the hips and lower extremities. These patients show restricted range of motion in the affected segment due to muscle spasm. There is tenderness to percussion over the involved spinous process. There may be fluctuant swelling in the posterior triangle of the neck, an abdominal mass, or an inguinal mass associated with a cold abscess. Cervical tuberculous osteomyelitis can present with a change in the voice, throat discomfort, or a mass in the neck.

The most devastating presenting symptoms are paraparesis or paraplegia. This may be complete or incomplete, with varying degrees of sensory loss, motor weakness, and bowel and bladder dysfunction. The patient will show an upper motor neuron lesion below the level of involvement and a lower motor neuron lesion at the level of disease. These are distinguishable in the cervical and lumbar spine.

Late presentation can include progressive kyphosis with or without pain. Patients may present with the paraplegia of healed disease.

Laboratory Findings

There is usually an increase in the erythrocyte sedimentation rate, which may be associated with moderate lymphocytosis and anemia. The Mantoux test will be positive except in cases of very active disease, in which there may be anergy.

When tuberculosis is suspected, laboratory evaluation should include sputum and gastric washings for acid-fast bacilli, urinalysis with culture for tuberculosis, and a chest radiograph for pulmonary disease.

Roentgenographic examination may make the diagnosis in advanced cases. Studies should include plain films of the involved area, including anteroposterior and lateral views, and possibly tomograms (laminagrams). Computed tomography scan is very helpful early in the disease for detecting small lesions and soft-tissue changes.[6] Magnetic resonance imaging will likely be an additional help. Bone scanning may detect multiple bony foci. Myelograms still play some role, especially in evaluating late deformity cases. Arteriography may be indicated in special circumstances, especially with late deformity.

Radiographic Features

Radiographic changes may not appear until several weeks after onset. Tomography, computed tomography, and magnetic resonance imaging may be especially helpful during the earliest stages of the disease. When changes do occur on plain films, they may be either soft-tissue or bony changes.

Soft-tissue changes in the cervical spine include a prevertebral soft-tissue swelling or mass with or without tracheal narrowing. With thoracic spine involvement, a paravertebral abscess may be present. This presents in many forms, including fusiform, pyramidal, unilateral, double, or fusiform pointed to one side, which indicates lung penetration.[33] Sequestra may be seen within the abscess shadow.

Bony changes are many; they include osteoporosis and erosion of the vertebral body on one or both sides of the intervertebral disk. This may progress to the point of total destruction of one or more vertebrae with a resulting kyphosis. The disk may be completely spared. There may be localized calcification. Other changes include concertina collapse (complete collapse of one vertebrae with radial protrusion of the vertebral body's granulation-filled body), aneurysmal syndrome (superficial, circumferential destruction of the vertebral body with erosions on the sides and anterior aspect of the vertebra), bony bridging, lateral deviation when the lower thoracic or lumbar spine

is involved, calcification or wedging of the intervertebral disk, reversal of the height:width ratio of the vertebral body, and changes in the ribs secondary to kyphosis and collapse.[37]

DIFFERENTIAL DIAGNOSIS

The differential diagnosis in tuberculosis of the spine includes pyogenic and fungal infections of the spine. The former is true primarily in cases of low-grade or chronic infection. Other entities to be considered are primary and secondary neoplasms, eosinophilic granuloma, multiple myeloma, hemangioma, leukemia, and Hodgkin's disease, as well as the benign lesions of Schmorl's nodules or Scheuermann's disease.

The diagnosis can be highly suspect, so pathologic and bacteriologic confirmation are critical. With a suspected tuberculosis, needle biopsies are not recommended. Because of the large amount of necrosis, biopsy specimens may be sterile or nondiagnostic, and there is considerable risk of hemorrhage. Open biopsy through an anterior cervical, transthoracic, or retroperitoneal approach is the preferred route. Only through these approaches can adequate specimens be harvested, débridement and drainage be established, and when indicated, anterior fusion be performed. Resistant strains are being found among the acid-fast bacilli, making sensitivity testing necessary.

TREATMENT

Treatment of spinal tuberculosis has fluctuated between nonoperative and operative over the years. The last major treatment shift was toward operative care, as pioneered by Hodgson and Stock in the mid 1950s.[35,36] This shift came in conjunction with the evolution of antituberculosis drug therapy, from the introduction of streptomycin sulfate injection in 1945 to the later development of aminosalicylic acid, isoniazid (INH), ethambutol hydrochloride, and rifampin. Current drug treatment recommendations will be discussed in the following section.

Surgical treatment today follows the principles of Hodgson and Stock, which are:

1. All the avascular contents of the abscess must be removed, including fluid or caseous pus, sloughs, avascular bone, and granulation tissue, so as to leave a raw bleeding bed
2. If this leaves the spine unstable, it should be stabilized with an anterior fusion of the anterior defect left by the disease and the débridement.

Hodgson and Stock felt that even though some cases would heal spontaneously or with drug therapy alone, anterior débridement and fusion would lead to the greatest percentage of cases healing in the shortest possible time. They felt that a conservative, nonoperative approach left the patient vulnerable to late kyphosis, paraplegia, or both.

The Medical Research Council Working Party on Tuberculosis of the Spine, formed in the 1960s, has evaluated various treatment regimens through controlled studies in parts of the world where tuberculosis is still a common malady. The studies were limited to thoracic and lumbar involvement without paraplegia; most of the cases were in children. The council defined a favorable result of treatment as radiologically healed disease with all sinuses and abscesses healed, full physical activity, and no central nervous system involvement.

The various study groups included ambulatory outpatient drug treatment with and without an initial 6 months of in-hospital bed rest (Masan, Korea); ambulatory outpatient drug treatment for all patients with and without plaster casting (Pusan, Korea); ambulatory outpatient drug therapy compared with simple surgical débridement alone (Bulawayo, Rhodesia), and compared with débridement alone versus débridement and bone grafting (Hong Kong). There were also some subgroups within the study, including some variation in the drug treatment.[56-61]

The ambulatory care groups in Masan, Pusan, and Bulawayo showed favorable results of 82% to 88%. These studies showed no significant alteration in results with the use of 6 months of bed rest, 9 months of casting, or simple surgical débridement.

When débridement alone vs. débridement and grafting were compared in Hong Kong at 5- and 10-year intervals, some statistically significant differences were found. By 3 years, in both groups 87% of the lesions were healed. At 5 years, there were significantly more solid bony fusions (93%) in the graft and débridement group, compared with 69% in the débridement alone group. By 10 years, both groups had again equalled out; however, the grafted group did so earlier. There was no evidence of recurrent disease in either group between years 5 and 10. The greatest difference between the two groups was that the grafted group showed less loss of vertical height and less kyphosis than the débridement alone group.

When fusion rates in the nonsurgical groups in Korea were compared with the Hong Kong and Rhodesia groups at 5 years, there was a significant difference, with 46% fusion in the nonoperated Korean patients vs. 69% with débridement alone and 93% with débridement and grafting.

The most significant finding was that only one patient in the Hong Kong group developed paraparesis, compared with 43 patients who developed paralysis while under treatment using other protocols at the other centers.

In summary, although one can expect healing in approximately 85% of patients with active disease treated in an ambulatory outpatient setting, there is a 15% chance that the tuberculosis will not be eradicated and that these patients may have further progression with or without paraplegia. This compares with a healing rate of 93% or higher by the addition of débridement and grafting with postoperative immobilization. The addition of surgical intervention can also help avoid the tragedy of neurologic compromise.

Rajasekaran and Shanmugasundaram have reported on prediction of the angle of gibbus deformity in tuberculosis of the spine.[67] In 90 cases they showed a statistically significant difference between patients treated with radical surgery vs. those treated with chemotherapy for 6 and 9 months. At a mean follow-up of 6 years, analysis of the amount of initial loss of vertebral body and the final angle of the gibbus deformity showed a correlation coefficient of 0.83. The authors devised a formula for predicting the final angle of deformity with 90% accuracy in nonsurgically treated patients. The results of this study may help select patients for radical resection and bone grafting to prevent severe kyphosis.

Current Recommendations of Treatment

Treatment for tuberculosis of the spine in patients with active disease is surgical, except in the unusual case of early, single-level involvement. In these selected cases, antibiotics should be started, in most cases with two drugs.[79] Immobilization with a brace or cast will normally make the patient more comfortable; these can be used as necessary during the early stages. Patients must be followed carefully for any future recurrence of the disease. With failure of this conservative treatment, surgery should be performed for adequate débridement and fusion as indicated. Continuance of drug therapy is recommended for 6 to 18 months.

With involvement of two or more vertebrae, surgery is indicated for optimal results. As was illustrated in the studies in Korea and Rhodesia, nonoperative treatment of *any* tuberculosis of the spine has an 85% success rate with drugs alone. These results are not acceptable except in situations in which there are no equipment or facilities for a surgical approach. When possible, the patient should have a short period of preoperative drug therapy, nutrition enhancement, and bed rest. With adequate facilities and personnel, the treatment should then consist of an anterior cervical, transthoracic, or retroperitoneal approach for decompression and débridement. For lesions at C-1–C-2, a transoral approach may be necessary, followed by anterior or posterior fusion with halo vest or Minerva jacket immobilization. Decompression at any level should include débridement of the abscess tissue and infected necrotic bone. The removal of affected tissue should continue to raw bleeding bone.[2,36]

This is combined with an anterior fusion utilizing struts of either autologous bone or bone chips (Fig. 20-4). For patients with significant disease involving the thoracic or lumbar spine, a second procedure, a posterior fusion with or without internal fixation, should follow to improve stability and to prevent progression of kyphosis in the fu-

ture.[25] This may be done at the same time or 10 days to 2 weeks following the initial procedure. No posterior fusion is necessary in the cervical spine except at C-1–C-2.[40] At this most proximal level, a transoral decompression may be necessary.[22] Postoperative immobilization with a brace or cast is necessary except in cases in which devices such as Luque rods with segmental fixation or Cotrel–Dubousset instrumentation were used.[9] Here the surgeon may feel that the construct and underlying bony quality are sufficient to avoid use of any immobilization.

Lifeso reported on 12 adult patients with atlanto-axial tuberculosis.[52] He proposed a classification system with treatment recommendations.

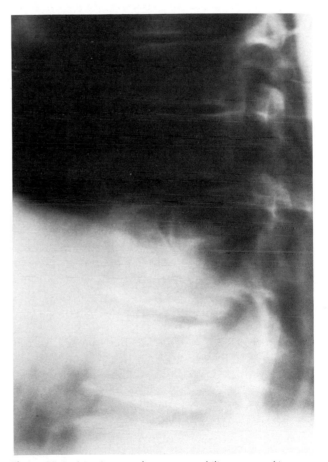

Figure 20-4. Anterior vertebrectomy and iliac strut grafting.

Stage I involvement has minimal ligamentous or bony destruction with no displacement of C-1 or C-2; stage II has ligamentous disruption and minimal bony destruction, but anterior displacement of C-1 on C-2; stage III has marked ligamentous and bony destruction with displacement of C-1 forward on C-2. Treatment for stage I disease consists of transoral biopsy and decompression followed by use of an orthosis; stage II treatment consists of transoral biopsy and decompression, and reduction by halo traction followed by a posterior C-1–C-2 fusion; stage III is the same as for stage II with the exception of the fusion, which is from the occiput to C-2 or C-3. All of Lifeso's patients went on to solid union with resolution of any neurologic deficit, with the exception of one patient, who died before treatment was begun. The author noted no reactivation of disease at an average follow-up period of 36 months.

In patients with neurologic involvement, surgical decompression is crucial in attempting to restore function. There are reports of patients improving their neurologic picture with bed rest, drug therapy, and casting alone; however, surgical patients tend to recover faster and more completely.[79] In patients with neurologic involvement, surgery is urgent, so the preoperative treatment is shortened. Decompression should be performed through the posterior longitudinal ligament, exposing the dura throughout the length of the decompression. If there has been penetration of the dura, or if there is loss of dural pulsations, the dura should be opened and inspected for tuberculous meningomyelitis or a tuberculoma in the cord itself. If encountered, the tuberculoma should be removed.[33]

With paralysis, the patient is kept on bed rest until there is neurologic recovery. In cases in which fusion has been performed, postoperative immobilization should be continued until the fusion is solid. If the paralysis has been long-standing, expect osteopenia. These patients are best served with postoperative immobilization regardless of which, if any, internal fixation device has been used. Recovery of neurologic function can be profound in these patients, even with an initial presentation of complete and long-standing paralysis.[11]

Louw has reported on 10 patients with paraplegia who were managed by anterior débridement and vascular rib pedicle bone graft, followed by a posterior fusion and Harrington compression instrumentation.[53] With an average of 22.6 months follow-up, he demonstrated bony consolidation of the vascular graft after an average 1.8 months, and bony fusion after an average of 4.9 months. Eight patients regained normal neurologic function and the remaining two were ambulatory with crutches.

Chemotherapy

Without proper and adequate drug therapy, even the most perfectly performed débridement and fusion is prone to failure. Eradication of the tuberculous organism is essential for eradication of infection. Proper treatment consists of multiple-drug therapy, taken in a regular and responsible fashion for a prolonged period of time. Poor compliance can lead to failure of treatment or, potentially worse, resistant strains of bacteria. Complete culture and sensitivity evaluations of infected tissue are necessary for the proper selection of drugs. An infectious disease specialist should be involved in the care of all patients with tuberculosis of the spine.

Traditionally, chemotherapy has been recommended with up to three drugs for 18 months. A recent report from the Medical Research Council's Working Party describes a controlled clinical trial of the treatment of more than 600 patients in Korea, India, and Hong Kong. With 3-three year follow-up, they showed that chemotherapy based on rifampin and isoniazid (INH) for 6 to 9 months was as effective as an 18-month course of isoniazid and aminosalicylic acid.[29]

Currently, the recommended drugs are streptomycin sulfate injection, isoniazid, and rifampin. Other drugs used on occasion, and with a consultation from an infectious disease specialist, are ethambutol hydrochloride and pyrazinamide.[41]

Use of streptomycin sulfate injection must be monitored with repeated hearing evaluations to avoid injury to the vestibular nerve. The dosage is 20 mg/kg, to a maximum of 1 g per day, for a maximum of 2 to 3 months or a total dose of 50 g. Isoniazid does not carry the toxic risk of streptomycin sulfate injection, but patients can become hypersensitive to this medication. The dosage is 10 mg/kg, to a maximum of 300 mg per day, for 6 to 9 months. Rifampin is administered in a dosage of 15 mg/kg, to a maximum of 600 mg per day, for 6 to 9 months. Regular laboratory work is necessary to identify thrombocytopenia, a possible side-effect.[41]

NONTUBERCULOUS INFECTION OF THE SPINE

Prior to the use of penicillin and other antibiotics, death from pyogenic osteomyelitis was common. Butler, Blusgen, and Perry, in 1941, reported on 15 deaths in 16 patients with pyogenic osteomyelitis of the spine.[8] Currently, widespread use of antibiotics has decreased the mortality rate. In a recent study of pyogenic and fungal vertebral osteomyelitis by Eismont and associates, 5 of 61 patients died with infection, but only 3 deaths were directly attributed to the infection.[20] This is a significant advance. However, that same study revealed an incidence of 31 of 61 patients with nontuberculous vertebral osteomyelitis who had some degree of paralysis. Regardless of our past gains in fighting this age-old problem, we have a great deal of work to do in decreasing the morbidity and mortality that still exists. Perhaps through better understanding, new diagnostic and therapeutic modalities, and a vigilant index of suspicion we will be able to diminish the serious sequelae of this disease.

INCIDENCE

The incidence of pyogenic spinal infection differs in various reports in the modern literature. It ranges from a low of 1.5% to a high of 3.94%.[45,68,77] More accurate methods of diagnosis, including Technetium 99m bone scanning, gallium scanning, indium white blood cell scanning,[55,66] magnetic resonance imaging, open and needle biopsy, computed tomography-guided biopsy,[66] have improved our ability to make an early accurate diagnosis.

SEX

Pyogenic spinal infections are more common in males in all series reviewed.[30,45,68,70] This may be a reflection of the fact that osteomyelitis is more common in males in general, or it may reflect the frequency of prostatic and urinary infections in the elderly male, with inevitable prostate hypertrophy.[31]

SITE AND LEVEL OF INVOLVEMENT

The vertebral body is the usual site of primary involvement, comprising 100% of cases in most series.[28,38,73] Involvement of the dens or posterior elements is described by several authors.[26,47,54] The majority of cases involve the lumbar spine; the thoracic spine is next likely to be affected, and the cervical (Fig. 20-5) and sacral segments are involved with the least frequency.

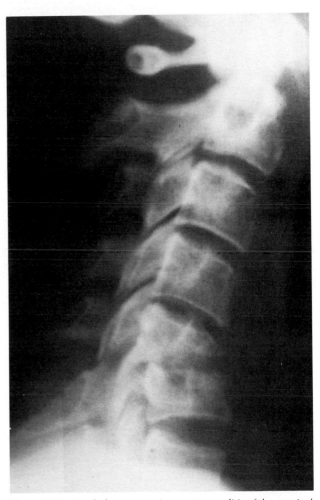

Figure 20-5. *Staphylococcus aureus* osteomyelitis of the cervical spine in an intravenous drug abuser.

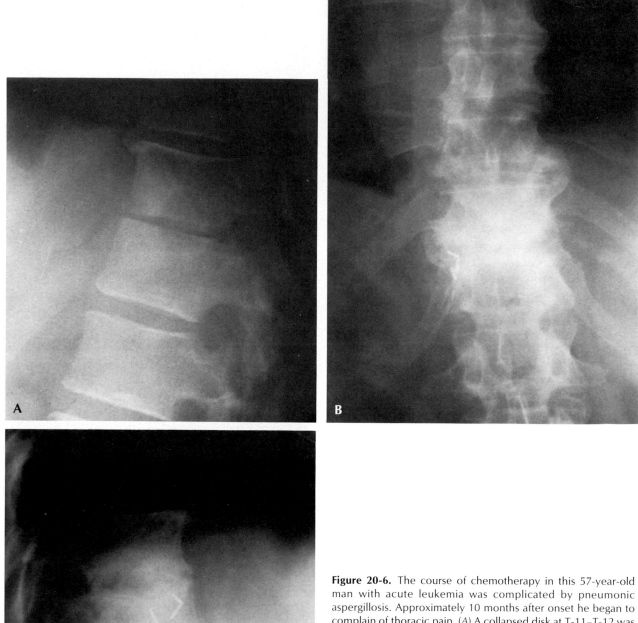

Figure 20-6. The course of chemotherapy in this 57-year-old man with acute leukemia was complicated by pneumonic aspergillosis. Approximately 10 months after onset he began to complain of thoracic pain. (*A*) A collapsed disk at T-11–T-12 was proven with biopsy to be secondary to an aspergillosis disk space infection. (*B, C*) Radiographs taken after débridement and fusion using rib chips.

ORGANISM

By far the most common causative organism worldwide is *Mycobacterium tuberculosis;* the most common nontuberculous organism is *Staphylococcus aureus.* The "popularity" of intravenous drug use has increased the incidence of pseudomonas vertebral osteomyelitis.[38,44,76] Gram-positive aerobic cocci dominated the cases in Sapico's series and literature review.[70] Those organisms were noted to be more than twice as frequent causative agents as gram-negative bacilli and anaerobic bacteria. An increase in the frequency of all types of osteomyelitis, including that of the spine, can be anticipated in the ever-growing numbers of immunocompromised patients with acquired immunodeficiency syndrome (AIDS) and other immunodeficiency syndromes, or in association with immunosuppressive therapy. Osteomyelitis due to organisms such as *Pneumocystis carinii* and other previously uncommon infective agents may be foreseen. Fungal infections can also lead to bony destruction and collapse (Fig. 20-6, Table 20-1).[7,20]

Table 20-1. Organisms[14,17,18,27,33,64,70] Causing Vertebral Osteomyelitis

---

Gram-positive aerobic cocci
  Staphylococcus aureus
  Streptococcus pneumoniae
  Group A streptococci
  Group B streptococci
  Non-group A, non-group B β-hemolytic streptococci
  Enterococci
  Coagulase-negative staphylococci
Gram-negative bacilli
  Escherichia coli
  Klebsiella organisms
  Enterobacter organisms
  Proteus organisms
  Pseudomonads
  Serratia organisms
  Salmonellae
  Neisseria meningitides
Anaerobic bacteria
  Bacteroides fragilis
  Peptostreptococcus organisms
  Propionibacterium organisms
  Clostridium perfringens
  Arachnia propionica
Fungi
  Candida organisms
  Blastomyces dermatitidis
  Mucor organisms

ASSOCIATED CONDITIONS AND PREDISPOSING FACTORS

It has been noted in several studies that infection, including that causing vertebral osteomyelitis, is more common in patients with insulin-dependent diabetes mellitus (Fig. 20-7).[15,20,28,70,73] Other chronic illnesses may also increase the incidence of infection. Therefore, patients with chronic renal disease who require hemodialysis,[50] patients with rheumatoid arthritis, and those on steroids or injecting intravenous drugs should be monitored closely (Fig. 20-8).[38,44,51,76]

Patients with penetrating neck or abdominal wounds also require close observation. Contamination of the spinal canal or column with hypopharyngeal or bowel contents may lead to osteomyelitis. A recent report of low velocity missile injuries to the abdomen noted infection in seven of eight cases when the colon was perforated, resulting in meningitis, paraspinal infection, or osteomyelitis.[69]

Iatrogenic introduction of infection through diskography, angiography, and surgery has been reported.[13] A recent report by Barr and associates describes a case of cervical osteomyelitis following a rigid esophagoscopy and injection sclerotherapy for esophageal varices.[3]

Siroky and associates studied metastatic infection related to sepsis from the genitourinary tract.[71] They noted that 87 of the 106 skeletal metastases (83%) involved the spine, and that males predominated in this subgroup. They noted an equal distribution of cases throughout the spine, with 39 at the lumbar level, 35 at the thoracic level, and 13 at the cervical level. One case was not classified. Other authors have noted a similar distribution. Numerous reports have described the frequency of urinary tract infections and instrumentation with vertebral osteomyelitis.[16,31,32,49,75]

In their literature review, Sapico and Montgomerie found cases secondary to soft-tissue infection, including furuncles, infected surgical sites, and post-traumatic wound infections. They also noted a connection to upper respiratory infection and pneumonia. Other conditions included spinal surgery, an infected intravenous site, diarrhea due to infection with salmonella, and infective endocarditis. In many cases no obvious source of infection was identified.[70]

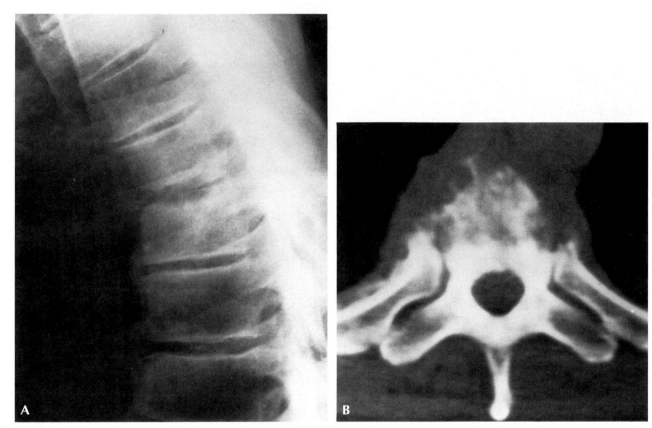

Figure 20-7. A 58-year-old insulin-dependent diabetic for 10 years developed a chronic low grade *Pseudomonas* infection of the foot. (*A*) Subsequently he developed thoracic pain. He was noted to have disk space destruction and involvement of T-5 and T-6. (*B*) A CT scan through the bottom of T-5 reveals the destruction of the vertebral body.

PARALYSIS

Paralysis is probably the most devastating of the possible complications of vertebral osteomyelitis. Eismont and associates reviewed 61 patients with vertebral osteomyelitis; 31 of these had some paralysis.[20] Factors predisposing to paralysis included increasing age (50 to 70 years) and more cephalad involvement in the spine. Cervical vertebral osteomyelitis carried a high incidence of paralysis. This was also noted by Messer.[62] Paralysis was uncommon in lumbar infections and somewhat greater in thoracic infections. Ten of 12 patients with diabetes mellitus or rheumatoid arthritis developed paralysis. This relationship was further noted in a series of seven patients with diabetes mellitus and vertebral osteomyelitis, four of whom developed paralysis.[15] Because seven of the eight patients with the most severe paralysis in Eismont's series had infection with *Staphylococcus aureus*, some question was raised as to whether the organism predisposed patients to paralysis.[20] Sapico did not show a statistically significant difference between infections with *Staphylococcus aureus* and gram-negative organisms in the development of paraplegia.[70]

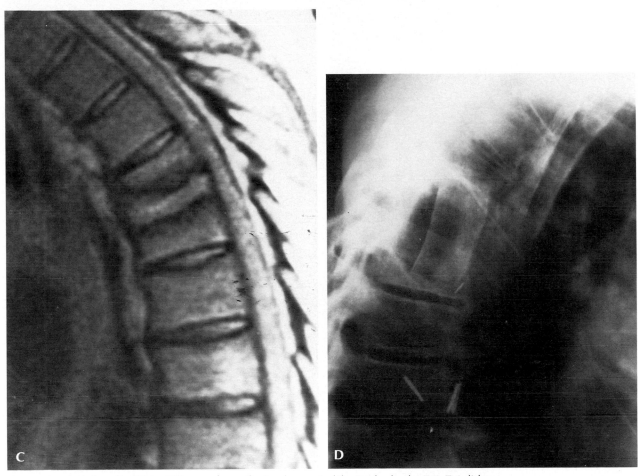

Figure 20-7. *(continued).* *(C)* An MRI scan shows the involvement of the T-5 body, the T-5–T-6 disk space, and the T-6 body. *(D)* Radiograph taken after débridement and fusion.

PATHOLOGY

Although there are a number of routes of infection to involve the spine, in the majority of pyogenic infections, the principal route of infection is hematogenous. Some debate exists as to whether the seeding is arterial or venous. Proponents of arterial seeding look to the work of Wiley and Trueta, who theorized that the bacteria were spread through the vertebral nutrient branches of the posterior spinal arteries.[78] This correlates with the observation that vertebral osteomyelitis often involves the end-plates of two adjoining vertebrae

simultaneously.[16,72] Other arterial blood supplies the vertebrae through nutrient vessels from the vertebral, intercostal, or lumbar arteries. Another argument for arterial spread is that in genitourinary-borne infections there is a fairly even dispersal between thoracic and lumbar foci. If a venous route were the sole source, then there should be a greater number of lumbar and lumbosacral infections.[70]

Batson,[4,5] in his much referenced works, demonstrated the abundant intercommunications between the veins draining the pelvic organs (lateral sacral veins) and the valveless external venous

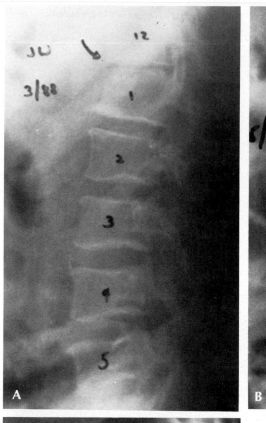

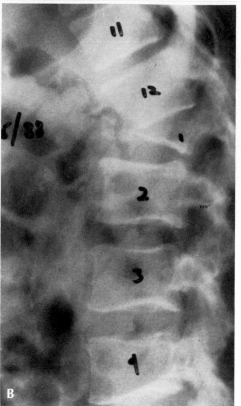

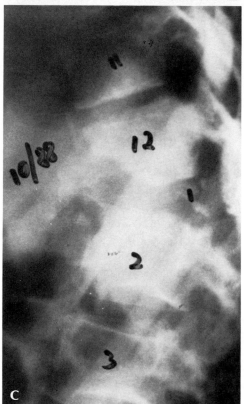

Figure 20-8. (*A*) This intravenous drug abuser was noted to have vertebral osteomyelitis of T-12–L-1 secondary to *Staphylococcus aureus*. He was treated with 6 weeks of intravenous antibiotic therapy. (*B*) Two months later, despite the antibiotic therapy, the lesion had gone on to destroy most of the body of L-1. He refused surgical intervention. Repeat needle biopsy confirmed the diagnosis, culture, and sensitivities. A repeat course of intravenous antibiotics was given. (*C*) Five months later, further destruction had occurred, resulting in almost complete absence of the body of L-1 and further involvement of T-12.

plexus, which drains the valveless internal venous plexus on the spinal canal. These veins join the interosseus vertebral veins, and through frequent anastomoses, a venous ring is formed around each vertebral body. This extends throughout the entire vertebral column. "Batson's plexus" is made of these vessels and their communication with the ascending lumbar and intercostal veins, as well as the lateral sacral veins. Spread has been implicated through this vast communication network of valveless veins.

One interesting observation by Siroky and associates was that in 14 of 16 patients in whom the upper urinary tract was the primary focus of infection, the problem originated in the left kidney.[71] In only two patients was the original site in the right kidney; neither of these patients developed vertebral osteomyelitis. Siroky's explanation was that in 70% of the normal population the left renal vein communicates with the lumbar or vertebral veins, whereas in the right side, the renal vein empties into the inferior vena cava.

Regardless of the hematogenous origin, the infectious agent is felt to remain in the low-flow vascular arcades, which communicate with both the arterial and venous trees at the level of the subchondral plate of the vertebra. It is in this capillary sinusoidal space of the cancellous bone that the organism can grow, much like in the metaphysis of long bones in growing children.

If the growth of the organism is not halted by the host's natural defense barriers, it begins to proliferate. With the host's leukocyte response comes lysosomal activity, which, together with the erosive nature of the infection, causes destruction of bony trabeculae and penetration of the cartilaginous end-plate, thus involving the intervertebral disk. There is also localized osteopenia as a result of the hyperemic response to the infection. The bone is weakened; this insult, together with the direct bony destruction, is the underlying pathology that leads to the compression fractures of the involved segments, with collapse and deformity.

The disk itself may be the primary site of infection from hematogenous spread.[42] This occurs less commonly than vertebral osteomyelitis. At one time the disk was felt to be avascular; however, the work of Wiley and Trueta showed that the same vessels responsible for supplying the vertebrae also contributed to the circumferential supply, which supplies the disk from the periphery. This blood supply was shown to be patent in intervertebral disks until the age of 30 years. After that age there are disk degeneration and changes in the vertebral end-plate with ingrowth of new vessels. At any point there appears to be adequate access to the disk from a vascular route.

CLINICAL PRESENTATION

Spinal osteomyelitis usually presents as back pain in the affected area, sometimes accompanied by radicular pain from compression or irritation of a segmental nerve. In a review of the literature, Sapico and associates noted that the presenting symptoms in 92% of 250 patients were back or neck pain, with or without fever.[70]

Acute signs of sepsis are usually absent. In most series an elevated temperature of greater than 100°F was noted in only 52% of the cases.[70] In Garcia's study of 100 patients,[28] two thirds of the patients had temperatures of less than 100°F. The malaise often seen with infection is usually absent. Pain is relatively constant, with aggravation by activity; this can progress to the point of incapacitating the patient. Because the onset of pain is usually gradual, diagnosis may be delayed for weeks or months.[1] This contrasts with osteomyelitis of the spine in infants, who are systemically ill.[21]

Because some segmental nerves give rise to somatic pain, patients with spinal osteomyelitis are sometimes misdiagnosed with a variety of ailments. In Sapico and associates'[70] review of the literature, 15% of the patients presented with atypical symptoms such as chronic chest pain, abdominal pain, occipital pain, and leg pain. Some patients were diagnosed during exploratory laparotomy; others were diagnosed while undergoing other studies during a gastrointestinal workup for the pain.

The physical examination usually reveals localized tenderness to the involved segment. There is normally restriction of motion and muscle spasm, and a small kyphosis may be present. Straight leg raising test may be positive for radicular pain. Patients previously treated in a cast or brace may be pain-free, only to become symptomatic once mobilization is discontinued.[42]

Laboratory Findings

In keeping with the subacute insidious nature of the presentation, the laboratory findings are not impressive according to the usual parameters of evaluating an acute infection. The white blood cell count is often normal, though it can be mildly elevated. The characteristic shift to the left seen in acute infections is not present. Blood cultures are likely to be positive in patients with a more specific reaction to the infection, such as the typical chills and fever.

Frequently, the erythrocyte sedimentation rate is elevated to levels greater than 70 mm/hour. This rate is a helpful index to a patient's response to treatment, with a decrease indicating success. Where determinations were available, Sapico and associates[70] showed that in patients who underwent successful treatment this rate dropped to less than two thirds of its presenting value. The authors stressed that this measurement is nonspecific and it should be seen in the context of other clinical, historical, roentgenographic, and laboratory parameters.

Radiographic Features

The common radiographic features of nontuberculous vertebral osteomyelitis may take 4 weeks to develop enough to be seen with plain radiographs. Tomograms may yield information as early as 2 weeks. Newer investigative procedures such as magnetic resonance imaging and computed tomography may allow us to see changes sooner.[6] Paravertebral abscesses can be visualized this way. Nuclear scanning can be very helpful.[55,66]

When the infection primarily involves the vertebrae, the radiologic findings lag behind the pathologic changes by 4 to 8 weeks. Vertebral changes seen on radiographs are rarefaction or loss of trabecular density, usually in the superior or inferior part of the vertebral body close to the cartilaginous end-plate, often followed by disk space narrowing. There is subsequent bony destruction with loss of vertebral height, followed by proliferation of bone. Occasionally there is spontaneous fusion across the disk space.

When the intervertebral disk is the site of primary involvement, the earliest change noted is narrowing. The initial bony feature is a decrease in bony density in the affected area on both sides of

the disk. In time, this decrease in density can give rise to increased density, the result of compressed and necrotic bone. The next stage occurs over the following 2 to 3 months. There is an increase in density or sclerosis of the subchondral bone in the adjacent areas of the two vertebrae involved. This increase has been attributed to deposition of new bone on existing trabeculae and subperiosteal new bone formation.[42] By the third month there is usually reactive new bone within the vertebrae, progressive osteophyte formation, or both. The hypertrophic response in pyogenic infections occurs sooner than similar changes in tuberculosis. As the disease progresses in the disk space, there is a progressive irregularity of the vertebral end-

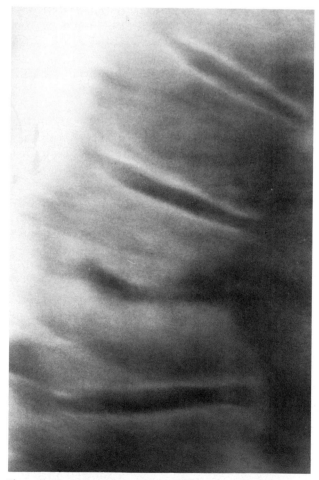

Figure 20-9. Destruction of the end-plates above and below the disk space. This characteristic involvement of two vertebral bodies helps to differentiate from metastatic disease.

plates (Fig. 20-9). Spontaneous fusion across the infected disk often occurs, or there may be development of a stable fibrous union. When the primary source of the infection is in the intervertebral disk, fusion is actually the result of the formation of bone circumferentially around the annulus fibrosus, not the formation of bone across the disk space, as is seen in vertebral osteomyelitis.[42]

DIFFERENTIAL DIAGNOSIS

The differential diagnosis includes entities with an infective etiology, primary or secondary osteoporotic compression, and other metabolic pathologic fractures. The infectious etiologies include pyogenic, tuberculous, and fungal osteomyelitis, disk space infections, perinephric abscess, meningitis, suppurative arthritis of the hip, and osteoporotic compression fractures. Other entities to be considered are primary and secondary neoplasms, eosinophilic granuloma, multiple myeloma, hemangioma, leukemia, and Hodgkin's disease, as well as the benign lesions of Schmorl's nodules and Scheuermann's disease.

The workup should include a complete blood count with differential white blood cell count, erythrocyte sedimentation rate, and urinalysis. In order to rule out tuberculosis, the evaluation should include the Mantoux test, sputum and gastric washings for tuberculosis, a urine culture for tuberculosis, and a chest radiograph to look for characteristic changes.

Radiographic evaluation should include supine anteroposterior and lateral views of the spine with tomography, computed tomography, or, in some cases, magnetic resonance imaging. Nuclear scanning techniques are becoming increasingly sophisticated and can be helpful in early or difficult cases.[55,66]

While all of the above studies are helpful, diagnosis is made only by bacteriologic documentation. With positive blood cultures and a clinical and radiographic picture that is characteristic for infection, treatment can begin based on the cultural results. In any other situation, a tissue diagnosis is critical for proper diagnosis and treatment. In and around the spine, needle or trocar biopsy is possible. This is more risky in the thoracic spine, where needle biopsy can cause a pneumothorax.

Computed tomography-guided biopsy has improved the ability to safely direct a needle into an area, but there is still the risk of hemorrhage. In order to ensure an adequate sample using the safest possible approach, an open biopsy through the anterior cervical, transthoracic, or retroperitoneal approach is preferable. Adequate drainage and débridement, as necessary, is possible through the same approach. Definitive treatment, including reduction of deformity, stabilization, and fusion, may also be carried out through one of these surgical approaches. An adequate tissue sample can be obtained for histologic examination, as well as for use in Gram's stain, aerobic and anaerobic cultures, tuberculosis cultures, and fungal studies where appropriate.

TREATMENT

Once the diagnosis has been established, treatment proceeds along one of two lines: operative or nonoperative. The goals of treatment are eradication of the sepsis, prevention or correction of instability or deformity, and preservation or recovery of neurologic function.

Once the causative organism is identified, treatment should consist of the proper parenteral antibiotic administered for 4 to 6 weeks.[20,70,72,76] This is emphasized throughout the literature. Studies have shown a higher incidence of recurrence in patients treated for less than 4 weeks with parenteral antibiotics.[46,70]

Achievement of the second and third goals are intimately tied together, since preservation or recovery of neurologic function is dependent on the stability and minimal deformity of the spine. In patients presenting with a normal neurologic examination and no deformity or significant bony destruction, bed rest, immobilization, and antibiotics may be all that is necessary. This may be the case in lesions of and near the intervertebral disks. Various braces as well as casting will be of help here. Where there is more significant involvement, with bony loss and deformity, as seen with central and multiple lesions, a surgical approach is indicated. Preoperative and postoperative immobilization need to be maintained to prevent further deformity and neurologic loss. Treatment principles used in spinal trauma are useful here. Skeletal traction including halo or tongs is helpful in the cervical spine. Postoperatively the patient may be maintained in a halo vest or other cervical orthosis, depending on the specific aspects of the infection, bony loss and deformity, and stability.

The indications for surgery include the need for open biopsy and cultures in cases not amenable to needle aspiration and for drainage of an abscess. Principles of stabilization and correction of deformity applicable to trauma and tumor are the guidelines for treatment of these fractures due to infection. The approach is anterior and cervical, transthoracic, thoracoabdominal, or retroperitoneal. Where stability is in question, stabilization with a strut of iliac crest bone is preferred (Fig. 20-10). Rib can also be used, although shorter segment fusions will not provide the stability of the crest graft. With longer segments, the fibula can provide a long strut; however, the fibula, with its cortical bone, takes longer than the iliac crest or ribs to fully incorporate.

In cases with significant bony loss and instability, the anterior procedure should be followed by a posterior instrumentation and fusion with postoperative bracing (Fig. 20-11). This should be a cast or custom-molded brace in the thoracic and lumbar spine, and a halo vest or cervical orthosis in the cervical spine.

With neurologic involvement, the principles and goals of treatment are the same as those applied with instability and deformity in trauma cases with neurologic involvement. Neurologic loss is the result of instability and deformity, with the added problem of possible direct involvement of the epidural space or meninges with infection.[46] Inflammatory tissue can have a mass effect with pressure on the spinal cord or nerve roots. This is

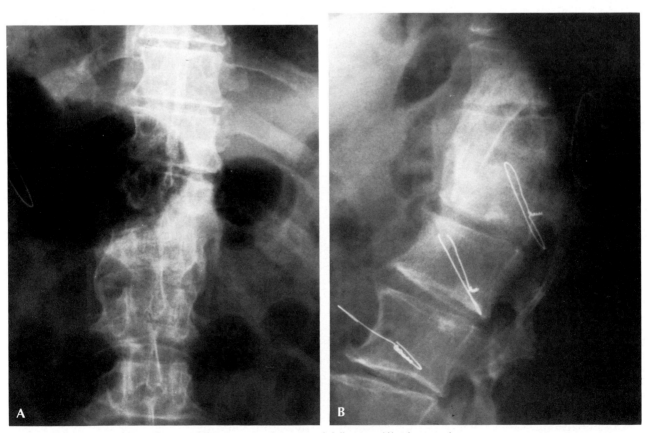

Figure 20-10. (*A, B*) Tricortical strut of iliac crest graft is placed following débridement down to bleeding bone above and below.

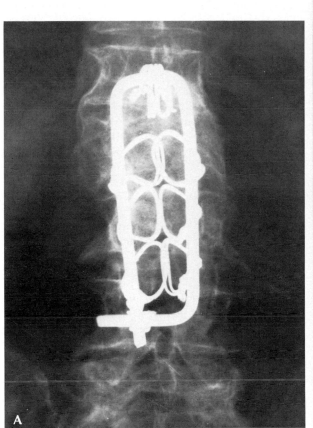
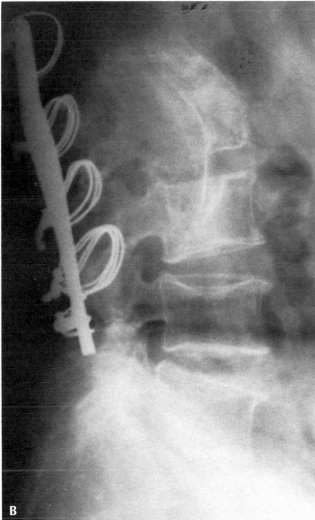

Figure 20-11. (*A, B*) This elderly woman had resection of two vertebral segments secondary to osteomyelitis due to *Pseudomonas*. A second-stage Luque instrumentation was performed to stabilize the lesion.

especially true with tuberculous infection, in which granulation tissue is typically more abundant than in pyogenic disease. The mass effect can compromise the vascular supply by direct pressure or through thrombosis and myeloradicular ischemia.[46] When these factors are responsible for the neurologic loss, time plays an important role in treatment and subsequent recovery. The extent of the recovery depends on the degree of permanent injury at the time of decompression.

Laminectomy is definitely not appropriate for the treatment of anterior disease. As with anterior trauma and instability, posterior approaches with decompression only further destabilize the spine, leaving it increasingly vulnerable to further devastation. This has been noted in the past by various authors and should no longer occur.[24,43,46] Involvement of the posterior elements with vertebral osteomyelitis is extremely rare, and a posterior approach should be limited to these highly unusual cases. Where there is circumferential disease, the anterior approach should be performed first, followed by posterior decompression with internal fixation and fusion to render the spine stable.

SUMMARY

Osteomyelitis of the spine, regardless of its etiology, is a serious problem that must be considered in any patient presenting with back or neck pain. A high index of suspicion is necessary so as not to miss this curable problem before it results in serious complications, including paralysis. Though previously an uncommon problem in developed countries, tuberculosis has become more prevalent. Its presence continues in much of the less developed world. Bacterial osteomyelitis of the spine carries with it similar risks. Regardless of the underlying organism, treatment is directed by culture and sensitivity reports on infected tissue. Surgery is frequently necessary for correct diagnosis, and débridement and stabilization are required for proper treatment and prevention of future recurrence and deformity. With paralysis, surgical decompression is necessary for restoration and preservation of maximum function.

REFERENCES

1. Ambrose GB, Alpert M, Neer CS: Vertebral osteomyelitis. JAMA 197:101-104, 1966
2. Bailey HL, Gabriel M, Hodgeon AR, Shin JS: Tuberculosis of the spine in children: Operative findings and results in 100 consecutive patients treated by removal of the lesion and anterior grafting. J Bone Joint Surg [Am] 54:1633-1657, 1972
3. Barr RJ, Hannon DG, Adair IV, McCoy GF: Cervical osteomyelitis after rigid oesophagoscopy: Brief report. J Bone Joint Surg [Br] 70:147-148, 1988
4. Batson OV: The vertebral veins and their role in the spread of metastasis. Ann Surg 112:138-149, 1940
5. Batson OV: The vertebral vein system. AJR 78:195-212, 1957
6. Brant-Zawadski M, Burke VD, Jeffry RB: CT in the evaluation of spine infection. Spine 8:358-364, 1983
7. Buruma OJS, Crane H, Kunst MW: Vertebral osteomyelitis epidural abscess due to mucormycosisi: A case report. Clin Neurol Neurosurg 81:39-44, 1979
8. Butler ECB, Blugger IN, Perry KMA: Staphylococcal osteomyelitis of the spine. Lancet 1:480, 1941
9. Cardoso A, Flores A, Galvam R: Segmental instrumentation in Pott's disease. Orthopaedic Transactions 9:125, 1985
10. Centers for Disease Control, Tuberculosis Division: Tuberculosis statistics: States and cities. DHEW Publication No. 79-8294. Atlanta, US Department of Health, Education and Welfare, 1979
10a. Centers for Disease Control: Summary of notifiable diseases, United States. Morbidity and Mortality Weekly Report 37(54), 1988
11. Chahal AS, Jyoti SP: The radical treatment of tuberculosis of the spine. Int Orthop 4:93-99, 1980
12. Cleveland M, Bosworth DM: The pathology of tuberculosis of the spine. J Bone Joint Surg [Am] 24:527, 1942
13. Cloward RB: Metastatic disc infection and osteomyelitis of the cervical spine: Surgical treatment. Spine 3:194-201, 1978
14. Conrad SE, Breivis J, Fried MA: Vertebral osteomyelitis, caused by Arachnia propionica and resembling actinomycosis: Report of a case. J Bone Joint Surg [Am] 60:549-553, 1978
15. Cooppan R, Schoenbau MS, Younger MD et al: Vertebral osteomyelitis in insulin dependent diabetics. S Afr Med J 50:1993-1996, 1976
16. Coventry MB, Ghormley RK, Kernohan JW: The intervertebral disc: Its microscopic anatomy and pathology: I. Anatomy, development, and physiology. J Bone Joint Surg [Am] 27:105-112, 1945
17. Derry OG: Pott's disease in ancient Egypt. Medical Press and Circular 197:196-200, 1938
18. Detrisac DA, Harding WG, Greinger AL et al: Vertebral North American blastomycosis. Surg Neurol 13:311-312, 1980
19. Digby JM, Kersley JB: Pyogenic non-tuberculous spinal infection: An analysis of thirty cases. J Bone Joint Surg [Br] 61:47-55, 1979
20. Eismont FJ, Bohlman HH, Soni PL et al: Pyogenic and fungal vertebral osteomyelitis with paralysis. J Bone Joint Surg [Am] 65:19-29, 1983
21. Eismont FJ, Bohlman HH, Soni PL et al: Vertebral osteomyelitis in infants. J Bone Joint Surg [Br] 64:32-35, 1982
22. Fang D, Leong JCY, Fang HSY: Tuberculosis of the upper cervical spine. J Bone Joint Surg [Br] 65:47-50, 1983

23. Fang HSY, Ong GB, Hodgson AR: Anterior spinal fusion: The operative approaches. Clin Orthop: 35:16-33, 1964

24. Fellander M: Paraplegia in spondylitis: Results of operative treatment. Paraplegia 13:75-88, 1975

25. Fountain SC, Hsu LCS, Yau ACMD, Hodgson AR: Progressive kyphosis following solid anterior spine fusion in children with tuberculosis of the spine. J Bone Joint Surg [Am] 57:1103, 1975

26. Frank TJF: Osteomyelitis of the odontoid process of the axis (dens of the epistropheus). Medical Journal of Australia 1:198-201, 1944

27. Freehafer AA, Heiser DP, Saunders AP: Infection of the lower lumbar spine with Neisseria meningitides: A case report. J Bone Joint Surg [Am] 60:1001-1002, 1978

28. Garcia A Jr, Grantham SA: Hematogenous pyogenic vertebral osteomyelitis. J Bone Joint Surg [Am] 42:429-436, 1960

29. Griffiths D: Short course chemotherapy in the treatment of spinal tuberculosis: A report from the Medical Research Council's Working Party. J Bone Joint Surg [Br] 68:158, 1986

30. Griffiths HED, Jones DM: Pyogenic infection of the spine. J Bone Joint Surg [Br] 53:383-391, 1971

31. Henriques CQ: Osteomyelitis as a complication of urology. Br J Surg 46:29-28, 1958

32. Henson SW Jr, Coventry MB: Osteomyelitis of the vertebrae as a result of infection of the urinary tract. Surg Gynecol Obstet 102:207, 1956

33. Hodgson AR: Infectious disease of the spine. In Rothman RH, Simeone FA (eds): The Spine, pp 507-598. Philadelphia, WB Saunders, 1975

34. Hodgson AR, Skinsnes CK, Leong CY: The pathogenesis of Pott's paraplegia. J Bone Joint Surg [Am] 49:1147, 1967

35. Hodgson AR, Stock FE: Anterior spinal fusion: A preliminary communication on the radical treatment of Pott's disease and Pott's paraplegia. Br J Surg 44:266-275, 1956

36. Hodgson AR, Stock FE, Fang HSY, Ong GB: Anterior spinal fusion: The operative approach and pathologic findings in 412 patients with Pott's disease of the spine. Br J Surg 48:172-178, 1960

37. Hodgson AR, Wong W, Yau ACMC: X-ray appearances of tuberculosis of the spine. Springfield, IL, Charles C Thomas, 1969

38. Holzman RS, Bishko F: Osteomyelitis in heroin addicts. Ann Intern Med 75:693-696, 1971

39. Hsu LCS, Cheng CL, Leong JCY: Pott's paraplegia of late onset. J Bone Joint Surg [Br] 70:534-538, 1988

40. Hsu LCS, Leong JCY: Tuberculosis of the lower cervical spine (C2-C7): A report on 40 cases. J Bone Joint Surg [Br] 66:1-5, 1984

41. Hsu LCS, Yau ACMC: Tuberculosis in the cervical spine. In The Cervical Spine Research Society (eds): The Cervical Spine, pp 336–342. Philadelphia, JB Lippincott, 1983

42. Kemp HBS, Jackson JW, Jeremiah JD, Hall AJ: Pyogenic infections occuring primarily in intervertebral discs. J Bone Joint Surg [Br] 55:698-714, 1973

43. Kemp HBS, Jackson JW, Shaw NC: Laminectomy in paraplegia due to infective spondylosis. Br J Surg 61:66, 1974

44. Kido D, Bryan D, Halpern M: Haematogenous osteomyelitis in drug addicts. AJR 118:356-363, 1973

45. Kulowski J: Pyogenic osteomyelitis of the spine: An analysis and discussion of 102 cases. J Bone Joint Surg [Am] 18:343-364, 1936

46. La Rocca SH, Eismont FJ: Other infectious diseases in the cervical spine. In The Cervical Spine Research Society (eds): The Cervical Spine, pp 343–355. Philadelphia, JB Lippincott, 1983

47. Leach RE, Goldstein H, Younger D: Osteomyelitis of the odontoid process. J Bone Joint Surg [Am] 49:369, 1967

48. Leff A, Leter TW, Addington WW: Tuberculosis: A chemotherapeutic triumph but a persistent socioeconomic problem. Arch Intern Med 139:1375-1379, 1979

49. Leigh TF, Kelly RP, Weens HS: Spinal osteomyelitis associated with urinary tract infections. Radiology 65:334-342, 1955

50. Leonard A, Comty CM, Shapiro FL, Rail L: Osteomyelitis in hemodialysis patients. Ann Intern Med 78:561-658, 1973

51. Lewis R, Gorbach SE, Altner P: Spinal pseudomonas chondroosteomyelitis in heroin users. N Engl J Med 286:1303, 1972

52. Lifeso R: Atlanto-axial tuberculosis in adults. J Bone Joint Surg [Br] 69:183-187, 1987

53. Louw JA: Anterior vascular rib pedicle bone graft and posterior fusion and instrumentation in tuberculosis of the spine. J Bone Joint Surg [Br] 69:684, 1987

54. Mankins GH, Abbot FC: An acute primary osteomyelitis of the vertebrae. Ann Surg 23:150-539, 1896

55. McDougall IR, Keeling CA: Complications of fractures and their healing. Semin Nucl Med 18:113-125, 1988

56. Medical Research Council Working Party on Tuberculosis of the Spine: A controlled trial of ambulatory out-patient treatment and in-patient rest in bed in the management of tuberculosis of the spine in young Korean patients on standard chemotherapy: A study in Masan, Korea. J Bone Joint Surg [Br] 55:678-697, 1973

57. Medical Research Council Working Party on Tuberculosis of the Spine: A controlled trial of anterior spinal fusion and debridement in the surgical management of tuberculosis of the spine in patients on standard chemotherapy: A study in Hong Kong. Br J Surg 61:853-866, 1974

58. Medical Research Council Working Party on Tuberculosis of the Spine: A controlled trial of debridement and ambulatory treatment in the management of tuberculosis of the spine in patients on standard chemotherapy: A study in Bulawayo, Rhodesia. J Trop Med Hyg 77:72-92, 1974

59. Medical Research Council Working Party on Tuberculosis of the Spine: A controlled trial of plaster of paris jackets in the management of ambulant out-patient treatment of tuberculosis of the spine in children on standard chemotherapy: A study in Pusan, Korea. Tubercule 54:261-282, 1973

60. Medical Research Council Working Party on Tuberculosis of the Spine: A five year assessment of controlled trials of in-patient and out-patient treatment in plaster of paris jackets for tuberculosis of the spine in children on standard chemotherapy. J Bone Joint Surg [Br] 58:399, 1976

61. Medical Research Council Working Party on Tuberculosis of the Spine: A 10 year assessment of a controlled trial comparing debridement and anterior spinal fusion in the management of tuberculosis of the spine in patients on standard chemotherapy in Hong Kong. J Bone Joint Surg [Br] 64:393-398, 1982

62. Messer HD, Litvinoff J: Pyogenic cervical osteomyelitis: Chondro-osteomyelitis of the cervical spine frequently associated with parenteral drug use. Arch Neurol 33:571-576, 1976

63. O'Brian JD: Kyphosis secondary to infectious disease. Clin Orthop 128:56-64, 1977

64. O'Connell CJ, Cherry AU, Zoll JG: Osteomyelitis of the cervical spine: Candida guilliermondii. Ann Intern Med 79:748, 1973

65. Pott P: Remarks on that kind of palsy of the lower limbs which is frequently found to accompany a curvature of the spine. London, J Johnson, 1779

66. Probst-Proctor SL, Dillingham MD, McDougall IR et al: The white blood cell scan in orthopaedics. Clin Orthop 168:157-165, 1982

67. Rajasekaran S, Shanmugasundaram MS: Prediction of the angle of gibbus deformity in tuberculosis of the spine. J Bone Joint Surg [Am] 69:503-509, 1987

68. Robinson BHB, Lessof MH: Osteomyelitis of the spine. Guy's Hospital Reports 110:303, 1961

69. Romanick PC, Smith TK, Kopaniky DR, Oldfield D: Infection about the spine associated with a low-velocity missile injury to the abdomen. J Bone Joint Surg [Am] 67:1195-1201, 1985

70. Sapico FL, Montgomerie JZ: Pyogenic vertebral osteomyelitis: Report of nine cases and review of the literature. Rev Infect Dis 1(5):754-776, 1979

71. Siroky MB, Moylan RA, Austen G, Olsson CA: Metastatic infection secondary to genitourinary tract sepsis. Am J Med 61:351-360, 1976

72. Stauffer RN: Pyogenic vertebral osteomyelitis. Orthop Clin North Am 6:1015-1027, 1975

73. Stone DB, Bonfiglio M: Pyogenic vertebral osteomyelitis. Arch Intern Med 112:491-500, 1963

74. Swett PP, Bennett GE, Street DM: Pott's disease: The initial lesion, the relative infrequency of extension by contiguity, the nature and type of healing, the role of the abscess and the merits of operative and non-operative treatment. J Bone Joint Surg [Am] 22:878, 1940

75. Turner P: Acute infective osteomyelitis of the spine. Br J Surg 26:17, 1938

76. Weisseman GJ, Wood VE, Kroll LL: Pseudomonas vertebral osteomyelitis in heroin addicts: Report of five cases. J Bone Joint Surg [Am] 55:1416-1424, 1973

77. Wilensky AO: Osteomyelitis of the vertebrae. Ann Surg 89:561, 1929

78. Wiley AM, Trueta J: The vascular anatomy of the spine and its relationship to pyogenic vertebral osteomyelitis. J Bone Joint Surg [Br] 41:796-809, 1959

79. Winter RB: Osteomyelitis. In Bradford DS, Longstein JE, Ogilvie JW, Winter RB (eds): Moe's Textbook of Scoliosis and Other Spinal Deformities, 2nd ed, pp 568-576. Philadelphia, WB Saunders, 1987

21

PENETRATING SPINAL INJURIES

Ismael Montane

The management of high-velocity gunshot wounds to the spine occurring during wartime has been well documented in the neurosurgical and orthopedic literature.[7,17,20,22,24,31,35] In the past 20 years, there has been a steady increase of gunshot spinal injuries in the civilian population of the larger urban communities. These injuries, in contrast to those occurring during wartime, are usually produced by low-velocity handguns. Most civilian handguns and rifles (.22-, .38-, .25-, and .45-caliber) are low-velocity weapons, that is, they have a muzzle velocity of less than 600 to 700 m/sec. Only certain hunting rifles and military weapons have muzzle velocities of greater than 700 m/sec. These high-velocity projectiles cause more extensive soft-tissue damage and distant tissue necrosis than their low-velocity counterparts.

The pathophysiology of gunshot injuries is complex. Several theories have been proposed in an attempt to explain the wounding capacity of gunshot wounds. Of these, the kinetic energy theory is the most widely accepted.[4,8] Kinetic energy may be calculated from the formula: $Ek = \frac{1}{2}MV^2$. Simply stated, doubling the mass doubles the kinetic energy, while doubling the velocity quadruples the kinetic energy. Therefore, small increments in missile velocity greatly increase the kinetic energy imparted to the soft tissues, and consequently greatly increase the wounding capacity of gunshot wounds.

A permanent wound tract with well-defined borders is created by the bullet as it pierces the soft tissues. Concomitantly, a larger, ill-defined temporary cavity is formed. This temporary cavitation is produced by the kinetic energy expended as the bullet passes through the body. Significant neurologic injury ranging from incomplete paraparesis to complete paraplegia may be caused by the wave of kinetic energy produced as the projectile passes close to the spinal cord or conus medullaris or impacts the vertebral column.

The past two decades have noted an increased incidence of civilians with gunshot wounds to the spine. In 1970, Yashon and associates[38] reported on 65 patients who sustained low-velocity gunshot wounds to the spine. They found that the major determinant for recovery of neural function was the extent of the initial injury. Thirty-five patients with complete paralysis remained paraplegic whether or not laminectomy was performed. The removal of bone or metal fragments from the spinal canal did not improve recovery in those patients who sustained incomplete spinal cord injury.

In 1975, Heiden and associates[16] reported on 38 civilian patients who sustained cervical gunshot wounds. The 25 patients with complete spinal cord injuries failed to improve regardless of whether surgical or nonsurgical treatment was performed. The 13 patients with incomplete injuries showed progressive recovery. Laminectomy was not found to be beneficial in either group. They concluded that the ultimate prognosis depended on the initial neurologic injury.

In 1979, Stauffer and associates[33] reviewed 185 patients treated at the spinal cord injury center in Rancho Los Amigos, California. The 106 patients with complete spinal cord injury failed to improve with or without laminectomy. Patients with incomplete injuries were divided into surgical and nonsurgical groups. Of the 45 patients treated with laminectomy, 71% showed significant neurologic recovery. The remaining 34 patients with incomplete spinal cord injury were treated nonsurgically. Of these, 76.5% showed some return of neural function.

CERVICAL INJURIES

The management of gunshot wounds to the cervical spine has been well described and the surgical indications for neck exploration well delineated.[28] Patients whose entry wounds are located in the anterior or anterolateral neck must be carefully evaluated. With continued bleeding from the wound or the presence of an expanding hematoma, major arterial or venous bleeding should be suspected and wound exploration must follow. Anterior penetrating wounds with perforation of the

pharynx or trachea should be considered infected. Esophageal perforations have an especially high incidence of bacterial contamination. These wounds must be thoroughly débrided, and concurrent intravenous antibiotics must be administered to diminish the possibility of vertebral osteomyelitis or spinal meningitis.

Decompressive laminectomy of cervical gunshot wounds has not improved neurologic recovery in patients with either complete or incomplete spinal cord injuries (Fig 21-1).[16] However, patients with persistent compression of spinal nerve roots exiting above the level of the lesion may benefit from surgical decompression. Removal of the offending bony fragments or foreign objects may make the difference between a patient who is an independent wheelchair ambulator and one who is dependent for bed-to-chair transfers.

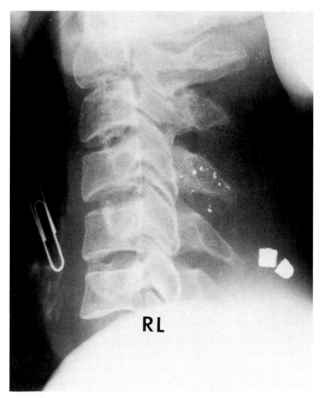

Figure 21-1. This 24-year-old man sustained a gunshot wound to the neck that resulted in complete quadriplegia. The paper clip marks the entry wound. Note the bullet fragments at C-4.

THORACIC INJURIES

Gunshot wounds to the spine between T-1 and T-10 usually result in complete paraplegia (Fig 21-2). The mechanism of injury is either anatomic cord transection or spinal concussion with transient ischemic cord injury. As in other causes of traumatic paraplegia involving the thoracic spine, instability and late deformity rarely become problems unless a decompressive laminectomy is performed.[14] Immobilization with a thoracolumbosacral orthosis for 3 to 4 months allows rapid patient mobilization while osseous healing occurs.

CONUS MEDULLARIS AND CAUDA EQUINA INJURIES

Gunshot wounds between T-11 and L-2 may injure the conus medullaris. This may result in incomplete paraparesis with sparing of the more peripheral sacral roots.[27] Direct injury to the neural elements from the bullet may occur, or the injury may be caused by concussion from the kinetic injury of the bullet traversing near the spinal canal or impacting against the osseous encasement of the neural elements (Fig. 21-3). Recovery of neural function in patients who sustain incomplete paraparesis may occur, with evidence of continued improvement 12 to 18 months after injury (Fig 21-4).

Gunshot wounds to the lumbar spine have a better prognosis than those occurring at either the cervical or thoracic levels. Injuries of the cauda equina may result in monoparesis or isolated root lesions. Removal of bullet and bony fragments decompresses the affected nerve roots and reduces postinjury scarring.[37]

Spinal infections rarely follow abdominal gunshot wounds unless there has been a violation of the intestinal tract. Romanick and associates,[29] in a review of 20 patients with abdominal gunshot wounds and lumbar spine injuries, reported no infections in patients without bowel penetration or with bowel penetration that involved only the stomach or small intestines. Perforation of the colon occurred in eight patients, and of these, seven subsequently developed meningitis, paraspinal infections, or vertebral osteomyelitis. The author has had a similar experience in the management of these patients. Thorough débridement of the spinal injuries and appropriate antibiotic coverage decreases the likelihood of infection.

GUNSHOT WOUNDS IN CHILDREN

Gunshot wounds to the spine in children merit special consideration. The vertebral components in children are smaller than those in adults. Therefore, the kinetic energy produced by low-velocity gunshot wounds in children may result in a greater amount of soft-tissue and osseous destruction than that produced in adults by similar-caliber projectiles. The degree of osseous destruction parallels that produced by high-velocity gunshot wounds in adults. Consequently, while low-velocity gunshot wounds rarely cause spinal instability in adults, unstable spinal injuries are not uncommon in children. Early detection of spinal instability and prompt treatment is mandatory to avoid future deformity.

Additionally, a greater number of gunshot wounds to the spine in children result in complete paraplegia. As in other causes of traumatic paraplegia in skeletally immature individuals, the development of paralytic scoliosis below the level of the lesion approaches 100%. Laminectomy further complicates the deformity by increasing the possibility of development of kyphosis at the level of the lesion. For these reasons, close follow-up of children with serial radiographs is necessary. Prolonged bracing or early fusion of progressive deformities is advised.

COMPLICATIONS

INTRASPINAL MIGRATION OF BULLETS

Spontaneous migration of bullet fragments within the central nervous system has been reported.[2,19,34,36] Arasil[2] reported on the spontaneous migration of an intracranial bullet fragment to the cervical spinal cord. The patient subsequently developed paresthesia in her right hand and foot. After excision of the bullet from the subarachnoid space, the neurologic deficit completely resolved.

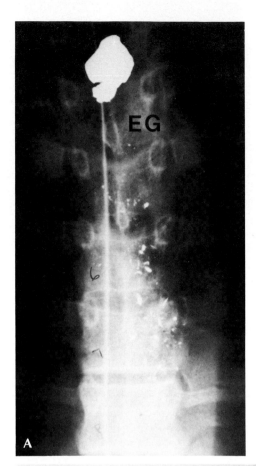

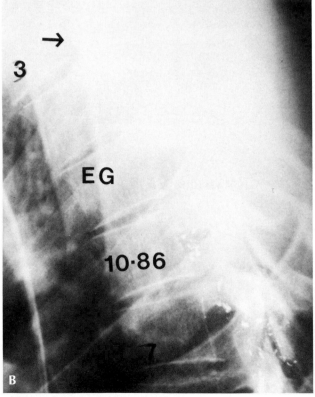

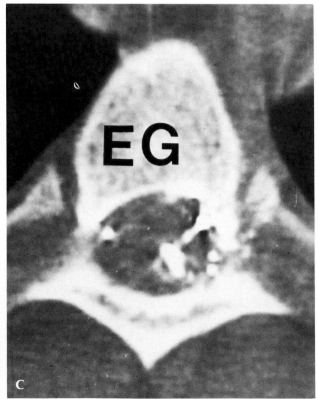

Figure 21-2. This 30-year-old man sustained a gunshot wound to the thoracic spine. (*A, B*) The bullet entered at T-8 and traveled cephaladly with the spinal canal to become lodged at T-3 (*B—arrow*). (*C*) A CT scan shows bullet fragments within the thoracic canal.

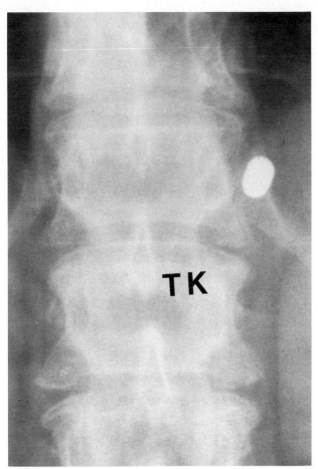

Figure 21-3. This 25-year-old man sustained a gunshot wound to the abdomen and a concurrent complete paraplegia below T-12. The neurologic injury was the result of the kinetic energy expended when the bullet impacted T-12.

radiographs should be taken immediately prior to laminectomy to determine the exact location of the bullet. Most frequently the bullet is located within the subarachnoid space. Following bullet removal, meticulous dural repair decreases postoperative complications.[30]

SUBARACHNOID–PLEURAL FISTULA

Traumatic subarachnoid–pleural fistula is a rare complication of gunshot wounds to the spine, with only six cases reported in the English literature.[5,6,9,21,25,26] The presence of a subarachnoid–pleural fistula should be considered in a patient with traumatic paraplegia and a persistent concomitant pleural effusion. With a penetrating injury to the spine and chest, simultaneous perforation of both the dura mater and pleurae may occur, resulting in a persistent communication between these two structures. Cerebrospinal fluid then flows from the relatively high-pressured subarachnoid space into the low-pressured pleural cavity.

The diagnosis of a subarachnoid–pleural fistula is made by myelographic demonstration of dye leakage from the subarachnoid space into the pleural cavities. Radioisotope scanning may also show cerebrospinal fluid flow into the pleural cavities. Initial treatment should be conservative. Thoracentesis may be indicated for larger effusions. Chest tubes should not be removed until drainage is negligible. Persistent or recurrent effusions may require surgical repair of the dural defect.

Tanguy and associates[34] reported on a patient who sustained a gunshot wound to the cervical spine. Initial radiographs showed a bullet within the spinal cord at C-7. Repeat radiographs taken 3 months after injury showed the bullet at S-2.

Encroachment on spinal nerve roots or the spinal cord from bullets or bullet fragments may produce radicular pain, paresthesia, and motor weakness (Fig 21-5).[1,19] Spontaneous migration of these foreign bodies may occur, resulting in variable neurologic deficits. Excision of the bullet via laminectomy may be required to relieve pressure from the compressed neural structures. Intraoperative

POST-TRAUMATIC SPINAL CORD CYST

Rarely, a post-traumatic spinal cord cyst may develop in patients who have sustained gunshot injuries to the spine. The cyst develops either from ischemic necrosis of neural tissue or possibly from lysosomal destruction of the spinal cord.[3,18] The presence of a syrinx should be suspected in a patient with a stable spinal cord injury who suddenly develops progressive motor weakness, sensory loss, hyperhidrosis, or increasing spasticity. Metrizamide myelography with delayed computed tomography allows visualization of the cyst. Magnetic resonance imaging delineates its location and

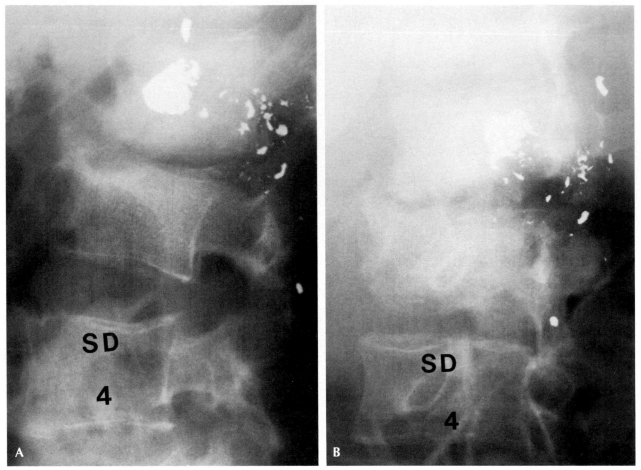

Figure 21-4. *(A, B)* This 40-year-old man sustained a gunshot wound that resulted in an incomplete neurologic deficit. Note the bullet fragments along the spinal canal.

extent. Shunting of the cyst to the subarachnoid space may significantly improve the symptoms.[10]

POST-TRAUMATIC ARACHNOIDITIS

Focal arachnoiditis has been described as a late complication of penetrating injuries to the spine. Its occurrence has been reported years after a gunshot wound to the spine.[1,32,37] Irritation of the cauda equina is not directly produced by the foreign body itself. It is the reactive formation of an extradural or intradural fibrotic mass that causes displacement, stretching, or constriction of the affected nerve roots. Alternatively, ischemia of the

neural tissues may be the source of radicular pain and progressive neurogenic claudication. Surgical excision of the fibrotic mass may ameliorate the symptoms.

ACUTE LEAD INTOXICATION

Lead intoxication has been reported years after gunshot wounds. Prolonged bathing of the retained bullet fragments by either joint or body fluids allows systemic absorption of lead. Grogan and Bucholz[13] reported on a patient who developed acute lead intoxication 12 years after injury. At surgery, the bullet, retained within the inter-

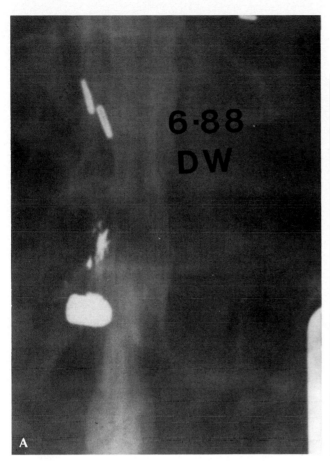

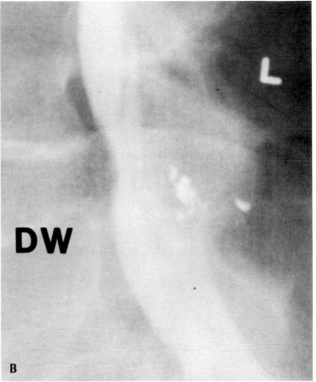

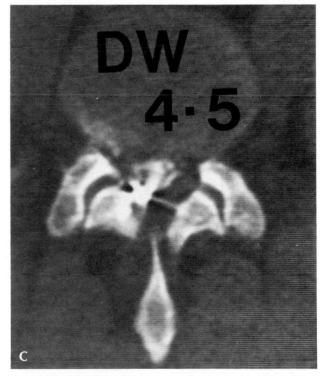

Figure 21-5. This 45-year-old man sustained an intra-abdominal gunshot wound that required an exploratory laparotomy. Twenty years postinjury the patient developed a right radiculopathy. (*A, B*) Myelograms showed a bullet fragment encroaching on the dural elements posteriorly at the L-4–L-5 level. (*C*) A CT scan confirmed the location of the bullet fragment. At surgery, a large amount of scar tissue surrounding the fragment was found, which had resulted in a localized spinal stenosis. Following excision of the reactive scar tissue, the patient's pain and neurologic deficit resolved.

vertebral space, was found to communicate with a retroperitoneal cyst. A large surface area of lead increases the probability of developing lead intoxication. Elevated serum and urine lead levels support the diagnosis. Chelation therapy helps lower lead levels. Surgical removal of the lead source constitutes definitive treatment.

LATE PAIN

The onset of late pain after gunshot injuries is not uncommon. Rarely, pain may be mechanical in nature and related to instability of the affected intervertebral motion segments. More commonly, pain is of spinal cord or nerve root origin. The pain is dysesthetic in nature, and is often produced by lightly stroking the skin. Characteristically, this pain is described as burning and may follow a dermatomal distribution. The pain is constant and becomes exacerbated at night, often interfering with sleep.

The most distressing problem in the management of these patients is the intractability of the pain. Narcotic analgesics are not beneficial and only create dependency. Carbamazepine and phenytoin (Diphenylhydantoin) have been used in an attempt to control the pain; however, results with these medications are unpredictable and are only rarely beneficial. Cordotomy above the level of injury has been recommended.[11] This may only provide temporary pain relief; recurrence of pain has been reported months after surgical transection of the cord.

Percutaneously inserted epidural spinal cord stimulators are presently under trial and show promising results. Finally, a comprehensive, rehabilitation program with elimination of narcotic analgesics and patient reeducation on how to manage intractable pain is being employed with variable success.

KNIFE STAB WOUNDS

Knife stab wounds have become infrequent causes of spinal cord injury. They usually are the consequence of stab wounds to the posterior thorax or abdomen. One third of patients sustain a complete cord transection and permanent paraplegia.[12]

More commonly, a Brown–Séquard syndrome or nonspecific neurologic deficit results. The neurologic deficit may result from intrinsic cord damage secondary to direct cord hemisection or vascular injury. Although complete motor and sensory recovery rarely occurs, the prognosis for recovery of bladder function and ambulation is favorable.[23]

REFERENCES

1. Amitani K, Tsuyuguchi Y, Hukuda S: Delayed cervical myelopathy caused by bomb shell fragment. J Neurosurg 44:626-627, 1976
2. Arasil E, Tascioglu AO: Spontaneous migration of an intracranial bullet to the cervical spinal canal causing Lhermitte's sign. J Neurosurg 56:158-159, 1982
3. Barnett HJM, Jousse AT, Ball MJ: Pathology and pathogenesis of progressive cystic myelopathy as a late sequela to spinal cord injury. In Barnett HJM, Foster JB, Hudgson P: Syringomyelia, pp 179-219. Philadelphia, WB Saunders, 1973
4. Berman AT, Salter F: Low-velocity gunshot wounds in police officers. Clin Orthop 192:113-119, 1985
5. Beutel EW, Roberts JD, Langston HT, Barker WL: Subarachnoid-pleural fistula. J Thorac Cardiovasc Surg 80:21-24, 1980
6. Bramwit DN, Schmelka DD: Traumatic subarachnoid-pleural fistula. Radiology 89:737-738, 1967
7. Comarr AE, Kaufman AA: A survey of the neurological results of 858 spinal cord Injuries: A comparison of patients treated with and without laminectomy. J Neurosurg 13:95-106, 1956
8. DeMuth WE: Bullet velocity and design as determinants of wounding capability: An experimental study. J Trauma 6:222-232, 1966
9. Djergaian RS, Roberts JD, Ditunno JF, Angstadt J: Subarachnoid-pleural fistula in traumatic paraplegia. Arch Phys Med Rehabil 63:488-489, 1982
10. Eismont FI, Green BA, Quencer RM: Post-traumatic spinal-cord cyst. J Bone Joint Surg [Am] 66:614-618, 1984
11. Freeman LW, Heimburger RF: Surgical relief of pain in paraplegic patients. Arch Surg 55:433-440, 1947
12. Gentleman D, Harrington M: Penetrating injury of the spinal cord. Injury 16:7-8, 1984
13. Grogan DP, Bucholz RW: Acute lead intoxication from a bullet in an intervertebral disc space. J Bone Joint Surg [Am] 63:1180-1182, 1981

14. Guttmann SL: Spinal deformities in traumatic paraplegics and tetraplegics following surgical procedures. Paraplegia 7:38-49, 1968

15. Hagan RE: Early complications following penetrating wounds of the brain. J Neurosurg 34:132-141, 1971

16. Heiden JS, Weiss MH, Rosenberg AW et al: Penetrating gunshot wounds of the cervical spine in civilians: Review of 38 cases. J Neurosurg 42:575-579, 1975

17. Jacobson SA, Bors E: Spinal cord injury in Vietnamese combat. Paraplegia 7:263-281, 1970

18. Kao CC, Chang LW: The mechanism of spinal cord cavitation following spinal cord transection: Part 1. A correlated histochemical study. J Neurosurg 46:197-209, 1977

19. Karim NO, Nabors MW, Golocovsky M, Cooney FD: Spontaneous migration of a bullet in the spinal subarachnoid space causing delayed radicular symptoms. Neurosurgery 18:97-100, 1986

20. Kennedy F, Denker PG, Osborne R: Early laminectomy for spinal cord injury not due to subluxation. Am J Surg 60:13-21, 1943

21. Lovaas ME, Castillo RG, Deutschman MS: Traumatic subarachnoid-pleural fistula. Neurosurgery 17:650-652, 1985

22. Matson DD: Treatment of compound spine injuries in forward army hospitals. J Neurosurg 3:114-119, 1946

23. Maynard FM, Reynolds GG, Fountain S et al: Neurological prognosis after traumatic quadriplegia. J Neurosurg 50:611-616, 1979

24. Meirowsky AM: Penetrating wounds of the spinal canal: Problems of paraplegia and notes on autonomic hyperreflexia and sympathetic blockade. Clin Orthop 27:90-107, 1963

25. Milloy FJ, Correl NO, Langston HT: Persistent subarachnoid-pleural space fistula: Report of a case. JAMA 169:1467, 1959

26. Ozer H, Barki Y, Bertran V: Traumatic arachnoido-pleural fistula: Report of a case. J Can Assoc Radiol 23:287-289, 1972

27. Ransohoff J: Lesions of the cauda equina. Clin Neurosurg 8:157-183, 1962

28. Rao PD, Bhatti FK, Gaudino J et al: Penetrating injuries of the neck: Criteria for exploration. J Trauma 23:47-49, 1983

29. Romanick PC, Smith TK: Infection about the spine associated with low-velocity-missile injury to the abdomen. J Bone Joint Surg [Am] 67:1195-1201, 1985

30. Sanford RA, Romfh JH: Closure of large traumatic lumbosacral defects. Neurosurgery 11:235-238, 1982

31. Schneider RC, Webster JE, Lofstrom JE: A Follow-up report of spinal cord injuries in a Group of World War II patients. J Neurosurg 6:118-126, 1949

32. Stamforth P, Watt I: Extradural "plumboma": A rare cause of acquired spinal stenosis. Br J Radiol 55:772-774, 1982

33. Stauffer ES, Wood RW, Kelly EG: Gunshot wounds of the spine: The effects of laminectomy. J Bone Joint Surg [Am] 61:389-392, 1979

34. Tanguy A, Chabannes J, Deubelle A et al: Intraspinal migration of a bullet with subsequent meningitis. J Bone Joint Surg [Am] 64:1244-1245, 1982

35. Wannamakur GT: Spinal cord injuries: A review of the early treatment in 300 consecutive cases during the Korean conflict. J Neurosurg 11:517-524, 1954

36. Wasserman SM, Cohen JA: Spontaneous migration of an intracranial bullet fragment. Mt Sinai J Med 46:512-515, 1979

37. Wu WO: Delayed effects from retained foreign bodies in the spine and spinal cord. Surg Neurol 25:214-218, 1986

38. Yashon D, Jane JA, White RJ: Prognosis and management of spinal cord and cauda equina bullet injuries in sixty-five civilians. J Neurosurg 32:163-170, 1970

22

LATE SEQUELAE OF SPINAL TRAUMA

Thomas F. Gleason
Timothy H. Massey

The late sequelae of spinal trauma consist of complications of the injury itself as well as iatrogenic complications. In some instances the clinical manifestations may be the same, as, for example, in progressive kyphosis in a conservatively treated fracture and progressive kyphosis following implant failure. Whether due to complications of injury or complications of treatment, late problems result from failure of immediate treatment.

As there does not appear to be a published time-related definition of early or late complications, in the following discussion we will define late sequelae of fractures as failures and complications of initial treatment, surgical or otherwise, and failure to prevent the natural progression of associated disease processes, such as decubiti and sepsis.[30]

Complications may be classified according to the organ system involved, whether they result from the initial injury or are iatrogenic. Examples of organ system complications include respiratory (pneumonia), gastrointestinal (ileus, stress ulcers), genitourinary (urinary tract infections, calculi),[50] integumentary (ulcers, negative nitrogen balance), osseous (static or progressive deformity, pain), muscular, and neurologic (static or progressive) problems. The orthopedic surgeon is most familiar with skeletal and neurologic problems. The multisystem problems listed emphasize the importance of a team approach to spinal trauma. It is important to include physicians whose interest and expertise in these areas exceeds that of the average orthopedic surgeon or neurosurgeon.[20]

We hope that a discussion of these and other potential problems will allow the physician to foresee and avoid the late sequelae of spinal injuries.[55]

CERVICAL SPINE

ANATOMY

The cervical spine is a mobile structure containing the cervical portion of the spinal cord. Paired on each side of the cervical spine are the vertebral arteries, providing the blood supply for the cervical cord and brain stem.

The cervical spine can be divided into two distinct mechanical complexes. The occiput–atlantoaxial articulation is a transition between the vertebral joint structure and the skull that provides support to the head while allowing significant degrees of flexion, extension, and rotation.[96,97] The lower cervical spine is different anatomically, and therefore unique biomechanically.[60]

INSTABILITY

The avoidance of late sequelae of spinal trauma may depend on the prompt and proper treatment of instability patterns. The stability of C-1 injuries is dictated by the integrity of the transverse alar ligament.[32] As determined by Spence, when, in an anteroposterior open-mouth radiograph, transverse measurement of the atlas exceeds that of the axial lateral masses by 7 mm or more, the fracture is unstable and requires fixation.[88]

There is a frequent risk of iatrogenic instability in cervical spine fractures treated with laminectomy, especially in hyperflexion or flexion–compression injuries. Shields and Stauffer[87] reported that one third of patients treated with laminectomy later required a fusion due to the instability this procedure introduced. Flexion–rotation injuries are notoriously unstable, and require operative stabilization to prevent progressive deformity. Operative intervention does not influence the neurologic outcome of these injuries.[28]

Progression of spinal deformity, instability, and progression of neurologic deficit are often seen when the unstable cervical spine is treated by anterior bone block or dowel fusions. Stauffer and Kelly[89] reviewed all Ranchos Los Amigos, California patients with cervical spine fracture-dislocations treated by anterior dowel interbody fusions. All had progression of their deformity, and three had progression of their neurologic deficit. Thir-

teen of 16 required two or more attempts at fusion. Bohler reported a similar experience, and resorted to additional posterior fusion to provide stability. Whitehill and Schmidt[99] reported excellent results using posterior intraspinous wiring in patients with significant posterior ligamentous disruption. Fusion occurred in all 22 patients. No patient deteriorated, and overall recovery was 32%. They did note, however, an adjacent flexible kyphosis, which averaged 16 degrees in 22 patients.

SYRINGOMYELIA

Syringomyelia is an unusual cause of late neurologic deterioration after spinal injury. Syringomyelia may or may not communicate with the cerebrospinal fluid. Barnett[6] suggested that traumatic myelomalacia, hematomyelia, or ischemic necrosis results in noncommunicating syrinx formation. Kao and Chany[47] suggested that lysosomal action, presumably related to the above process, would cause cystic cord degeneration. Serial magnetic resonance imaging following trauma may better elucidate this process in the near future, and may differentiate edema with the potential for neurologic recovery from hemorrhage and eventual syrinx formation with permanent deficits (Fig. 22-1).

Cysts typically form in the ventral portion of the dorsal columns and in the medial aspects of the dorsal horns. This may be related to the vascularity of the region, which makes it more susceptible to hemorrhage, or to the relatively greater elasticity of this tissue compared with the more rigid white matter. Barnett[6] postulated that body motion produces fluid pressure gradients that cause dissection of cyst fluid along tissue planes of least resistance. Pressures are increased if adhesions prevent free motion of the cord.

Gardner[36] suggested an alternative explanation. He proposed a presyringomyelic population with an asymptomatic communicating syrinx. Severe cord trauma leads to subarachnoid adhesions. Normal intracranial vascular pulsations can then no longer be dissipated along the subarachnoid space and are redirected into the spinal cord through a developmental defect near the fourth ventricle. This would most commonly result in a

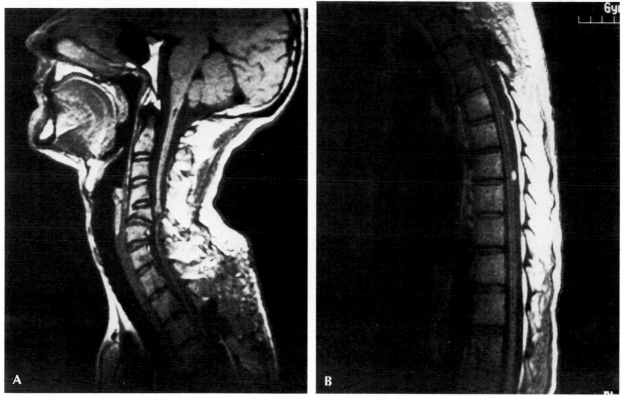

Figure 22-1. (*A*) Magnetic resonance image of a complete C-6 spinal cord injury. (*B*) Formation of a post-traumatic syringomyelia in the thoracic spine below the injury level is seen via MRI.

cervical syrinx formation, although brain stem symptoms in the trigeminal nerve distribution and signs of asymmetrical tongue weakness have been described.

Symptoms suggestive of syrinx formation include new pain, increased spasticity, progressive motor and sensory loss, hyperhidrosis, persistent postural hypotension, and autonomic dysreflexia. These may occur alone or in combination. The diagnosis of syringomyelia has previously been made by computed tomography–myelography. A 4-hour delay is recommended to allow the soluble contrast to demonstrate the syrinx.[29] Magnetic resonance imaging, if available, is now the diagnostic tool of choice.

Syringomyelia usually presents as a late sequelae between 2 and 15 years after injury, as reported by Laha[54] and by Barnett.[5] Mudge[73] identified two cases among 520 spinal cord in-

jured patients reviewed at Ranchos Los Amigos, California. If this series is considered with Barnett's, the likelihood of developing post-traumatic syringomyelia is 19 out of 1907 cases, or about 1%. Only seven of Barnett's patients required surgical decompression for disabling or progressive symptoms. Curiously, two had a remission suggestive of spontaneous decompression.

Surgical treatment of syringomyelia is dictated by fluid dynamics. A normotensive syrinx may be simply incised either with a scalpel or by laser. The thinnest region of the wall is determined by intraoperative ultrasound. A syrinx characterized by elevated pressure may be treated by syringo-subarachnoid or syringoperitoneal shunting, as described by Anton.[2] Approximately 50% of surgically treated patients will have improved motor function and relief of pain, which is often dramatic.

SYSTEMIC COMPLICATIONS

Systemic complications can be a significant problem in cervical spine injuries. These include cardiopulmonary dysfunction, vasomotor instability, autonomic dysreflexia, and hypercalcemia.

Neurologic pulmonary edema associated with central nervous system injuries above T-4 to T-6 has been reported by several authors.[8,50,76] It is attributed to a massive centrally mediated sympathetic discharge that is distinct from autonomic dysreflexia.[8] Treatment requires mechanical ventilation.

Aberration of cardiac reflexes is a self-limited but significant problem within the first 2 months of injury, accounting for 66% of mortality due to cervical spinal cord injury in one series.[103]

The usual response to hypoxia in a neurologically intact patient is tachycardia; in cervical spinal cord injured patients, the response is bradycardia.[63] This appears to be due to a vagovagal reflex for both afferent and efferent limbs of the vagus nerve. Contributing factors are absent sympathetic activity, hypoxia, and the inability to breathe spontaneously. This response can be prevented by oxygenation or can be treated with atropine.

Hyperhidrosis is another common sympathetic complication of cervical spine injuries. It rarely occurs with lesions below the T-8 to T-10 level. It may be precipitated by afferent stimuli from the bladder, rectum, and other sources. When these sources have been eliminated as a cause, α-adrenergic blocking agents such as phenoxybenzamine hydrochloride can be effective.[86]

Hypercalcemia of immobilization is a self-limited disorder that may persist for up to 14 months if left untreated.[66] It is most commonly seen in cervical spine injuries, with onset within 3 months of injury. The serum calcium concentration may rise to 11 to 15.8 mg/dl. Males aged 15 to 19 years who have complete high cervical lesions, dehydration, and immobilization are at greatest risk. Nausea, vomiting, polydipsia, polyuria, and lethargy are presenting complaints. The differential diagnosis in older patients must include preinjury Pagets disease or primary hyperparathyroidism. These must by evaluated by appropriate laboratory studies. Renal function is reduced during the hypercalcemia, but returns to normal as serum calcium levels decline. Treatment includes reduced calcium intake, rehydration, sodium infusion, and furosemide administration.[67]

THORACOLUMBAR SPINE

ANATOMY

The thoracolumbar spine is defined as the region from T-1 to L-5. At the various levels, skeletal and neural structures range considerably in function, mechanical properties, and response to injury. The thoracic spine is a rigid structure whose major role is protecting the dura mater and spinal cord. This is contrasted with the more mobile thoracolumbar junction and lumbar spine, whose major role is weight bearing. The change in functional emphasis, from rigid, protective thoracic spine to mobile, less protective lumbar spine makes teleologic sense in that the cauda equina, being a peripheral nervous system, is more resistant to injury than the spinal cord.

The neural axis likewise changes considerably, from central gray and white matter to peripheral nerve; each tissue type responds differently to injury. The neural transition zone corresponds to the skeletal transition zone between T-12 and L-1.

Trauma to the thoracolumbar spine can produce varied and complex bony or neural injury. Treatment can therefore be difficult.

SKELETAL COMPLICATIONS

Skeletal complications of spinal trauma are related to deformity, which can be static or progressive, and pain, which can originate at the fracture site from bone or soft tissue. Later, degenerative changes above or below the injured level may cause deformity and pain.

Spinal Deformity

An understanding of spinal stability* and spinal balance is a prerequisite to a discussion of spinal

---

* Reference numbers 25, 26, 41, 42, 57, 69, 70, 83, 98, 100.

deformity. Any definition of stability should incorporate patient complaints, such as pain, neurologic compromise, or cosmetics. White defined a stable spine as one in which "there is neither damage nor irritation to the spinal cord or the nerve routes with the spine under physiologic loads."[98]

Nicoll[74] was among the earliest authors to equate disruption of posterior ligaments, posterior joints, and facet capsules with recurrence of deformity. Holdsworth[41] likewise emphasized posterior structural integrity when he described stable and unstable fractures. Holdsworth recognized, but did not see clinically, a theoretical method of neurologic injury related to failure of the middle column. Middle column failure was later described by Denis as when a vertebral body fragment is displaced posteriorly into the neural elements.

Denis[25,26] defined acute spinal instability as disruption of the third or middle spinal column. This consists of the posterior longitudinal ligament and its attachments to the posterior annulus fibrosus, disk, and posterior vertebral body. The importance of the middle column was further investigated by McAfee,[68] who identified three different methods of middle column failure: compression, distraction, and translation. In each type of failure a different mechanical stabilizing procedure was required to avoid late complications. Roy-Camille[83] similarly noted the importance of the middle column in spinal stability.

Spinal balance refers to sagittal and coronal alignment of the spinal axis. It must also consider the amount of curve displacement from the C-7 to S-1 plumb line. Although a clearly stated definition of spinal balance is difficult to find in the literature, general guidelines exist. Intuitively, balance implies that the head is centered over the center of gravity, that is, just anterior to S-1. This, however, does not consider sagittal or coronal deformity, such as kyphosis related to trauma with a compensatory distal lordosis or a compensatory scoliosis. These may progress—that is, they are unstable, even when C-7 is above S-1 and the spine is balanced.

The initial treatment of thoracolumbar spine trauma must restore both spinal stability and balance to avoid present and future deformity[24] (Fig. 22-2). Significant deformity following thoraco-

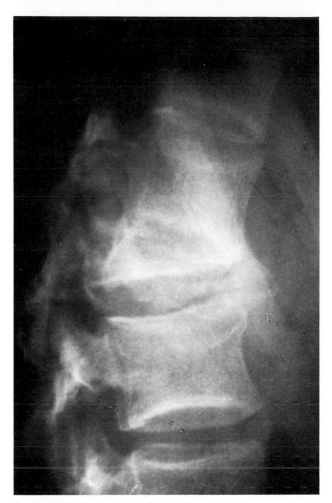

Figure 22-2. Progressive collapse of an L-1 fracture as seen 1 year after injury.

lumbar spine trauma does not appear to be a common problem, especially in the thoracic spine, because of the stability afforded by the ribs.[35]

Leidholt[56] reviewed 204 paraplegic patients after fractures and fracture-dislocations. He arbitrarily selected patients with a kyphosis of 30 degrees or greater and a lateral angulation of 10 degrees or greater. Subgroups consisted of injuries from T-1 to T-10, T-11 to L-1, and L-2 to L-5. It should be noted that the inherent stability of T-1 through T-10 is greater than the other subgroups, and a 30-degree kyphos of L-2 to L-5 is a significantly greater deformity than a 30-degree kyphos elsewhere, as the lumbar spine has a normal lordosis. Leidholt was unable to demonstrate clinically significant problems with these arbitrarily selected limits, although he cautioned against significant lateral angulation leading to pelvic obliquity and ischial ulceration.

Malcolm and associates[61] reviewed 48 patients treated surgically for post-traumatic kyphosis. All thoracic deformities were greater than 45 degrees, with an average of 74 degrees; thoracolumbar kyphosis averaged 46 degrees, with a range of 18 to 72 degrees; and lumbar kyphosis averaged 31 degrees, with a range of 5 to 79 degrees. Patients initially treated with laminectomy had greater deformity. All 48 patients were treated with anterior, posterior, or combined fusions, using iliac, rib, and fibular grafts with posterior Harrington instrumentation in compression or distraction. Postoperative immobilization averaged 9.3 months. The average spinal correction was 26%.

Bradford[15] suggested that anterior rib grafts be placed no further than 4 cm anterior to the kyphotic apex to minimize the risk of graft fracture. He also described a vascularized rib graft.[14]

Pain

Musculoskeletal pain is a frequent late sequela of thoracolumbar spine trauma, and may be related to fracture,[101,102] deformity, instability, pseudarthrosis, spinal stenosis,[40] disk degeneration above or below the injured level,[3] facet degeneration, facet fracture, facet synovial or other cysts, myositis ossificans, or infection subsequent to penetrating trauma, as in stab or gunshot wounds.

Leidholt[56] found that pain related to deformity was not a major problem for his patients; however, this may be because none of the patients in his series had significant deformity. Holdsworth[41] reported that spontaneous anterior fusion almost always occurred when the disk and body were destroyed, and pain was present for minor periods. Nicoll[74] reported spontaneous fusions in all 10 patients. Kaufer[48] noted that four out of nine patients without fusion developed severe back pain, while none of the patients with fusion had significant pain. He attributed successful relief of pain to a solid fusion.

Malcolm[61] reported a significant improvement or elimination of back pain in his patients who were successfully fused. He felt that a solid arthrodesis was more important than the correction of deformity obtained. The pain successfully treated by fusion was typically constant, aching in character, and increased with activity or prolonged sitting or standing. It was located at the apex of the deformity. Bed rest often relieved this pain.

In conclusion, mechanical pain related to thoracolumbar fractures appears to be related to significant deformity, as reported by Malcolm, or to instability. It is successfully treated by arthrodesis. Reduction of deformity in the presence of solid fusion is of secondary importance.

Pain may also be related to compensatory changes above and below the injured segment. Swiderski[92] reported that 35% of 120 patients had pain at a location other than the fracture site. This was attributed to pathologic changes such as instability, stenosis, and collapse or degeneration of intervertebral disks at uninjured levels.

A compensatory excessive lordosis, which presents with symptoms typical of mechanical back pain or degenerative disease, has been reported to produce accelerated degenerative changes.[53] Evaluation should include diskography, saline, acceptance or stress tests, and facet blocks to define the structures affected. Treatment often requires anterior, posterior, or combined single or staged procedures, as outlined by Kostuik.[52]

Pain originating from facet joints may be related to degenerative changes, facet fractures, facet impingement syndrome, or, rarely, to facet cysts.

Facet fractures may occur at the time of initial injury or following surgical decompression.[108] Rothman[82] noted 25 inferior facet fractures in 400 computed tomographic scans taken postoperatively to evaluate new symptoms of pain in the back or leg after a period of well-being. Typically, a new pain pattern consisting of local pain and tenderness, pain with unusual motion, and relief with rest suggested the diagnosis. Facet fractures may present with asymmetrical joint space widening or motion segment subluxation.

Various types of facet cysts have been reported to cause pain after thoracolumbar trauma. Synovial cysts of lumbar facets are rare, but recognized, deformities presenting as degenerative back pain.[77] Their etiology has not been determined, but is probably related to apophyseal joint degeneration, capsular tears, and synovial tissue herniation. In addition to pain associated with degenerative changes, they may present with root or cord compression symptoms, depending on size, location, or associated intraspinal pathology—for example, post-traumatic stenosis. Polivy[77] has reported two such cases and Franck,[34] one such case.

Juxtafacet ganglionic cysts may present in a similar fashion. Histologically, they consist of a loose vascular collagenous wall around a viscous, gelatinous material. Ganglionic cysts lack a synovial lining. Their presumed origin is myxoid degeneration of connective tissue associated with hyaluronic acid production, possibly synovial fluid extrusion from injured facet joints, and pleuripotential mesenchymal cell proliferation.

Granulomatous lesions have been described in inflammatory arthropathies such as ankylosing spondylitis following trauma.[46] They present with localized back pain with or without sensory motor changes. They are felt to be inflammatory lesions. Kanefield[46] believed that granulomatous lesions may represent a response of delayed union or nonunion of fractures in inflammatory spondylitis.

Recently, a facet impingement syndrome has been proposed to explain pain above or below a fused segment.[85] This syndrome produces localized pain due to impingement of the mobile facet by the solid fusion mass.

Myositis ossificans has been reported as a complication following thoracolumbar trauma.[44] It presented with painful motion and a hypertrophic callus around a slightly displaced transverse fracture. A pseudarthrosis was evident within the mass of hypertrophic bone. Pain was relieved by excision of the pseudarthrosis and physical therapy. The authors attributed pain relief to local denervation, increased lumbar motion, and development of a new pseudarthrosis after physical therapy that permitted unrestricted lumbar motion.[44]

NEUROLOGIC COMPROMISE

Late neurologic compromise from thoracolumbar fractures can be related to a number of factors.[62] Kyphosis with or without progression may place traction on the spinal cord, conus medullaris,[78] or nerve roots in the cauda equina. Spinal stenosis, either central, lateral recess, or foraminal, may result sometime after the original injury. Perineural cysts have also been described.

In Malcolm's study[61] of 48 patients treated surgically for post-traumatic kyphosis, 13 required surgery due to a late progressive neurologic deficit related to the kyphosis. Eight of the 13 had initially been treated by laminectomy; this undoubtedly contributed to their progression. The majority of these patients, 11 out of 13, plus three patients with static neurologic findings, for a total of 14 patients, were treated by an anterior decompression and fusion. One third of these improved, one third were unchanged, and one third worsened.

Roberson[80] reviewed 34 patients with kyphosis after fracture. All patients were treated at least 3 months, the majority 1 year or more, after fracture. Eighteen patients with incomplete neurologic findings or progression were treated with anterior decompression and fusion. Five were improved and none were worse. Roberson attributes these positive results to the fact that none of the decompressions was in Dommissee's critical vascular zone, from T-5 to T-9, as were three of four of Malcolm's patients who did deteriorate. Roberson also credits his technique of decompression, from anterior to posterior, with clear visualization of the dura, neural foramina, and nerve roots for his success.

Bohlman[11-13] has recently reported his results in late decompression of patients with neurologic complaints related to thoracolumbar fractures. These patients were treated with posterolateral or anterior decompression between 3 months and 20 years after injury. Two out of 37 patients who presented with leg complaints were not improved. Six out of 30 patients with paralysis were not significantly improved with a follow-up of 6 months to 8 years. He concluded that patients who presented with continued, progressive, or late neurologic sequelae will benefit from an appropriate decompressive procedure.

The neurologic sequelae of thoracolumbar trauma have been compared to the more commonly seen problem of degenerative stenosis.[84,95] Weisz discussed the concept of spinal reserve capacity in 10 patients who presented with a progressive spinal stenosis. He attributes the stenosis to ossification of soft tissues around the injured motion segment, which ultimately causes nerve root or cauda equina compression. Early after injury, neural elements are freely mobile despite canal compromise by fracture fragments. As the normal tissue responses of inflammation, fibrosis, and callus formation progress, eventual mechanical constriction of the canal occurs.

Late neurologic sequelae can result from either intradural or extradural cystic degeneration. Synovial cysts are rare but recognized[77] causes of root or cord decompression. They are likely related to facet degeneration, capsular tears, or synovial herniations. Perineural cysts have been described on sacral roots, causing radicular pain or paresthesias. They originated between the perineurium and endoneurium, and may be related to trauma.[29]

Although dural defects are not uncommon when acute spinal fractures are explored posteriorly, there do not appear to be any reports of symptomatic pseudomeningocele or significant arachnoiditis related to these injuries. This may be due to the large "blood patch" applied to these cerebrospinal fluid leaks in the form of fracture hematoma.

PENETRATING TRAUMA

Penetrating trauma to the thoracolumbar spine is relatively unusual in civilians. In addition to complications related to closed spine injury, open or penetrating injuries may result in fistula formation, osteomyelitis, or central nervous system lead toxicity.

Subarachnoid pleural fistulas are rare. The first reported case was by Langston in 1959.[9] The diagnosis is suggested by recurrent or persistent pleural effusions in a patient with either blunt or penetrating thoracic spine trauma. Laboratory comparison of pleural and spinal fluid may confirm the diagnosis, as may the pleural aspiration of a dye such as indigo carmine injected into the spinal canal. Myelography may confirm the diagnosis and establish the site of the fistula. Surgical treatment can then be considered.

The risk of meningitis, paraspinal abscess, or osteomyelitis after gunshot wounds to the spine is low.

Several authors[21,39,72,94,104] discussed spinal injuries related to military gunshot wounds. Open fractures of the spine, as elsewhere, are treated with prompt operative débridement and antibiotics. As with other open fractures, they have an increased risk of osteomyelitis.[81]

Systemic lead toxicity following gunshot wounds to the spine is rarely reported.[38] Plumbism is promoted by the presence of an appropriate solvent, such as synovial fluid, bursal fluid, and, presumably, cerebrospinal fluid. Additional factors are the surface area and size of the bullet and the length of time in contact with body fluids. Most cases develop many years (i.e., 9 to 17 years) after injury.

Routine decompressive laminectomy is no longer a controversial issue in the management of gunshot wounds to the spine. Such a procedure should only be performed in the presence of compressive signs or symptoms. Compression of the cord or roots may be by the missile itself, or from displaced fracture fragments (Fig. 22-3). Bullets should be removed from the canal to prevent late lead intoxication. The timing of decompression is not critical unless the neurologic deficit is incomplete and progressing. If the foreign body is removed immediately and the neural deficit has progressed after surgery, one does not know if the deficit was related to the initial injury or to the procedure itself. Stauffer, therefore, recommends removal at 3 or 4 days after surgery.[90]

An extensive historical experience with routine decompressive laminectomy has failed to show significant improvement in neurologic status, and has demonstrated many problems related to iatrogenic destabilization following penetrating trauma to the spine.

Wanamaker[94] reported on his experience with the early treatment of 300 patients with spinal cord injuries. The majority of these patients were casualties from the Korean War. Both penetrating and closed spine injuries were reviewed. Of 254 patients with penetrating trauma, 121 were improved. He concluded that perioperative mortality related to laminectomy was low, and in careful

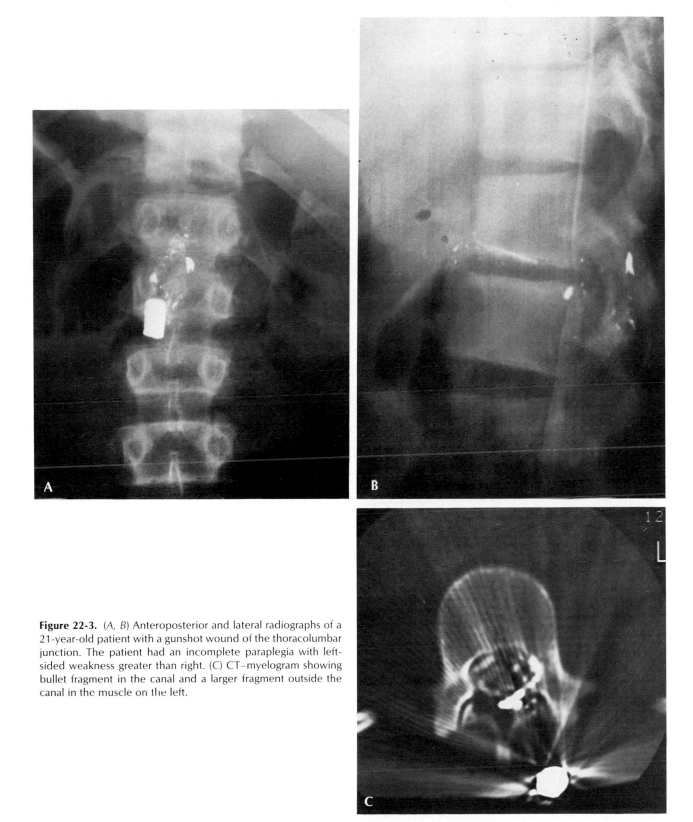

Figure 22-3. (*A, B*) Anteroposterior and lateral radiographs of a 21-year-old patient with a gunshot wound of the thoracolumbar junction. The patient had an incomplete paraplegia with left-sided weakness greater than right. (*C*) CT–myelogram showing bullet fragment in the canal and a larger fragment outside the canal in the muscle on the left.

hands, quite rewarding. His data are difficult to evaluate, as detailed neurologic status before or following surgery is not reported, nor does he report on evidence of cord or root compression on preoperative studies. Likewise, fewer than 50% of his patients were decompressed within 24 hours. This was due to other life-threatening problems or delayed evacuation. He does not report on late iatrogenic instability.

Stauffer[90] addressed these issues in a review of 185 cases of gunshot wounds to the spine among patients admitted to Ranchos Los Amigos, California between 1966 and 1973. One hundred six patients presented with complete neurologic deficit. Fifty-six were treated with laminectomy, and of these one patient improved; the 50 patients treated without laminectomy did not improve. Forty-five patients who presented with incomplete lesions underwent laminectomy. Of these, 32 patients, or 71%, improved. Thirty-four patients who presented with incomplete lesions were not decompressed. Of these, 26 patients, or 76%, likewise showed improvement. There was a 10% incidence of wound infection or spinal fistula complicating operative treatment. In addition, six patients developed instability related to decompression. Stauffer also analyzed the interval from injury to decompression, and felt that this had no bearing on neurologic outcome. He concluded that the neurologic outcome of low-velocity missile wounds to the spine was not related to laminectomy. He did make a special case for rapidly progressing neurologic deterioration as an indication for prompt decompression. Several other authors[22,23,64] support these conclusions based on mixed series of spinal cord injured patients.

PEDIATRIC SPINE

The growth potential and mechanical properties of the pediatric or adolescent spine present management problems unique to this age group. Younger tissue, being more viscoelastic, allows displacement of the spinal column sufficient to cause severe and permanent neurologic injury, even without fracture. The pediatric spine may suffer a central or lateral Salter–Harris type fracture of vertebral apophyses.[18] A third factor that distinguishes pediatric spine trauma from adult is the development of scoliosis, kyphosis, lordosis, or combinations of these deformities related to paralysis in continued growth.[7] Finally, children have a greater risk of kyphosis after laminectomy as compared to adults.[105]

Nerve root impingement in children or adolescents is rare without trauma. When it occurs, it is related to vertebral end-plate apophyseal fracture rather than degeneration of disk or annulus fibrosus. Apophyseal fractures are commonly seen with trauma.[16] Computed tomography or computed tomography–myelography, and now perhaps magnetic resonance imaging, are more likely to demonstrate this injury than routine radiographs. Technetium 99m bone scans are less clear in demonstrating these fractures, unless back pain without neurologic complaints or hamstring spasm is the presenting complaint.

McPhee[71] discussed some of these issues in a review of 42 pediatric spine fractures or dislocations. Multilevel injury, usually thoracic, was seen more often than in adults, which was defined as older than 15 years in this series. He found it difficult to predict stability, noting late spontaneous progression of unstable injuries as well as progression of apparently stable injuries. This may be analogous to kyphosis after laminectomy, and may be aggravated by secondary support from immature muscular and posterior ligaments. In addition, growth disturbance from vertebral crush and apophyseal injury may cause a progressive deformity. Vertebral height is not uniformly reestablished after injury.

Hubbard[43] noted a similar inability of the pediatric vertebral body to remodel, although several of his cases demonstrated some reconstitution of vertebral body height. This usually occurred in younger patients with wedge compression fractures.

Late pain is unusual in pediatric spine fractures. McPhee[71] attributed this to the ability of juvenile disks to withstand injury. As a general rule, the intervertebral disk and joint are preserved. He noted that spontaneous interbody fusion is rare, and recommended surgical fusion for grossly unstable injuries.

Paralytic spinal deformity is the most devastating problem unique to pediatric and adolescent spinal trauma. It is almost universal in children injured prior to their growth spurt. It is also related to the level of the lesion: its frequency and severity increase with the level of injury. Children younger than 10 years with a lesion above T-10 are at greatest risk. Scoliosis is the most frequent primary spinal deformity reported, with kyphosis and lordosis, in that order, less frequently seen.[19]

Paralytic scoliosis results from muscle imbalance. It most frequently occurs in the rotator muscle groups of the erector spinal group and in the postural muscles.[79] Treatment of paralytic deformities often proceeds to spinal fusion. Wheelchair modifications and orthotics should be used initially in an effort to gain trunk height maturity, and to free the upper extremities for daily activities. Orthotic treatment can be difficult in patients with insensate skin, who may already have pressure sores. A thoracic suspension orthosis may be useful in cooperative patients with mild or moderate spasticity.

Mayfield[65] reviewed a large series of children (younger than 18 years of age), and noted that orthotic management was difficult in preadolescence, but successfully delayed surgical fusion. Sixty-eight percent of his patients ultimately did require fusion. The deformities treated included thoracic kyphosis and excessive lumbar lordosis, which were aggravated by muscle imbalance, the effects of gravity, and, according to Kilfoyle,[51] the typical tripod stance used by paraplegics for crutch walking. These spinal deformities may contribute to pelvic obliquity, hip dislocation, difficulty with sitting balance, or pressure sores. It is to prevent these complications as well as to prevent progressive spinal deformity and respiratory compromise that most authors recommend spinal fusion when the curve cannot be controlled orthotically. Fusion should be performed while the curve is fairly supple.[4,17,19,51,65]

Surgical treatment consists of fusing the paralytic segment to the sacrum. This will maintain a balanced pelvis, prevent hip subluxation, maximize sitting balance, prevent decubiti, and free the upper extremities for daily activities. Mayfield[65] noted that 68% of his patients whose injury occurred prior to the adolescent growth spurt had progression of their curve and required fusion. His rate of complications was high—83%. Babcock[4]

likewise reported that paralytic spinal deformities were resistant to surgical correction. In Burke's study[17] 10 out of 29 patients with injury prior to age 13 required one or more fusion procedures. Soft-tissue procedures to correct paralytic curves are rarely helpful, as noted by Kilfoyle.[51]

COMPLICATIONS ASSOCIATED WITH INSTRUMENTATION

The goals of surgical treatment of spinal injuries are to prevent progressive neurologic loss, to permit neurologic recovery when possible, to reestablish the mechanical integrity of the spine, and to promptly mobilize the patient, thus preventing the problems of incumbency and the cost of prolonged bed rest. Pursuit of these goals was difficult in the past because the fixation devices available were unable to bear the forces applied to them. The history of operative treatment of spinal trauma is one, therefore, checkered by many iatrogenic implant-related complications. With recent metallurgic improvements and improved implant design, spinal instrumentation systems have entered a new era. Historically, combinations of plates, screws, springs, rods, hooks, and wires have been used, each with their own specific complications. Complications can be generally categorized as related to infection; compression of structure, such as dura, cord, nerve routes, and vessels; superficially prominent hardware; delayed union, nonunion, or malunion due to distraction or hardware failure; and iatrogenic fracture.

Systems can be categorized as anterior (e.g., Harrington–Kostuik, Dunn, Kaneda, and AO plates), posterior (e.g., Harrington and Luque instrumentation or spinous process plates),[41,93] or those that utilize pedicle screws. Complications occur with every newly introduced instrumentation system while its indications for proper use are defined.

RODS

Harrington rods with or without sublaminar wires have become the classic method to reduce, stabilize, and fuse the unstable spine.[102,107] After a difficult initial experience, Dickson[27] reported on a series of 95 patients with spinal fracture-dislocations treated with Harrington rod instrumentation. Twenty-six out of 95 patients had complications related to the operation. These included incorrect placement of instrumentation, broken rods, pseudarthrosis, loss of angular correction, hook displacement, infection, and persistent pain.

The error in placement of instrumentation consisted of insufficient length of fusion. Dickson recommended placement two interspaces above and below the fracture level. Rod breakage did not invariably result in pseudarthrosis or recurrent deformity. Six patients experienced rod fracture (Fig. 22-4). Two of these lost all correction within 18 months of surgery, two had a minimal loss of correction, and two had no important change. An additional six patients had their hooks disengage. This occurred at both the upper and lower hooks in five patients. These patients lost their correction in the immediate postoperative period. The sixth suffered a single hook disengagement without loss of correction. Two deep infections occurred, one early and the second 2½ years after injury. Postoperative pain was reported by five patients. In one, this was attributed to a psychological problem; the others were felt to have pain related to cauda equina injury.[27]

Aebi[1] treated 35 patients with a variety of instrumentation systems. He had four hook or rod dislodgements, which required operative removal in all cases. Three patients required rod shortening or removal because of skin irritation after rod migration. This occurred because rods or sublaminar wires broke.

Gertzbeim[37] noted similar problems with Harrington rod instrumentation (Fig. 22-5). He emphasized securing the upper hook to the rod to prevent caudal migration. He recommended seating the hooks under the laminar notch between the facets to prevent lateral hook migration. He also cautioned against excessive removal of laminar bone, as 10% of his patients fractured a lamina. Half of these lost correction as a result.

The experience of Yosipovich[106] was similar with respect to local irritation caused by prominent rods. He reported an average loss of correction of 5 degrees and one case of cast-related pressure necrosis. Both Svensson[91] and Flesch[33]

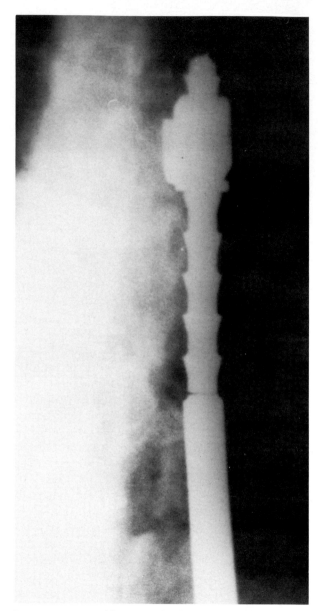

Figure 22-4. Typical location of rod fracture at the junction of the smooth portion of the rod and the first rachet.

reported a complication rate of approximately 50% with Harrington rod instrumentation. The complications included decubiti, pseudarthrosis, rod breakage, rod dislodgement, thromboembolus, painful bursae, cardiac arrest, wound hematoma, pneumonia, transitory paresthesia, su-

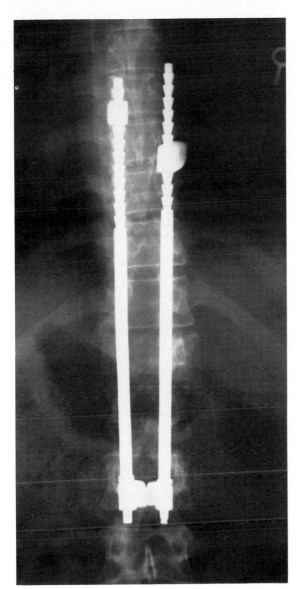

Figure 22-5. Note the dislodged top right hook on this dual Harrington rod instrumentation of an L-1 fracture.

WIRES

The addition of sublaminar wires considerably reduced the incidence of complications in rod instrumentation.[58,59] Bryant[16] did not observe residual gibbus or hook dislodgement in 15 patients followed an average of 19 months. His sole instrument-related failure was a rod reversal, which could have been prevented by square-ended rods and laminar hooks (Fig. 22-6). He emphasized the fracture reduction, stability, absence of late deformity, low pseudarthrosis rate, and early mobilization made possible with this combination.

Harrington rod instrumentation can cause overdistraction at the fracture site in an unstable fracture-dislocation with disruption of all three

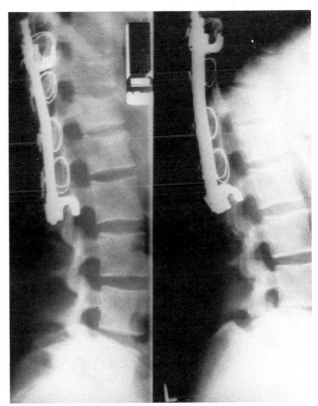

Figure 22-6. Example of "rod reversal" despite use of sublaminar wires. The initial postoperative reduction is shown on the left. The radiograph on the right shows how the rods have spun around 180 degrees. This complication might have been prevented by the use of square-ended rods and laminar hooks.

perficial wound infection, and cerebrospinal fluid fistulas. Soreff[45] reviewed 147 compression fractures 8 years after treatment, and noted that in this relatively stable fracture, the best results were obtained with Harrington rod instrumentation. However, anatomic reduction was accomplished and maintained in only two thirds of cases.

columns. This is a complication related to misapplication of the Harrington rod distraction but it has, nevertheless, been reported by Esposito.[31] Because the patient was a paraplegic, he suffered no further neurologic deterioration as a result. However, in a less neurologically compromised patient, this could have had catastrophic consequences. It should be emphasized that intraoperative and early postoperative radiographs demonstrated a near anatomic reduction in this patient. It was not until films taken on the 10th day after surgery that the error was evident.

PEDICLE SCREWS

Several pedicle screw instrumentation systems are now in the process of laboratory and clinical investigation. This technology has been available and used in Europe for many years. The results of this European experience are now being reviewed in an effort to introduce these techniques into the United States.

Some early results from the use of pedicle screw systems are available in this country. White[98] has recently evaluated 76 patients with instabilities from a variety of causes treated with pedicle screws and plates. There was a 5% incidence of deep infection, which he attributed to prolonged surgical time and the large surface area of the implant. Twenty-three percent of the screws fractured; some of these required reoperation. Three patients complained of prominent hardware. Eight of the first 30 reported some leg pain related to nerve root irritation. This could have been related to hardware outside the pedicle, intraoperative or postoperative pedicle fracture with root compression, or an induced foraminal stenosis from distraction across the fractured segment. These problems were treated with nerve root blocks, epidural injections, corsets, and braces. White also offered the caveat that stress transfer to either end of the instrumented segment may create further problems with disk degeneration, facet syndromes, or hypermobility. Despite a 30% reoperation rate and 10% failed fusion rate, he felt that the system was useful in some cases of marked spinal instability. One would expect results to improve with time and familiarity with the system.

Aebi[1] has reported his results in 30 patients treated with the internal spinal skeletal fixation system. This system is based on bilateral transpedicular Schanz screws attached by hinged coupling clamps to square-ended, treaded spanning rods. Like the vertebral spinal plate (VSP) system, this is considerably more rigid than Harrington rod instrumentation. Maintenance of reduction achieved with this system was excellent as measured by kyphosis, anterior and posterior height 12 months after surgery. One patient required repeat surgery for lost fixation early in the series. No other complications were reported. These results appear to represent the spectrum of results obtainable with pedicle fixation systems. White and associates[80] pointed out that their series represents learning curve and utilizes modified implants.

The use of sublaminar wires carries with it a risk of perioperative neurologic injury in up to 15% of the cases in some series,[7] with 4% consisting of major paraparesis. Late complications are rare but occur in scoliosis patients. Late wire breakage should be considered a failure of the surgeon's fusion technique, and it may result in neurologic complaints and pseudomeningocele. The risk of late sublaminar wire breakage and additional neurologic injury in trauma is unknown but should be explored.

Spasticity and the mass reflex following spinal cord injury is often useful to the patient in rehabilitation, transfers, and bladder function. In some instances, spasticity is sufficiently severe that it interrupts rehabilitation. Changes in both central synaptic excitability and hyperactive stretch reflexes have been implicated in the development of spasticity after trauma. Management consists of removal of nociceptive stimuli, and passive stretch to minimize joint contracture.

SUMMARY

Spinal surgery has entered a period of rapid technological advancement. Metallurgy and implant design has matured sufficiently so that surgical stabilization, neurologic decompression, and early mobilization are realistic goals in the spinal cord injured patient. Early mobilization avoids sequelae of long-term illness and spinal injuries associated with bed rest or casting over insensate skin. However, surgical treatment and instrumentation introduce a plethora of new problems. It is hoped that awareness of the complications discussed in this chapter will allow the physician to anticipate and prevent their occurrence, thus maximizing the likelihood of a stable spine without deformity or pain, and a patient whose maximum neurologic recovery is achieved.

REFERENCES

1. Aebi M, Mohler J, Koch G, Movscher E: Analysis of 75 operated thoraco-lumbar fractures and fracture-dislocations with and without neurological deficit. Arch Orthop Trauma Surg 105:100, 1986
2. Anton HA, Schweigel JF: Post-traumatic syringomyelia: The British Columbia experience. Spine 11:865, 1986
3. Arminio JA: Trauma in the lumbar disc lesion: Post-traumatic sequelae. Del Med J 39:198, 1967
4. Babcock JL, Albright JE: Spine trauma in children and adolescents. J Bone Joint Surg [Am] 58:728, 1976
5. Barnett HJM, Jousse AT, Ball MJ: Pathology and pathogenesis of progressive cystic myelopathy as a late sequela to spinal cord injury. In Barnett HJM, Foster JB, Hudgson P (eds): Syringomyelia, p 179. Philadelphia, WB Saunders, 1973
6. Berk JL, Levy MD: Profound reflex bradycardia produced by transient hypoxia of hypercapnia in man. Eur Surg Res 9:75, 1977
7. Beutel EW, Roberts JD, Langston HT, Barker WT: Subarachnoid pleural fistula. J Thorac Cardiovasc Surg 80:21, 1980
8. Bohler J, Gaudernak T: Anterior plate stabilization for fracture dislocations of the lower cervical spine. J Trauma 20:203, 1980
9. Bohlman HH: Late pain and paralysis following fracture of the thoraco-lumbar spine: The long term results of anterior decompression and fusion in T1 patients. Orthopaedic Transaction 12:60, 1988
10. Bohlman HH: Late progressive paralysis and pain following fractures of the thoraco-lumbar spine. J Bone Joint Surg [Am] 58:728, 1976
11. Bohlman HH, Freehafer A, Dejak J: The results of treatment of acute injuries of the upper thoracic spine with paralysis. J Bone Joint Surg [Am] 67:360, 1985
12. Bradford DS, Daher YH: Vascularized rib grafts for stabilization of kyphosis. J Bone Joint Surg [Br] 68:357, 1986
13. Bradford DS, Ganjavian S, Antonious D et al: Anterior strut grafting for the treatment of kyphosis. J Bone Joint Surg [Am] 64:680, 1982
14. Bryant CE, Sullivan JA: Management of thoracic and lumbar spine fractures with Harrington distraction rods supplemented with segmental wiring. Spine 8:532, 1983
15. Burke DC: Traumatic spinal paralysis in children. Paraplegia 11:268, 1974
16. Callahan DJ, Pack LL, Bream RC, Hensinger RN: Intervertebral disc impingement syndrome in a child: Report of a case and suggested pathology. Spine 11:402, 1986
17. Campbell J, Bonnett C: Spinal cord injury in children. Clin Orthop 112:113, 1975
18. Chou SN: The treatment of paralysis associated with kyphosis. Clin Orthop 128:149, 1977
19. Comarr AE, Kaufman AA: A survey of neurologic results. J Neurosurg 13:95, 1956
20. Covalt DA, Cooper IS, Hoen TI, Rusle IIA: Spinal cord injury. JAMA 151:89, 1953
21. Davidoff LM: Spinal cord injuries. Surg Clin North Am 21:433, 1941
22. Davies WE, Morris JH, Hill V, Phty B: An analysis of conservative (non-surgical) management of thoraco-lumbar fractures and fracture-dislocations with neural damage. J Bone Joint Surg [Am] 62.1324, 1980
23. Denis F: Spinal instability of defused by the three column spine concept in acute spine trauma. Clin Orthop 189:65, 1984
24. Denis F: The three column spine and its significance in the classification of acute thoraco-lumbar spine injuries. Spine 8:817, 1983
25. Dickson JH, Harrington PR, Erwin WD: Results of reduction and stabilization of the severely fractured thoracic and lumbar spine. J Bone Joint Surg [Am] 60:799, 1978
26. Dorr LD, Harvey JP Jr, Nickel VL: Clinical review of the early stability of spine injuries. Spine 7:545, 1982
27. Eismont FJ, Green BA, Quence RM: Post-traumatic spinal cord cyst: A case report. J Bone Joint Surg [Am] 66:614, 1984
28. Epps CH: Complications in Orthopedic Surgery. Philadelphia, JB Lippincott, 1986
29. Esposito PW, Alexander AH, Lichtman DM: De-

layed overdistraction of a surgically treated unstable thoraco-lumbar fracture: A case report. Spine 10:393, 1985

30. Fielding JW, Cockvau GVB, Lawsing JF, Hohl M: Tears of the transverse ligament of the atlas. J Bone Joint Surg [Am] 56:1683, 1974

31. Flesch JR, Leider LL, Erickson DL et al: Unstable fractures and fracture-dislocations of the thoracic and lumbar spine. J Bone Joint Surg [Am] 59:143, 1977

32. Franck JI, King RG, Petro GR, Kanzer MD: A post-traumatic lumbar spinal synovial cyst: Case report. J Neurosurg 66:293, 1987

33. Frankel HL, Hancock DO, Hysop G et al: The value of postural reduction in the initial management of closed injuries of the spine with paraplegia and tetraplegia: Part one. Paraplegia 7:139, 1969

34. Gardner WJ, McMurray FG: Non-communicating syringomyelia: A non-existent entity. Surg Neurol 6:251, 1976

35. Gertzbein SD, MacMichael D, Tile M: Harrington instrumentation as a method of fixation in fractures of the spine. J Bone Joint Surg [Br] 64:526, 1982

36. Grogan DP, Bucholz RW: Acute lead intoxication from a bullet in an intervertebral disc space. J Bone Joint Surg [Am] 63:1180, 1981

37. Guttman LJ: Surgical aspects of the treatment of traumatic paraplegia. J Bone Joint Surg [Br] 31:389, 1949

38. Hasue M, Kikuehi S, Inoue K, Miura H: Post-traumatic spinal stenosis of the lumbar spine: Report of a case caused by hyperextension. Review of the literature. Spine 5:259, 1980

39. Holdsworth FW: Fractures, dislocations and fracture-dislocations of the spine. J Bone Joint Surg [Am] 52:1534, 1970

40. Holdsworth FW, Hardy A: Early treatment of paraplegia from fractures of the thoraco-lumbar spine. J Bone Joint Surg [Br] 35:540, 1953

41. Hubbard DD: Injuries of the spine in children and adolescents. Clin Orthop 100:56, 1974

42. Jackson DW: Unilateral osseous bridging of the lumbar transverse process following trauma: Case report. J Bone Joint Surg [Am] 57:125, 1975

43. Jacobs RR, Asher MA, Snider RR: Thoraco-lumbar spinal injuries. Spine 5:463, 1980

44. Kanefield DG, Mullins WP, Freehafer AA et al: Ankylosing spondylitis. J Bone Joint Surg [Am] 61A:1369, 1979

45. Kao CC: The mechanism of spinal cord cavitation following spinal cord transection: Part I. A correlated chemical study. J Neurol 6:251, 1976

46. Kaufer H, Hayes JT: Lumbar fracture dislocation. J Bone Joint Surg [Am] 38:712, 1966

47. Keene JS, Goletz TYH, Benson RC: Undetected genito-urinary dysfunction in vertebral fractures. J Bone Joint Surg [Am] 62:997, 1980

48. Kicker JD, Woodside JR, Jelinek GE: Neurogenic pulmonary edema associated with autonomic dysreflexia. J Urol 128:1038, 1982

49. Kilfoyle RM, Foley JJ, Norton PL: Spine and pelvic deformity in childhood and adolescent paraplegia. J Bone Joint Surg [Am] 47:659, 1965

50. Kostuik JP: Anterior Kostuik-Harrington distraction systems for treatment of kyphotic deformities. Scientific exhibit at the 52nd annual meeting of the American Academy of Orthopaedic Surgeons, Las Vegas, Nevada, January 1984

51. Kostuik JP, Errico TJ, Gleason TF: Techniques of internal fixation for degenerative conditions of the lumbar spine. Clin Orthop 203:219, 1986

52. Laha RK, Malik HG, Langille RA: Post traumatic syringomyelia. Surg Neurol 4:519, 1975

53. Levine AM, Edwards CC: Complications in the treatment of acute spinal injuries. Orthop Clin North Am 17:183, 1986

54. Liedholt JD, Young JJ, Hahn HR et al: Fracture dislocations of the dorsal and lumbar spine in paraplegics. Paraplegia 7:16, 1969

55. Louis R: Surgery of the Spine. New York, Springer-Verlag, 1983

56. Luque ER: Segmental spinal instrumentation. Thorofare, NJ, Slack, 1984

57. Luque ER, Cassis N, Ramirez-Wiella G: Segmental spinal instrumentation in the treatment of fractures of the thoraco-lumbar spine. Spine 7:312, 1982

58. Lysell E: Motion in the cervical spine. Acta Orthop Scand 123(suppl), 1969

59. Malcolm BW, Bradford DS, Winter RB, Chou SN: Post-traumatic kyphosis. J Bone Joint Surg [Am] 63:891, 1981

60. Marshall LF, Knowlton S, Garfin SR et al: Deterioration following spinal cord injury: A multicenter study. J Neurosurg 66:4000, 1987

61. Mathias CJ: Bradycardia and cardiac arrest during tracheal suction: Mechanism in tetraplegic patients. European Journal of Intensive Care Medicine 2:147, 1976

62. Matson DD: Craniocerebral Trauma: Surgery of Trauma. Philadelphia, JB Lippincott, 1953

63. Mayfield JK, Erkkila JC, Winder RB: Spine deformities subsequent to acquired childhood spinal cord injury. J Bone Joint Surg [Am] 63:1401, 1981

64. Maynard FM: Immobilization hypercalcemia fol-

lowing spinal cord injury. Arch Phys Med Rehabil 67:41, 1986

65. Maynard FM, Imai K: Immobilization hypercalcemia in spinal cord injury. Arch Phys Med Rehabil 58:16, 1977

66. McAfee PC, Hanson AY, Fredrickson BE, Lubicky JP: The value of computed tomography in thoraco-lumbar fractures. J Bone Joint Surg [Am] 65:461, 1983

67. McAfee PC, Werner FW, Glisson RR: Biomechanical analysis of spinal instrumentation systems in thoraco-lumbar fractures: Comparison with traditional Harrington distraction instrumentation with segmental spinal fixation. Spine 10:204, 1985

68. McAfee PC, Yuan HA, Lasda NA: The unstable burst fracture. Spine 7:365, 1982

69. McPhee IB: Spinal fractures and dislocations in children and adolescents. Spine 6:533, 1981

70. Morgan TH, Wharton GW, Austin GN: The results of laminectomy in patients with incomplete spinal cord injuries. Paraplegia 9:14, 1971

71. Mudgle K, Van Dolson L, Lake AS: Progressive cystic degeneration of the spinal cord following spinal cord injury. Spine 9:253, 1984

72. Nicoll EA: Fractures of the dorso-lumbar spine. J Bone Joint Surg [Br] 31:376, 1949

73. Poe RH, Reisman JL, Rodenhouse TG: Pulmonary edema in cervical spinal cord injury. J Trauma 18:71, 1978

74. Polivy KD, Hamelon J, Boyd RJ: Synovial facet joint cyst causing extra-dural compression. Spine 12:412, 1987

75. Ragnarsson TS, Durward QJ, Nordgren RE: Spinal cord tethering after traumatic paraplegia with late neurologic deterioration. J Neurosurg 64:397, 1986

76. Roaf F: Scoliosis secondary to paraplegia. Paraplegia 8:42, 1970

77. Roberson JR, Whitesides TE: Surgical reconstruction of late post-traumatic thoraco-lumbar kyphosis. Spine 10:307, 1985

78. Rothman RH, Simeone FA: The Spine. Philadelphia, WB Saunders, 1982

79. Rothman SL, Glenn WV, Kerher CW: Post-operative fractures of the lumbar articular facets: Occult case of radiculopathy. AJR 145:779, 1985

80. Roy-Camille R: Management of fresh fractures of thoracic and lumbar spine. Presented at the 46th annual convention of the American Academy of Orthopaedic Surgeons, San Francisco, California, 1979

81. Schnaid E, Eisenstein SM, Drummond J: Delayed

82. Schwartz AM, Nash CL: Spinal impingement syndrome: Another cause for the failed spinal fusion. Orthopaedic Transaction 11:93, 1987

83. Shessel FS, Corrian HM, Politano VA: Pheuoxybenzamine and sweating in the spinal cord injury patient. J Urol 120:60, 1978

84. Shields CL Jr, Stauffers ES: Late instability in cervical spine fractures secondary to laminectomy. Clin Orthop 119:144, 1976

85. Spence KF, Decker S, Sell KW: Bursting atlantal fracture associated with rupture of the transverse ligament. J Bone Joint Surg [Am] 52:543, 1970

86. Stauffer ES, Kelly EG: Fracture dislocations of the cervical spine. J Bone Joint Surg [Am] 59:45, 1977

87. Stauffer ES, Wood RW, Kelly EG: Gunshot wounds of the spine: Effects of laminectomy. J Bone Joint Surg [Am] 61:389, 1979

88. Svensson O, Aaro S, Ohlen G: Harrington instrumentation for thoracic and lumbar vertebral-fractures. Acta Orthop Scand 55:38, 1984

89. Swiderski O, Daab J: Treatment of late sequelae of fractures of lumbar vertebrae. Acta Chir Orthop Traumatol Cech 42:497, 1975

90. Tertsch D, Otto W: Surgical stabilization of fractures of the thoracic and lumbar portion of the spine using para-spinal metal plates. Zentralbl Neurochir 45:55, 1984

91. Wannamaker GT: Spinal cord injuries. J Neurosurg 11:517, 1954

92. Weisz GM: Post-traumatic spinal stenosis. Arch Orthop Trauma Surg 106:57, 1986

93. Werne S: Studies in spontaneous atlas dislocation. Acta Orthop Scand 23(suppl), 1957

94. White AH, Johnson RM, Panjabi MM, Southwick WO: Biomechaincal analysis of clinical stability in the cervical spine. Clin Orthop 109:85, 1975

95. White AH, Rothman RH, Ray CD: Lumbar Spine Surgery. St. Louis, CV Mosby, 1987

96. Whitehill R, Schmidt R: The posterior interspinous fusion in the treatment of quadriplegia. Spine 8:733, 1983

97. Whitesides TE: Traumatic kyphosis of the thoraco-lumbar spine. Clin Orthop 128:78, 1977

98. Wilkinson HA: The Failed Back Syndrome. Philadelphia, JB Lippincott, 1986

99. Willen J, Lindahl S, Nordwell A: Unstable thoraco-lumbar fractures: A comparative clinical study of conservative treatment and Harrington instrumentation. Spine 10:111, 1985

100. Winslow EB, Lesch M, Talano JV, Meyer PR Jr:

Spinal cord injuries associated with cardiopulmonary complications. Spine 11:809, 1986

101. Yashon D, Jane JA, White RJ: Prognosis and management of spinal cord and cauda equina bullet injuries in 65 civilians. J Neurosurg 32:163, 1970

102. Yaskuouka S, Peterson HA, MacCarthy CS: Incidents of spinal column deformity after multi-level laminectomy in children and adults. J Neurosurg 57:441, 1982

103. Yosipovitch S, Robin GC, Makin M: Open reduction of unstable thoraco-lumbar spinal injuries and fixation with Harrington rods. J Bone Joint Surg [Am] 59:1003, 1977

104. Young B, Brooks SWH, Tibbs PA: Anterior decompression of fusion for thoraco-lumbar fractures with neurologic deficits. Acta Neurochir 57:287, 1981

105. Zakrevskii LK: Zygapophyseal joint and compression fractures of vertebrae and their sequelae. Ortop Travmatol Protez 8:68, 1982

23

UNIQUE ASPECTS OF PEDIATRIC SPINE INJURIES

Andrew E. Price

CERVICAL SPINE TRAUMA

GENERAL CONSIDERATIONS

The cervical spine in children is unique in that it reaches most of its adult characteristics prior to the extremities and the rest of the axial skeleton. Ligamentous laxity, which contributes to hypermobility in the young child, resolves by the age of 8 years.[308] With the exception of the ring apophysis and the tip of the odontoid, complete ossification occurs at between 8 and 10 years.[15,279] Vertebral bodies reach half of their adult height by the age of 2 years, and little longitudinal growth occurs after age 10. Much of the disproportionate head-to-body size diminishes by age 8.[133] Therefore, pediatric cervical injuries have unique features with respect to diagnosis and treatment prior to age 10, after which management is similar to that of adults. This discussion of pediatric cervical injuries will primarily deal with children under the age of 10 years.

Incidence

Cervical spine injuries are much less common in children than adults. Henrys and associates[127] reported that only 1.9% of cervical spine injuries are in children younger than 12 years old. Rang pinpointed greater mobility and flexibility of the child's spine and its ability to absorb more force over a greater number of segments as the reason for the relative infrequency of cervical injuries.[252] Among vertebral fractures in children, cervical injuries occur relatively infrequently.[143,198,269] When they do occur they usually involve the upper cervical segments, whereas in the adult, injuries from C-4 through C-7 are more common.[7,46,127,129,143,230,240] Funk and Wells showed that 84% of cervical spine injuries in children are found in the upper level.[96] This is probably due to the disproportionate size of the head, weaker neck muscles, and the increased angular mobility of the upper segments.[133]

Injuries among neonates and infants are exceedingly rare, and primarily result from obstetric trauma.[127] Fractures of the pedicles of C-2 in this age group do not result from obstetric trauma, but from vigorous shaking or a fall onto the face. These should be investigated for possible child abuse.[10] Falls and motor vehicle accidents are the major causes of cervical injury in 3- to 5 year olds, and athletic trauma and motor vehicle accidents in 6- to 15 year olds.[127] Most cervical injuries are the result of force transmitted through trauma to the face or scalp.[224] Any child with injuries to the head should be carefully evaluated for cervical fracture or dislocation. In a brain injured child, any of the following findings warrants investigation for spinal injury:

Neck pain
Dermatomic pattern of sensory loss
Absence of movement and reflexes in either both arms or both legs with preservation in the remaining extremities
Flaccidity
Absence of sacral reflexes
Diaphragmatic breathing using accessory respiratory muscles
Bradycardia with hypotension
Autonomic hyperreflexia
Temperature instability
Unexplained urinary retention
Unexplained ileus
Priapism
Clonus in an unconscious patient without decerebrate rigidity[283]

In suspected cervical injury, initial management should be rigid immobilization with the neck in a neutral position on a straight backboard, with tape or sandbags to secure the head.[5,144] In children younger than than 8 years, placement of the proportionately large head on a flat backboard causes flexion of the neck, which could lead to further displacement, injury, or compromise to the spinal cord. Thus, a modified backboard with a recess, or use of pads under the shoulders has been suggested for neutral positioning of the neck in a child (Fig. 23-1).[133] In the child with a neck injury resulting from major trauma, a complete assessment of the child should be performed to rule out other fractures and systemic injuries.

Diagnosis

In a child with a suspected cervical injury, accurate diagnosis is one the most difficult problems facing the orthopedist and radiologist. The young child may be limited in his ability to communicate and unwilling to cooperate during physical examination and roentgenographic studies.[80] Rachesky and associates reported that only 1.2% of cervical radiographs in children were positive for injury. After analyzing their series, they discovered a clinical marker with 100% sensitivity: Either complaint of neck pain or head trauma from a motor vehicle accident was present in all positive cervical radiographs.[251]

When cervical injury is suspected, standard radiographs are rather limited tools for accurate diagnosis. The advent of computed tomography and magnetic resonance imaging, which requires procedural sedation, has been of tremendous importance in evaluating an area of the body that does not have a contralateral extremity for comparison. These modalities have eliminated the need for passive positioning of the neck for flexion–extension, which is dangerous in a patient with instability.[285]

Anatomy

Children have a unique vertebral architecture with hypermobility and a changing pattern of ossification and epiphyseal lines.[46] Prior to fusion, synchondroses may be confused with fractures. Misinterpretation of a normal variant as a fracture or instability can occur.[15,46,83,125,191,193,274,279] Thus, knowledge of anatomy, ossification patterns, and normal limits of mobility can obviate unnecessary treatment.

The atlas and axis are different in both form and function from the lower cervical vertebrae.[139] Along with the occiput, the atlas and axis move as a unit in flexion and extension.[271] The odontoid articulates against the posterior rim of the atlas and, together with the transverse and alar ligaments, forms an arthrodial joint.[139,156] Second articulations occur between the lateral masses of the axis, which are like shoulders—convex and sloping outward, and the inferior articular facets of the atlas.[139,156,234,324] The atlanto-axial lateral apophyseal joints are horizontal and saddle-shaped, and

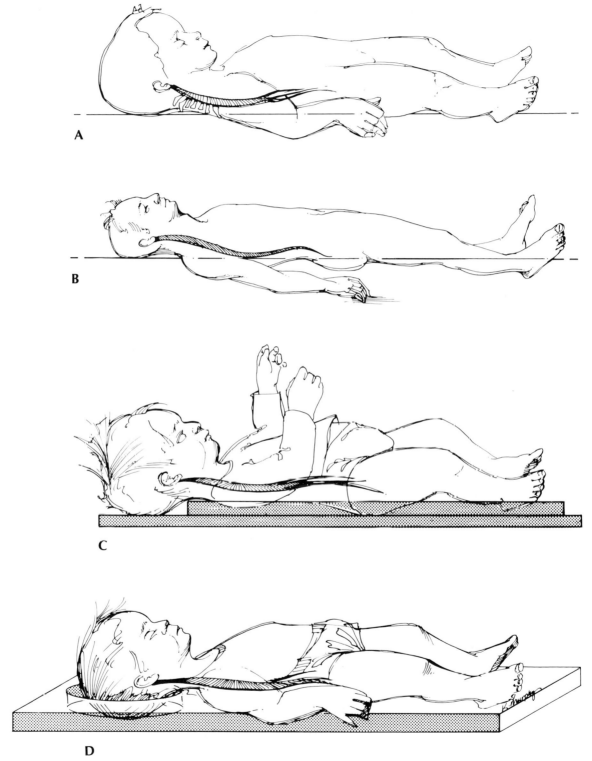

Figure 23-1. Modified backboard and positioning of child younger than 8 years for immobilization of suspected cervical injury. (*A*) Resultant neck flexion when a young child is immobilized on a flat surface. (*B*) Proper position of neck when an adult or older child is positioned on a flat surface. (*C*) and (*D*) Alternative methods of immobilization in a child younger than 8 years.

resist anterior and posterior displacement less than lower cervical articulations,[285] which have paired facets angled obliquely in an anteroposterior direction 45 degrees.[139,234] The atlanto-axial articulations and their architecture allow for greater rotational motion, accounting for as much as 50% of this motion in the cervical spine.[77] Relative horizontal posture of the facet joint is seen in the articulation of C-2 and C-3 and occasionally in that of C-3–C-4, and as a result, increased sagittal motion in these segments may occur.[46,79,297]

In children, the cervical spine is hypermobile as compared with adults.[15,79,185] The increased mobility is caused by a combination of ligamentous laxity,[46] underdevelopment of Luschka's joint,[42] and horizontal alignment of immature facets.[80,127,297] It may be very difficult to distinguish normal from abnormal mobility in the upper cervical spine of a child. In adults, an atlas–dens distance on full flexion of 3 mm is thought to be the upper limit of normal.[137] Roentgenographic interpretation of the pediatric cervical spine does not follow rigid numerical guidelines. Cattell and Filtzer found that 20% of children younger than 8 years demonstrated an overriding of the atlas on the odontoid, seen on lateral views in extension, and a distance of greater than 3 mm between these two structures, seen on flexion.[46] Fielding and associates studied the anteroposterior displacement in adult cadavers and determined that anterior displacement of up to 3 mm is normal, displacement of between 3 and 5 mm indicates rupture of the transverse ligament, and displacement of greater than 10 mm indicates failure of all ligaments.[81] They feel that these data can be extrapolated to children. With clinical signs and symptoms, greater than 5 mm of anterior displacement should be considered pathologic in children.

Pseudosubluxation of the C-2–C-3 and, to a lesser extent, C-3–C-4 articulations has also been reported.[46,297] This increased mobility tends to appear in the younger child or infant, and diminishes at the age of 4 or 5 years, when the facets become more vertically oriented (Fig. 23-2).[80,83]

Variations in curvature of the cervical spine may be associated with injury and accompanying muscle spasm. Irregular angulation of the interspaces can result from sprain of the interspinous ligaments.[46] However, several authors have shown that absence of a lordotic curve in the cervical spine is not necessarily an indication of injury.[46,47,83,319] Lateral radiographs of children show that 16% will have a kyphotic angulation at a single interspace.[46] Absence of the cervical lordosis, uniform angulation between adjacent vertebrae, or the presence of significant kyphosis at one interspace can be seen in a child at any age.

Ossification and Development

Epiphyseal plates and synchondroses appear on radiographs as smooth, regular images in predicted locations, with a subchondral sclerotic line. They can be distinguished from fractures, which have irregular borders and no sclerotic line, and appear in unusual positions.[129] Apophyseal and epiphyseal cartilage are weaker than bone, and the disk–end-plate junction is the weakest point under torsional or shear stresses.[98] Therefore, in the face of a "normal" radiographic appearance, stability in children must be carefully assessed. In very young children, fracture may occur through such weaker, radiolucent areas after minor falls or trivial injuries.[285]

The atlas forms from three primary ossification centers, two for each neural arch and one for the body. In the 7th week of fetal life, ossification of the neural arches occurs; however, the body will not appear radiographically until the child is about 1 year old. Three variations may occur:

1. Two separate ossification centers fuse to form the body, which in turn fuses with the lateral masses.
2. The ossification center for the body fails to appear and the lateral masses extend and then fuse anteriorly.
3. The ossification center for the body does not form, and the lateral masses fail to extend and fuse, resulting in anterior spondyloschisis.[98]

Posterior spondyloschisis is more commonly seen and is usually clinically insignificant.[46,193,212,276] Cervical anatomic anomalies have clinical significance only when combined with trauma or other congenital abnormalities to create an unstable spine.[212,276] The posterior synchondrosis normally fuses by the age of 3 years, while the anterior synchondroses fuse by the age of 7

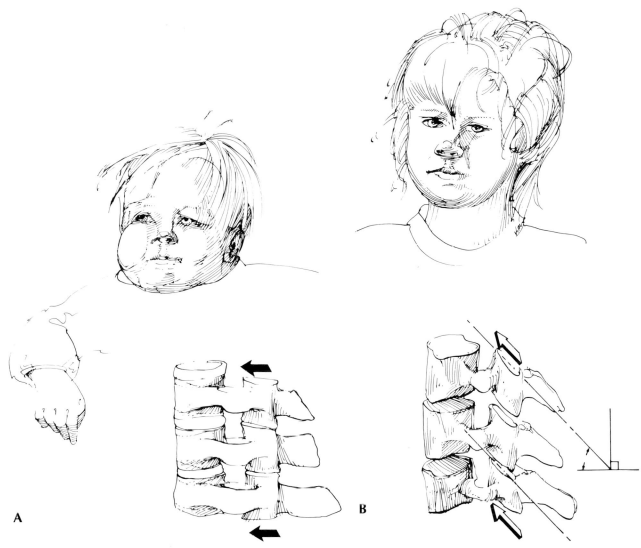

Figure 23-2. Difference in orientation of upper cervical facet joints between an infant and 4 year old, demonstrating the reason for relative hypermobility of the cervical spine in the infant.

years (Fig. 23-3). The latter are seen on the open-mouth radiographic view and should not be confused with fractures.[15,46,83,125,191,212,274,279] When the atlas fails to separate from the occiput, narrowing of the foramen magnum can occur; this may cause neurologic compromise. These symptoms may be progressive and may lead to death during the 2nd or third decade of life.[47,123,211-213] Such a deformity renders a child more vulnerable to spinal cord injury.[129]

The axis consists of four ossification centers, which appear between the 5th and 7th month of fetal life. The four centers consist of one each for the neural arches, one for the odontoid, and one (or two) for the body (Fig. 23-4). The ossification center of the odontoid forms from two cartilaginous anlagen. A vertical line may persist, and should not be confused with a fracture.[80] The tip or summit ossification center is derived from the fourth occipital sclerotome. This ossifies between

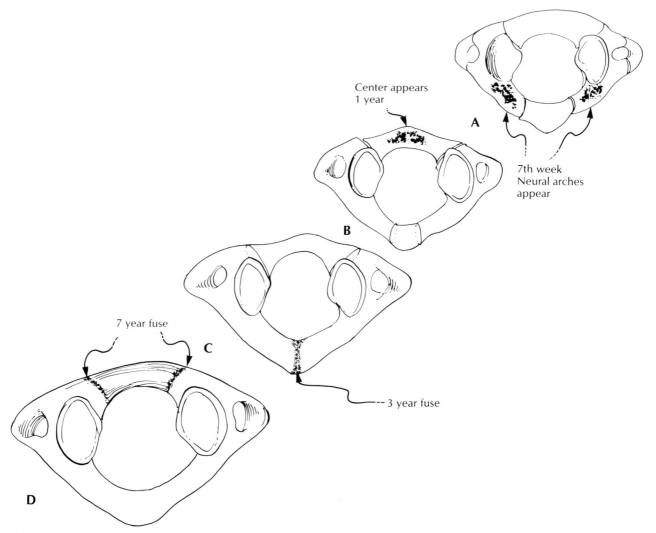

Figure 23-3. (*A*) The neural arches are the first to appear at the seventh fetal week. (*B*) The body appears radiographically during the first year after birth. (*C*) Synchrondrosis of the spinous processes fuse by the third year. (*D*) Neurocentral synchondrosis between body and neural arches unite during the seventh year. (Adapted from Bailey DK: The normal cervical spine in infants and children. Radiology 59:712, 1952)

the ages of 3 and 6 years. Thus the tip of the odontoid has a V-shaped appearance for the first several years of life. It will fuse with the body of the dens at about age 12. When it fails to fuse, it is called an ossiculum terminale.[123] The odontoid sits between the neural arches and is connected with the body of the axis by the epiphyseal plate, which sits well below the level of the articulating facets of the axis (Fig. 23-5).[80] This epiphyseal line and the synchondroses between the body and neural arches form an "H" on the open-mouth view (Fig. 23-6). All synchondroses fuse between the age of 3 and 6 years, and therefore all portions of the "H" disappear by age 6.[15,42] The odontoid epiphysis will occasionally persist as late as age 11, appearing as a thin line at the base of the dens; this can be mistaken for an acute fracture.[127] The inferior ring apophysis of the axis will ossify in late childhood and fuse with the body at age 25.[15,42]

The lower cervical vertebrae are fairly similar in form, function, and development. As with the atlas, each forms from three ossification centers,

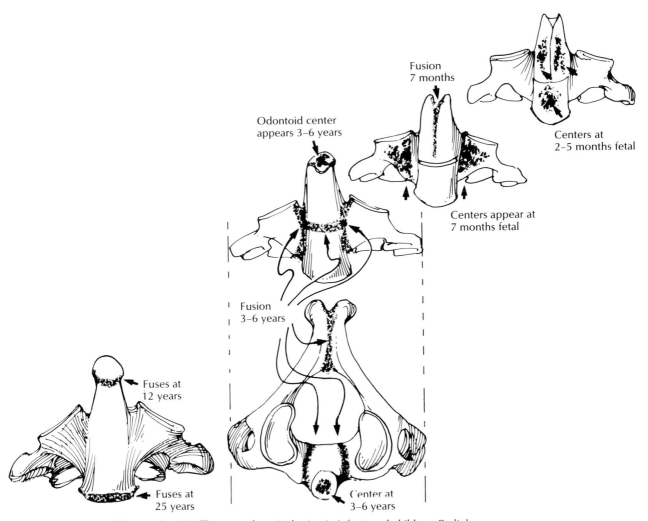

Fusion
7 months

Centers at
2–5 months fetal

Odontoid center
appears 3–6 years

Centers appear at
7 months fetal

Fusion
3–6 years

Fuses at
12 years

Fuses at
25 years

Center at
3–6 years

Figure 23-4. (Adapted from Bailey DK: The normal cervical spine in infants and children. Radiology 59:712, 1952)

two for each neural arch and one for the body (Fig. 23-7). The body appears during the 5th fetal month, and the neural arches appear between the 7th and 9th fetal months. The synchondroses located posteriorly at the spinous processes fuse between the 2nd and 3rd year; the anterior neurocentral synchondroses fuse at 3 to 6 years. The anterior portion of the transverse processes may develop from a separate ossification center that appears during the 6th fetal month and fuses with the neural arch at 6 years. On lateral radiographic

views, the vertebral bodies initially are wedge-shaped, and with growth become squared off by the age of 7 years.[15,46,129,236] The apophyseal rings appear prior to adolescence and fuse with the body at age 25.[15,42,236] The seventh cervical spinous process is thicker, longer, and nonbifid; more anteroposterior mobility may appear at the C-3–C-4 junction. Otherwise, the lower cervical vertebrae are fairly uniform. The entire cervical spine reaches an adult radiographic and clinical character by age 8.

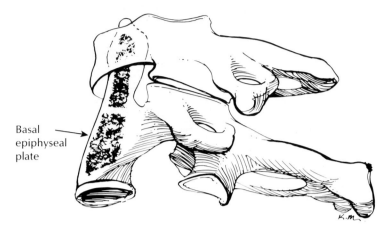

Figure 23-5. Basal epiphyseal plate of the odontoid sitting well below the articulating facets of C-1–C-2.

Basal epiphyseal plate

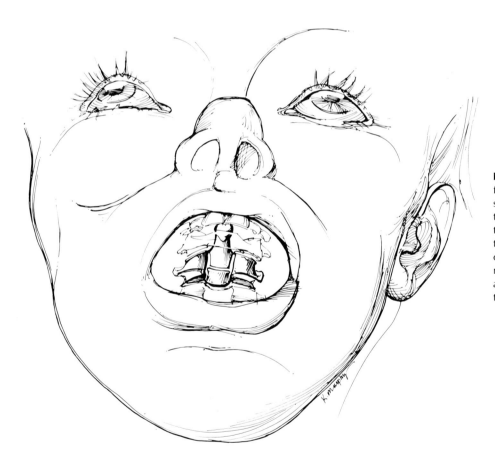

Figure 23-6. An ''H'' is formed by the basal epiphyseal plate of the odontoid and the synchondroses between the body and neural arches of the axis. The ''H'' appears on open-mouth anteroposterior radiographs until the age of about 6 years, when fusion of these synchondroses occur.

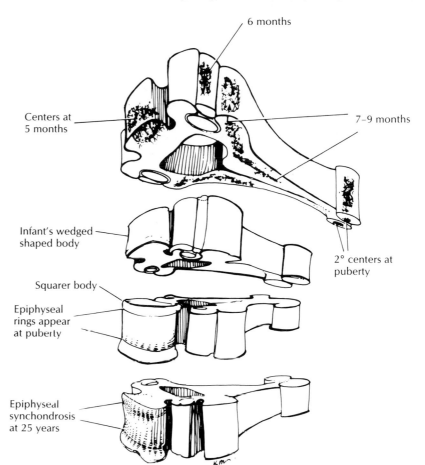

Figure 23-7. Development of the cervical vertebrae, C-3 to C-7:
- Neural arches appear by the seventh to ninth fetal week.
- The body appears by the fifth fetal month.
- The costal portion of the transverse process develops from a separate center by the sixth fetal month and joins the arch by the sixth year.
- Synchondrosis of the spinous process fuses by the second or third year.
- Physeal rings appear at puberty and fuse with the body by 25 years.

(Adapted from Bailey DK: The normal cervical spine in infants and children. Radiology 59:712, 1952)

Radiographic Signs

Some radiographic clues may be helpful in distinguishing a traumatic injury or instability from congenital anomalies or normal variants. The retropharyngeal soft tissues measured on lateral roentgenograms of the spine have been used to detect hemorrhage or edema after fracture. Wholey and associates stated that 3.5 mm is the average width of the retropharyngeal space, measured at the anteroinferior border of C-2.[325] Weir reported that the normal width of this space measured at the same location on C-3 is 5 mm.[319] These guidelines are subject to variations that occur simply through inspiration and expiration; the pharyngeal wall lies close to the vertebrae on inspiration and is pushed away during expiration.[10] This can be magnified in a crying child, in whom significant forward displacement of the hyoid and pharynx will dramatically increase the width of the shadow.[15,80,279] One series reported that almost 36% of patients with cervical fracture did not have prevertebral swelling as measured on lateral radiographs.[241] Therefore, the presence or absence of an enlarged prevertebral shadow should not be relied on to determine the existence of significant trauma.

Fielding listed several normal radiographic findings that can be misinterpreted as fracture or instability:[78]

The apical ossification center of the dens, which appears between 3 and 6 months and usually, but not always (as in ossiculum terminale), fuses with the body at 12 years

The secondary ossification center of the transverse process, which appears in fetal life and fuses at puberty, and the secondary ossification centers of the spinous processes, which appear during puberty and fuse with their adjacent elements at 25 years

Pseudosubluxation superiorly on lateral extension view of the atlas on an incompletely ossified odontoid

Angulation of the odontoid, noted to occur in 4% of children

Persistence of the epiphyseal line at the base of the dens, which has been reported as late as 11 years

The hypermobility at C-2–C-3 and occasionally at C-3–C-4, which may be misinterpreted as instability

An increased atlas–dens interval on lateral flexion view of up to 4 mm, which may be misinterpreted as instability

Physiologic variations in the prevertebral soft-tissue shadow, which may be mistaken for hemorrhage or edema

The "normal" delay in radiographic appearance of the body of the atlas until the age of 1 year, which can look like posterior subluxation of the atlas on the axis

The "wedging" of the cervical vertebral bodies until age 7, which can be confused with a compression fracture

The horizontal posture of the facets in the infant or young child, which may be misread as a pillar fracture

The superimposed shadows of the ears, braided hair, teeth, or hyoid, which may form false fracture lines over the cervical vertebrae

Os odontoideum, spina bifida, nonsegmentation, or other congenital abnormalities, which may be confused with trauma

Wackenheim's five signs can help to distinguish the normal from the traumatic in the upper cervical spine:

1. Condylo–atlantal diastasis—when one side is twice the width of the other, definite abnormality is diagnosed.
2. Increase of the axis foramen diameter. Normally, the anteroposterior diameter of the atlas is 1 to 3 mm greater than the axis. Reverse is abnormal.
3. Transverse dislocation of the cervico-occipital joint manifested by loss of symmetry of the atlanto-occipital atlanto-axial joint.
4. A functional block of the atlanto-occipital or atlantoaxial joint creating a constant relationship with the atlanto-occipital or atlantoaxial joint, with flexion, extension, or neutral position of the neck.
5. Differentiation of an odontoid fracture from an os odontoid, with a congenital anomaly* showing evidence of reduction only with flexion, from a fracture of base showing reduction usually with extension[127]

NEONATAL INJURY

Trauma may occur to a newborn during a difficult delivery, especially if the presentation is breech. The most common injuries, in order of decreasing frequency, are fractures of the clavicle, humeral shaft, femoral shaft, proximal and distal humeral physes, and proximal and distal femoral physes.[300] Although relatively uncommon, injuries to the spine and spinal cord may also occur. Spinal cord damage may vary from tetraparesis, respiratory compromise, and death to minimal or transient deficits.[289] A series of autopsies performed after neonatal death revealed a 30% to 50% incidence of spinal cord trauma.[4] If injury occurs above the level of C-5, death secondary to respiratory paralysis will ensue. If the injury occurs below C-5, diaphragmatic function is preserved.

Neurologic damage may or may not be accompanied by vertebral injury. Since newborn spines are composed of a large amount of preosseous cartilage, radiographic evaluation is pretty limited in determining whether or not osseous injury occurred. Nevertheless, some authors report that the most common obstetric injury is anterior dislocation of the cervical spine with fracture

---

* Os odontoideum is currently believed to result from antecedent trauma, rather than being a congenital anomaly.

through the superior plate of a vertebral body.[70,244,289] The upper cervical spine is more frequently injured in difficult cephalic deliveries, presenting as stillbirth or death.[91,227,279,282,289,293] Injuries to the lower cervical spine are the result of excessive traction with breech deliveries.[1,34,55,56,153,244] After breech delivery of a "star-gazing" fetus with intrauterine cervical hyperextension, the incidence of neurologic damage is 25%.[1,34,55] Therefore, cesarean section is indicated. Thoracic injuries have also been recorded with breech deliveries.[55]

Spinal cord injuries can occur without "bony" injury.[39,89,111,184] The mechanism of injury is thought to be longitudinal traction combined with lateral flexion or torsion.[289] The cervical spine is the most susceptible to birth injury.[317] The newborn neck has weak musculature and lax ligaments incapable of supporting the head until the age of 3 months.[21] Thus, it is unable to resist the forces of torsion or traction. While the spine itself is capable of elongating 2 inches, the cord's elastic limit is about ¼ inch.[188] The inablity of the relatively lax cervical spine to protect this inelastic cord can explain the incidence of cord injury without osseous or ligamentous damage. The pathologic damage to the spinal cord in obstetric injury usually spans several segments and includes laceration, congestion, edema, and hemorrhage.[307] With the cervical cord anchored by the tectorial ligament at the foramen magnum and horizontally directed nerve roots, other intrathecal damage may include avulsion of nerve roots, meningeal tearing with hemorrhage, and laceration or occlusion of vessels, including vertebral artery damage, which is cited as one of the causes of cerebral palsy.[337]

The weak infantile neck is susceptible to vigorous shaking. This type of child abuse may lead to intracranial and intraocular hemorrhage, cerebral injury and retardation, visual or hearing deficits, spinal fractures, or spinal cord lesions with or without bony injury.[43,299] Spontaneous reduction of severe injuries can occur in the face of such neurologic damage. Subluxation and dislocation in an infantile cervical spine may be more frequent than is generally thought. They may escape detection due to the following:

1. Spontaneous reduction without neurologic deficit
2. Deficiency of radiographs to fully visualize preosseous cartilage and facets until later childhood
3. Neonatal death erroneously attributed to other factors[185]

Neurologic damage, neonatal respiratory distress, and complicated deliveries should be investigated for cervical spine injury. Such injuries should be managed conservatively, with gentle reduction and immobilization. Should instability persist into infancy, single-level fusion with limited exposure is warranted.[209]

TORTICOLLIS

When a young child presents with torticollis, or wryneck, proper treatment requires that the exact etiology of the deformity be determined. Torticollis may result from trauma of variable severity. Fracture or instability of any segment of the occipital–atlanto-axial complex may cause a child to hold his head in the wryneck posture. Minor trauma or extreme physiologic motion superimposed on a congenital anomaly of the upper cervical spine can cause torticollis.

Other causes may be easily distinguished from a traumatic etiology. Congenital muscular torticollis will demonstrate tightness in the sternocleidomastoid muscles opposite to the side of rotation. Between 4 and 6 weeks of age, one may appreciate a mass in the belly of the muscle, which should disappear by 6 months. With rotatory atlanto-axial instability, the ipsilateral sternocleidomastoid muscle is in spasm; some authors believe this to be the body's attempt to reduce the deformity.[49,82,118,243] Congenital anomalies can be seen on standard radiographs.[84] Benign paroxysmal torticollis is an infantile neurologic condition in which there is the periodic appearance of torticollis.[266] Unilateral palsy of the trochlear nerve (cranial nerve IV) will cause a child to hold the head in a posture like torticollis in order to minimize the double vision.[21,243] Syringomyelia, Arnold–Chiari malformation, infection, or tumor of cervical bone may cause torticollis.[203] The deformity may result from tumors of the posterior fossa or upper cervical cord, and thus intracranial and medullary evaluation must not be overlooked.[298] Dystonia and myositis ossificans can be associated with abnormal positioning of the head.[21]

With standard radiographs it may be difficult to interpret changes in cervical rotation caused by any of the conditions mentioned. Computed tomography, both static and dynamic, has become the preferred method for ruling out non-neurologic etiologies. Once the exact etiology is determined, the appropriate treatment can be instituted.

ATLANTO-OCCIPITAL TRAUMA

Atlanto-occipital instability may be post-traumatic or nontraumatic in origin, and can range from mild subluxation to frank dislocation. Atlanto-occipital dislocation, which is rare, is the result of severe trauma[3,28] that is nearly always fatal.[3,37,59] This type of cervical injury is seen in 8% of fatal motor vehicle accidents.[37] Only 15 cases of long-term survival are reported in the English literature.[50]

Instability has been associated with upper congenital cervical fusions[326] and linked with one theory of crib death.[109] Atlanto-occipital instability can also be caused by rheumatic diseases or pharyngitis in children.

The clinical presentation may vary widely, ranging from mild to catastrophic. Patients may present in cardiopulmonary arrest with partial to complete paralysis and cranial nerve lesions. If traumatic in origin, the patient usually was in a motor vehicle accident and presents with submental laceration or mandibular fracture. If nontraumatic in origin, a child may present with torticollis, neck pain, or neurologic deficit, or with vertebral basilar symptoms such as nausea, vertigo, and projectile vomiting.[106]

Hyperextension of the occiput is limited by the tectorial membrane, which is an extension of the posterior longitudinal ligament. The mechanism of atlanto-occipital dislocation is believed to be hyperextension and distraction, resulting in rupture of this membrane.[37,94,97] This is borne out by the association of submental laceration and mandibular fracture with traumatic dislocation. Instability is more common in children because of the shallow cranio-cervical junction, namely, smaller occipital condyles and more horizontal atlanto-occipital joints.[73,204]

In adults, the diagnosis of instability can be made on a lateral roentgenogram of the cervical spine. The dens should line up with the basion,[15] and the distance between the two should be 4 to 5 mm (Fig. 23-8).[325,326] However, the use of the dens–basion distance has been disputed due to extreme variations and unreliability.[50] The most sensitive indicator of atlanto-occipital instability is the ratio of Powers and associates, BC:OA, where B = basion, O = opisthion, A = anterior arch of atlas, and C = posterior arch of atlas. This ratio is less than 1.0 unless the patient has a dislocation (Fig. 23-9).[50] However, it is unreliable with atlantal fractures or congenital anomalies of the foramen magnum. Computed tomography is thought to be the best tool for evaluating the atlanto-occipital joint,[107] especially since no studies of the normal distances and translation have been done on children.

Initial treatment of traumatic injury focuses on resolving cardiorespiratory problems while stabilizing the cervical spine. During reduction, care must be taken to apply traction gently in order to avoid further neurologic compromise with overdistraction. The choice between immobilization and surgical stabilization has been somewhat controversial. Immobilization, using a halo or Minerva cast, may require between 6 weeks and 4 months. One series reported failure of immobilization and recommended surgical fusion from the occiput to the atlas, with occasional extension to lower vertebrae when necessary.[106]

INJURY TO THE ATLANTO-AXIAL COMPLEX

The atlanto-axial articulation consists of a unique architecture combined with a complex of ligamentous and capsular attachments that allow for great motion in one plane while dramatically restricting motion in another. There are four synovial articulations between the atlas and the axis: the dens and the anterior ring of the atlas, the dens and the transverse ligament, and the two lateral facets. The dens prevents posterior translation of the atlas–occiput complex. The transverse ligament prevents excessive anterior shift of the atlas, while

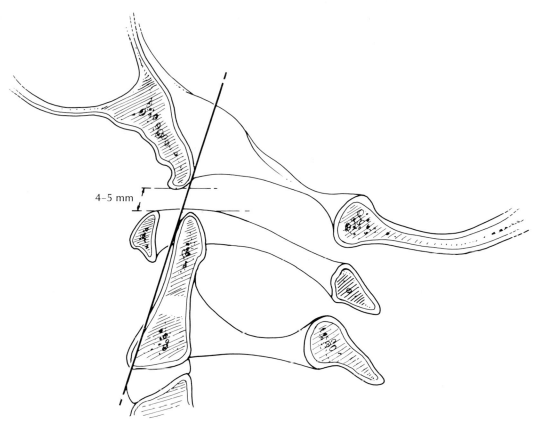

Figure 23-8. Normal relationships of the occiput–atlanto-axial complex seen on lateral view of the cervical spine. (*A*) The dens to basion distance is between 4 and 5 mm. (*B*) The anterior aspect of the dens lies even with basion.

4–5 mm

allowing rotation (Fig. 23-10). The normal rotation of the atlas over the axis is approximately 50% of cervical rotation.[77] During occipital rotation, the lateral masses of the atlas pivot about the dens, relatively unrestricted by the shoulder-shaped facets of the axis. Rotational stability is provided by the alar ligaments and the capsules of the facet joints. The alar ligaments, which extend superiorly and laterally from the tip of the dens and are anchored in the occipital condyles, become taut at 45 degrees, limiting further rotation. Lateral flexion of the head will relax the ipsilateral alar ligament and allow another 20 degrees of rotation. At this extreme of rotation the facets are disengaged and rotational stability is maintained by the facet capsules.[41,77,81]

The ring of the atlas has the largest diameter of any cervical vertebra. Steel's "rule of thirds" applies to the diameter of the atlantal foramen, which is shared equally by the spinal cord, the odontoid, and free space.[291] The free space is like "elbow room" for the spinal cord should any displacement of the atlas occur. Without it, the cord would be crushed between the odontoid and the posterior ring of the atlas. This portion of the cord contains the center for respiration, thus any significant displacement puts the patient's life at risk.[48] Furthermore, such a displacement can occlude the vertebral arteries, which are anchored in the transverse foramen of C-1 and C-2; the interupted

(*Text continued on p. 596*)

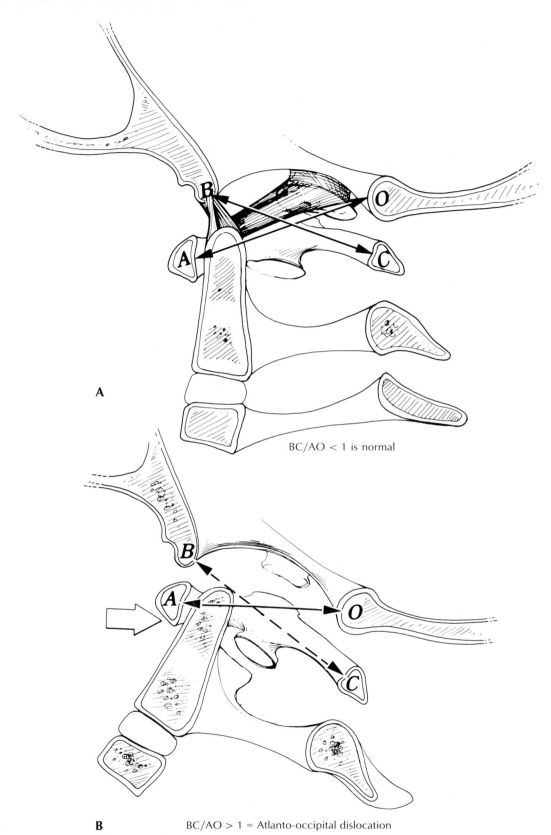

A

BC/AO < 1 is normal

B   BC/AO > 1 = Atlanto-occipital dislocation

Figure 23-9. The ratio BC:OA, the most sensitive indicator of occipito-atlantal instability, is less than 1.0 unless the patient has a dislocation. (B = basion O = opisthion A = anterior arch of atlas C = posterior arch of atlas)

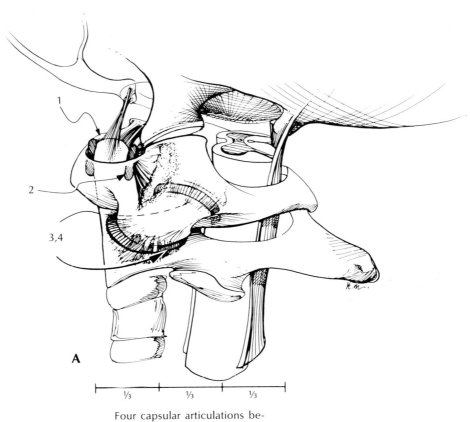

Figure 23-10. The dens–atlas articulation, including the transverse and alar ligaments. The transverse ligament is the primary stabilizer in the sagittal plane, preventing excessive anterior shift of the atlas while allowing rotation. The alar ligaments control the limits of rotation, becoming taut at 45 degrees; lateral tilt will relax the ipsilateral alar ligament, allowing another 20 degrees of rotation.

Four capsular articulations between axis and atlas

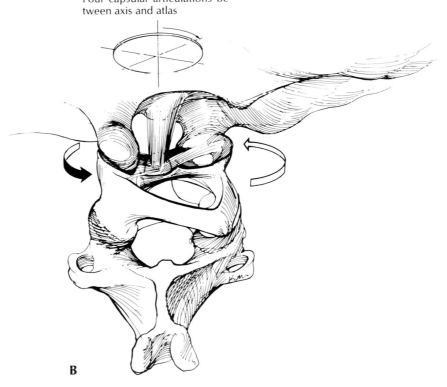

blood supply can cause a brain stem and cerebellar infarct.[78]

The atlanto-axial joint may be affected in four major ways in children:

1. Acquired atlanto-axial instability
2. Atlanto-axial rotatory subluxation
3. Traumatic ligamentous injury
4. Odontoid fractures

The first two may result from minimal trauma or may appear spontaneously; the latter two require major trauma, usually a motor vehicle accident or a fall. All may have catastrophic effects, and require careful investigation and treatment.

Acquired Atlanto-axial Instability

Instability patterns of the atlanto-axial complex may result from congenital or acquired disease processes that affect the bone or soft tissue.[116,132] Children with such instability will present with torticollis, neck pain, or paracervical spasm of spontaneous origin or due to mild trauma.

Nontraumatic atlanto-axial subluxation may occur concomitantly or may follow any inflammation of adjacent cervical soft tissue. This affliction is referred to as Grisel's syndrome.[235] It is mainly associated with children, although cases have been reported in adults.[203,294,328] A combination of many factors probably is responsible for this phenomenon. The drainage of the posterior nasopharynx via the pharyngovertebral veins provides a lymphovenous route for the spread of pathologic processes to the venous plexus around the atlanto-axial articulations (Fig. 23-11). The resultant inflammation and hyperemia causes decalcification of the adjacent vertebrae and the sites of ligamentous and capsular attachments.[235] Simple physiologic motion under these circumstances can lead to translation, rotatory subluxation, and even dislocation.[77,82,152,335] This condition may also be precipitated by surgery such as tonsillectomy, adenoidectomy, or mastoidectomy.[46] Children under the age of 15 have more frequent upper respiratory infections and often have hypertrophic peripharyngeal lymphoid tissue. The inflammatory-induced laxity superimposed on the physiologic hypermobility of the pediatric cervical spine

explains the predominance of this condition in children. Nonsuppurative infection such as tuberculosis or inflammatory disorders such rheumatoid arthritis can cause instability through destruction of the synovial joints and adjacent capsular and ligamentous restraints.[51,54,100,276] The occurence of inflammatory-induced instability is decreasing, probably due to the improved medical treatment of these diseases.[78,263]

Clinically, these patients will present with torticollis, diminished motion, paracervical spasm, and pain, varying from mild to severe, either during or

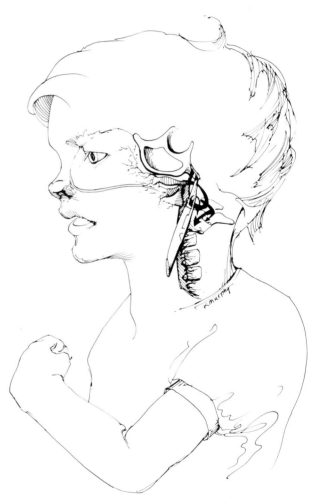

Figure 23-11. Schematic representation of the route of drainage of the posterior nasopharynx and its connection to the upper cervical spine. The posterior nasopharynx communicates via the pharyngovertebral veins with the periodontoidal plexus and the epidural veins; this is the mechanism by which inflammation spreads in Grisel's syndrome.

shortly after the abatement of inflammation. Routine radiographs may be difficult to interpret due to the problems of positioning in a patient with wryneck. Thus, computed tomography and magnetic resonance imaging are playing an increasingly important role in evaluation of the atlanto-axial complex.[243] The treatment is similar to that of rotatory subluxation.

Other conditions exist that also render the atlanto-axial complex unstable. Instability can occur from diseases, like osteogenesis imperfecta, rickets, Paget's disease, or renal osteodystrophy, in which there is pathologic remodeling of abnormal bone.[100,132] Congenital abnormalities, such as Morquio syndrome, Klippel–Feil syndrome, neurofibromatosis, Down's syndrome, spondyloepiphyseal dysplasia, and achondroplasic or metatrophic dwarfism, are associated with atlanto-axial instability due to characterisic ligamentous laxity or odontoid hypoplasia.[12,13,63,100,139,182,205,275,319] In hemophiliacs, recurrent hemarthroses will initially cause attenuation of the capsular ligaments. Eventually, the soft tissues become thickened and fibrotic; the resultant ligamentous stiffening gives the cervical spine more stability, allowing less osteoarthritic change.[11,51,260] After reduction, these conditions may warrant surgical fusion of unstable segments to prevent recurrence or serious complications.

Atlanto-axial Rotatory Subluxation

Atlanto-axial rotatory subluxation from mild trauma is probably the most common cause of torticollis in children. More severe trauma is required to produce the lesion in adults.[169,255,335] The atlas rotates on the axis and becomes fixed with or without an associated anterior or posterior shift. Many theories exist as to the pathogenesis, but the most likely explanation is that capsular and synovial interposition produces pain, spasm, and resultant torticollis.[78] This has been substantiated by the discovery of meniscuslike synovial folds in the atlanto-occipital and atlanto-axial facet joints of infants and small children.[162] When acute, the child will complain of pain and resist any movement of the head. Unlike congenital muscular torticollis, the muscle spasm or tightness is in the sternocleidomastoid muscle on the side where the head is rotated. Occasionally, the deformity may persist and develop fixed contracture, hence the term rotatory fixation; if this occurs, the pain and spasm may diminish over time, but the torticollis and limited motion will remain.

With atlanto-axial abnormalities, standard radiographs may be difficult to interpret because of changes in cervical rotation, problems positioning the patient due to pain and spasm, and the potential existence of congenital anomalies.[79,237,243,297] Cineradiography has been helpful in detecting these lesions,[77,79,134] although it requires a good deal of cooperation and exposes the patient to high levels of radiation.[84,243] Computed tomography and magnetic resonance imaging are especially helpful for evaluating the atlanto-axial complex because they readily demonstrate facet disengagement, as well as fractures or congenital anomalies.[71,78,81,82,86,243] Dynamic computed tomography offers a more accurate and easily interpreted method of evaluation.[68,175,232,243,255] Three-millimeter axial cuts parallel to the ring of C-1 are taken from the occiput to the area just below the atlanto-axial articulation, with the head maximally rotated to each side. With a fixed rotatory deformity, the computed tomographic scan will show eccentric positioning of C-1 relative to C-2, and limited or no motion between C-1 and C-2.[243]

Fielding and Hawkins[82] classified atlanto axial rotatory displacement into four types (Fig. 23-12):

Type I- Rotatory fixation without anterior displacement of the atlas on the axis. The atlas pivots about the dens and the transverse ligament remains intact. This is the most common type seen in children. The prognosis is good and there are no significant potential complications.

Type II- Unilateral anterior shift of one lateral mass while the other acts as pivot. There is 3 to 5 mm of anterior shift.

Type III- Anterior displacement of both lateral masses of the atlas and deficiency of transverse and alar ligaments. The displacement is greater than 5 mm.

Type IV- A deficiency of the dens allowing posterior shift of one or both lateral masses on the atlas

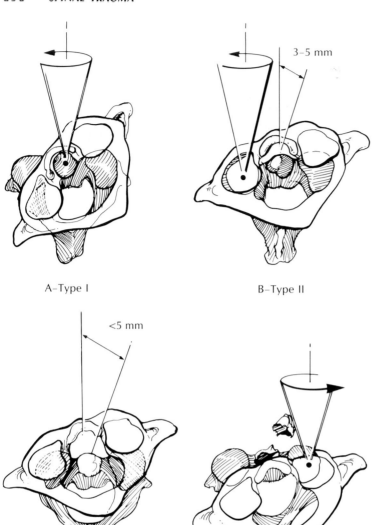

A–Type I

B–Type II

3–5 mm

<5 mm

C–Type III

D–Type IV

Figure 23-12. Fielding and Hawkins' classification of atlanto-axial rotary displacement.

Types III and IV are rare, but are quite dangerous because of the potential risk to the spinal cord; therefore, they must be managed with great caution.

With atlanto-axial rotatory displacement, treatment varies according to the severity and duration of symptoms prior to diagnosis. Mild cases, with symptoms prior to diagnosis of mild stiffness and slight torticollis of a few days' duration, may resolve spontaneously when treated with bed rest and a soft collar.[84,231,243] For patients who do not resolve spontaneously, head halter traction with 3

to 5 lb after administration of analgesics and mild sedation will usually be successful.[114,154,158,243,296,321] For patients who do not respond to these simple regimens or who have had symptoms for more than a week but less than a month, hospital admission and skeletal skull traction is recommended.

The weight used for traction depends on the age of the patient; younger children may begin with about 7½ lb, adults with 15 lb. The traction may be increased 1 or 2 lb every 3 or 4 days to a maximum of 15 lb in children and 20 lb in adults.[82] The traction is maintained until rotation to each side is equal. The patient is then kept in a cervical collar for 4 to 6 more weeks.[243]

The success of traction and the length of traction time necessary are directly related to the duration of symptoms prior to initiation of treatment.[243] If symptoms have been present for longer than 1 month, a 3-week attempt at halo traction can be made.[41] Longstanding subluxations, particularly of longer than 3 months, are less likely to repond to conservative management; Fielding and Hawkins recommended atlanto-axial fusion without attempt at reduction, due to the inherent risks.[82]

Indications for atlanto-axial fusion include neurologic involvement, anterior displacement, deformity present for longer than 3 months, and recurrence of deformity after a trial of conservative management.[78] Fusion should be preceded by 2 to 3 weeks of traction to obtain the best reduction possible, and should be followed by 6 weeks of immobilization either by traction or halo cast.[82] Manipulative reduction has been attempted in cases resistant to conservative measures; limited success and higher risks have narrowed the patient selection for this method.[243]

Burkus and Deponte felt that risk to the cord and vertebral arteries from the scarring and fibrosis that occurs with longstanding subluxation could be minimized using the right technique of reduction. They report a case of a 13-year-old boy with fixed rotatory subluxation of 8 weeks' duration. Successful reduction was achieved using graduated axial halter traction under fluoroscopic control, with constant neurologic monitoring in a sedated yet awake patient.[41]

After reduction by any means, a period of cervical collar immobilization should be adhered to until soft tissues have healed. Stability should be assessed by flexion–extension lateral radiographs. If stable, a physical therapy program can be instituted. When a painless full range of motion is achieved, immobilization can be discontinued.

Traumatic Ligamentous Injury

Injuries to the ligaments of the C-1–C-2 junction are quite rare. Diagnosis and treatment is different between adults and children. On flexion lateral radiographs, the atlas–dens interval in children is usually between 4 and 4.5 mm. Greater than 5 mm implies transverse ligament damage; in adults greater than 3 mm implies damage.[81,135,151,192,219] If any doubt about the diagnosis exists, computed tomography is valuable in delineating the amount of displacement or subluxation or the presence of a C-1 fracture.[18] While treatment in adults is mainly by fusion, conservative methods are preferred initially in children.[52,78,190,215,268] The displacement should be reduced in extension and held in halo or Minerva immobilization for 8 to 12 weeks. Flexion radiographs should be repeated after this to assess displacement; if instability is still present, atlanto-axial fusion is indicated.[78]

Odontoid Fracture

Fractures of the odontoid in children are usually the result of falls or motor vehicle accidents. They are often associated with injuries to the skull, mandible, and other cervical vertebrae.[7,224,239,290] Odontoid fractures are more common in children than in adults, and do not always require a violent force. In young children these fractures may be seen after a minor fall or trivial injury.[285] In an infant or very young child who cries when an attempt is made to sit them up without supporting the head, fracture of the odontoid should be suspected, no matter how trivial the injury.[272]

Clinical features include pain and spasm aggravated by the slightest motion. Neurologic deficit may be immediate or late secondary to gradual subluxation. On physical examination, the patient may present with upper cervical tenderness, spasm, and severe limitation of motion. Neural loss is variable, from high tetraplegia with respiratory center involvement to mild sensory and motor loss secondary to nerve root loss.[285] A high index of suspicion is important when symptoms, specifically torticollis and resistance to motion, persist.

This injury is best discovered using computed tomography or magnetic resonance imaging, which do not require manipulation or positioning of the head. The fracture usually occurs at the basilar odontoid epiphysis, which does not fuse until after the age of 7 years. This cartilaginous plate has excellent healing properties, and thus the difficulty in healing seen in similar type II odontoid fractures in adults is not seen in children younger than 10 years of age.[8] Despite any vascular injury to the ascending arteries of the axis, this epiphyseal separation easily unites and, if necessary, remodels.[25]

While the pathomechanics are a mystery, fracture of the odontoid usually displaces anteriorly. Reduction is accomplished by either recumbency in hyperextension or gentle traction and manipulation of the head in extension. Immobilization for approximately 12 weeks by any of several methods will achieve good results.* The rare case of posterior displacement is treated with gentle traction and immobilization in flexion.[254]

Os Odontoideum

Os odontoideum is an oval or round ossicle of variable size with a smooth cortical border, located either in the normal position of the odontoid process (orthotopic) or near the base of the occipital bone in the area of the foramen magnum (dystopic), where it may fuse with the clivus.[85] It is a very rare condition that may cause atlanto-axial instability. When symptomatic, pain is the most common complaint. Patients may also complain of weakness, numbness, and, less frequently, gait disturbance, neck stiffness, and headaches. Torticollis and neural compromise may be appreciated on clinical examination.

Patients with congenital aplasia or hypoplasia of the odontoid, particularly patients with Down's syndrome, Klippel–Feil syndrome, multiple epiphyseal dysplasia, and other skeletal dysplasias, may have similar symptoms.[58,69,205,277,287] However, true os odontoideum is now believed to be caused by prior trauma,[85,145,334] although two case reports exist that purport the etiology to be tuberculosis and rheumatoid disease, respectively.[159] Fielding and associates feel that the etiology is an unrecognized fracture or damage to the blood supply of the developing dens, followed by retraction of the proximal fragment by the alar ligaments.[85]

Os odontoideum may not become symptomatic for a significant period of time, as long as 10 years. Diagnosis is made on flexion–extension lateral radiographs, which reveal the round or oval ossicle and demonstrate the magnitude of the instability. Computed tomography is not useful for detecting

os odontoideum because it can miss defects in the transverse plane due to partial volume averaging of adjacent bone.[67] For patients who are symptomatic or unstable, Gallie-type surgical fusion of C-1–C-2 with wire is indicated. Fusion in children will usually occur within 2 months. Patients without symptoms or instability may be treated conservatively by observation and avoidance of sports.

Hangman's Fracture

Fractures of the pedicles of the axis are very rare.[105,320] They have been reported in very young children or infants to result from motor vehicle accidents, minor falls, or vigorous shaking secondary to child abuse.[124,208,245] These fractures are not seen in obstetric trauma. Several mechanisms of injury have been suggested, including extension and distraction,[53,201,271] axial loading with extension,[90,201,261,303] and flexion.[61,202,303]

The fracture may be seen on the lateral view of the spine; a flexion lateral view should also be taken to evaluate stability. Diagnosis is clarified using magnetic resonance imaging or computed tomography with sagittal reconstruction.[18,67] Initial treatment should be conservative with immobilization after gentle traction in extension. A Minerva jacket or halo cast is the preferred mode of immobilization, although neck braces, cervical collars, and traction have all led to good results.[241,245] These fractures will usually unite in 4 weeks. If any instability persists or nonunion occurs, a C-1 to C-3 fusion can be performed.[245]

INJURIES BELOW C-2

Injuries below C-2 are very uncommon in children; they consist of either ligamentous injuries or physeal injuries. Ligamentous injuries at the level of C-2–C-3 and occasionally C-3–C-4 can be particularly difficult from a diagnostic standpoint, due to the intrinsic hypermobility of these levels at a young age. Persistence of symptoms beyond several days may clarify the situation. However, Fielding noted that true ligamentous injuries are usually preceded by significant trauma and are followed by pain, spasm, tenderness over the upper spinous processes, and diminished range of motion, which do not abate despite conservative treatment.

---

* Reference numbers 22, 25, 74, 95, 117, 236, 278.

Radiographically, clues to ligamentous instability include ossification of posterior longitudinal or interspinous ligaments, fractures at the tips of the spinous processes, failure of reduction of instability by extension, or formation of a compensatory lordosis below the subluxation.[80] Roy-Camille's indicators of ligamentous instability in the cervical spine below C-2 have been shown to be quite reliable.[239] They include:

1. Widening of the interspinous space
2. Loss of parallelism of the articular facets
3. Widening of the posterior portion of the disk

A normal cervical interspinous distance on anteroposterior radiographs may be up to 1½ times the interspinous distance of an adjacent level. This has been called Naidich's law; it is a reliable guideline for detecting ligamentous instability.[238]

The biomechanics of the vertebral bodies are similar to those of long bones in that the weakest area is at the junction of the physis and metaphysis. Fractures in the cervical spine take two distinct forms, a Salter–Harris type I injury of the inferior physeal end-plate and a Salter–Harris type III injury, posteriorly (Fig. 23-13).

The type I injury involves a complete separation through the entire end-plate, which is the

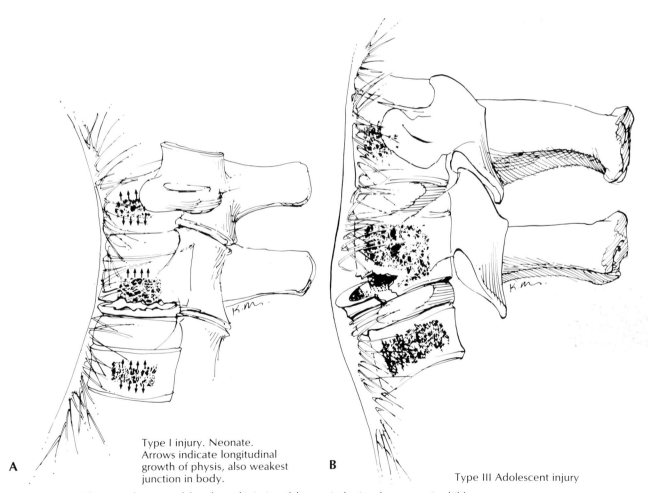

A   Type I injury. Neonate. Arrows indicate longitudinal growth of physis, also weakest junction in body.

B   Type III Adolescent injury

Figure 23-13. Schematic diagrams of the physeal injuries of the cervical spine that appear in children. (*A*) Salter–Harris type I injury seen in infants and young children. (*B*) Salter–Harris type III injury seen mainly in adolescents.

weakest link in the cervical spine with respect to fracture; the superior end-plate is protected by the uncinate process and therefore is rarely involved.[13,183,289] The type I injury occurs in the lower cervical and occasionally the upper thoracic vertebrae of infants and very young children.[78,183] It may result from child abuse.[231,310] Because the cartilaginous end-plate is radiolucent, this fracture is difficult to detect and probably occurs more often than reported. With type I injuries, longitudinal growth may be slowed or interrupted by vertebral growth plate injury.[231] The cervical spine, which reaches a mature state at an earlier age, has relatively limited potential for restoration of vertebral deformity[163,183] as compared to the thoracolumbar spine.[78,127,231] With adequate immobilization, these injuries heal within 2 to 3 weeks due to the excellent healing properties of growth plate injuries.*

Type III injuries occur mainly in the adolescent population at the anterior part of the inferior vertebral epiphysis. Similar injuries are reported more commonly in the lumbar spine. These fractures heal spontaneously and rapidly within 2 to 3 weeks. The osteogenic periosteum is lifted from the inferior portion of the vertebrae adjacent to the anterior longitudinal ligament, often forming anterior healing osteophytes. Premature growth plate closure and angular deformity have not been reported from this injury.[163]

APPLICATION OF A HALO DEVICE

The halo apparatus is a very effective device for immobilization of the cervical spine.† Halo fixation has been shown to restrict 75% of atlanto-axial motion, while the standard neck braces restrict only 45%.[155] Since the introduction of the halo by Perry and Nickel in 1959,[242] many improvements have been introduced, such as radiolucent rings, adjustable rings, convertible tong-to-ring devices, and light adjustable plastic jackets; these have made application and use of the halo much easier and effective. Through biomechanical

* Fielding JW: personal communication, 1988.

† Reference numbers 52, 103, 160, 170, 173, 174, 248, 304, 339, 340.

analysis, Garfin and associates[101] have developed a bullet-shaped pin with a broad shoulder that gives more rigid fixation at the bone–pin interface than the standard pins.

In the young child treated for longer than 4 weeks, the application and maintenance of the halo has a complication rate of over 40%, including pain, loosening, pin migration, and infection.[186] Children have smaller and thinner skulls with softer bone than adults, and therefore require delicate care during the application and maintenance of the halo.[102,186] Manual force is capable of causing penetration of the normal adult skull. The potential for this complication is enhanced by differences between people in load application and variations in friction of the pin–halo interface; thus, there is greater danger in the infant and young child for pin penetration and its sequelae, such as sepsis, hemorrhage, or neurologic injury.[186]

The child's skull attains 94% of its adult length and 89% of its adult width by 3 to 5 years of age.[121] During this period of growth and development, until the age of 6, there is great variability with age and sex in the thickness of skulls at the usual sites of pin placement; furthermore, there are undulations of topography in the inner table of the calverium.[186] A limited skull computed tomographic scan prior to application of the halo is recommended for pin site selection or relocation.[102,186]

In the infant younger than 2 years, braces attached to helmets or a Minerva-type apparatus has been used. Mubarak and associates reported good success with their multiple-pin halo technique, using a custom-made halo and polyethylene jacket and 10 to 12 pins applied with 2 in/lb of torque (Fig. 23-14).[222] The young child between 2 and 6 years of age should have 6 to 8 pins placed with 4 to 6 in/lb of torque. This "crown of thorns" fixation obviates the need for deep insertion of pins and reduces the chance of penetration or loosening.[186] In older children and adults, the usual 4 pins applied with 8 in/lb of torque in the standard anterolateral and posterolateral positions is satisfactory. An excellent discussion of the principles of halo application is presented by Botte and associates.[29]

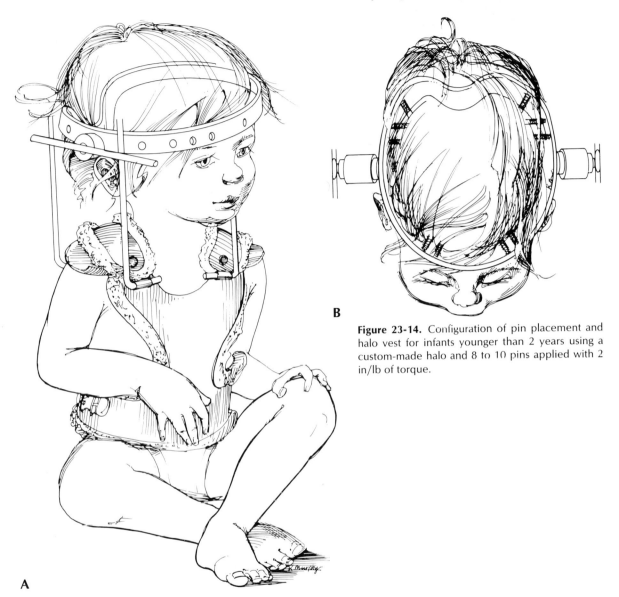

A

B

Figure 23-14. Configuration of pin placement and halo vest for infants younger than 2 years using a custom-made halo and 8 to 10 pins applied with 2 in/lb of torque.

SURGICAL FUSION

Surgery of the cervical spine is generally reserved for cases of documented instability with or without neural involvement. An arthrodesis is indicated if there is greater than 5 mm of upper cervical translational instability at any single level, documented progression, or cervical symptoms or neural deficits secondary to the instability.[172]

The surgical technique is similar to adults, with some important differences. Children's spines fuse readily and rapidly. Exposure must be limited to the specific vertebrae to be fused; otherwise, extended fusion to adjacent laminae will occur. For atlanto-axial instability, Gallie's technique is preferred: this involves passing a wire loop under the posterior arch of the atlas and through the spinous process of the axis while locking in corticocancellous interposition graft.[99,225,280] Cadaveric bone is contraindicated in posterior cervical fusion in children; autogenous bone is preferred.[288] The vertebral arteries in the infant or young child are situated in a groove along the posterosuperior arch to the atlas, 1 cm from the midline; extreme caution must be exercised during C-1 exposure.[78] Upper cervical arthrodesis with wire fixation may not be feasible in children with vertebral anomalies. Koop and associates describe a method of delicate exposure: occipital periosteal flap coverage with air drill decortication and autogenous onlay graft.[172]

ATHLETIC INJURIES TO THE CERVICAL SPINE

Athletic injuries to the cervical spine are more prominent in the older child and adolescent. They appear most prominently in children engaged in football, diving, gymnastics, hockey, and rugby. Clinical and laboratory studies have demonstrated that cervical spine injuries that result in fracture-dislocation and severe neural damage occur with axial loading. With the head flexed to 20 degrees, the normal cervical lordosis is eliminated; the straight segmented column, when put under maximal compressive load, will fail in the flexed direction, leading to fracture or unilateral or bilateral dislocation. In severe injuries, the cervical spine is compressed between the body and the rapidly decelerated head.

Elimination of "spearing" or head-first hitting techniques in football, "boarding" in hockey, and the use of trampolines in gymnastics has significantly reduced the incidence of catastrophic neck injuries. All children should be restricted from use of trampolines. Proper instruction in diving technique in designated diving areas of adequate depth will also decrease the incidence of cervical spine trauma. Proper instruction and education is the key to prevention of serious neck injuries.[306]

THORACOLUMBAR TRAUMA

GENERAL CONSIDERATIONS

Relative to adults, children sustain fewer spinal fractures and dislocations. This is due to greater flexibility of the immature spine and decreased exposure to automobile and industrial acci-

dents.[127] With a relatively smaller mass, a child's skeleton is subjected to less energy transfer during rapid deceleration, such as a fall or motor vehicle accident.[198] Only 2% to 3% of reported spinal injuries occur in children.[13,14,122] In neonates and infants, cervical spine injuries, resulting from obstetric trauma or child abuse, are more likely. In the child younger than 10 years, spinal injuries result from either falls from a height or motor vehicle accidents; in the second decade of life, sports and motor vehicle accidents are the primary causes of spinal trauma.

Other unique aspects of spinal trauma in children are related to the presence of the growth plate and the relatively strong disk–end-plate complex. Most spinal injuries are the result of compression with varying amounts of flexion.[140] The cartilaginous end-plate acts as shock absorber and protects the growth plate.[167,270] With compression, the end-plate bulges and blood is squeezed out of the cancellous portion of the vertebrae.[257] With increasing compressive force, the shock-absorbing capacity will be overcome, and injury of the end-plate or compression or burst fracture will occur, depending on the severity and acceleration of applied force.[142,257] Distraction and torsion in severe trauma may cause separation of the end-plate with or without dislocation.[13] As in the cervical spine, the weak link in the thoracolumbar spine is often the growth plate and epiphyseal end-plate.[13,210] The growth potential of the child acts as a two-edged sword: severe trauma can lead to growth disturbance or biomechanically induced progressive deformity.[195] With milder injury to the vertebral body, the immature spine can remodel the normal shape and height of the vertebral body; no remodeling capabilities exist in the posterior elements.

The nucleus pulposus is a secondary shock absorber, converting compressive vertical forces to horizontal forces absorbed by the annulus fibrosus.[270] In children, the intervertebral disk is strong enough to withstand the forces generated in spinal fractures; thus, the intervertebral joint and disk is usually preserved in children, and herniated disks and spontaneous interbody fusion are rare.[38,44,110,129,143,161,165,179,250,257,281,318]

Anatomy and Development

In utero, thoracic and lumbar ossification of the vertebral bodies begins in the lower thoracic spine and extends both proximally and distally. Ossification in the neural arches begins in the lower cervical spine and progresses caudally. These centers of ossification enlarge by appositional growth until birth, when the residual cartilage on the cranial and caudal surfaces becomes the upper and lower growth plates. These persist until the child reaches maturity.[198]

From birth, spinal growth is fairly steady until the adolescent growth spurt occurs; in girls, this growth spurt occurs sooner and over a shorter period of time.[248] The growth plates are attached to the interverbral disks through the cartilaginous end-plates. The thicker periphery of these end-plates is formed by the vertebral apophyses, secondary ossification centers that appear between the 8th and 12th years and fuse with the vertebral bodies beginning in the 14th year and ending in the 24th year.[65,129,198] This ring apophysis plays no part in longitudinal growth and is simply the peripherally ossified part of the end-plate, to which the ligament and periosteum attach.[23] Until fusion occurs, the weak cartilage–bone interface is susceptible to injury. Traumatic separation of the ring apophysis or the vertebral growth plate is a unique aspect of spinal trauma in children.

STABLE INJURIES

Compression Fractures

The most common injury in the thoracic or lumbar spine in children is the compression fracture.[198] Compression fractures are generally stable injuries that can vary in severity and radiologic appearance. The disc–end-plate complex is intact, and the vertebral spongiosa is crushed by the compressive force. The radiographic appearance may vary from mild flattening of the end-plate or a radiodense line in the vertebral metaphysis to gross wedging of the body.[122,126,140]

The wedged vertebra consists of compacted spongiosa and a fractured anterior cortex; the posterior cortex, posterior elements, ligaments, and joints are intact; thus a true compression fracture is a stable injury. In an infant, the normal radiographic notching in the anterior and posterior vertebral bodies may be confused with a compression fracture.[315]

In the child's spine, compressive force is distributed over several levels, and multiple compression fractures may occur.[143,165,257,281] Multiple fractures usually occur in the thoracolumbar region. They have been reported in as many as 50% of spinal injuries in children.[140]

Wedging may occur in the sagittal or frontal planes.[129,198] Since the growth plate is intact, the vertebral body will remodel and reconstitute its normal shape. Thus, in a child younger than 12 years of age, persistent kyphosis or scoliosis, regardless of the number of fractures, will not occur.[140,142,143] Even with more extensive damage involving the growth plate, subsequent uneven vertebral growth will be compensated for by adjacent segments, and deformity rarely occurs.[143]

Compression fractures heal rather quickly and rarely develop deformity. They can be treated simply by bed rest for 1 to 2 weeks; cast or brace immobilization has not been shown to affect the outcome and is unnecessary.[140,143]

Compression fractures may occur with child abuse; less commonly reported are disk herniations and fracture-dislocations.[57,66,171,299] Compression fracture in children may occur with minor trauma; it may also occur spontaneously in certain pathologic conditions. The combination of prolonged bed rest and violent muscle spasm associated with tetanus has led to compression fractures at multiple levels, primarily between T-4 and T-6. Rarely, burst fractures have also been reported.[126,295] Tetanus-induced fractures will heal adequately through conservative measures.[129]

Vertebral collapse may be seen in eosinophilic granuloma, which usually involves a single level in a child younger than 6 years of age. The classic radiographic appearance is vertebra plana, the waferlike complete collapse of a single body, in which the posterior elements are rarely involved (Fig. 23-15). Multiple adjacent levels, a variable

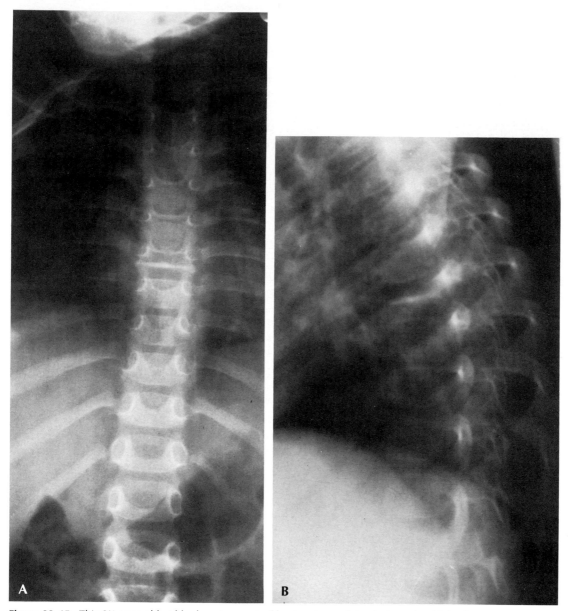

Figure 23-15. This 2½-year-old girl had acute onset of back pain resolving in 1 week with bedrest. Radiograph demonstrates classic appearance of the vertebra plana seen in eosinophilic granuloma.

amount of collapse, and, occasionally, lytic lesions can be seen. The intervertebral disk is uninvolved, and no adjacent soft-tissue mass is present, thus distinguishing eosinophilic granuloma from tuberculous or bacterial spondylitis. The clinical and laboratory presentation includes leukocytosis, mild eosinophilia, an elevated erythrocyte sedimentation rate, and mild hyperpyrexia, usually accompanied by pain. If asymptomatic, vertebra plana need not be treated. Conservative treatment in conjunction with medical therapy is advised for symptomatic patients or those at risk for further collapse. Partial restoration of the involved vertebra usually occurs regardless of the degree of collapse.[6,226]

Multiple compression fractures can occur in Gaucher's disease, the mucopolysaccharidoses, lymphoma, osteogenesis imperfecta, malignant metastatic lesions,[226] and idiopathic juvenile osteoporosis.[157] Gaucher's disease, the mucopolysaccharidoses, lymphoma, and metastatic lesions are similar in that abnormal cells infiltrate the vertebral body, causing structural weakness and, ultimately, collapse (Fig. 24-16). Diagnosis can be made with bone marrow aspiration or a biopsy of another lesion in conjunction with the clinical signs and symptoms; when the vertebral lesion is the only presenting sign of the disease, direct biopsy may be necessary.[226]

Children with osteogenesis imperfecta typically present with blue sclera, fragile skin, brittle long bones, a history of multiple fractures and deformity, and, occasionally, the development of scoliosis.[300] Idiopathic juvenile osteoporosis may be confused with osteogenesis imperfecta; the former lasts only 1 to 4 years, and primarily affects those between the ages of 8 and 15 years.[157] It is characterized by profound diffuse osteoporosis in a prepubertal child with no family history of the disease. The initial symptom is back pain from the compression fractures, which were sustained in minimal trauma. Idiopathic juvenile osteoporosis is effectively treated by bracing to prevent permanent kyphosis.[157]

Fractures of the Transverse Process

Fractures of the transverse process are rare yet stable injuries that occur primarily in the lumbar spine; they represent avulsion fractures of the insertion of either the greater psoas or the quadratus lumborum muscle during a violent contraction or by direct trauma in a Malgaigne fracture of the pelvis.[198] Treatment does not require any specific measures in the face of severe pelvic injuries. Isolated transverse process fractures are treated by initial bed rest and progression of activity as tolerated, combined with a physical therapy program.

UNSTABLE INJURIES

Instability in the thoracolumbar spine may result from burst fractures, fracture-dislocations, or distraction injuries. Burst injuries and fracture-dislocations often involve damage to the vertebral growth plate; therefore, growth disturbance and deformity can occur later. Unstable fracture-dislocations occur less frequently in the thoracic spine than in other areas, probably due to the stabilizing influence of the rib cage.[198] Distraction fractures of the Chance variety are rare in children; they result from severe distraction when the body is rapidly decelerated around a seat belt.[24,88,119,141] They usually occur between L-1 and L-3, and may be associated with traumatic pancreatitis, ruptured viscus, transient ileus, ruptured kidney or diaphragm, and seat belt burns on the abdomen.[119]

The goal of treatment should be coaptation of the fracture surfaces. If adequate reduction can be obtained through extension, a body cast is sufficient; otherwise, internal fixation with single-level fusion is recommended.[119] The selection of surgical vs. nonsurgical treatment depends on the type of fracture and the incidence of neurologic injury. Burst fractures without neurologic injury can be treated by bed rest in a plaster shell for 6 to 8 weeks until bony consolidation occurs, followed by mobilization in a body cast or brace for another 6 weeks.[198] As in adults, the indications for immediate surgical treatment of spinal injuries include: compound wound, progressive neurologic deficits in a incomplete lesion, and unstable fracture-dislocation.[45]

The methods of reduction or decompression follow the same principles as in the adult.[129,143,323] Following reduction, the spine is fused one or two segments above and below the injury level with

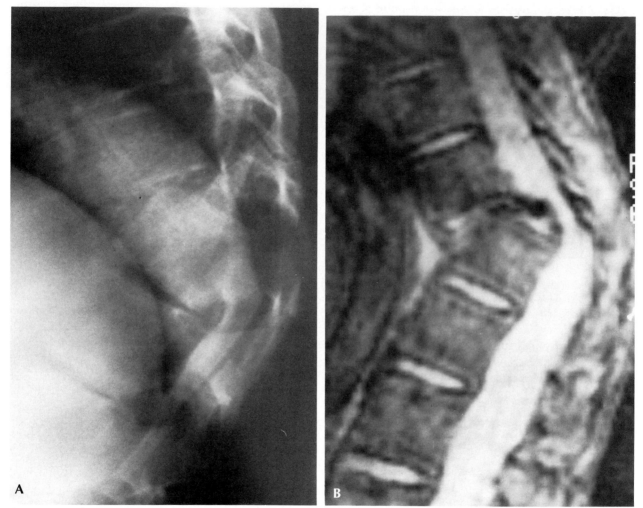

Figure 23-16. This 13-year-old boy with Gaucher's disease presented with destruction and absence of T-10, dislocation of T-9 on T-11, and incipient myelopathy. (*A*) Preoperative radiograph. (*B*) Magnetic resonance image shows kyphus and cord compression.

posterior instrumentation. Satisfactory results with Harrington rods and Luque instrumentation have been reported.[87,181,206] Newer techniques, such as Cotrel–Dubousset instrumentation, seem promising for reduction and rigid internal fixation. Adequate reduction and stabilization will prevent late complications (see Chapter 22). Laminectomy provides little neural benefit in children with spinal cord injury, and has been shown to have a

definite deleterious effect in postadolescent children.[206]

SPINAL CORD INJURY

Between 1% and 5% of all spinal cord injuries occur in children.[165] While disagreements exist as to its prevalence in the cervical spine vs. the tho-

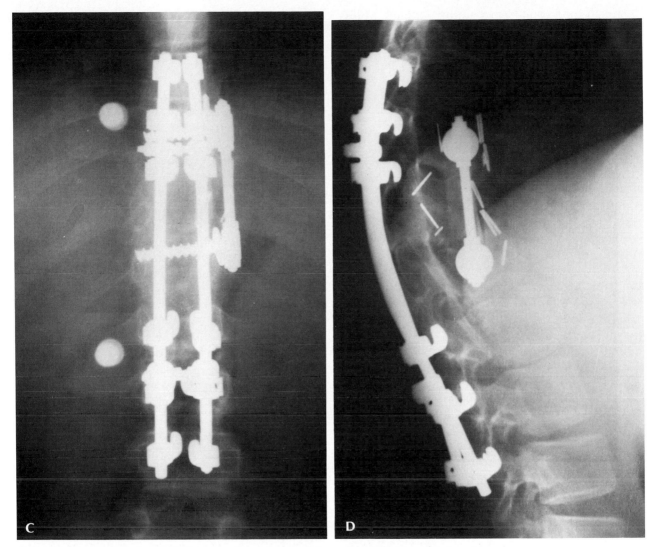

Figure 23-16. *(continued).* (*C, D*) Postoperative anteroposterior and lateral views after two-stage anterior decompression, fusion, and instrumentation and posterior fusion and instrumentation.

racolumbar region and its sex predominance, there is agreement that motor vehicle accidents and firearm injuries are the major causes of spinal cord injury in the first decade of life. After age 11, sports and recreation and motor vehicle accidents are the leading causes.[165,338] High risk is reported with use of all-terrain vehicles by children.[284]

In children younger than 10 years, tetraplegia occurred 2½ times more frequently than paraple-gia; in the 10 to 15 year age group, the ratio was somewhat reversed, with paraplegia twice as prev-alent as tetraplegia.[165] Children's recuperative powers from spinal cord injury may be better than adults', with the exception of complete lesions, which in all ages generally do not improve.[19,143]

Spinal cord injury can occur with or without bony or apparent ligamentous injury.[9,112,127,210,248] In a review of the literature, 19% of the cases demonstrated spinal cord injury without radiographic abnormality,[165] and a delay in diagnosis is reported in many of these cases varying from 30 minutes to 4 days.[233] In a comparison of spinal cord injuries with and without osseus fracture, Yngve and associates noted several characteristics in those with the fracture. They tended to be older (averaging 16 years of age), the fracture involved the lower cervical spine, and they had a higher percentage of complete lesions (44% vs. 31%); those without an osseus fracture averaged 6 years of age and the cervicothoracic junction was the major area of neurologic damage.[338]

Damage to the spinal cord from osseus injuries probably involves direct compression or tension after great displacement at an unstable fracture site.[338] In cord injuries without bony fractures, the mechanism of injury may be vascular compromise,[338] tension or compression,[112] or damage from multiple displacements of injured vertebral end-plates.[13]

Acute management of spinal cord injury usually involves a multiple trauma regimen with particular attention paid to pulmonary complications that may result from chest trauma or high cervical lesions. After the acute stage, a decrease in movement can lead to complications in bedridden or immobilized patients, which include cardiopulmonary, gastrointestinal, genitourinary, and musculoskeletal problems. Kinetic therapy, stabilization, and rapid mobilization will help to reduce the incidence of these complications.[115,338] When a spinal cord injury is suspected in the face of a negative radiographic examination, myelography is useful in localizing cord injury and in diagnosing end-plate damage or displacement. Extravasation of the dye out of the spinal canal indicates a high probability of complete lesion.[338] Computed tomography and magnetic resonance imaging are useful tools for evaluating cartilaginous and soft-tissue injury. When spinal cord compromise is associated with instability, surgical reduction, decompression, and stabilization is required. When neural damage occurs without bony injury, no instability is found and surgery is rarely indicated.[338]

POST-TRAUMATIC SPINAL DEFORMITY

Progressive deformity of a post-traumatic pediatric spine can result from a combination of four factors. Development or worsening of a deformity can be prevented with prompt and appropriate treatment.

1. Primary traumatic deformity. Stable burst or wedge compression fractures will produce a mild kyphosis or scoliosis of up to 10 degrees owing to anterior compression for stable burst fractures or lateral compression for wedge compression fractures. This deformity is stable and nonprogressive and may develop a compensatory curve.[210] However, unstable burst fractures, severe wedge compression, and multiple compression fractures can result in immediate, extensive curves in both planes, which will progress if not effectively reduced and stabilized surgically.[210,248,311] Posterior element disruption or ligamentous lesions such as an interspinous ligament sprain is often the cause of late development of kyphosis.[200,248] In the cervical spine, paracervical muscle spasm may mask or reverse the kyphosis and instability; as pain and spasm diminish, deformity will develop.[248] The sequelae of post-traumatic kyphosis include worsening neurologic deficits[194,199] and mechanical problems such as pain, abnormal mobility, back pressure sores, and abnormal sitting or standing balance.[200] Post-traumatic deformity and its sequelae can be eliminated by early surgical reduction, instrumentation, and adequate fusion of the unstable spine.[30,64,87]

2. Growth plate injuries. Hyperflexion and compression may crush the anterior growth plate cartilage producing a Salter-Harris type IV or type V lesion to the vertebral body.[210] If the lesion is anteriorly located, kyphosis will ensue; if it is laterally located, a scoliotic component will develop. Progression in trauma-induced deformities is less rapid than in neurologically induced deformities; however, if the injury occurs at an early age, the deformity may be severe.[248] A Salter-Harris type VI lesion as described by Rang[253] may act like a congenital unsegmented bar leading to a rapidly developing rigid angular deformity. Secondary spontaneous progression of deformity may occur after a crush to the vertebral body and end-

plate in which altered compressive forces will asymmetrically suppress growth according to the Heuter-Volkmann law.[231] This sequence usually results from an untreated initial deformity.[195,248] This complication can be avoided by early reduction and fusion for stabilization.

3. Laminectomy. Laminectomies have little neurologic benefit,[206,248] render the spine more unstable, and lead to progressive kyphotic deformity.[28,120,164,206,220,221,265,314] The spinal canal is often compromised from retropulsed anterior fragments, and wide posterior decompression only induces further posterior column instability. Mayfield and associates reported that only one out of 40 children had improved conus or cauda equina syndromes after laminectomy.[206] Therefore, because there is little chance of neurologic improvement and definite destabilization, laminectomy without concomitant stabilization has no role in modern management. Patients with incomplete neurologic deficits associated with anterior compressive lesions will be better managed with anterior decompression and stabilization.

4. Neurologic lesions. In a complete lesion, the loss of muscle tone in the spine, chest, and abdomen in a child leaves the bony arch and ligaments of the spine incapable of maintaining normal alignment against the forces of gravity.[36,168,181,206,248] Paralysis, spasticity, and muscle contractures with paraplegia or tetraplegia will contribute to the forces and lack of support in the development of spinal deformity. As the curve progresses, asymmetric forces on the vertebral end-plate may result in permanent changes in the disk, vertebral body, and facet joint.[36] The deformity is generally progressive, unrelated to growth spurts, and usually a single-long curve. It may be scoliosis, kyphosis, a combination, or occasionally lordosis.[20,40,45,181,206] If left untreated, severe disability and cosmetic deformity can develop including pulmonary function compromise, joint contractures, poor sitting balance and head position that results in pelvic obliquity, hip dislocation, pressure sores, and greater patient dependence.

The response of the spine to complete cord injury is different for the preadolescent and the postadolescent child. For the child younger than 14 years, spinal deformity developed after paraplegia or tetraplegia in 91% to 100% of cases.[36,45,168,206] Postadolescents, like adults, rarely develop paralytic spinal deformity; however, deformity may result from the configuration of the fracture and the instability of the injury, but is limited to the segments involved.[31,87,138,206] Several authors have demonstrated that the younger the patient is at the time of injury, the greater the paralytic deformity.[35,36,45,111,168,181,214,248,257,301] The severity of the curve is also increased by the presence of spasticity.[83] Higher lesions are more likely to develop progressive deformity than distal injuries.[16,45,214]

Treatment in the preadolescent child should be geared toward delaying spinal fusion for as long as possible to maximize spinal growth.[36] Bracing within 6 months of injury may lessen the incidence, extent, and progression of deformity and is effective in delaying spine fusion.[20,35,36,45,103,168,181,206,229] Ultimately 68% of these patients will require spine fusion.[205] An underarm plastic orthosis is used until the curve reaches 45 to 50 degrees, at which time a long fusion from the upper thorax to the sacrum with posterior instrumentation is performed.[20,181,206]

In the postadolescent patient, spinal deformity is usually the result of fracture—dislocation and treatment should be dictated by the stability of the injury. If the injury is stable, bed rest is required followed by a cast or orthosis until the spine is healed; if the injury is unstable, posterior fusion is ordered with instrumentation limited to one or two segments above and below.[206]

BACK PAIN IN CHILDREN

During growth, especially the adolescent growth spurt, some children tend to develop hyperlordosis or "sway back" of the lumbar spine. This is based on a relatively greater vertebral body growth coupled with posterior tethering by the lumbodorsal fascia.[217] With worsening lordosis, a postural pattern develops that includes hip flexion contractures, tight hamstrings, and compensatory thoracic or thoracolumbar kyphosis. With increased lumbar lordosis, the pars interarticularis and intervertebral disk are at greater risk for failure.[176] Clinically, three distinct entities are seen:

1. Spondylolysis, or fracture of the pars interarticularis
2. Disk herniation
3. Hyperlordotic lumbar strain[218]

A fourth entity that will produce back pain is an atypical form of Scheuermann's kyphosis, which involves the lumbar spine or the thoracolumbar junction.

TRAUMATIC SPONDYLOLYSIS

While the cause of a pars defect has been rather controversial in the past,[322] recent studies seem to point to a traumatic etiology.[187,267,313,322,333,336] A hereditary component may exist, as familial cases have been reported.[92,93,187,273,305,329-333] Because no fetal dissections have ever uncovered neural arch defects,[17,92,93,136,262,322] and because the incidence of spondylolysis among nonambulatory patients is zero,[261] spondylolysis is considered an acquired deformity, reaching a peak incidence in adulthood of between 5% and 5.8%.[305,322] The incidence is higher in Alaskan natives[294] and in adolescent athletes in such competitive sports as gymnastics, football, power lifting, figure skating, and hockey.[113,187,316] Spina bifida occulta occurs more frequently in patients with spondylolysis.[92] While males outnumber females two to one in most series,[92,259] an incidence of 11% has been reported in female gymnasts.[149]

While significant trauma can produce spondylolysis, the defect is usually the result of stress fracture.[322] Stress analysis has shown that the greatest concentration of stress is located in the pars interarticularis, and that in vitro cyclical stress loading will produce a fracture of the pars.[146,147,177,322] Trauma or fatigue loading will result in stress that exceeds the ultimate strength of bone at the pars.[180,187] Repetitive flexion–extension causes microfractures with attempts at repair; ultimately a fatigue fracture will occur, thereby overloading the contralateral side. If bilateral defects are produced, the disk alone resists shear loading, predisposing the lumbar spine to spondylolisthesis.[187]

The typical clinical presentation includes localized low back pain that is related in occurrence and severity to specific activity. The straight leg raising test is negative, and toe touching is limber when compared with an acute lumbar strain that presents with spasm and stiffness.[113,316] Pain is elicited on lateral bending, hyperextension while lying prone, and the single leg stance with the lumbar spine in extension, maneuvers that create compressive force across the pars.[113,316] There is no radiculopathy, and neurologic examination is normal.

The onset of symptoms may precede the radiographic changes observable on lateral or oblique views. Radionuclide skeletal scintigraphy is a valuable tool for detecting early lesions or stress fractures equivocal on standard radiographs.* An increased uptake on a bone scan may precede the radiographic appearance of a stress fracture.[104,246] However, one series reported that 74% of spondylolysis proven on standard radiographs had normal scintigraphic findings.[313] Therefore, a bone scan will be cold (negative) when nonunion is established.[62] The scintigraphic uptake with a spondylolytic lesion is dependent on the age, stability, and biologic healing of the injury; thus, a discrepancy may exist between radiographs and the bone scan.[130,148,197] Five radiologic situations may exist, each with its own pathologic interpretation:

1. Negative radiograph, negative bone scan: other etiology of back pain
2. Positive radiograph, negative bone scan: established nonunion
3. Positive radiograph, positive bone scan: healing progressing
4. Positive radiograph unilaterally, contralateral positive bone scan with negative radiograph: imminent bilateral spondylolysis
5. Negative radiograph, positive bone scan: imminent spondylolysis possible, but in light of the high sensitivity and low specificity of scintigraphy, must rule out other lesion[313]

Computed tomography is able to show subtle changes not evident on plain radiographs (Fig. 23-17). Single photon emission computed tomography provides sectional and multiplanar imaging.

* Reference numbers 76, 130, 150, 197, 247.

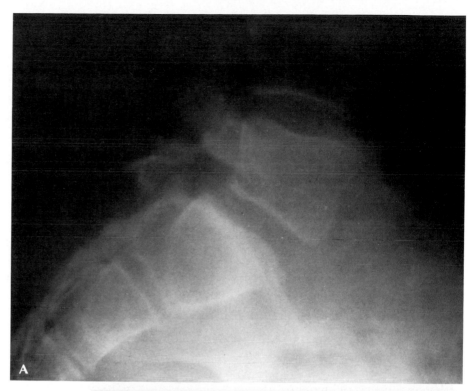

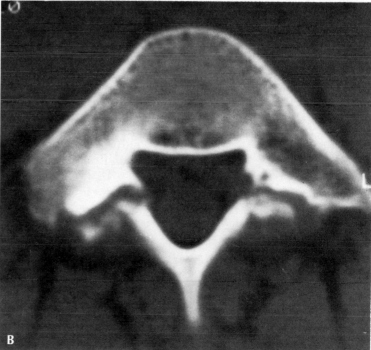

Figure 23-17. This 14-year-old boy presented with a 3-month history of low back pain associated with activity. (*A*) Lateral radiograph shows pars defect. (*B*) Computed tomography demonstrates bilateral pars defects.

This is a more sensitive study for detecting subtle changes in metabolic activity in complex anatomic structures such as the spine.[27,149,178] It is more sensitive than planar scintigraphy, and possesses the ability to localize an active lesion within the elements of a vertebral segment.[27]

Increased scintigraphic uptake is an indication for brace treatment in the young athlete.[148,150,217,218] Bracing will encourage healing and prevent chronic symptomatic pars pseudarthrosis or progression of contralateral reactive hypertrophy to stress fracture.[312,327,331,332] Acute pars stress fractures may heal,[2,218,223,258,312] especially if treated early with bracing.[187,292] Immobilization in an underarm brace in antilordotic posturing will decrease the shear stress across the pars.[75,309] With bracing for 3 to 6 months followed by a low back program of hamstring and lumbodorsal fascia stretching and abdominal and trunk strengthening, healing of the stress fracture is more likely to occur.[292] Although healing may not occur, the patient may become asymptomatic and return to his or her previous level of competition, with the exception of the competitive gymnast.[113,187] Yearly follow-up radiographs are recommended. If bilateral defects appear, athletes should be educated about the possibility of spondylolisthesis and advised to change their sport or activity.[187]

DISK DISEASE

The intervertebral disk is quite sturdy and is rarely the site of pathology. When involved, it may generate a clinical constellation that is similar to disk disease in adults. There are three distinct pathologic entities relating to the disk in children, in whom the lumbar spine is almost exclusively involved.

The first is the *classic herniated disk.* Patients younger than 20 years represent between 1% and 2.5% of all patients with disk herniation.[38,110,196,250,318] Very few cases are reported in the literature in children younger than 12 years.[44] Either acute or repetitive trauma plays an important role in the etiology of disk disease in the pediatric population; antecedent trauma has been reported in 30% to 60% of cases.[44,72,179,228] Multilevel disk pathology has been reported in

herniated disk disease on magnetic resonance imaging in adolescents, implying that underlying disk pathology may precede herniation, which would possibly explain failure of treatment in certain cases.[108] Thirty-three percent of pediatric patients with a herniated disk had associated structural anomalies, such as spina bifida occulta or hemisacralization of L-5, as compared to 10% in adults. Structural anomalies may place undue stress on disks in children, predisposing them to premature herniation.[161] The levels of disk herniation are similar to those reported in adults, primarily the L-4–L-5 and L-5–S-1 disks.

Children usually present with leg pain of sciatic distribution, and much less often with the concomitant back pain so characteristic in adults.[161,339] Gait disturbance, pain on forward flexion, scoliosis, spasm with scoliosis or listing, and a positive straight leg raising test are common signs. Some reports note that neurologic changes are less common in children, although others found a higher incidence of objective motor deficits in children.[161]

The water content of the disk is 88% in the fetus. This decreases to 80% at 12 years and to 70% by age 72.[44] With magnetic resonance imaging, T2 weighted images show the nucleus pulposus and are sensitive to the changes in water content, reflected by a reduction in intensity and an irregular outline of the nucleus pulposus.[108] In older patients, disk disease is more difficult to assess due to signal changes with aging. In adolescents, little degeneration has occurred and any abnormality is likely to be pathologic; magnetic resonance imaging is therefore an excellent tool in diagnosis of disk disease in children.[108]

Initial treatment should be conservative, with bed rest followed by a low back physical therapy program. Most patients will not require surgery. Some authors believe that children do not do as well with conservative therapy as adults; at the same time, several studies show that young surgical patients fare better than adults, yielding better than 90% excellent or good results.[38,60,72,161,264] Surgically, a tightly bulging disk impinging on the nerve root is most commonly found; sequestration is less likely seen in children than adults.[38,161,166,264] Results are not affected by the addition of fusion to the diskectomy. Therefore fusion has no role in disk surgery in the pediatric population.[32]

A *fracture of the posterior ring apophysis* may produce the symptoms of disk herniation. With the advent of computed tomography, more of these lesions are being diagnosed; many of these fracture are not appreciated on plain radiographs.[302] The pathogenesis is probably traumatic or sports-related, although a significant number of cases have no antecedent trauma.[286,302]

Takata and associates reported on 31 fractures of the posterior ring apophysis for which they established a three-type classification (Fig. 23-18). All type I fractures, an arcuate rim of cartilage, occur in children between the ages of 11 and 13 years. Type II is an avulsion fracture at the posterior rim, with bone. It appears in slightly older children. Type III is a localized fracture behind a defect in the end-plate in patients aged 15 to 56 years. These patients usually present with back pain and sciatica. Fractures of the cephalad rim of the body are associated with a positive straight leg raising test; fractures of the caudad rim are less consistent in presenting with this sign.[302] When present, the straight leg raising test may appear out of proportion with other signs.[286] Treatment usually requires surgical removal of the offending fragment.[44,302]

Acute traumatic intraosseous disk herniation is an uncommon post-traumatic syndrome resulting from a vertical compression injury. The patient will present with prolonged localized back pain and radiographic evidence of vertebral end-plate fracture.[207] The pain is immediate in onset and is localized to the low back, with occasional radiation to the thigh. The patient will complain of significant disability and restriction of activities lasting from 6 months to 11 years.[207] The injury involves a lower thoracic or upper lumbar vertebra; the initial changes are subtle and not well defined, with disk space narrowing and flattening of the anterosuperior edge of the vertebra. With time, a radiolucent defect appears and localized kyphosis at the anterior edge of the superior aspect of the vertebral body develops.[207] Diskography will demonstrate the herniation of disk material through the end-plate and will reproduce the pain during injection.

The end-plate is the weakest part of the pediatric vertebral body, especially during adolescent growth.[207] The occurrence of this injury and the appearance of Schmorl's nodes correspond to the

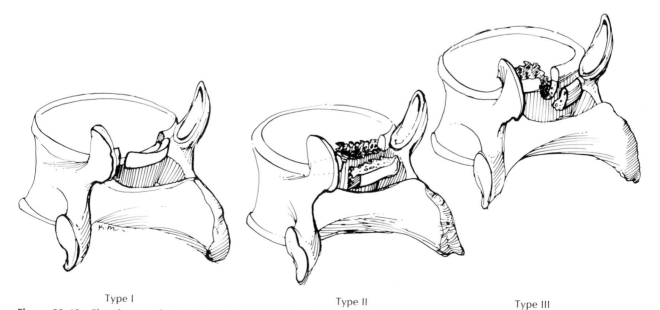

Type I   Type II   Type III

Figure 23-18. Classification describing the three types of fractures that involve the posterior rim apophysis of the vertebral body and clinically mimic disk herniation.

onset of adolescence. The traumatic intraosseus disk herniations are located in the marginal area of the body, while the classic Schmorl's node is central; both represent a herniation of the disk material through the end-plate and growth plate. The acute intraosseus disk herniation will be hot (positive) on the bone scan, whereas the central Schmorl's node will not.[26,207]

Treatment of the condition requires prolonged immobilization and administration of analgesics; slow improvement in the condition is the typical course of the injury.

ATYPICAL SCHEUERMANN'S KYPHOSIS

Typical Scheuermann's kyphosis involves the thoracic spine. Diagnosis requires 5 degrees of wedging in three or more adjacent vertebrae. It is usually asymptomatic. It results from hereditary factors, and is associated with Schmorl's nodes, disk narrowing, and end-plate irregularity.[33,207] Atypical Scheuermann's kyphosis, also called "apprentice kyphosis," occurs most commonly at multiple levels of the thoracolumbar junction in adolescent boys. It is associated with heavy labor or a repetitive sports activity.[129,216,217] The pathogenesis is probably repetitive microfractures at the anterior margin of the vertebral end-plates.[128] Early recognition and bracing is helpful in eliminating pain and eradicating the deformity with growth.

SUMMARY

Pediatric spine injuries present some of the greatest challenges in orthopedics. They are rare problems that can present spontaneously or with minor trauma, or may result from major falls or motor vehicle accidents replete with multiple fractures and spinal cord and visceral injuries. The variable characteristics of the immature spine in an often uncooperative, uncommunicative child create a difficult diagnostic problem. The advent of computed tomography and magnetic resonance imaging has improved the accuracy and, in some cases, expanded our awareness of spinal pathology in children. The growing spine will respond to trauma differently depending on its stage of development. This changing clinical picture, combined with a wide variation of unique effects in children, requires an extensive knowledge of the anatomy and development of the growing spine.

REFERENCES

1. Abroms IF, Bresnan MJ, Zuckerman JE et al: Cervical cord injuries secondary to hyperextension of the head in breech presentation. Obstet Gynecol 41:369, 1973
2. Ahlgren S: Spontaneous healing of spondylolisthesis. Acta Orthop Scand 28:306, 1959
3. Alker GJ, Oh YS, Leslie EV: High cervical spine and craniocervical junction injuries in fatal traffic accidents: A radiological study. Orthop Clin North Am 9:1003, 1978
4. Allen JP: Birth injury to the spinal cord. Northwest Medicine, 69:323, 1970
5. American Academy of Orthopaedic Surgeons, Committee on Allied Health: Emergency Care and Transportation of the Sick and Injured, 3rd ed. Chicago, American Academy of Orthopaedic Surgeons, 1981
6. Amstutz HC, Carey EJ: Skeletal manifestations and treatment of Gaucher's disease. J Bone Joint Surg [Am] 48:670, 1966
7. Anderson JM, Schutt AH: Spinal injury in children: A review of 156 cases seen from 1950 through 1978. Mayo Clin Proc 55:499, 1980
8. Anderson LD, D'Alonzo RT: Fractures of the odontoid process of the axis. J Bone Joint Surg [Am] 56:1663, 1974
9. Andrews LG, Jung SK: Spinal cord injuries in children in British Columbia. Paraplegia 17:442, 1979
10. Ardran GM, Kemp FH: The mechanism of changes in form of the cervical airway in infancy. Med Radiogr Photogr 44:26, 1968
11. Arnold WD, Hilgartner MW: Hemophilic arthropathy: Current concepts of pathogenesis and management. J Bone Joint Surg [Am] 59:287, 1977
12. Audic B, Maury M: Secondary vertebral deformities in childhood and adolescence. Paraplegia 7:11, 1969
13. Aufdermaur M: Spinal injuries in juveniles. J Bone Joint Surg [Br] 56:513, 1974
14. Babcock JL: Spinal injuries in children. Pediatr Clin North Am 22:487, 1975

15. Bailey DK: The normal cervical spine in infants and children. Radiology 59:712, 1952

16. Banniza von Bazan UK, Paeslack V: Scoliotic growth in children with acquired paraplegia. Paraplegia 15:65, 1977-1978

17. Batts M Jr: The etiology of spondylolisthesis. J Bone Joint Surg 21:879, 1939

18. Baumgarten M, Mouradian W, Boger D, Watkins R: Computed axial tomography in C1–C2 trauma. Spine 10:187, 1985

19. Beatson T: Fractures and dislocations of the cervical spine. J Bone Joint Surg [Br] 45:21, 1963

20. Bedbrook GM: Correction of scoliosis due to paraplegia sustained in paediatric age-group. Paraplegia 15:90, 1977

21. Behrman RE, Vaughn VC III (eds): Nelson's Textbook of Pediatrics, 13th ed. Philadelphia, WB Saunders, 1987

22. Bhattacharyya SK: Fracture and displacement of the odontoid process in a child. J Bone Joint Surg [Am] 56:1071, 1974

23. Bick EM, Copel FW: The ring apophysis of the human vertebra: Contribution to human osteogeny. II. J Bone Joint Surg [Am] 33:783, 1951

24. Blasier RD, LaMont RL: Chance fracture in a child: A case report with nonoperative treatment. J Pediatr Orthop 5:92, 1985

25. Blockey NJ, Purser DW: Fractures of the odontoid process of the axis. J Bone Joint Surg [Br] 38:794, 1956

26. Blumenthal SL, Roach J, Herring JA: Lumbar Scheuermann's: A clinical series and classification. Spine 12:929, 1987

27. Bodner RJ, Heyman S, Drummond DS, Gregg JR: The use of single photon emission computed tomography (SPECT) in the diagnosis of low-back pain in young patients. Spine 13:1155, 1988

28. Bohlman HH: Acute fractures and dislocations of the cervical spine: An analysis of three hundred hospitalized patients and review of the literature. J Bone Joint Surg [Am] 61:1119, 1979

29. Botte MJ, Garfin SR, Byrne TP et al: The halo skeletal fixator: Principles of application and maintenance. Clin Orthop 239:12, 1989

30. Bradford DS: Role of internal fixation and spine fusion in thoracic and lumbar spine fractures. In Chou SN, Seljeskog EL (eds): Spinal Deformities and Neurological Dysfunction, p 155. New York, Raven Press, 1978

31. Bradford DS, Akbarnia BA, Winter RB, Seljeskog EL: Surgical stabilization of fracture and fracture dislocations of the thoracic spine. Spine 2:185, 1977

32. Bradford DS, Garcia A: Herniations of the lumbar intervertebral disc in children and adolescents. JAMA 210:2045, 1969

33. Bradford DS, Moe JH, Montalvo FJ, Winter RB: Scheuermann's kyphosis and roundback deformity. J Bone Joint Surg [Am] 56:740, 1974

34. Bresnan MJ, Abroms IF: Neonatal spinal cord transection secondary to intrauterine hyperextension of the neck in breech presentation. J Pediatr 84:734, 1974

35. Brown HP, Bonnett CC: Spine deformity subsequent to spinal cord injury: Proceedings of the Scoliosis Research Society. J Bone Joint Surg [Am] 55:441, 1973

36. Brown JC, Swank SM, Matta J, Barras DM: Late spinal deformity in quadriplegic children and adolescents. J Pediatr Orthop 4:456, 1984

37. Bucholz RW, Burkhead WZ: The pathological anatomy of fatal atlanto-occipital dislocations. J Bone Joint Surg [Am] 61:248, 1979

38. Bulos S: Herniated intervertebral lumbar disc in the teenager. J Bone Joint Surg [Br] 55:273, 1973

39. Burke DC: Injuries of the spinal cord in children. In Vinken PJ, Bruyn GW (eds): Handbook of Clinical Neurology, Vol 25, p 175. Amsterdam, North Holland Publishing Co, 1976

40. Burke DC: Traumatic spinal paralysis in children. Paraplegia 11:268, 1974

41. Burkus JK, Deponte RJ: Chronic atlantoaxial rotatory fixation correction by cervical traction, manipulation, and bracing. J Pediatr Orthop 6:631, 1986

42. Caffey J: Paediatric X-ray Diagnosis. Chicago, Year Book Medical Publishers, 1985

43. Caffey J: The whiplash shaken infant syndrome. Pediatrics 54:396, 1974

44. Callahan DJ, Pack LL, Bream RC, Hensinger RN: Intervertebral disc impingement syndrome in a child: Report of a case and suggested pathology. Spine 11:402, 1986

45. Campbell J, Bonnett C: Spinal cord injury in children. Clin Orthop 112:114, 1975

46. Cattell HS, Filtzer DL: Pseudosubluxation and other normal variations in the cervical spine in children. J Bone Joint Surg [Am] 47:1295, 1965

47. Chamberlain WE: Basilar impression (platybasia): Bizarre developmental anatomy of occipital bone and upper cervical spine with striking and misleading neurologic manifestations. Yale J Biol Med 11:487, 1939

48. Chusid JG: Correlative Neuroanatomy and Functional Neuroanatomy. Los Altos, Lange Medical Publications, 1985

49. Clark RN: Diagnosis and management of torticollis. Pediatr Ann 5:43, 1976

50. Collalto PM, DeMuth WW, Schwentker EP, Boal DK: Traumatic atlanto-occipital dislocation. J Bone Joint Surg [Am] 68:1106, 1986

51. Coneon PW, Isdale IC, Rose BS: Rheumatoid arthritis of the cervical spine. Ann Rheum Dis 25:120, 1966

52. Cooper PR, Maravilla KR, Sklar FH et al: Halo immobilization of cervical spine fractures: Indications and results. J Neurosurg 50:603, 1979

53. Cornish BL: Traumatic spondylolisthesis of the axis. J Bone Joint Surg [Br] 50:31, 1968

54. Crellin RQ, MacCalee JJ, Hamilton EBD: Severe subluxation of the cervical spine in rheumatoid arthritis. J Bone Joint Surg [Br] 52:244, 1970

55. Crothers B: Injury of the spinal cord in breech extraction as important cause of fetal death and paraplegia in childhood. Am J Med Sci 165:94, 1923

56. Crothers B, Putnam MC: Obstetrical injuries of the spinal cord. Medicine 6:41, 1927

57. Cullen JC: Spinal lesions in battered babies. J Bone Joint Surg [Br] 57:364, 1975

58. Curtis BH, Blank S, Fisher RL: Atlantoaxial dislocation in Down's syndrome: Report of two patients requiring surgical correction. JAMA 205:464, 1968

59. Davis D, Bohlman H, Waker AE et al: The pathological findings in fatal craniospinal injuries. J Neurosurg 34:603, 1971

60. Day PL: The teenage disc syndrome. South Med J 60:247, 1967

61. Delorme TL: Axis-pedicle fractures: Proceedings of the American Orthopaedic Association. J Bone Joint Surg [Am] 49:1472, 1967

62. Deutsch SD, Gandsman EJ: The use of bone scanning for the diagnosis and management of musculoskeletal trauma. Surg Clin North Am 63:567, 1983

63. Diaw ME, Langer LO: Spinal cord compression in the Morquio-Brailsford's disease. J Pediatr 74:593, 1969

64. Dickson JH, Harrington PR, Erwin WD: Results of reduction and stabilization of the severely fractured thoracic and lumbar spine. J Bone Joint Surg [Am] 60:799, 1978

65. Dickson RA, Deacon P: Annotation: Spinal growth. J Bone Joint Surg [Br] 69:690, 1987

66. Dickson RA, Leatherman KD: Spinal injuries in child abuse: Case report. J Trauma 18:811, 1978

67. Dorwart RH, LaMasters DL: Applications of computed tomographic scanning of the cervical spine. Orthop Clin North Am 16:381, 1985

68. Dvorak J, Hayek J, Zehnder R: CT-functional diagnostics of the rotatory instability of the upper cervical spine: Part 2. An evaluation on healthy adults and patients with suspected instability. Spine 12:726, 1987

69. Dzenitis AJ: Spontaneous atlanto-axial dislocation in mongoloid child with spinal cord compression: Case report. J Neurosurg 25:458, 1966

70. Ehrenfest H: Injuries of the vertebral column and spinal cord in birth injuries of the child. New York, Appleton, 1931

71. El-Khoury GY, Clark CR, Gravett AW: Acute traumatic rotatory atlanto-axial dislocation in children: A report of three cases. J Bone Joint Surg [Am] 66:774, 1984

72. Epstein JA, Lavine LS: Herniated lumbar intervertebral discs in teenage children. J Neurosurg 21:1070, 1964

73. Evarts CM: Traumatic occipito-atlantal dislocation: Report of a case with survival. J Bone Joint Surg [Am] 52:1653, 1970

74. Ewald FC: Fracture of the odontoid process in a seventeen-month-old infant treated with a halo. J Bone Joint Surg [Am] 53:1636, 1971

75. Farfan JF, Osteria V, Lamy C: The mechanical etiology of spondylolysis and spondylolisthesis. Clin Orthop 117:40, 1976

76. Fidler MW, Hoefnagel CA: Lateral and computerized transverse 99m Tc-MDP bone scintigrams to supplement the anteroposterior bone scintigram for spinal hot spot localization. Spine 6:665, 1984

77. Fielding JW: Cineroentgenography of the normal cervical spine. J Bone Joint Surg [Am] 39:1281, 1957

78. Fielding JW: Injuries of the cervical spine. In Rockwood CA Jr, Wilkins KE, King RE (eds): Fractures in Children. Philadelphia, JB Lippincott, 1984

79. Fielding JW: Normal and selected abnormal motion of the cervical spine from the second cervical vertebra to the seventh cervical vertebra based on cineroentgenography. J Bone Joint Surg [Am] 46:1779, 1964

80. Fielding JW: Selected observations on the cervical spine in the child. In Ahstrom JP Jr (ed): Current Practice in Orthopaedic Surgery, Vol 5, p 31. St. Louis, CV Mosby, 1973

81. Fielding JW, Cochran GVB, Lawsing JF III, Hohl M: Tears of the transverse ligament of the atlas: A clinical and biomechanical study. J Bone Joint Surg [Am] 56:1683, 1974

82. Fielding JW, Hawkins RJ: Atlanto-axial rotatory fixation (fixed rotatory subluxation of the atlanto-axial joint). J Bone Joint Surg [Am] 59:37, 1977

83. Fielding JW, Hawkins RJ: Roentgenographic diagnosis of the injured neck. Instr Course Lect 25:149, 1976

84. Fielding JW, Hawkins RJ, Hensinger RN, Francis WR: Atlantoaxial rotary deformities. Orthop Clin North Am 9:955, 1978

85. Fielding JW, Hensinger RN, Hawkins RJ: Os odontoideum. J Bone Joint Surg [Am] 62:376, 1980

86. Fielding JW, Stilwell WT, Chynn KY, Spyropoulos EC: The use of computed tomography for the diagnosis of atlanto-axial rotatory fixation. J Bone Joint Surg [Am] 60:1102, 1978

87. Flesch JR, Leider LL, Erickson DL et al: Harrington instrumentation and spine fusion for unstable fractures and fracture-dislocations of the thoracic and lumbar spine. J Bone Joint Surg [Am] 59:143, 1977

88. Fletcher BD, Brogdon BG: Seat belt fractures of the spine and sternum. JAMA 200:167, 1967

89. Ford FR: Breech delivery in its possible relations to injury of the spinal cord. Arch Neurol Psychiatr 14:742, 1925

90. Francis WR, Fielding JW, Hawkins RJ et al: Traumatic spondylolisthesis of the axis. J Bone Joint Surg [Br] 63:313, 1981

91. Franken EA Jr: Spinal cord injury in the newborn infant. Pediatr Radiol 3:101, 1975

92. Fredrickson BE, Baker D, McHolick WJ et al: The natural history of spondylolysis and spondylolisthesis. J Bone Joint Surg [Am] 66:699, 1984

93. Friberg S: Studies on spondylolisthesis. Acta Chir Scand 82 [Suppl 55]:1, 1939

94. Fruin AH, Pirotte TP: Traumatic atlanto-occipital dislocation: Case report. J Neurosurg 46:663, 1977

95. Fujii E, Kobayashi K, Hirabayashi K: Treatment in fractures of the odontoid process. Spine 13:604, 1988

96. Funk FJ, Wells RE: Injuries to the cervical spine in football. Clin Orthop 109:50, 1975

97. Gabrielsen TO, Maxwell JA: Traumatic atlanto-occipital dislocation: With case report of a patient who survived. AJR 97:624, 1966

98. Galindo MJ Jr, Francis WR: Atlantal fracture in a child through congenital anterior and posterior arch defects: A case report. Clin Orthop 178:220, 1983

99. Gallie WE: Fractures and dislocation of the cervical spine. Am J Surg 46:495, 1939

100. Garber JN: Abnormalities of the atlas and axis vertebrae: Congenital and traumatic. J Bone Joint Surg [Am] 46:1782, 1964

101. Garfin SR, Lee TO, Roux RD et al: Structural be-havior of the halo orthosis pin-bone interface: Biomechanical evaluation of standard and newly designed stainless steel halo fixation pins. Spine 11:977, 1986

102. Garfin SR, Roux R, Botte MJ et al: Skull osteology as it affects halo pin placement. J Pediatr Orthop 6:434, 1986

103. Garrett AL, Perry J, Nickel VL: Stabilization of the collapsing spine. J Bone Joint Surg [Am] 43:474, 1961

104. Garrick JG, Anderson PW, Rudd TG, Johnson C: Early diagnosis of stress fractures and their precursors. J Bone Joint Surg [Am] 58:733, 1976

105. Gaufin LM, Goodman SJ: Cervical spine injuries in infants: Problems in management. J Neurosurg 42:179, 1975

106. Georgopoulos G, Pizzutillo PD, Lee MS: Occipito-atlantal instability in children: A report of five cases and review of the literature. J Bone Joint Surg [Am] 69:429, 1987

107. Gerlock AJ, Mirfakhraee M, Benqel EC: Computed tomography of traumatic atlanto-occipital dislocation. Neurosurgery 13:316, 1983

108. Gibson MJ, Szypryt EP, Buckley JH et al: Magnetic resonance imaging of adolescent disc herniation. J Bone Joint Surg [Br] 69:699, 1987

109. Gilles FH, Bina M, Sotrel A: Infantile atlantooccipital instability: The potential danger of extreme extension. Am J Dis Child 133:30, 1979

110. Giroux JC, Leclerq TA: Lumbar disc excision in the second decade. Spine 7:168, 1982

111. Glasauer FE, Cares HL: Biomechanical features of traumatic paraplegia in infancy. J Trauma 13:166, 1973

112. Glasauer FE, Cares HL: Traumatic paraplegia in infancy. JAMA 219:38, 1972

113. Goldberg MJ: Gymnastic injuries. Orthop Clin North Am 11:717, 1980

114. Greeley PW: Bilateral (ninety degrees) rotatory dislocation of the atlas upon the axis. J Bone Joint Surg 12:958, 1930

115. Green BA, Green KL, Klose KJ: Kinetic therapy for spinal cord injury. Spine 8:722, 1983

116. Greenberg AD: Atlanto-axial dislocations. Brain 91:655, 1968

117. Griffiths SC: Fracture of odontoid process in children. J Pediatr Surg 7:680, 1972

118. Grisel P: Enucleation de l'Atlas et torticolis nasopharyngien. Presse Med 38:50, 1930

119. Gumley G, Taylor TK, Ryan MD: Distraction fractures of the lumbar spine. J Bone Joint Surg [Br] 64:520, 1982

120. Guttman L: Spinal deformities in traumatic para-

plegics and tetraplegics following surgical procedures. Paraplegia 7:38, 1969

121. Haas LL: Roentgenological skull measurements and their diagnostic application. AJR 67:197, 1952

122. Hachen HJ: Spinal cord injury in children and adolescents: Diagnostic pitfalls and therapeutic considerations in the acute stage. Paraplegia in infancy. Paraplegia 15:55, 1977-1978

123. Hadley LA: The Spine. Springfield, IL, Charles C Thomas, 1956

124. Hadley MN, Sonntag VK, Grahm TW et al: Axis fractures resulting from motor vehicle accidents: The need for occupant restraints. Spine 11:861, 1986

125. Handel SF, Lee Y: Computed tomography of spinal fractures. Radiol Clin North Am 19:69, 1981

126. Hegenbarth R, Ebel KD: Roentgen findings in fractures of the vertebral column in childhood: Examination of 35 patients and its results. Pediatr Radiol 5:34, 1976

127. Henrys P, Lyne ED, Lifton C, Salciccioli G: Clinical review of cervical spine injuries in children. Clin Orthop 129:172, 1977

128. Hensinger RN: Back pain and vertebral changes similating Scheuermann's disease. Orthop Trans 6:1, 1982

129. Hensinger RN: Fractures of the thoracic and lumbar spine. In Rockwood CA Jr, Wilkins KE, King RE (eds): Fractures in Children. Philadelphia, JB Lippincott, 1984

130. Hensinger RN: Spondylolysis and spondylolisthesis: Part I. Spondlylolysis and spondylolisthesis in children. Instr Course Lect 32:132, 1983

131. Hensinger RM, Lang FE, MacEwen GD: The Klippel-Feil syndrome: A constellation of associated anomalies. J Bone Joint Surg [Am] 56:1246, 1974

132. Hensinger RN, MacEwen GC: Congenital abnormalities of the cervical spine. Spine 1:189, 1982

133. Herzenberg JE, Hensinger RN, Dedrick DK, Phillips WA: Emergency transport and positioning of young children who have an injury of the cervical spine. J Bone Joint Surg [Am] 71:15, 1989

134. Hess JH, Bronstein IP, Abelson SM: Atlantoaxial dislocations unassociated with trauma and secondary to inflammatory foci of the neck. Am J Dis Child 49:1137, 1935

135. Hinck VC, Hopkins CE: Measurement of the atlanto-dens interval in the adult. AJR 84:945, 1960

136. Hitchcock HH: Spondylolisthesis: Observations on its development, progression, and genesis. J Bone Joint Surg 22:1, 1940

137. Hohl M: Normal motions in the upper portion of the cervical spine. J Bone Joint Surg [Am] 46:1777, 1964

138. Holdsworth RW: Fractures, dislocations and fracture-dislocations of the spine. J Bone Joint Surg [Br] 45:6, 1963

139. Hollinshead WH: Anatomy of Surgeons, Vol 3: The Back and Limbs. New York, Harper & Row, 1981

140. Horal J, Nachemson A, Scheller S: Clinical and radiological long term follow-up of vertebral fractures in children. Acta Orthop Scand 43:491, 1972

141. Howland WJ, Curry FL, Buffington CB: Fulcrum fractures of the lumbar spine. JAMA 193:240, 1965

142. Hubbard DD: Fractures of the dorsal and lumbar spine. Orthop Clin North Am 7:605, 1976

143. Hubbard DD: Injuries of the spine in children and adolescents. Clin Orthop 100:56, 1974

144. Huerta C, Griffith R, Joyce SM: Ann Emerg Med 16:1121, 1987

145. Hukuda S, Oga H, Okabe N, Tazima K: Traumatic atlantoaxial dislocation causing os odontoideum in infants. Spine 5:207, 1980

146. Hutton WC, Cyron BM: Spondylolysis. Acta Orthop Scand 49:604, 1978

147. Hutton WC, Stott FRR, Cyron BM: Is spondylolysis a fatigue fracture? Spine 2:202, 1977

148. Jackson DW: Low-back pain in young athletes: Evaluation of stress reaction and discogenic problems. Am J Sports Med 4:314, 1979

149. Jackson DW, Wiltse LL, Cirincione RJ: Spondylolysis in the female gymnast. Clin Orthop 117:68, 1976

150. Jackson DW, Wiltse LL, Dingeman RD, Hayes M: Stress reaction involving the pars intra-articularis in young athletes. Am J Sports Med 9:304, 1981

151. Jackson H: Diagnosis of minimal atlanto-axial subluxation. Br J Radiol 23:672, 1950

152. Jacobson G, Adler DC: Examination of the atlanto-axial joint following injury, with particular emphasis on rotational subluxation. AJR 76:1081, 1956

153. Jellinger K, Schwingshackl A: Birth injury of the spinal cord. Neuropediatrics 4:111, 1973

154. Johnson DP, Fergusson CM: Early diagnosis of atlanto-axial rotatory fixation. J Bone Joint Surg [Br] 68:698, 1986

155. Johnson RM, Hart DL, Simmons EF et al: Cervical orthoses: A study comparing the effectiveness in restricting cervical motion in normal subjects. J Bone Joint Surg [Am] 59:332, 1977

156. Johnson RM, Southwick WO: Functional and surgical anatomy of the neck. Spine 7:67, 1982

157. Jones ET, Hensinger RN: Spinal deformity in idiopathic juvenile osteoporosis. Spine 6:1, 1981

158. Jones RN: Rotatory dislocation of both atlanto-axial joints. J Bone Joint Surg [Br] 66:6, 1984

159. Juhl M, Seerup KK: Os odontoideum: A cause of atlanto-axial instability. Acta Orthop Scand 54:113-118, 1983

160. Kalamchi A, Yau ACMC, O'Brien JP, Hodgson AR: Halo-pelvic distraction apparatus: An analysis of one hundred and fifty consecutive patients. J Bone Joint Surg [Am] 58:1119, 1976

161. Kamel M, Rosman M: Disc protrusion in the growing child. Clin Orthop 185:46, 1984

162. Kawabe N, Hirotani H, Tanaka O: Pathomechanism of atlantoaxial rotatory fixation in children. J Pediatr Orthop 9:569, 1989

163. Keller RH: Traumatic displacement of the cartilaginous vertebral rim: A sign of intervertebral disc prolapse. Radiology 110:21, 1974

164. Kelly RP, Whitesides TE Jr: Treatment of lumbodorsal fracture-dislocations. Ann Surg 167:705, 1968

165. Kewalramani LS, Tori JA: Spinal cord trauma in children: Neurologic patterns, radiologic features, and pathomechanics of injury. Spine 5:11, 1980

166. Key JA: Intervertebral disc lesions in children and adolescents. J Bone Joint Surg [Am] 32:97, 1950

167. Keyes DC, Compere EL: The normal and pathological physiology of the nucleus pulposus of the intervertebral disc: An anatomical, clinical, and experimental study. J Bone Joint Surg 14:897, 1932

168. Kilfoyle RM, Foley JJ, Norton PL: Spine and pelvic deformity in childhood and adolescent paraplegia. J Bone Joint Surg [Am] 47:659, 1965

169. Klein DM, Kuhn JP: Problems in the radiographic diagnosis of atlanto-axial rotation deformity. Concepts in Pediatric Neurosurgery 5:26, 1985

170. Koch RA, Nickel VL: The halo vest: An evaluation of motion and forces across the neck. Spine 3:103, 1978

171. Kogutt MS, Swischuk LE, Fagan GJ: Patterns of injury and significance of uncommon fractures in the battered child syndrome. AJR 121:143, 1974

172. Koop SE, Winter RB, Lonstein JE: The surgical treatment of instability of the upper part of the cervical spine in children and adolescents. J Bone Joint Surg [Am] 66:403, 1984

173. Kopits SE, Steinglass MH: Experience with the "halo cast" in small children. Surg Clin North Am 50:935, 1970

174. Kostuik JP: Indications for the use of the halo immobilization. Clin Orthop 154:46, 1981

175. Kowalski HM, Cohen WA, Cooper P, Wisoff JH: Pitfalls in the CT diagnosis of atlantoaxial rotary subluxation. AJR 149:595, 1987

176. Kraus H: Effect of lordosis on the stress in the lumbar spine. Clin Orthop 117:56, 1976

177. Krenz J, Troup JDG: The structure of the pars interarticularis of the lower lumbar vertebrae and its relation to the etiology of spondylolysis: With a report of a healing fracture in the neural arch of a fourth lumbar vertebra. J Bone Joint Surg [Br] 55:735, 1973

178. Kuhl DE, Edwards RO: Image separation radioisotope scanning. Radiology 80:653, 1963

179. Kurihara A, Kataoka O: Lumbar disc herniation in children and adolescents: A review of 70 operated cases and their minimum 5-year follow-up studies. Spine 5:443, 1980

180. Lafferty JF, Winter WG, Gambaro SA, Lexington MS: Fatigue characterisiics of posterior elements of vertebrae. J Bone Joint Surg [Am] 59:154, 1977

181. Lancourt FE, Dickson JH, Carter RE: Paralytic spinal deformity following traumatic spinal cord injury in children and adolescents. J Bone Joint Surg [Am] 63:47, 1981

182. Langer LO Jr: Spondyloepiphyseal dysplasia tarda: Hereditary chondrodysplasia with characteristic vertebral configuration in the adult. Radiology 82:833, 1964

183. Lawson JP, Ogden JA, Bucholz RW, Hughes SA: Physeal injuries of the cervical spine. J Pediatr Orthop 7:428, 1987

184. LeBlanc HJ, Nadell J: Spinal cord injuries in children. Surg Neurol 2:411, 1974

185. Lester DK, Skinner SR: Unilateral synostosis of C3-C4 facet in subluxated position: A case report. Spine 9:322, 1984

186. Letts M, Kaylor D, Gouw G: A biomechanical analysis of halo fixation in children. J Bone Joint Surg [Br] 70:277, 1988

187. Letts M, Smallman T, Afanasiev R, Gouw G: Fracture of the pars interarticularis in adolescent athletes: A clinical-biomechanical analysis. J Pediatr Orthop 6:40, 1986

188. Leventhal HR: Birth injuries of the spinal cord. J Pediatr 56:447, 1960

189. Lippitt AB: Fracture of a vertebral body end plate and disk protrusion causing subarachnoid block in an adolescent. Clin Orthop 116:112, 1976

190. Lipscomb PR: Cervical occipital fusion for congenital and post traumatic anomalies of the atlas and axis. J Bone Joint Surg [Am] 39:1289, 1957

191. Lipson SJ, Mazur J: Anteroposterior spondyloschisis of the atlas revealed by computerized tomography scanning. J Bone Joint Surg [Am] 60:1104, 1978

192. Locke GR, Gardner JI, Van Epps EF: Atlas-dens

interval (ADI) in children: A survey based on 200 normal cervical spines. AJR 97:135, 1966

193. Logan WW, Stuard ID: Absent posterior arch of the atlas. AJR 118:670, 1973

194. Lonstein FE, Winter RB, Moe JH et al: Neurologic deficits secondary to spinal deformity: A review of the literature and report of 43 cases. Spine 5:331, 1980

195. Lonstein J: Post-laminectomy kyphosis. Clin Orthop 128:93, 1977

196. Love JG: The disc factor in low-back pain with or without sciatica. J Bone Joint Surg 29:438, 1947

197. Lowe J, Schochner E, Hirschberg E et al: Significance of bone scintigraphy in symptomatic spondylolysis. Spine 6:653, 1984

198. Magerl F, Brunner C, Zoch K, Berreux P: Fractures and dislocations of the vertebral column. In Weber BG, Brenner C, Freuler F (eds): Treatment of Fractures in Children and Adolescents, p 226. New York, Springer-Verlag, 1980

199. Malcolm BW: Spinal deformity secondary to spinal injury. Orthop Clin North Am 10:943, 1979

200. Malcolm BW, Bradford DS, Winter RB, Chou SN: Post-traumatic kyphosis: A review of 48 surgically treated patients. J Bone Joint Surg [Am] 63:891, 1981

201. Marar BC: Fracture of the axis arch: "Hangman's fracture" of the cervical spine. Clin Orthop 106:155, 1975

202. Marar BC: The pattern of neurological damage as an aid to the diagnosis of the mechanism in cervical spine injuries. J Bone Joint Surg [Am] 56:1648, 1974

203. Marar BC, Balachandran N: Non-traumatic atlanto-axial dislocation in children. Clin Orthop 92:220, 1973

204. Martel W: The occipito-atlanto-axial joints in rheumatoid arthritis and ankylosing spondylitis. AJR 86:223, 1961

205. Martel W, Tishler JM: Observations of the spine in mongolism. AJR 97:630, 1966

206. Mayfield JK, Erkkila JC, Winter RB: Spine deformity subsequent to acquired childhood spinal cord injury. J Bone Joint Surg [Am] 63:1401, 1981

207. McCall IW, Park WM, O'Brien JP, Seal V: Acute traumatic intraosseous disc herniation. Spine 10:134, 1985

208. McGrory BE, Fenichel GM: Hangman's fracture subsequent to shaking in an infant. Ann Neurol 2:82, 1977

209. McLain RF, Clark CR, El-Khoury GY: C6-7 dislocation in a neurologically intact neonate: A case report. Spine 14:125–127, 1989

210. McPhee IB: Spinal fractures and dislocations in children and adolescents. Spine 6:533, 1981

211. McRae DL: Bony abnormalities in the region of the foramen magnum: Correlations of the anatomic and neurologic findings. Acta Radiologica [Diagn] 40:335, 1953

212. McRae DL: The significance of abnormalities of the cervical spine. AJR 84:3, 1960

213. McRae DL, Barnum AS: Occipitalization of the atlas. AJR 70:23, 1953

214. McSweeney T: Spinal deformity after spinal cord injury. Paraplegia 6:212, 1969

215. McWhorter J, Alexander E Jr, Davis CH, Kelly DL Jr: Posterior cervical fusion in children. J Neurosurg 45:211, 1976

216. Micheli LJ: Low back pain in the adolescent: Differential diagnosis. Am J Sports Med 7:362, 1979

217. Micheli LJ: Overuse injuries in children's sports: The growth factor. Orthop Clin North Am 14:337, 1983

218. Micheli LJ, Hall JE, Miller ME: Use of modified Boston brace for back injuries in athletes. Am J Sports Med 8:351, 1980

219. Minderhoud JM, Braakman R, Penning L: Os odontoideum: Clinical, radiological and therapeutic aspects. J Neurol Sci 8:521, 1969

220. Moe JH, Winter RB, Bradford DS, Lonstein JE: Scoliosis and Other Spinal Deformities. Philadelphia, WB Saunders, 1978

221. Morgan TH, Wharton GW, Austin GN: The results of laminectomy in patients with incomplete spinal cord injuries. Paraplegia 9:14, 1971

222. Mubarak SJ, Camp JF, Vuletich W et al: Halo application in the infant. J. Pediatr Orthop 9:612, 1989

223. Munster JK, Troup JDG: The structure of the pars interaricularis of the lower lumbar vertebrae and its relation to the etiology of spondylolisthesis. J Bone Joint Surg [Br] 55:735, 1973

224. Nachemson A: Fracture of the odontoid process of the axis: A clinical study based on 26 cases. Acta Orthop Scand 29:185, 1960

225. Nerubay J, Lin E, Weiss J et al: Posttraumatic atlantoaxial rotatory fixation. J Pediatr Orthop 5:734, 1985

226. Nesbit ME, Kieffer S, D'Angio GJ: Reconstitution of vertebral height in histiocytosis X: A long-term follow-up. J Bone Joint Surg [Am] 51:1360, 1969

227. Norman MG, Wedderburn LC: Fetal spinal cord injury with cephalic delivery. Obstet Gynecol 42:355, 1973

228. O'Connell JEA: Protrusions of the lumbar intervertebral discs. J Bone Joint Surg [Br] 33:8, 1951

229. Odom JA, Brown CW, Jackson RR et al: Scoliosis in paraplegia. Paraplegia 11:290, 1974

230. Ogden JA: Postnatal development of the cervical spine. Orthopaedic Transactions 6:89, 1982

231. Ogden JA: Skeletal Injury in the Child. Philadelphia, Lea & Febiger, 1982

232. Ono K, Yonenobu K, Fuji T, Okada K: Atlantoaxial rotatory fixation: Radiographic study of its mechanism. Spine 10:602, 1985

233. Pang D, Wilberger JE: Spinal cord injury without radiographic abnormalities in children. J Neurosurg 57:114, 1982

234. Parke WW: Applied anatomy of the spine. Spine 1:19, 1982

235. Parke WW, Rothman RH, Brown MD: The pharyngovertebral veins: An anatomical rationale for Grisel's syndrome. J Bone Joint Surg [Am] 66:568, 1984

236. Parke WW, Schiff DCM: The applied anatomy of the intervertebral disc. Orthop Clin North Am 22:309, 1971

237. Paul LW, Moir WW: Non-pathologic variations in relationship of the upper cervical vertebrae. AJR 62:519, 1949

238. Pennecot GF, Gouraud D, Hardy JR, Pouliquen JC: Roentgenographic study of the stability of the cervical spine in children. J Pediatr Orthop 4:346, 1984

239. Pennecot GF, Leonard P, Peyrot Des Gachons S et al: Traumatic ligamentous instability of the cervical spine in children. J Pediatr Orthop 4:339, 1984

240. Penning L: Normal movements of the cervical spine. AJR 130:317, 1978

241. Pepin JW, Hawkins RJ: Traumatic spondylolisthesis of the axis: Hangman's fracture. Clin Orthop 157:133, 1981

242. Perry J, Nickel VL: Total cervical-spine fusion for neck paralysis. J Bone Joint Surg [Am] 41:37, 1959

243. Phillips WA, Hensinger RN: The management of rotatory atlanto-axial subluxation in children. J Bone Joint Surg [Am] 71:664, 1989

244. Pierson RN: Spinal and cranial injuries of the baby in breech deliveries. Surg Gynecol Obstet 37:802, 1923

245. Pizzutillo PD, Rocha EF, D'Astous J et al: Bilateral fractures of the pedicle of the second cervical vertebra in the young child. J Bone Joint Surg [Am] 68:892, 1986

246. Porter RW, Hibbert CS: Symptoms associated with lysis of the pars interarticularis. Spine 9:755, 1984

247. Porter RW, Park W: Unilateral spondylolysis. J Bone Joint Surg [Br] 64:344, 1982

248. Pouliquen JC, Pennecot GF: Progressive spinal deformity after spinal injury in children. In Houghton GR, Thompson GH (eds): Problematic Musculoskeletal Injuries in Children, p 32. London, Butterworth & Co, 1983

249. Prolo DJ, Runnels JB, Jameson RM: The injured cervical spine: Immediate and long-term immobilization with the halo. JAMA 224:591, 1973

250. Raaf J: Some observations regarding 905 patients operated upon for protruded lumbar intervertebral disc. Am J Surg 97:388, 1959

251. Rachesky I, Boyce WT, Duncan B et al: Clinical prediction of cervical spine injuries in children. Am J Dis Child 141:199-201, 1987

252. Rang MC: Children's Fractures. Philadelphia, JB Lippincott, 1974

253. Rang MC: The Growth Plate and Its Disorders. Baltimore, Williams & Wilkins, 1969

254. Ries MD, Ray S: Posterior displacement of an odontoid fracture in a child. Spine 11:1043, 1986

255. Rinaldi I, Mullins WJ Jr, Delaney WF et al: Computerized tomographic demonstration of rotational atlanto-axial fixation: Case report. J Neurosurg 50:115, 1979

256. Roaf R: Scoliosis secondary to paraplegia. Paraplegia 8:42, 1970

257. Roaf R: A study of the mechanics of spinal injuries. J Bone Joint Surg [Br] 42:810, 1960

258. Roche MB: Healing of bilateral fracture of the pars interarticularis of a lumbar neural arch. J Bone Joint Surg [Am] 30:1005, 1948

259. Roche MB, Rowe GG: The incidence of separate neural arch and coincident bone variations: A survey of 4,200 skeletons. Anat Rec 109:233, 1951

260. Romeyn RL, Herkowitz HN: The cervical spine in hemophilia. Clin Orthop 210:113, 1986

261. Rosenberg NJ, Bargar WL, Friedman B: The incidence of spondylolysis and spondylolisthesis in non-ambulatory patients. Spine 6:35, 1981

262. Rowe GG, Roche MB: The etiology of separate neural arch. J Bone Joint Surg [Am] 35:102, 1953

263. Roy-Camille R, Saillant G, Bisserie M: Rachis cervical traumatologique non-neurologique. In Journee d'Orthopedie de la Pitie, p 134. Paris, Masson, 1979

264. Rugtveit A: Juvenile lumbar disc herniations. Acta Orthop Scand 37:348, 1966

265. Sampson P: Editorial: Laminectomy: The "wrong" treatment for fracture dislocations of spine. JAMA 239:1597, 1978

266. Sanner G, Bergstrom B: Benign paroxysmal torticollis in infancy. Acta Paediatr Scand 68:219, 1979

267. Saraste H: The etiology of spondylolysis: A retrospective radiographic study. Acta Orthop Scand 56:253, 1985

268. Sassard WR, Heinig CF, Pitts WR: Posterior at-

lanto-axial dislocation without fracture: Case report with successful conservative treatment. J Bone Joint Surg [Am] 56:625, 1974

269. Scher AT: Trauma of the spinal cord in children. S Afr Med J 50:2023, 1976

270. Schmorl G, Junghanns H: The Human Spine in Health and Disease, 2nd ed. New York, Grune & Stratton, 1971

271. Schneider RC, Livingston KE, Cave AJE, Hamilton G: "Hangman's fracture" of the cervical spine. J Neurosurg 22:141, 1965

272. Seimon LP: Fracture of the odontoid process in young children. J Bone Joint Surg [Am] 59:943, 1977

273. Shahriaree H, Harkess JW: A family with spondylolisthesis. Radiology 94:631, 1970

274. Shapiro R, Youngberg AS, Rothman SLG: The differential diagnosis of traumatic lesions of the occipito-atlanto-axial segment. Radiol Clin North Am 11:505, 1973

275. Sherk HH: Atlantoaxial instability and acquired basilar invagination in rheumatoid arthritis. Orthop Clin North Am 9:1053, 1978

276. Sherk HH: Lesions of the atlas and axis. Clin Orthop 109:33, 1975

277. Sherk HH, Nicholson JT: Rotatory atlanto-axial dislocation associated with ossiculum terminale and mongolism: A case report. J Bone Joint Surg [Am] 51:957, 1969

278. Sherk HH, Nicholson JT, Chung SMK: Fractures of the odontoid process in young children. J Bone Joint Surg [Am] 60:921, 1978

279. Sherk HH, Schut L, Lane J: Fractures and dislocations of the cervical spine in children. Orthop Clin North Am 7:593, 1976

280. Sherk HH, Snyder B: Posterior fusions of the upper cervical spine: Indications, techniques and prognosis. Orthop Clin North Am 9:1091, 1978

281. Shrosbree RD: Spinal cord injuries as a result of motorcycle accidents. Paraplegia 16:102, 1978

282. Shulman ST, Madden JD, Esterly JR, Shanklin DR: Transection of the spinal cord: A rare obstetrical complication of cephalic delivery. Arch Dis Child 46:291, 1971

283. Sneed RC, Stover SL: Undiagnosed spinal cord injuries in brain injured children. Am J Dis Child 142:965, 1988

284. Sneed RC, Stover SL, Fine PR: Spinal cord injury associated with all-terrain vehicle accidents. Pediatrics 77:271, 1986

285. Southwick WO: Management of fractures of the dens (odontoid process). J Bone Joint Surg [Am] 62:482, 1980

286. Sovio OM, Bell HM, Beauchamp RD, Tredwell SJ: Fracture of the lumbar vertebral apophysis. J Pediatr Orthop 5:550, 1985

287. Spitzer R, Rabinowitch JY, Wybar DC: A study of the abnormalities of the skull, teeth and lenses in mongolism. Can Med Assoc J 84:567, 1961

288. Stabler CL, Eismont FJ, Brown MD et al: Failure of posterior cervical fusions using cadaveric bone graft in children. J Bone Joint Surg [Am] 67:371, 1985

289. Stanley P, Duncan AW, Isaacson J, Isaacson AS: Radiology of fracture-dislocation of the cervical spine during delivery. AJR 145:621, 1985

290. Stauffer ES, Mazur JM: Cervical spine injuries in children. Pediatr Ann 11:502, 1982

291. Steel HH: Anatomical and mechanical consideration of the atlanto-axial articulation: Proceedings of the American Orthopedic Association. J Bone Joint Surg [Am] 50:1481, 1968

292. Steiner ME, Micheli LJ: Treatment of symptomatic spondylolysis and spondylolisthesis with the modified Boston brace. Spine 10:937, 1985

293. Stern WE, Rand RW: Birth injuries to the spinal cord. Am J Obstet Gynecol 78:498, 1959

294. Stewart TD: The age incidence of neural-arch defects in Alaskan natives, considered from the standpoint of etiology. J Bone Joint Surg [Am] 35:937, 1953

295. Sujoy E: Spinal lesions in tetanus in children. Pediatrics 29:629, 1962

296. Sullivan AW: Subluxation of the atlanto-axial joint: Sequel to inflammatory processes of the neck. J Pediatr 35:451, 1949

297. Sullivan CR, Bruwer AJ, Harris LE: Hypermobility of the cervical spine in children: A pitfall in the diagnosis of cervical dislocation. Am J Surg 95:636, 1958

298. Sutton LN, Schut L, Bruce DA, Luerssen TG: Acquired torticollis in childhood. Concepts in Pediatric Neurosurgery 5:13, 1985

299. Swischuk LE: Spine and spinal cord trauma in the battered child syndrome. Radiology 92:733, 1969

300. Tachdjian MO: Pediatric Orthopedics. Philadelphia, WB Saunders, 1972

301. Tachdjian MO, Matson DD: Orthopaedic aspects of intraspinal tumors in infants and children. J Bone Joint Surg [Am] 47:223, 1965

302. Takata K, Inoue S, Takahashi K, Ohtsuka Y: Fracture of the posterior margin of a lumbar vertebral body. J Bone Joint Surg [Am] 70:589, 1988

303. Termansen NB: Hangman's fracture. Acta Orthop Scand 45:529, 1974

304. Thompson H: Halo traction apparatus: A method of external splinting of the cervical spine after surgery. J Bone Joint Surg [Br] 44:655, 1962

305. Toland JJ: Spondylolisthesis in identical twins. Clin Orthop 5:184, 1955

306. Torg J: Epidemiology, pathomechanics, and prevention of athletic injuries to the cervical spine. In Cervical Spine Research Society Editors Committee [eds]: The Cervical Spine, p 442. Philadelphia, JB Lippincott, 1989

307. Towbin A: Spinal cord and brainstem injury at birth. Arch Pathol Lab Med 77:620, 1964

308. Townsend EH Jr, Rowe ML: Mobility of the upper cervical spine in health and disease. Pediatrics 10:567, 1952

309. Troup JDG: Mechanical factors in spondylolisthesis and spondylolysis. Clin Orthop 117:59, 1976

310. Truesdell E: Birth Fractures and Epiphyseal Dislocations, pp 53-57. New York, Paul B Hoeber, 1917

311. Tupper JW, Gunn DR: Factors influencing stability of spine fractures. Orthopaedic Transactions 1:132, 1977

312. Turner RH, Bianco AJ Jr: Spondylolysis and spondylolisthesis in children and teenagers. J Bone Joint Surg [Am] 53:1298, 1971

313. van den Oever M, Merrick MV, Scott JH: Bone scintigraphy in symptomatic spondylolysis. J Bone Joint Surg [Br] 69:453, 1987

314. Verbiest H: Results of surgical treatment of idiopathic developmental stenosis of the lumbar vertebral canal: A review of 27 years' experience. J Bone Joint Surg [Br] 59:181, 1977

315. Wagoner G, Pendergrass EP: The anterior and posterior "notch" shadows seen in lateral roentgenograms of the vertebrae of infants: An anatomic explanation. AJR 42:663, 1939

316. Walsh WM, Huurman WW, Shelton GL: Overuse injuries of the knee and spine in girls' gymnastics. Orthop Clin North Am 16:329, 1985

317. Warwick M: Necropsy findings in newborn infants. Am J Dis Child 21:488, 1921

318. Webb JH, Svien HJ, Kennedy RLJ: Protruded lumbar intervertebral discs in children. JAMA 154:1153, 1954

319. Weir DC: Roentgenographic signs of cervical injury. Clin Orthop 109:9, 1975

320. Weiss MH, Kaufman B: Hangman's fracture in an infant. Am J Dis Child 126:268, 1973

321. Werne S: Studies in spontaneous atlas dislocation. Acta Orthop Scand [Suppl] 23:1, 1957

322. Wertzberger KL, Peterson HA: Acquired spondylolysis and spondylolisthesis in the young child. Spine 5:437, 1980

323. Westerborn A, Olsson O: Mechanics, treatment and prognosis of fractures of the dorso-lumbar spine. Acta Chir Scand 102:59, 1953

324. White AA III, Panjabi MD: The clinical biomechanics of the occipitoatlantoaxial complex. Orthop Clin North Am 9:868, 1978

325. Wholey MH, Brewer AJ, Baker HL Jr: The lateral roentgenogram of the neck (with comments on the atlanto-odontoid-basion relationship). Radiology 71:350, 1958

326. Wiesel SW, Rothman RH: Occipitoatlantal hypermobility. Spine 4:187, 1979

327. Wilkinson RH, Hall JE: The sclerotic pedicle: Tumor or pseudotumor? Radiology 111:683, 1974

328. Wilson MJ, Michele AA, Jacobson EW: Spontaneous dislocation of the atlanto-axial articulation, including a report of a case with quadriplegia. J Bone Joint Surg 22:698, 1940

329. Wiltse LL: Etiology of spondylolisthesis. Clin Orthop 10:45, 1957

330. Wiltse LL: The etiology of spondylolisthesis. J Bone Joint Surg [Am] 44:539, 1962

331. Wiltse LL: Spondylolisthesis in children. Clin Orthop 21:156, 1961

332. Wiltse LL, Newman PH, Macnab I: Classification of spondylolysis and spondylolisthesis. Clin Orthop 117:23, 1976

333. Wiltse LL, Widell EH Jr, Jackson DW: Fatigue fracture: The basic lesion in isthmic spondylolisthesis. J Bone Joint Surg [Am] 57:17, 1975

334. Wollin DG: The os odontoideum: Separate odontoid process. J Bone Joint Surg [Am] 45:1459, 1963

335. Wortzman G, Dewar FP: Rotary fixation of the atlantoaxial subluxation. Radiology 90:479, 1968

336. Wynne-Davies R, Scott JHS: Inheritance and spondylolisthesis: A radiographic family survey. J Bone Joint Surg [Br] 61:301, 1979

337. Yates PO: Birth trauma to the vertebral arteries. Arch Dis Child 311:436, 1959

338. Yngve DA, Harris WP, Herndon WA et al: Spinal cord injury without spine fracture. J Pediatr Orthop 8:153, 1988

339. Zamani MH, MacEwan GD: Herniation of the lumbar disc in children and adolescents. J Pediatr Orthop 2:528, 1982

340. Zwerling MT, Riggins RS: Use of the halo apparatus in acute injuries of the cervical spine. Surg Gynecol Obstet 138:189, 1974

24

GENERAL CONSIDERATIONS OF REHABILITATION OF SPINAL CORD INJURED PATIENTS

Jung H. Ahn

In the rehabilitation of spinal cord injured patients the physiatrist is concerned not only with the physical disability, but also with the medical, psychological, and social consequences of the injury.

The degree of neurologic deficit following spinal cord injury (SCI) depends on the level and extent of the lesion. Muscular paralysis can cause respiratory insufficiency, immobility, osteoporosis, and deep venous thrombosis of the lower extremities. Sensory loss and prolonged local pressure can cause decubitus ulcers over the bony prominences. Autonomic dysfunction can lead to neurogenic bladder, neurogenic bowel, sexual dysfunction, and, in quadriplegia, autonomic hyperreflexia. As a rule of thumb, the less the cord damage and the lower the neurologic level, the better the functional outcome and the fewer the medical complications.

Over the past two decades, medical management of spinal cord injured patients and rehabilitation engineering for the disabled have made substantial progress. Life expectancy has markedly improved following SCI, and a wider variety of rehabilitation equipment is available to meet the specific requirements of each patient.

RESTRICTIVE PULMONARY FUNCTION

Morbidity and mortality during the first 4 weeks following SCI are most often related to paralysis of the respiratory muscles. Pulmonary function parameters following quadriplegia and high paraplegia are consistent with a restrictive pattern on spirometry and lung volume testing (Fig. 24-1).[16]

Paralysis of the diaphragm in quadriplegia due to injury above C-5 brings an immediate threat to life, and often requires artificial ventilation. In cases in which phrenic nerves are intact, electrophrenic stimulation is sufficient to maintain respiration.[3,9] In most cases, however, a mechanical respirator is necessary. Where electrical pacing of the diaphragm is used, continuous bilateral low-

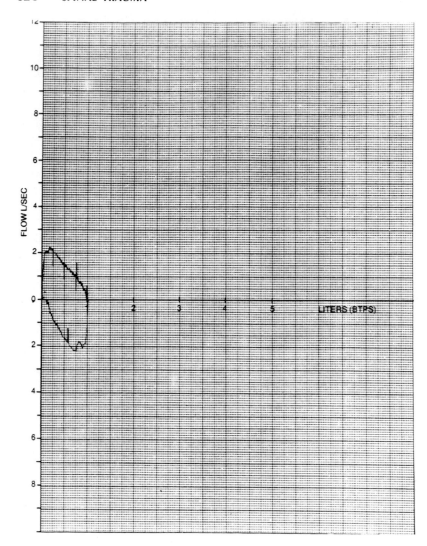

Figure 24-1. Abnormal flow–volume loop of a C-5 quadriplegic patient with a typical restrictive pulmonary function due to paralysis of the intercostal, parasternal, and abdominal muscles.

frequency stimulation at a slow rate of respiration is most efficient and causes less fatigue of the diaphragm muscle fibers, compared to unilateral high-frequency stimulation.[9]

While C-4 and C-5 quadriplegics, who have intact sternocleidomastoid muscles but a weak diaphragm, may initially suffer from respiratory insufficiency, they can usually be weaned off the respirator. By performing active breathing exercises, their inspiratory capacity significantly improves. With adequate conditioning they may reach the point where they are able to breathe comfortably while at rest, with basal tidal volumes maintaining adequate arterial oxygen tension.

Patients whose injury is at or below C-6 can not only improve their inspiratory capacity by using an inspirometer, but can also increase their expiratory reserve volume by exercising the clavicular portion of the pectoralis major, which reportedly has a major role in the mechanism of active expiration in quadriplegia.[28]

In the past it was felt that a return of muscle tone in the intercostal and abdominal muscles would eventually improve quadriplegics' pulmonary function. Since expiration depends on the passive recoil of the lung, most quadriplegics and high paraplegics do not feel respiratory difficulty during quiet breathing. They are potentially susceptible, however, to acute respiratory distress and bronchopulmonary complications when excessive secretions develop in the respiratory tract. Because the paralyzed expiratory muscles impair the patient's cough mechanism, mucous plugging in the respiratory tract can lead to sudden respiratory distress or arrest. Therefore, prophylactic measures, including intermittent positive pressure breathing and chest physical therapy, should be carried out as early as clinically permitted. Upon discharge from a rehabilitation hospital, continued incentive spirometry or even intermittent positive pressure breathing is recommended.

CARDIOVASCULAR COMPLICATIONS

During the acute stage of traumatic quadriplegia, severe bradycardia or prolonged asystole may be noted on cardiac monitoring due to a sudden loss of supraspinal sympathetic cardiac modulation, but with normal vagal parasympathetic discharges to the heart. For bradycardia, an oral anticholinergic agent is useful. Significant pauses should be managed by intravenous injection of atropin 0.5 mg on a p.r.n. basis or by use of a temporary cardiac pacemaker.

At the beginning of rehabilitative training, orthostatic hypotension may develop due to a slow return of the venous blood to the heart while sitting upright in a wheelchair. The patient complains of dizziness and looks pale. When this occurs, the head should be tilted down immediately. For frequent episodes of dizziness interfering with rehabilitation, oral sympathomimetics may be tried. However, the decision to use sympathomimetics in quadriplegia should be made with care because of the potential to worsen autonomic hyperreflexia. In order to prevent a hypotensive episode, a semi-reclining wheelchair should be used until the patient tolerates 65 degrees of upright positioning on a tilt table. A pair of elastic stockings and an abdominal binder are helpful in prevention of orthostatic hypotension.

The patient suffering from acute SCI is at high risk for developing deep venous thrombosis (DVT),[4,21,27,30] as muscular paralysis of the lower extremities, local pressure of the calf against the bed, and impaired sympathetic vasomotor control may lead to venous stasis distally. A hypercoagulable state associated with changes in factor VIII activities following SCI is also considered to play an important role in the development of venous thrombosis.[23] To prevent DVT, low-dose heparin, elastic stockings, and intermittent pneumatic compression cuffs may be used. Electrical stimulation of the paralyzed calf muscles has been proposed as a potentially effective modality in prevention of DVT in patients with SCI, but this approach is not yet in general use.

Deep venous thrombosis is most often diagnosed within the first 6 weeks after injury. Its incidence ranges from 16% to 100%, depending on the diagnostic method employed.[4,21,27] No apparent correlation is found between quadriplegia and paraplegia in the development of DVT, although these patients are more susceptible to clot formation than those with paresis. Approximately 20% of patients with SCI admitted to the Rusk Institute of Rehabilitation Medicine in New York suffer from DVT.[4]

Accurate diagnosis of DVT is critical to prevent pulmonary embolism and unnecessary anticoagulant therapy. Contrast venography is recognized as the highest standard for the diagnosis of DVT (Fig. 24-2). Currently, the Doppler ultrasound flowmetry and venous plethysmography are commonly used. Experienced examiners have combined these noninvasive procedures with clinical examination,[4] leading to a favorable degree of accuracy, patient safety and comfort, and economy. When results are equivocal, venography is indicated.

Once the diagnosis of DVT is made, anticoagulant therapy with intravenous heparin is initiated, followed by warfarin sodium (Coumadin) for about 3 months. When anticoagulation is contraindicated, insertion of a vena caval filter or umbrella should be considered to prevent pulmonary embolism. The treatment plan should include elevation of the affected leg, warm soaks, and bed rest until swelling resolves.

As a consequence of DVT, pulmonary embolism is relatively common following SCI.[21,30] Its incidence has been reported to be as high as 12%.[30] It sometimes presents as sudden death without the warning of venous thrombosis. In quadriplegia the absence of subjective feelings of chest pain masks

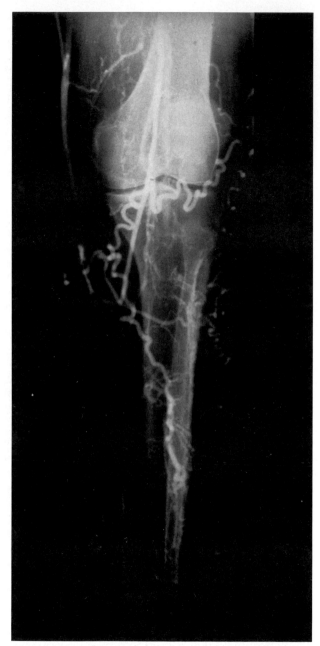

Figure 24-2. Multiple extensive filling defects in the posterior tibial and popliteal veins, consistent with deep venous thrombosis.

the progression of pulmonary embolism, until shortness of breath, hemoptysis, or even sudden death occurs. When pulmonary embolism is suspected clinically, measurement of blood gases and ventilation perfusion lung scans should be done as soon as possible to confirm the diagnosis, so that appropriate medical management may be initiated.

AUTONOMIC HYPERREFLEXIA

Spinal cord injury above T-5 results in interruption of normal supraspinal control on splanchnic sympathetic outflow, whereas the vagal parasympathetic pathway remains entirely intact. In quadriplegia and high paraplegia, therefore, any noxious afferent stimuli entering the thoracolumbar cord from organs or body parts below the injury may cause imbalanced reflex activity of the autonomic nervous system.[13] This situation results in the syndrome of autonomic hyperreflexia or dysreflexia, clinically characterized by pounding headaches, sweating, paroxysmal hypertension, anisocoria,[12] and changes of heart rate. Accelerated hypertension is potentially serious and could be complicated by a cerebrovascular accident. During autonomic hyperreflexia, arterial dopamine–hydroxylase activity is elevated.[18] A significant rise of plasma norepinephrine[15] is also reported, which supports a sympathetic mechanism for paroxysmal hypertension in quadriplegia.

Although the precise pathophysiology of autonomic hyperreflexia remains unknown, the most common precipitating condition is distension of the urinary bladder,[13] which irritates the sympathetic receptors of the bladder, which in turn fire sympathetic discharges via the hypogastric plexus and the isolated thoracolumbar cord. Other common recognizable causes include fecal impaction, hemorrhoids, urinary tract infection, transurethral resection of the external sphincter, cystography, vaginal delivery in females, decubiti, ingrown toenails, and passive stretching of joints.

In conservative management of autonomic hyperreflexia, the precipitating factor is removed;[8] this causes the syndrome to improve dramatically in most cases. If symptoms, hypertension in particular, persist despite appropriate conservative measures, pharmacologic therapy should be considered. In the author's experience, intravenous administration of a ganglionic blocker or a direct arteriolar vasodilator has not been necessary, although an oral ganglionic blocker such as mecamylamine hydrochloride (Inversine) has been successfully used to treat reflex sweating and mild hypertension. Diazepam seems to be helpful in reducing the patient's anxiety level during autonomic hyperreflexia.

NEUROGENIC BLADDER

Micturition is a highly integrated neuromuscular and physiologic phenomenon that empties the urinary bladder.[2] The bladder (the detrusor muscle) is innervated by the hypogastric plexus (which is sympathetic, and originates from the spinal cord between T-12 and L-2) and by the pelvic nerves (which are parasympathetic, and originate from the S-2 to S-4 cord segments). The external urethral sphincter is innervated mainly by the pudendal nerves (which are somatic, and originate from the S-2 to S-4 cord segments) and partly by the hypogastric and pelvic nerve fibers. Normal micturition requires a synergistic behavior between the detrusor and the external sphincter. Voiding of urine can be assisted by Valsalva's maneuver, and holding of urine by volitional tightness of the pelvic floor musculature.

When the bladder is felt to be full and is ready for voiding, the parasympathetic motor fibers are activated and release acetylcholine at the neuroeffector sites in the detrusor to stimulate contraction.[1] Simultaneously, the internal sphincter (bladder neck) opens and allows the urine to flow through (Fig. 24-3). At this point, the external sphincter, which has been in a state of tonic contraction, is inhibited by afferent sensory impulses from the bladder and becomes less tonic. After the bladder is emptied, the sympathetic nerve fibers are activated, releasing norepinephrine and stimulating sympathetic receptors in the detrusor to relax.[1] Simultaneously, the internal sphincter

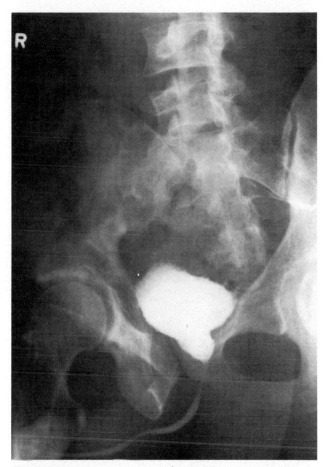

Figure 24-3. A voiding cystourethrogram shows contraction of the bladder dome and simultaneous opening of the bladder neck.

closes, and the external sphincter returns to its original tonic state.

Spinal cord injury above the level of the conus medullaris interrupts proprioceptive sensory feedback from the detrusor and urethra, leading to a loss of normal supraspinal autonomic control on the detrusor and sphincters. Immediately following the injury, the bladder is totally flaccid (Fig. 24-4), resulting in urinary retention. Intermittent catheterization[11] should start as soon as intravenous fluids are discontinued. With the passage of time, however, the detrusor begins to contract independently of supraspinal influence, and the ex-

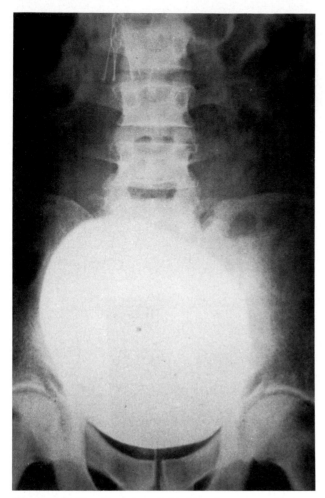

Figure 24-4. Flaccid neurogenic bladder, demonstrated by cystography, immediately following spinal cord or lower motor neuron injury.

ternal sphincter also becomes hypertonic (spastic). At this time, hyperreflexic detrusor–external sphincter dyssynergia is noted on urodynamic testing (Fig. 24-5).When the contraction of the detrusor is stronger than the uninhibited tone of the external sphincter, incontinence (spontaneous voiding) occurs.

For males with SCI, spontaneous voiding via an external catheter with low residuals is an ideal goal. In males who experience urinary retention due to hyperreflexic detrusor–external sphincter dyssynergia, trials of phenoxybenzamine hydrochloride (a sympatholytic agent) and baclofen (a chlorophenyl derivative of τ-aminobutyric acid) have been tried to reduce outlet resistance for spontaneous voiding, but were deemed to be ineffective. External sphincterotomy is sometimes necessary in males[14] who have developed vesicoureteral reflux (Fig. 24-6) or who frequently suffer from autonomic hyperreflexia due to urinary retention.

Incontinence should be prevented by catheterization in females with SCI; application of an external catheter is too difficult. In order to prevent urinary incontinence during either intermittent catheterizations or indwelling catheterization, use of a parasympatholytic agent such as oxybutynin chloride or propantheline bromide should be considered. A sympathomimetic drug such as ephedrine or pseudoephedrine hydrochloride may be added to increase outlet resistance.

Lower motor neuron injury (LMNI), such as an injury to the conus medullaris or cauda equina, results in parasympathetic denervation of the detrusor and, therefore, in a flaccid neurogenic bladder (see Fig. 24-4). The external sphincter is also denervated. Accordingly, urodynamic findings are consistent with areflexia of the bladder and external sphincter (Fig. 24-7). This is the lower motor neuron type of neurogenic bladder. Patients with LMNI suffering from urinary retention are prone to develop vesicoureteral reflux from loss of muscle tone, and are usually managed by self-intermittent catheterizations. Some patients, however, prefer noninvasive methods of emptying the bladder such as Credé's method and Valsalva's maneuver, which are done four to six times daily. If the lower urinary tract is partially denervated and there is no evidence of outlet obstruction, bethanechol chloride (a parasympathomimetic) may be tried to assist contractions of the detrusor. When patients use diuretics or alcoholic beverages, precautions should be taken to prevent overdistension of the bladder.

During neurogenic bladder management, urinary tract infections (UTI) are often encountered.[17] The definition of UTI in patients with SCI is still controversial, unless accompanied by fever. Bacteriuria associated with more than 20 white blood cells per high power field in urinalysis may be called "asymptomatic UTI" when the patient is afebrile.

BROWNE CORPORATION
K.S.: T4 paraplegia
Flow: 100 cc/min
Vol.: 200 cc
>8cm
BROWNE CORPORATION

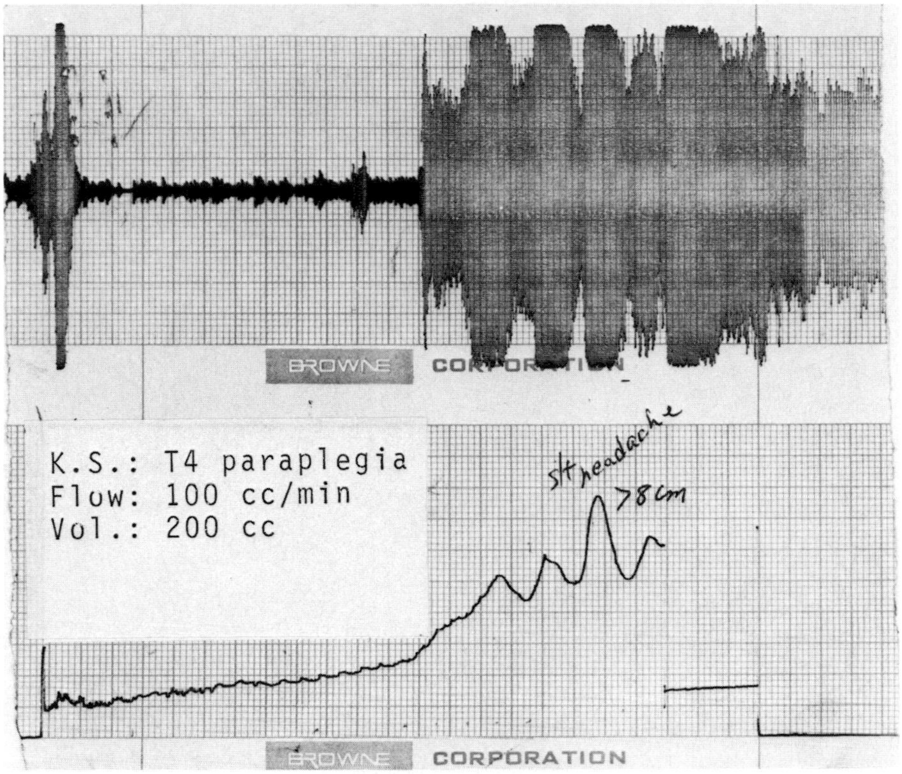

Figure 24-5. Typical urodynamic findings indicating hyperreflexic detrusor–external sphincter dyssynergia in a C-5 quadriplegic patient.

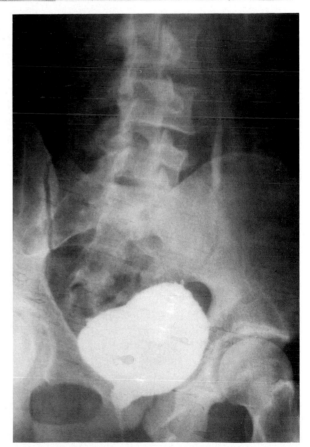

Figure 24-6. Vesicoureteral reflux on the left side is demonstrated on a cystogram in a C-6 quadriplegic patient.

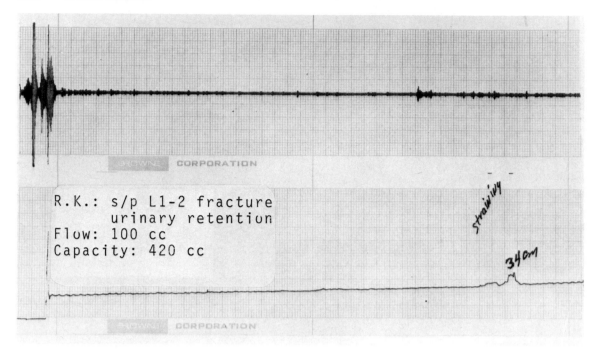

Figure 24-7. Areflexic detrusor and external sphincter in mixed injuries involving the conus medullaris and cauda equina secondary to L-1–L-2 fracture-dislocation.

A UTI with high grade fever should be treated immediately by intravenous antibiotics, hydration, and indwelling catheterization. A UTI with low grade fever may be treated by oral antibiotics. An asymptomatic UTI that occurs during use of an external catheter or intermittent catheterization program is presently treated at the Rusk Institute with oral antibiotics to prevent symptomatic UTI. Urinalysis and urine culture and sensitivities are checked on admission; urinalysis is repeated weekly during early hospitalization and less frequently later on, depending on medical status.

The selection of antibiotics can be difficult for asymptomatic UTI, but is usually based on the most recent urine culture and sensitivities report. A dilemma arises when the organisms are resistant to all oral antibiotics. In this case, the question is whether to treat afebrile UTIs with intravenous antibiotics or broad-spectrum oral antibiotics, or with acidifying agents, clinical observation, and follow-up urinalysis. In the author's experience, species of microorganisms often change, and findings from the urinalysis improve with nonantibio-

tic measures, including oral hydration and temporary indwelling catheterization. When the urine looks cloudy and has lots of sediment, the bladder may be irrigated. Asymptomatic UTI associated with indwelling catheterization is managed by changing the catheter, irrigating the bladder with normal saline, and increasing oral fluid intake. Antibiotic irrigation has been reported to have no decisive effect on the rate of acquisition of catheter-associated UTIs.[29]

In the past, renal failure was a major cause of death following SCI. In recent years, however, renal failure has been reported much less frequently; in fact, mortality rates from genitourinary diseases among SCI patients declined to 3.2%, according to the National Spinal Cord Injury Statistical Center.[25] Long-term urologic follow-up is undoubtedly one of the reasons for the decrease in renal mortality. The urologic evaluation comprises the measurement of residual urine, urinalysis, urine culture and sensitivities, urodynamics, KUB, cystography, voiding cystourethrography, intravenous pyelography, blood tests for blood urea nitrogen and creatinine, and cystoscopy. Renal ultrasonography is used, when intravenous pyelograms cannot be taken, to discover the presence of stones or other anatomic abnormalities of the urinary tract. When indwelling catheterization has been clinically employed, particularly by females, asymptomatic bladder stones are frequently found on follow-up cystoscopy. The frequency of comprehensive urologic follow-up for patients without complications is controversial. At the present time, it is recommended every year.

NEUROGENIC BOWEL

Sensory feedback that carries the desire to defecate from the rectum to the brain is lost following an injury to the spinal cord, conus medullaris, or cauda equina. Clinical problems, however, differ depending on the neurologic level of injury.[5] In SCI above the conus medullaris, the submucosal and myenteric plexus in the colon are intact. The pudendal nerve in the external anal sphincter is also intact, but supraspinal control is lost. In LMNI, on the other hand, the colon, except for the ascending portion, the rectosigmoid and anal sphincters, is denervated. As a result, insufficient water absorption and absent peristalsis occur in the colon, leading to frequent fecal oozing as well as persistent unsatisfactory evacuation of the feces in daily bowel rehabilitation.

From a pharmacologic standpoint, a colonic stimulant is anticipated to be effective in inducing peristalsis of the colon around the designated time for bowel routine in patients with SCI, but not in those with LMNI. Fecal incontinence is less likely to be problematic in SCI because of spasticity of the anal sphincter, but it can be serious in LMNI because of the flaccidity of the sphincter. In SCI the bowel routine is initiated by digital stimulation or rectal suppositories at the designated time.[5] In LMNI, the routine is usually initiated by enemas, manual abdominal compressions, and Valsalva's maneuver, and is often followed by another enema to clean the rectum. Table 24-1 summarizes laxatives commonly used for the management of the neurogenic bowel.

SEXUAL DYSFUNCTION

Sexual function, like micturition and defecation, is also affected following SCI or cauda equina injury because of disturbed autonomic functions in the genital and reproductive organs. The prognosis for sexual complications depends on the level of injury, completeness of the lesion, and gender of the patient.

In males with SCI above the conus medullaris, reflexogenic erections are frequently observed while preparing the penis for urinary catheterization. In LMNI, reflexogenic erection is not possi-

Table 24-1. Laxatives Commonly Used for Management of the Neurogenic Bowel

GENERIC NAME	TRADE NAME	PHARMACOLOGIC ACTION
Docusate sodium	Colace	Surface-active stool softener
Casanthranol and docusate sodium	Peri-colace	Mild stimulant and stool softener
Magnesium hydroxide	Milk of Magnesia	Nonabsorbable salt, holding water in the intestine in amounts sufficient to maintain its isotonic concentration
Psyllium hydrophilic mucilloid	Metamucil	Highly efficient dietary fiber, nonirritating bulk producer
Castor oil		Hydrolized like other fats in the upper small intestine to form irritating ricinoleic acid, which acts locally to increase intestinal motility
Bisacodyl	Dulcolax	Synthetic compound chemically similar to phenolphthalein, which is a powerful stimulant of the large bowel
Senna	Senokot	Glycosides converted to agycones in the colon, stimulating Auerbach's plexus to induce peristalsis
Lactulose	Chronulac	Poorly absorbed from the gastrointestinal tract, broken down primarily to lactic acid and also to small amounts of formic and acetic acids by colonic bacteria. This results in increased osmotic pressure and stool water content

ble; however, psychogenic erections may be possible in a minority of this group. For neurogenic impotence, particularly that due to LMNI, penile prostheses can be implanted. The majority of males with either SCI or LMNI are unable to ejaculate or feel an orgasm. Fertility was reported in 1% of cases with complete SCI, 5.6% with complete LMNI, 6% with incomplete SCI, and 10% with incomplete LMNI.[6] For ejaculation, intrathecal neostigmine methylsulfate (Prostigmin) was tried cautiously in the past, but this had poor results in term of successful live births. Presently, an intrarectal electroejaculator is used to obtain specimens with qualified spermatozoa. Because autonomic hyperreflexia may occur during electrostimulation, the procedure requires close observation and pharmacologic preparation for paroxysmal hypertension. As a rule, patients with incomplete lesions have better chances of having erections and ejaculations[7] and of fathering than do patients with complete lesions.

In females, transient amenorrhea occurs in 50% following SCI, with spontaneous return of the normal menstrual cycle after a period of 2 to 6 months. All premenopausal SCI women can conceive and carry to full term; however, they are unable to feel an orgasm. Paraplegia alone is usually not an indication for cesarean section,[20] and an uncomplicated vaginal delivery is possible.[10] It should be kept in mind, however, that there is a high risk of paroxysmal hypertension secondary to autonomic hyperreflexia during labor and vaginal delivery.[20] Daily medications throughout pregnancy should be reviewed by the obstetrician to avoid a teratogenic effect. Urinary tract infections, decubitus ulcers, anemia, hypoproteinemia, autonomic hyperreflexia (with SCI above T-5), and DVT may develop during pregnancy and postpartum. In SCI above T-10, labor may not be detected, and thus repeated sterile examinations of the cervix from the 28th week of pregnancy are advisable.[20] In terms of the hormonal status, there is no interference with the effects of estrogen and progesterone on uterine contractions in full-term pregnant females with SCI.

DECUBITUS ULCERS

One of the major causes of morbidity among patients with SCI is pressure sores (Fig. 24-8). They commonly develop over the sacrum, posterior

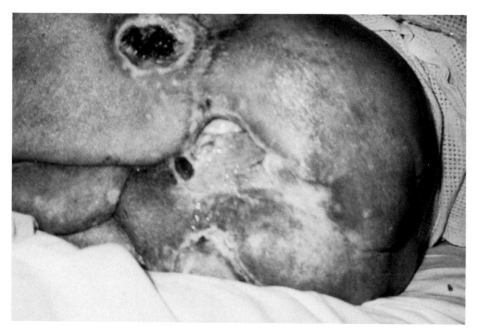

Figure 24-8. Multiple grade III and IV decubitus ulcers.

calcaneus, ischial tuberosity, greater trochanter, and lateral malleolus secondary to local soft-tissue ischemia. Prolonged pressure exceeding the supracapillary pressure that occurs on the soft tissue over bony prominences below the level of injury results in local ischemia and subsequent tissue breakdown. The ischemia is frequently associated with hyperemia in the surrounding tissue, which further increases local oxygen consumption.

Decubitus ulcers are often classified as:

Grade I: With erythema, blistering, or a superficial dermal breakdown
Grade II: With subcutaneous tissue involvement
Grade III: With muscle damage
Grade IV: With evidence of local osteomyelitis

Grade I and II and small grade III ulcers are conservatively treated by creating a healthy environment to enhance wound healing. Conservative measures include absolute removal of local pressure, application of topical antibiotic cream (preferably 1% silver sulfadiazine [Silvadene cream]) for superficial wound infection, and débridement of any thick eschar by simple surgery or use of a topical enzymatic agent. A hydrocolloidal dressing was recently introduced and is helpful in selected cases with clean and well-granulating ulcers. Vitamin C and zinc may be given orally for general wound healing. Grade IV ulcers should be surgically treated, but require conservative treatments preoperatively to prepare the ulcer for successful myocutaneous flap surgery and resection of the infected bony lesion.

SPASTICITY

Within a few months following SCI, muscle tone and tendon reflexes return gradually from the initial loss in a caudocephalic direction. In addition, the interruption of supraspinal control on local reflex activities of α- and τ-motor neuron systems below the level of SCI results in unchecked reflex contractions of the paralyzed limb muscles, that is, spasticity. Whether or not spasticity improves local hemodynamics and delays osteoporosis is unclear.

Some patients like spasticity and request not to be treated by anything more than physical therapy, which includes cold packs, hydrotherapy, and range of motion exercises to prevent joint contractures. When spasticity is clinically problematic, however, and interferes with the patient's functional activities of transfers, dressing, and wheelchair mobility, pharmacologic therapy[31] with single doses or combinations of baclofen, diazepam, and dantrolene sodium should be considered. Baclofen is a chlorophenyl derivative of τ-aminobutyric acid-ergic and has a direct depressing effect mainly on the presynaptic receptors. Diazepam is believed to increase τ-aminobutyric acid release presynaptically, and potentiates the effects of τ-aminobutyric acid postsynaptically. Dantrolene sodium supposedly has direct effects on the contractile mechanisms within the muscle, probably by interfering with Ca^{2+} release from the sacroplasmic reticulum.

Although the clinical result of these drugs is often unsatisfactory, spasticity worsens after discontinuation. If the pharmacologic approach fails to reduce spasticity, motor point or nerve blocks with a 5% or 7% phenol solution may be attempted to improve the range of motion. In order to prevent joint contractures, splinting or serial castings should be applied to the spastic elbow, wrist, knee, and ankle when preservation of range of motion is critical in rehabilitation.

HETEROTOPIC OSSIFICATION

Bone formation in the soft tissue adjacent to the hip joints (Fig. 24-9) is frequently noticed on radiographs during urologic workups. Heterotopic ossification of this sort can occur at any major joints below the level of the SCI. The pathogenesis of heterotopic ossification is unknown. This process, with or without warm soft-tissue swelling as seen in DVT, may begin during the first several months after injury in susceptible patients. When soft-tissue swelling of the paralyzed lower limb is found, DVT, cellulitis, intramuscular hemorrhage, and bone fracture should be ruled out for proper medical management.

Heterotopic ossification is benign in nature and usually evokes no clinical findings, but when se-

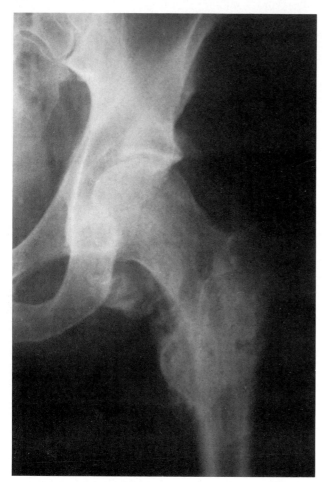

Figure 24-9. Heterotopic ossification about the hip without involvement of the joint space.

vere, can bridge from one bone to another across a joint, leading to a limitation of range of motion and ankylosis. The soft-tissue swelling, accompanied by an elevated serum alkaline phosphatase level and normal radiographs, is indicative of the earliest stage of heterotopic ossification.[19] The bone is gradually formed within muscle bundles, not in the joint space and capsule.

For uncomplicated heterotopic ossification, vigorous range of motion exercises with cold packs and oral administration of etidronate disodium[24] are recommended. The drug is usually given for a period of 3 months, during which time the alkaline phosphatase level is checked weekly to monitor osteoblastic activities. For severe extensive het-

erotopic ossification with resultant ankylosis of the involved joint, a surgical wedge resection of the ectopic bone can be useful to increase range of motion, but may have to be delayed until the ectopic bone is mature. Clinical methods to determine the maturity of heterotopic ossification include a blood test for the alkaline phosphatase level and serial bone scans. When the uptake ratio on the scans and the serum alkaline phosphatase level have decreased to normal, the ectopic bone is believed to be mature.[26] However, the sensitivity of these determinants is controversial. The prophylactic use of etidronate disodium immediately after injury or surgical resection was reported to be effective. If limited range of motion occurs, it can not only increase difficulties in personal daily care, but can further impair functional abilities that were already compromised.

PATHOLOGIC FRACTURES

Although osteoporosis in all skeletal bones below the lesion, particularly in the lower extremities, is a well-known sequela secondary to SCI, the incidence of bone fractures (Fig. 24-10) is relatively low, and has been reported in only 4% of patients.[22] A localized soft-tissue swelling, often associated with ecchymosis or a history of trauma, can be an important diagnostic clue and warrants radiographic investigation.

The method of treatment for closed pathologic fractures in SCI is generally nonsurgical. A circular well-padded plaster-of-Paris cast is most frequently employed, with close observation for the possible development of pressure sores.[22] A pillow splint or fracture brace may be applied. Pathologic fractures appear to heal sooner than would be expected for a similar fracture in patients without SCI. Passive range of motion exercises should begin as soon as orthopedically permitted to prevent contractures of the joint, which has been immobilized for healing.

PSYCHOLOGICAL REACTION

Following SCI, every patient will feel the psychological impact of the sudden onset of disability.

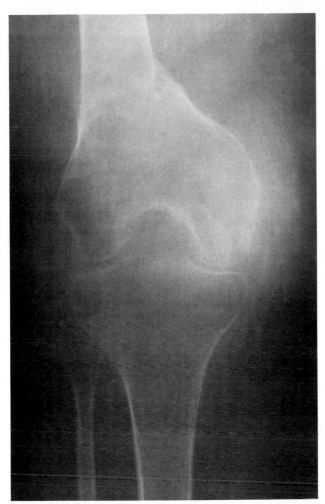

Figure 24-10. Severe osteoporosis in a chronic paraplegic woman, who suffered a supracondylar fracture from a fall out of a wheelchair.

maximum independence in activities of daily living. As comprehensive rehabilitation, which includes close medical supervision, nursing care, physical exercises, functional training, psychological support, vocational counseling, and social intervention, begins and progresses, patients notice that they can do a lot more things than they initially thought. At this point, the majority of patients are able to get out of their psychological slump and zero in on rehabilitation training. However, they may still experience frustrations from time to time.

DAILY REHABILITATION PROGRAM

A typical daily rehabilitation program for a patient with SCI consists of:

1. General medical care: vital signs, skin inspection, bowel routine, and urinary catheterizations
2. Tilt-table training
3. Passive range of motion exercises to the paralyzed extremities
4. Active range of motion and strengthening exercises to the unaffected or partially affected skeletal muscles and joints
5. Balance exercises on a mat
6. Functional training in the activities of daily living
7. Wheelchair class and, when feasible, ambulation training
8. Training with an environmental control unit for quadriplegics
9. Prevocational or vocational training
10. Driver training when indicated

REHABILITATION POTENTIAL

A rehabilitation outcome of functional independence depends primarily on the motivation of the patient and the neurologic level of the lesion. The patient's medical status, family support, home situation, and financial coverage undoubtedly play important roles as well. A person with quadriplegia above the level of C-4 is not only totally physically dependent, but is also respirator-dependent.

Some patients develop severe depression and continue to feel devastated about their neurologic deficits, while others may try to be realistic about the nature of the injury but experience underlying fears due to their uncertainties about the future. Patients with poor coping skills or who are severely depressed are likely to make slow progress in rehabilitation, and are prone to develop medical complications, particularly pain, joint contractures, pressure sores, and urologic complications. The better adjusted patient, however, adopts a more active role in his rehabilitation, achieving

Surgical implantation of a pair of phrenic nerve pacemakers for diaphragmatic paralysis in high quadriplegics with intact phrenic nerves has been successful in selected cases. In high quadriplegia, full-time nursing care is recommended for medical reasons.

Patients with C-4 quadriplegia have good function of the diaphragm and shoulder elevators (trapezius and levator scapulae muscles), and can breathe spontaneously. The tracheostomy tube that was initially inserted is removed, unless suctioning for upper airway secretions is necessary. The patient can use a sip/puff mouth control unit to drive a motorized wheelchair for moving around independently, to operate an environmental control unit at home, and to use a computer for vocational purposes. Attendant care is needed for other activities of daily living.

Individuals with C-5 quadriplegia can do self-feeding and light grooming by wearing an activities-of-daily-living cuff on the paralyzed hand. The patient is able to assist in upper-body dressing activities and can drive a motorized wheelchair with a hand control device (Fig. 24-11).

C-6 quadriplegics have functional wrist extensor muscles in addition to the normal shoulder abductor and elbow flexor muscles. Quadriplegics at this level have good rehabilitation potential for self-sufficiency with a wheelchair. Pushing a manual wheelchair that has vertical tips on the hand rims is a realistic goal. Without elbow flexion contractures the patient can reposition the pelvis and relieve local pressure on soft tissue over the ischeal tuberosities by pushing up on the wheels while sitting in a wheelchair. Independent transfers can be achieved by using a sliding board (Fig. 24-12). Simple writing and driving (using a modified van) are also anticipated.

C-7 quadriplegia is the neurologic level for becoming independent in activities of daily living with less difficulty at the wheelchair level because of functional elbow extensor and wrist flexor muscles. Limited help from attendants or nurses is justifiable for quadriplegia of the C-6 and C-7 levels when vocational requirements necessitate shortening the time and effort required in the morning routine. A motorized wheelchair can be used at school or work for convenience and efficiency.

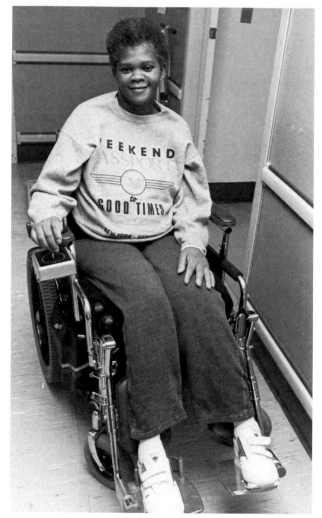

Figure 24-11. Driving a motorized wheelchair by using a hand control unit.

A person with C-8 quadriplegia has useful hand function despite paralysis of the hand intrinsics. He should be independent, and have decent activities-of-daily-living skills at the wheelchair level.

T-1 quadriplegia means that the patient has sensory loss in the proximal inner arm (at the T-2 dermatome), but minimal weakness, if not normal ability, of the hand intrinsics, with paralysis from the upper chest downward. Ambulation is still unrealistic in low quadriplegia of this level, and even in paraplegia from T-2 to T-9.

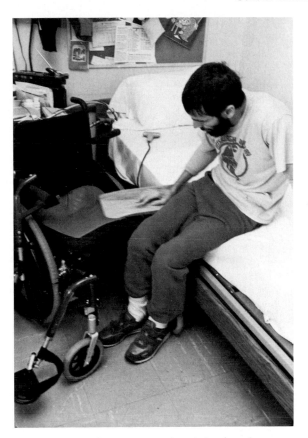

Figure 24-12. Transfer activities with a sliding board.

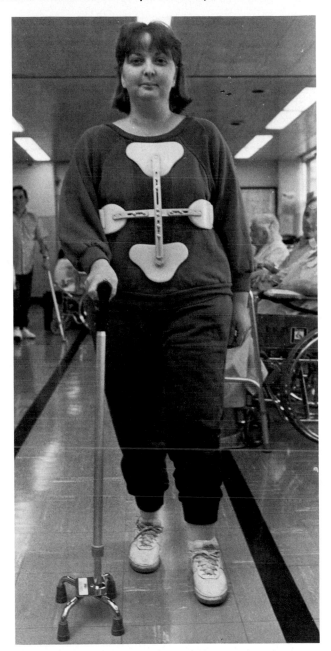

Figure 24-13. Ambulation training with a quadripod cane in mild paraparesis.

T-10 paraplegics are generally considered for limited ambulation with bilateral long-leg braces and crutches, but require a wheelchair for the activities of daily living. Paraplegics from T-10 to L-1 often fail to ambulate functionally because of the high energy expenditure necessary for the swing-through crutch gait.

L-2 paraplegia is the level for functional ambulation with a four-point alternate gait, using a walker or a pair of crutches. Bilateral long-leg braces should be worn to prevent knee buckling and ankle and foot instability.

Paraplegics at L-3 or lower can ambulate with bilateral ankle–foot orthoses and a walker, canes, or crutches. As the level of lesion lowers, the gait is smoother and requires less mechanical assistance (Fig. 24-13).

Obviously, rehabilitation training during hospitalization cannot anticipate every minor obstacle patients may encounter in the outside world. They will constantly be challenged by difficult tasks and will learn how to overcome them successfully. Despite occasional frustrations and disappointments, they can still enjoy a zest for living with appropriate medical and physiatric follow-ups.

REFERENCES

1. Bissada NK, Finkelbeiner AE: Pharmacology of continence and micturition. Am Fam Physician 20:28-136, 1979
2. Bradley WE: Innervation of the male urinary bladder. Urol Clin North Am 5:279-293, 1978
3. Carter RE: Medical management of pulmonary complications of spinal cord injury. Adv Neurol 22:261-269, 1979
4. Chu DA, Ahn JH, Ragnarsson KT et al: Deep venous thrombosis: Diagnosis in spinal cord injured patients. Arch Phys Med Rehabil 66:365-368, 1985
5. Comarr AE: Bowel regulation for patients with spinal cord injury. JAMA 167:18-21, 1958
6. Cressy JM, Comarr AE: Sexuality and spinal cord injury. Model Systems' SCI Digest 3:23-30, 1981
7. David A, Ohry A, Rozin R: Spinal cord injuries: Male infertility aspects. Paraplegia 15:11-14, 1977-1978
8. Erickson RP: Autonomic hyperreflexia pathophysiology and medical management. Arch Phys Med Rehabil 61:431-440, 1980
9. Glenn WWL, Hogan JF, Loke JSO et al: Ventilatory support by pacing of the conditioned diaphragm in quadriplegia. N Engl J Med 310:1150-1155, 1984
10. Griffith ER, Trieschmann RB: Sexual functioning in women with spinal cord injury. Arch Phys Med Rehabil 56:18-21, 1975
11. Guttmann L, Frankel H: The value of intermittent catheterization in the early management of traumatic paraplegia and quadriplegia. Paraplegia 4:63-83, 1965
12. Kline LB, McCluer SM, Bonikowski FP: Oculosympathetic spasms with cervical spinal cord injury. Arch Neurol 41:61-64, 1984
13. Kurnick NB: Autonomic hyperreflexia and its control in patients with spinal cord lesions. Ann Intern Med 44:678-686, 1956
14. Lee IY, Ragnarsson KT, Sell GH et al: Transurethral bladder neck surgery in spinal cord injured patients. Arch Phys Med Rehabil 59:80-83, 1978
15. Mathias CJ, Christensen NJ, Corbett JL et al: Plasma catecholamines during paroxysmal neurogenic hypertension in quadriplegic man. Circ Res 39:204-208, 1976
16. McMichan JC, Michel L, Westbrook PR: Pulmonary dysfunction following traumatic quadriplegia: Recognition, prevention and treatment. JAMA 243:528-531, 1980
17. Merritt JL: Urinary tract infections causes and managements with particular reference to the patient with spinal cord injury: A review. Arch Phys Med Rehabil 57:365-373, 1976
18. Nafchi NE, Demeny M, Lowman EW, Tuckman J: Hypertensive crises in quadriplegic patients: Change in cardiac output, blood volume, serum dopamine-B, hydroxylase activity and arterial prostaglandin PGE2. Circ Res 57:336-341, 1978
19. Nicholas JJ: Ectopic bone formation in patients with spinal cord injury. Arch Phys Med Rehabil 54:354-359, 1973
20. Ohry A, Peleg D, Goldman J et al: Sexual function, pregnancy and delivery in spinal cord injured women. Gynecol Obstet Invest 9:281-291, 1978
21. Perkash A, Perkash V, Perkash I: Experience with management of thromboembolism in patients with spinal cord injury: Part I. Incidence, diagnosis and role of some risk factors. Paraplegia 16:322-331, 1978-1979
22. Ragnarsson KT, Sell GH: Lower extremity fractures after spinal cord injury: A retrospective study. Arch Phys Med Rehabil 62:418-423, 1981
23. Rossi EC, Green D, Rosen JS et al: Sequential changes in factor VIII and platelets proceeding deep vein thrombosis in patients with spinal cord injury. Br J Haematol 45:143-151, 1980
24. Stover SL, Niemann KMW, Miller JM III: Disodium etidronate in the prevention of postoperative recurrence of heterotopic ossification in spinal cord injury patients. J Bone Joint Surg [Am] 58:683-688, 1976
25. Stover SL, Fine PR, Go BK et al: Spinal Cord Injury: The Facts and Figures. Birmingham: University of Alabama at Birmingham, 1986
26. Tibone J, Sakimura I, Nickel VL, Hsu JD: Heterotopic ossification around the hip in spinal cord injured patients. J Bone Joint Surg [Am] 60:769-775, 1978
27. Todd JW, Frisbie JH, Rossier AB et al: Deep venous

thrombosis in acute spinal cord injury: A comparison of 125 I fibrinogen leg scanning, impedance plethysmography and senography. Paraplegia 14:50-57, 1976

28. Troyer AD, Estenne M, Heilporn A: Mechanism of active expiration in tetraplegia subjects. N Engl J Med 314:740-744, 1986

29. Warren JW, Platt R, Thomas RJ et al: Antibiotic irrigation and catheter-associated urinary tract infections. N Engl J Med 299:570-573, 1978

30. Watson N: Anti-coagulant therapy in the prevention of venous thrombosis and pulmonary embolism in the spinal cord injury. Paraplegia 16:265-269, 1978-1979

31. Young RR, Delwaide PJ: Drug therapy: Spasticity. N Engl J Med, 304:28-33, 96-99, 1981

APPENDIX

Spinal Cord Injury Treatment Studies at the New York University-Bellevue Spinal Cord Injury Center

New York University-Bellevue (NYU-Bellevue) Spinal Cord Injury (SCI) Center has been committed to developing and evaluating SCI treatments for more than two decades. Funded by the National Institutes of Health (NIH) as a Clinical Center for SCI Studies since 1971, laboratory and clinical studies at the Center have emphasized pharmacologic treatments of acute SCI, surgical decompression, electromagnetic fields, and re-myelination. In 1973, the Center was designated a Regional Model SCI System by the Rehabilitation Services Administration of the Department of Education and the National Institute for Handicapped Research to improve health, vocational outcome, and reintegration of spinal-injured patients.

In 1978, the NYU-Bellevue SCI Center helped found the National Acute Spinal Cord Injury Study (NASCIS). Administered by Yale University and funded by NIH, NASCIS has since conducted several multicenter trials of SCI treatments. In 1983, NASCIS completed the first randomized clinical trial of SCI, finding no significant difference between patients treated with low (100 mg/day) and high (1 g/day) doses of methylprednisolone (MP) given to patients within 48 hours and for 10 days after SCI. In the meantime, laboratory studies indicated that the beneficial effects of MP are due to lipid peroxidation inhibition and that higher and earlier doses were necessary. Too little MP was given too late in the first NASCIS trial. Based on these data and reports that naloxone (10 mg/kg) improves functional recovery in animal SCI models, the Center initiated two Phase I trials demonstrating the safety of giving very high dose MP or naloxone to SCI patients. NASCIS carried out a randomized clinical trial from 1985 to 1989 of 487 patients, comparing naloxone (10 g/day), MP (10 g/day), and placebo given within 12 hours of SCI for one day.

The NYU-Bellevue SCI center is currently conducting a clinical trial on tirilazad (also called U74006F or Lazaroids). This steroid drug is 10 times more potent than MP as a lipid peroxidation inhibitor and has no corticosteroid receptor activity. Laboratory studies indicate that 0.03 to 10 mg/kg doses of tirilazad significantly improve neurologic recovery in spinal-injured animals when given within 8 hours of injury. In the trial, three doses (0.6, 2.0, and 6 mg/kg) of tirilazad will be randomized to SCI patients admitted to NYU-Bellevue within 8 hours of injury. If tirilazad is as effective as MP in humans, it would be preferred. Patients must be evaluated and treated as soon as possible after SCI.

The Center is also assessing new surgical approaches to correcting spinal fracture sites. The neurosurgery and orthopaedic departments have been using new internal fixation devices, including posterior and anterior plates, for rapid and secure stabilization of the spinal column. The effects of early decompressive surgery and fixation are being studied. Medical complications, hospitalization costs, and long term neurologic and orthopic outcome are being evaluated.

For referral of spine-injured patients preferably within 24 hours after injury to the Bellevue-NYU SCI Center, please call (212) 340-6413 and ask for Donna Whitam, RN (SCI Research Coordinator) or (212) 340-7182 and ask for the Spinal Fellow. For referral of spinal-injured patients for rehabilitation, call the New York Regional Spinal Cord Injury System at (212) 340-6090.

INDEX

Page numbers followed by *f* indicate figures; those followed by *t* indicate tabular material.

ISBN 0-397-50983-9

DATE DUE

AP 19 '96			
DE 3 '96			
AP 15 '97			
OC 8 '97			
JUN 1 1 1999			
MAR 1 4 2000			